SURGICAL TECHNIQUES

IN SPORTS MEDICINE

SURGICAL TECHNIQUES
IN SPORTS MEDICINE

■ NEAL S. ELATTRACHE, MD

Director Sports Medicine Fellowship
Kerlan-Jobe Orthopaedic Clinic
Associate Clinical Professor
Department of Orthopaedic Surgery
USC Keck School of Medicine
Los Angeles, California

■ RAFFY MIRZAYAN, MD

Co-Director of Sports Medicine
Director of Cartilage Restoration and Repair
Department of Orthopaedic Surgery
Kaiser Permanente
Baldwin Park, California
Associate Clinical Professor
Department of Orthopaedic Surgery
Keck School of Medicine
University of Southern California
Los Angeles, California

■ CHRISTOPHER D. HARNER, MD

Blue Cross of Western Pennsylvania Professor
Medical Director, Center for Sports Medicine
Department of Orthopaedic Surgery
University of Pittsburgh Medical Center
Pittsburgh, Pennsylvania

■ JON K. SEKIYA, MD

Assistant Professor
Center for Sports Medicine
Department of Orthopaedic Surgery
University of Pittsburgh Medical Center
Pittsburgh, Pennsylvania

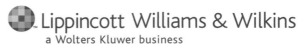

Lippincott Williams & Wilkins
a Wolters Kluwer business
Philadelphia · Baltimore · New York · London
Buenos Aires · Hong Kong · Sydney · Tokyo

Acquisitions Editor: Robert Hurley
Managing Editor: Jenny Koleth and Michelle LaPlante
Production Manager: Bridgett Dougherty
Senior Manufacturing Manager: Benjamin Rivera
Director of Marketing: Sharon Zinner
Design Coordinator: Doug Smock
Production Services: Techbooks
Printer: RRD Shenzhen, China

Printed in China

Library of Congress Cataloging-in-Publication Data
Surgical techniques in sports medicine / [edited by] Neal S. Elattrache . . . [et al.]. — 1st ed.
    p. ; cm.
  Includes bibliographical references and index.
  ISBN-13:978-0-7817-5427-9
  ISBN-10:0-7817-5427-5 (case)
  1. Sports injuries—Surgery. 2. Wounds and injuries—Surgery. 3. Sports medicine. I. Elattrache, Neal S. II. Title.
  [DNLM: 1. Athletic Injuries—surgery. 2. Arthroscopy—methods. 3. Elbow—surgery.
    4. Leg Injuries—surgery. 5. Orthopedic Procedures—methods. 6. Rotator Cuff—surgery.
    7. Shoulder—surgery.
QT 261 S961 2007]
RD97.S87 2007
617.1'027—dc22

2006015763

10 9 8 7 6 5 4 3 2 1

Dedication

To my wife, Tricia, and daughters, Nicole, Natalie, and Eva. Anything that I do that is good is dedicated to you, the heart of my world.

—Neal S. ElAttrache

To Cindy, Tiph, Andrew, and Nina – When I am not home, you know where I am.
To my parents Kay and Jim Harner for the intellectual and personal gifts you have given me to do my best.
To my dear friend George S. Paulus, may you always know the importance you had in my life.

—Christopher D. Harner

I would like to dedicate this book to my three boys, Zareh, Andre, and Raymond. They are the joy in my life and give me the strength to work harder.

—Raffy Mirzayan

To my wife, Jennie, thanks for your love and support through "another project." I really couldn't have done it without you. I love you!!!

—Jon K. Sekiya

Daniel C. Acevedo, B.S.
Medical Student
UCI School of Medicine
Irvine, California
UCI Medical Center
Orange, California

Christopher S. Ahmad, M.D.
Assistant Professor
Department of Orthopaedic Surgery
Columbia University
Attending Physician
Department of Orthopaedic Surgery
Columbia University Medical Center
New York, New York

J. Winslow Alford, M.D.
Orthopeadic Surgeon
Shoulder and Sports Medicine
West Bay Orthopaedics
Warwick, Rhode Island

Christina R. Allen, M.D.
Assistant Professor
Department of Orthopaedic Surgery
University of California, San Francisco
San Francisco, California

Annunziato Amendola, M.D., F.R.C.S.(C).
Professor
Department of Orthopaedic Surgery
University of Iowa
Director of Sports Medicine
Department of Orthopaedic Surgery
University of Iowa Hospitals and Clinics
Iowa City, Iowa

James R. Andrews, M.D.
Clinical Professor
Department of Orthopaedics and Sports Medicine
Birmingham School of Medicine—Department of Orthopaedic
  Surgery
Program Director
Orthopaedic Sports Medicine Fellowship
American Sports Medicine Institute
Orthopaedic Surgeon
Department of Orthopaedics
St. Vincent's Hospital
Birmingham, Alabama

Robert A. Arciero, M.D.
Director Orthopaedic Sports Medicine Fellowship
Department of Orthopaedics
University of Connecticut Health Center
Professor
Department of Orthopaedics
John Dempsey Hospital
Farmington, Connecticut

Bernard R. Bach, Jr., M.D.
The Claude Lambert—Helen S. Thomson Professor of
  Orthopaedic Surgery
Department of Orthopaedic Surgery
RUSH University Medical Center
Director, Division of Sports Medicine
RUSH Presbyterian St. Luke's Medical Center
Chicago, Illinois

Champ L. Baker, Jr., M.D.
Clinical Assistant Professor
Department of Orthopaedics
Medical College of Georgia
Augusta, Georgia
Staff Physician
The Hughston Clinic
Columbus, Georgia

Champ L. Baker III, M.D.
Resident
Department of Orthopaedic Surgery
University of Pittsburgh Medical Center
Pittsburgh, Pennsylvania

Troy L. Berg, M.D.
Chippewa Valley Orthopedics and Sports Medicine
Eau Claire, Wisconsin

Gregory C. Berlet, M.D.
Chief, Section of Foot and Ankle and Clinical Assistant
  Professor
Department of Orthopedics
Ohio State University
The Orthopedic Foot and Ankle Center
Columbus, Ohio

James Bicos, M.D.
JRSI Sports Medicine
St. Vincent Health Center
Indianapolis, Indiana

Louis U. Bigliani, M.D.
Frank E. Stinchfield Professor and Chairman
Department of Orthopaedic Surgery
Columbia University College of Physicians and Surgeons
Frank E. Stinchfield Professor and Chairman
Department of Orthopaedic Surgery
New York Presbyterian Hospital
New York, New York

Brant Blair, M.D.
Redondo Beach, California

James M. Bothwell, M.D.
Private Practice
Orthopedic Specialty Associates
Fort Worth, Texas

James P. Bradley, M.D.
Clinical Associate Professor
Department of Orthopaedic Surgery
University of Pittsburgh School of Medicine
Orthopaedic Surgeon
Department of Surgery
UPMC St. Margaret
Pittsburgh, Pennsylvania

Karen K. Briggs, M.B.A., M.P.H.
Director, Clinical Research
Steadman Hawkins Research Foundation
Clinical Research
Vail, Colorado

Matthew M. Buchanan, M.D.
Orthopaedic Foot and Ankle Surgery
Vail-Summit Orthopaedics
Vail, Colorado

Stephen S. Burkhart, M.D.
Clinical Associate Professor
Department of Orthopaedic Surgery
University of Texas Health Science Center
Director of Orthopaedic Education
The Orthopaedic Institute
San Antonio, Texas

Wayne Z. Burkhead, Jr., M.D.
Clinical Professor
Department of Orthopaedic Surgery
UT Southwestern Medical School
Attending Orthopaedic Surgeon
Department of Shoulder and Elbow Service
The Carrell Clinic
Dallas, Texas

Joseph P. Burns, M.D.
The Southern California Orthopedic Institute
Van Nuys, California
The Southern California Orthopedic Institute
Simi Valley, California

E. Lyle Cain, Jr., M.D.
Fellowship Director
Orthopaedic Sports Medicine Fellowship

American Sports Medicine Institute
Orthopaedic Surgeon
Alabama Sports Medicine and Orthopaedic Center
St. Vincent's Medical Center
Birmingham, Alabama

James E. Carpenter, M.D.
Associate Professor
Department of Orthopaedic Surgery
University of Michigan Medical School
Chairman
Department of Orthopaedic Surgery
University of Michigan
Ann Arbor, Michigan

Peter S. Cha, M.D.
Attending Surgeon
Beacon Orthopaedics and Sports Medicine
Cincinnati, Ohio

Michael G. Ciccotti, M.D.
Associate Professor
Department of Orthopaedic Surgery
Rothman Institute/Thomas Jefferson University
Chief, Division of Sports Medicine
Director, Orthopaedic Sports Medicine Fellowship
Department of Orthopaedic Surgery
Rothman Institute/Thomas Jefferson University
Philadelphia, Pennsylvania

Brian J. Cole, M.D., M.B.A.
Associate Professor
Departments of Orthopaedics and Anatomy and Cell Biology
Rush University Medical Center
Director
Cartilage Restoration Center at Rush
Rush University Medical Center
Chiago, Illinois

John E. Conway, M.D.
Private Practice
Orthopedic Specialty Associates
Forth Worth, Texas

John G. Costouros, M.D.
Clinical Instructor
Department of Orthopaedic Surgery
Harvard Medical School
Clinical Instructor
Department of Orthopedic Surgery
Massachusetts General Hospital
Boston, Massachusetts

William R. Creevy, M.D.
Assistant Professor
Department of Orthopaedic Surgery
Boston University School of Medicine
Vice Chairman
Department of Orthopaedic Surgery
Boston University Medical Center
Boston, Massachusetts

Brent W. d'Arc, M.D.
Resident
Department of Orthopaedic Surgery
LAC and USC Medical Center
Los Angeles, California

Ronald E. Delanois, M.D.
Assistant Professor
Department of Surgery/Orthopedics
Uniformed Services University of the Health Sciences
Bethesda, Maryland
Staff Orthopedics
Rubin Institute of Advanced Orthopedics
Sinai Hospital of Baltimore
Baltimore, Maryland

Peter A. J. de Leeuw, Fellow Ph.D.
Medical Student
University of Amsterdam
Fellow Ph.D.
Department of Orthopaedic Surgery
Academic Medical Center
Amsterdam, The Netherlands

Eugene J. DeMorat, M.D.
Orthopaedic Surgeon
Department of Orthopedic Surgery
Shore Memorial Hospital
Somers Point, New Jersey

Brian G. Donley, M.D.
Vice Chair
Department of Orthopaedic Surgery
Cleveland Clinic Foundation
Cleveland, Ohio

Pete Draovitch, P.T., A.T.
University of Pittsburgh Medical Center
Department of Rehabilitation
Center for Sports Medicine
Pittsburgh, Pennsylvania

James C. Dreese, M.D.
Assistant Professor
Department of Orthopedics
University of Maryland Medical Center
Baltimore, Maryland

Jeffrey R. Dugas, M.D.
Fellowship Director
Orthopaedic Sports Medicine Fellowship
American Sports Medicine Institute
Orthopaedic Surgeon
Alabama Sports Medicine and Orthopaedic Center
St. Vincent's Medical Center
Birmingham, Alabama

Neal S. ElAttrache, M.D.
Director Sports Medicine Fellowship
Kerlan-Jobe Orthopaedic Clinic
Associate Clinical Professor
Department of Orthopaedic Surgery

USC Keck School of Medicine
Los Angeles, California

Hussein A. Elkousy, M.D.
Fondren Orthopedic Group
Texas Orthopedic Hospital
Houston, Texas

Christopher I. Ellingson, M.D.
Chief Resident
Bone and Joint Sports Medicine Institute
Naval Medical Center Portsmouth
Portsmouth, Virginia

Keelan R. Enseki, M.S., M.P.T.
Adjunct Instructor
Department of Physical Therapy
University of Pittsburgh
Director, Orthopedic Physical Therapy Residency
CRS-UPMC Center for Sports Medicine
Pittsburgh, Pennsylvania

Richard Erhardt, Ph.D.
University of Pittsburgh Medical Center
Department of Rehabilitation
Center for Sports Medicine
Pittsburgh, Pennsylvania

Gregory C. Fanelli, M.D.
Fanelli Sports Injury Clinic
Orthopaedic Surgery
Geisinger Medical Center
Danville, Pennsylvania

Jonathan B. Feibel, M.D.
Director, Foot and Ankle Surgery and Assistant Program Director
Orthopedic Surgery Residency Program
Mount Carmel Health
The Cardinal Orthopaedic Institute
Columbus, Ohio

Larry D. Field, M.D.
Clinical Instructor
Department of Orthopaedic Surgery
University of Mississippi School of Medicine
Co-Director, Upper Extremity Service
Orthopaedic Department
Mississippi Sports Medicine and Orthopaedic Center
Jackson, Mississippi

Peter J. Fowler, M.D.
Professor
Department of Surgery
The University of Western Ontario
Medical Director
Fowler Kennedy Sport Medicine Clinic
The University of Western Ontario
London, Ontario, Canada

Austin T. Fragomen, M.D.
Instructor
Department of Orthopaedic Surgery

Weill Medical College of Cornell University
Assistant Attending
Department of Orthopaedic Surgery
Hospital for Special Surgery
New York, New York

Stephen J. French, M.D., F.R.C.S.C.
Fellow
Fowler Kennedy Sports Medicine Clinic
University of Western Ontario
London, Ontario, Canada
Orthopaedic Surgeon
Department of Surgery
Thunder Bay Regional Health Sciences Centre
Thunder Bay, Ontario, Canada

Freddie H. Fu, M.D., D.Sc. (Hon), D.Ps. (Hon)
Chairman
Department of Orthopaedic Surgery
University of Pittsburgh School of Medicine
Chief, Orthopaedic Surgery
UPMC Presbyterian-Shadyside
Pittsburgh, Pennsylvania

John P. Fulkerson, M.D.
Clinical Professor of Orthopedic Surgery
Sports Medicine Fellowship Co-Director
University of Connecticut School of Medicine
Orthopedic Associates of Hartford, P.C.
Farmington, Connecticut

Christian Gerber, M.D., F.R.C.S.E.d. (Hon)
Professor
Department of Orthopaedics
Balgrist University Hospital
Medical Director
Department of Orthopaedics
Balgrist University Hospital
Zurich, Switzerland

J. Robert Giffin, M.D.
Assistant Professor
Department of Surgery
University of Western Ontario
Fowler Kennedy Sport Medicine Clinic
Department of Surgery
University Hospital
London, Ontario, Canada

Michael K. Gilbart, M.D., F.R.C.S.(C).
Assistant Professor
Department of Orthopaedic Surgery
University of British Columbia
Assistant Professor
Department of Orthopaedic Surgery
University of British Columbia Hospital
Vancouver, British Columbia, Canada

Ronald E. Glousman, M.D.
Kerlan-Jobe Orthopaedic Clinic
Los Angeles, California

Carlos A. Guanche, M.D.
Southern California Orthopedic Institute
Van Nuys, California

Bryan T. Hanypsiak, M.D.
Hamptons Orthopaedic and Rehabilitation Institute
Peconic Bay Medical Center
Riverhead, New York

Christopher D. Harner, M.D.
Professor
Department of Orthopaedic Surgery
University of Pittsburgh
Medical Director
Department of Orthopaedic Surgery
University of Pittsburgh Medical Center for Sports Medicine
Pittsburgh, Pennsylvania

Forest T. Heis, M.D.
Partner
Greater Cincinnati Orthopaedic Center
Crestview Hills, Kentucky

Stephen M. Howell, M.D.
Adjunct Professor Mechanical Engineering
Member of Biomedical Graduate Group
University of California at Davis
Davis, California
Orthopedic Surgeon
Methodist Hospital
Sacramento, California

G. Russell Huffman, M.D., M.P.H.
Assistant Professor
Department of Orthopaedic Surgery Penn Sports Medicine Center
University of Pennsylvania
Philadelphia, Pennsylvania

Christopher F. Hyer, D.P.M.
Faculty, Surgical Residency
Department of Pediatric Surgery
Grant Medical Center
Medical Staff
Department of Pediatric Surgery
Grant Medical Center
Columbia, Ohio

Christopher M. Jobe, M.D.
Chairman
Department of Orthopedic Surgery
Loma Linda University Medical Center
Loma Linda, California

Frank W. Jobe, M.D.
Clinical Professor
Department of Orthopaedics
University of Southern California
Keck School of Medicine
Los Angeles, California
Director of Biomechanics Lab
Department of Orthopaedics
Centinela Freeman Health System
Inglewood, California

Darren L. Johnson, M.D.
Professor and Chairman
Department of Orthopaedic Surgery
Director of Sports Medicine
University of Kentucky School of Medicine
Lexington, Kentucky

Steve E. Jordan, M.D.
Adjunct Professor
Florida State University School of Medicine
Team Physician
Florida State University
Tallahassee, Florida

Jay D. Keener, M.D.
Assistant Professor
Department of Orthopaedic Surgery
University of North Carolina
Chapel Hill, North Carolina

Bryan T. Kelly, M.D.
Assistant Professor
Department of Orthopaedics
Weill Medical College of Cornell University
Orthopaedic Surgeon
Hospital for Special Surgery
New York, New York

David H. Kim, M.D.
Huntington Beach Orthopedics and Sports Medicine
Huntingon Beach, California
Department of Orthopedic Surgery
Hoag Memorial Hospital Presbyterian
Newport Beach, California

John R. Klein, M.D.
Shoulder Fellow
The San Antonio Orthopaedic Group
San Antonio, Texas

Mininder S. Kocher, M.D., M.P.H.
Assistant Professor of Orthopaedic Surgery
Harvard Medical School
Associate Director
Division of Sports Medicine
Children's Hospital Boston
Boston, Massachusetts

Melissa D. Koenig, M.D.
Fellow
Kaufmann Medical Building
Pittsburgh, Pennsylvania

Rover Krips, M.D., Ph.D.
Resident
Department of Orthopaedic Surgery
University of Amsterdam
Resident
Department of Orthopaedic Surgery
Academic Medical Center
Amsterdam, The Netherlands

Sumant G. Krishnan, M.D.
Clinical Assistant Professor
Department of Orthopaedic Surgery
University of Texas Southwestern
Attending Orthopaedic Surgeon
Department of Shoulder and Elbow Service
The Carrell Clinic
Dallas, Texas

Christopher A. Kurtz, M.D.
Assistant Professor
Department of Surgery
Uniformed Services University of the Health Sciences
Bethesda, Maryland
Head, Division of Sports Medicine
Department of Orthopaedic Surgery
Naval Medical Center Portsmouth
Portsmouth, Virginia

Keith W. Lawhorn, M.D., L.T.C., U.S.A.F., M.C.
Staff Orthopedic Surgeon
Advanced Orthopaedics and Sports Medicine Institute
Fair Oaks Hospital
Fairfax, Virginia

Thomas H. Lee, M.D.
Clinical Assistant Professor
Ohio State University
Orthopedic Foot and Ankle Center
Columbus, Ohio

Orr Limpisvasti, M.D.
Orthopaedic Surgeon
Kerlan-Jobe Orthopaedic Clinic
Los Angeles, California

Usha S. Mani, M.D.
Olympia Orthopaedics
Olympia, Washington

RobRoy L. Martin, Ph.D., P.T., C.S.C.S.
Assistant Professor
Department of Physical Therapy
Duquesne University
Staff Physical Therapist
Centers for Rehab Services/Center for Sports Medicine
Pittsburgh, Pennsylvania

Paul A. Martineau, M.D., F.R.C.S.C.
Clinical Fellow
Department of Orthopaedics
Cleveland Clinic Foundation
Cleveland, Ohio

Augustus D. Mazzocca, M.D.
Assistant Professor, Assistant Residency Director
Department of Orthopaedic Surgery
University of Connecticut Health Center
Sports Medicine Orthopaedic Surgeon
Department of Orthopaedic Surgery
John Dempsey Hospital
Farmington, Connecticut

Glen A. McClung, M.D.
Chief
Department of Orthopaedic Surgery
Samaritan Hospital
Lexington, Kentucky

Bruce S. Miller, M.D.
Assistant Professor
Division of Sports Medicine
Department of Orthopaedic Surgery
University of Michigan
Ann Arbor, Michigan

Mark D. Miller, M.D.
Professor
Department of Orthopaedic Surgery
University of Virginia
Professor of Orthopaedic Surgery
Head, Division of Sports Medicine
University of Virginia
Charlottesville, Virginia

Anthony Miniaci, M.D., F.R.C.S.C.
Professor
Department of Orthopaedic Surgery
Case Western Reserve University
Executive Director, Head Section
Cleveland Clinic Sports Health
Cleveland Clinic
Cleveland, Ohio

Raffy Mirzayan, M.D.
Associate Clinical Professor
Department of Orthopaedic Surgery
USC Keck School of Medicine
Los Angeles, California
Co-Director of Sports Medicine, Director of Cartilage
    Restoration and Repair
Department of Orthopaedic Surgery
Kaiser Permanente
Baldwin Park, California

Bernard F. Morrey, M.D.
Emeritus Chairman and Professor of Orthopedics
Department of Orthopedic Surgery
Mayo Medical School, Mayo Clinic
Rochester, Minnesota

Shawn W. O'Driscoll, M.D., Ph.D.
Professor of Orthopedic Surgery
Department of Orthopedics
Mayo Clinic College of Medicine
Professor of Orthopedic Surgery
Department of Orthopedics
Mayo Clinic
Rochester, Minnesota

Hans P. Olsen, M.D.
Associate
Department of Orthopaedics
Geisinger Wyoming Valley Medical Center
Wilkes-Barre, Pennsylvania

Maxwell C. Park, M.D.
Associate
Department of Orthopaedic Surgery
Southern California Permanente Medical Group
Woodland Hills Medical Center
Los Angeles, California

Richard D. Parker, M.D.
Professor of Surgery
Department of Orthopaedic Surgery
CCF Lerner College of Medicine
Education Director
Cleveland Clinic Sports Health
Cleveland Clinic
Cleveland, Ohio

Leon E. Paulos, M.D.
Professor
Department of Orthopedic Surgery
Baylor College of Medicine
Staff
Department of Orthopedic Surgery
The Methodist Hospital
Houston, Texas

Scott D. Pennington, M.D.
Shoulder Fellow
Department of Orthopaedic Surgery
Harvard School of Medicine
Clinical Instructor
Department of Orthopaedic Surgery
Massachusetts General Hospital
Boston, Massachusetts

Julio Petilon, M.D.
Resident
Department of Orthopaedics
Naval Medical Center Portsmouth
Portsmouth, Virginia

Terrence M. Philbin, D.O.
Clinical Assistant Professor
Ohio State University
Orthopedic Foot and Ankle Center
Columbus, Ohio

Marc J. Philippon, M.D.
Clinical Assistant Professor
Department of Orthopaedics
University of Pittsburgh Medical Center, Center for Sports
    Medicine
Pittsburgh, Pennsylvania
Partner/Orthopaedic Surgeon
Steadman Hawkins Clinic
Vail, Colorado

Christopher A. Radkowski, M.D.
Orthopaedic Surgery Sports Medicine Fellow
Department of Orthopaedic Surgery
University of Pittsburgh Medical Center
Pittsburgh, Pennsylvania

Jeffrey A. Rihn, M.D.
Resident Physician
Department of Orthopaedic Surgery
University of Pittsburgh
Pittsburgh, Pennsylvania

Reneé S. Riley, M.D.
Orthopaedic Surgeon
Department of Surgery
Trinity Medical Center
Birmingham, Alabama

William G. Rodkey, D.V.M., Diplomate A.C.V.S.
Director
Basic Science Research
Steadman Hawkins Research Foundation
Vail, Colorado

Anthony A. Romeo, M.D.
Orthopaedic Surgeon
RUSH Oak Park Hospital
Oak Park, Illinois
RUSH University Medical Center
Chicago, Illinois

Marc R. Safran, M.D.
Associate Professor
Department of Orthopaedic Surgery
University of California, San Francisco
Chief, Division of Sports Medicine
Department of Orthopaedic Surgery
University of California, San Francisco
San Francisco, California

William H. Satterfield, M.D.
Private Practice
Winston-Salem, North Carolina

Felix H. Savoie III, M.D.
Clinical Associate Professor
Department of Orthopaedic Surgery
University of Mississippi School of Medicine
Co-Director, Upper Extremity Service
Department of Orthopaedic Surgery
Mississippi Sports Medicine and Orthopaedic Center
Jackson, Mississippi

Anthony A. Schepsis, M.D.
Professor
Department of Orthopaedic Surgery
Boston University Medical Center
Director of Sports Medicine
Department of Orthopaedic Surgery
Boston University Medical Center
Boston, Massachusetts

Jon K. Sekiya, M.D.
Assistant Professor
Center for Sports Medicine
Department of Orthopaedic Surgery

University of Pittsburgh Medical Center
Pittsburgh, Pennsylvania

Kevin J. Setter, M.D.
Fellow
Department of Orthopaedics
New York Orthopaedic Hospital
Columbia-Presbyterian Medical Center
New York, New York

Steven B. Singleton, M.D., Ph.D.
Orthopaedic Surgeon
Steadman Hawkins Clinic of the Carolinas
Spartanburg, South Carolina

Andrew H. Smith, M.D.
Active Staff
Cape Cod Orthopaedics and Sports Medicine
Cape Code Hospital
Hyannis, Massachusetts

Steven J. Snyder, M.D.
Medical Director
Center for Learning Arthroscopic Skills
Southern California Orthopedic Institute
Van Nuys, California

Heleen Sonneveld, M.D.
Orthopaedic Surgeon
Department of Orthopaedic Surgery
Academic Medical Center
University of Amsterdam
Amsterdam, The Netherlands

Natalie A. Squires, M.D.
Resident
Department of Orthopaedic Surgery
University of Pittsburg
Resident
Department of Orthopaedic Surgery
University of Pittsburgh Medical Center
Pittsburgh, Pennsylvania

J. Richard Steadman, M.D.
Orthopaedic Surgeon
Steadman Hawkins Clinic
Steadman Hawkins Research Foundation
Clinical Research
Vail, Colorado

Michael A. Terry, M.D.
Assistant Professor
Department of Orthopaedic Surgery
University of Chicago Pritzker School of Medicine
Assistant Professor
Department of Orthopaedic Surgery
The University of Chicago Hospitals
Chicago, Illinois

Frank V. Thomas, M.D.
Professor
Department of Orthopaedics

University of Connecticut Health Center
Farmington, Connecticut

James E. Tibone, M.D.
Clinical Professor
Department of Orthopaedics
USC Keck School of Medicine
Orthopaedic Fellowship Director
Department of Orthopaedics
USC University Hospital
Los Angeles, California

Adrienne J. Towsen, M.D.
Orthopedic Surgeon, Sports Medicine
West Grove, Pennsylvania

C. Niek van Dijk, M.D., Ph.D.
Professor
Department of Orthopedic Surgery
University of Amsterdam
Chief
Department of Orthopedic Surgery
Academical Medical Center
Amsterdam, The Netherlands

Nikhil N. Verma, M.D.
Assistant Professor
Rush University Medical Center
Chicago, Illinois

Ilya Voloshin, M.D.
Assistant Professor
Department of Orthopaedic Surgery
Boston University School of Medicine
Department of Orthopaedic Surgery
Boston University Medical Center
Boston, Massachusetts

Jon J. P. Warner, M.D.
Chief, The Harvard Shoulder Service
Associate Professor of Orthopaedic Surgery
Harvard Medical School
Massachusetts General Hospital
Brigham and Women's Hospitals
Boston, Massachusetts

Russell F. Warren, M.D.
Professor
Department of Orthopaedics
Weill Medical College of Cornell University
Surgeon-In-Chief Emeritus
Department of Orthopaedics
Hospital for Special Surgery
New York, New York

Lisa Wasserman, M.D., F.R.C.S.(c).
Sports Medicine/Foot and Ankle Fellow
Department of Orthopaedic Surgery
University of Iowa Hospitals and Clinics
Iowa City, Iowa

Frederick J. Watson, M.D.
Orthopaedic Surgeon
Tribury Orthopaedics, P.C.
Waterbury, Connecticut

Robin V. West, M.D.
Assistant Professor
Department of Orthopaedics
University of Pittsburgh
Pittsburgh, Pennsylvania

Thomas L. Wickiewicz, M.D.
Professor of Clinical Orthopaedic Surgery
Weill Medical College of Cornell University
Department of Surgery
Attending Orthopaedic Surgeon
Department of Orthopaedic
Hospital for Special Surgery
New York, New York

Edward M. Wojtys, M.D.
Professor
Department of Orthopaedic Surgery
University of Michigan
Chief of Sports Medicine
Medical Director—Medsport
University of Michigan
Ann Arbor, Michigan

Eugene M. Wolf, M.D.
Fellowship Director, Sports Medicine and Shoulder
Department of Orthopaedics
St. Mary's Medical Center
San Francisco, California

Dane K. Wukich, M.D.
Assistant Professor
Department of Orthopaedic Surgery
University of Pittsburgh School of Medicine
Chief
Division of Foot and Ankle Surgery
University of Pittsburgh Medical Center
Pittsburgh, Pennsylvania

Ken Yamaguchi, M.D.
Professor
Department of Orthopaedic Surgery
Washington University
Chief Surgeon
Department of Orthopaedic Sugery
Barnes Jewish Hospital
St. Louis, Missouri

Chad T. Zehms, M.D.
Resident Physician
Bone and Joint Sports Medicine Institute
Naval Medical Center Portsmouth
Portsmouth, Virginia

When I began my career as an orthopaedic sports medicine physician in 1973, the American Orthopaedic Society for Sports Medicine was only one year old and had less than 100 members. In orthopaedics, the debate raged as to whether sports medicine was a legitimate subspeciality. Thirty-three years later that question has long since been answered in the affirmative.

The media are filled daily with the exploits of athletes who have been returned to their sport, at the same or improved skill level they enjoyed prior to their injury, by the skilled hands of orthopaedic sports medicine surgeons across the country.

This happy state of affairs was made possible by early pioneers such as Don O'Donoghue, Bob Kerlan, Frank Jobe, Don Slocum, Jack Hughston, Jim Nicholas, Jack Kennedy, Fred Allman, Frank McCue, Marcus Stewart, and Hugh Tullos. These clinical and basic science researchers recognized the special needs of athletes for medical and orthopaedic care. Following that, the arthroscope was introduced and has been the number one revolution in sports surgery in the last thirty years. This was pioneered by such greats as Lanny Johnson, Bob Jackson, Howard Sweeney, Dick Caspari, and others. Their efforts to define and provide understanding of athletic healthcare issues have allowed arthroscopic surgical technology to be applied to a wide range of acute and chronic problems. And now, a variety of previously career-ending pathologies are routinely resolved with minimal intervention.

Orthopaedic sports medicine continues to march along, and keeping up with recent advancement is a task unto itself. Previous authors have produced an abundance of excellent texts addressing topics such as anatomic regions, arthroscopy, and open procedures. Neal ElAttrache, Chris Harner, Raffy Mirzayan, Jon Sekiya, and their contributors have produced an outstanding body of updated knowledge with this current work: *Surgical Techniques in Sports Medicine*.

This comprehensive work will serve equally well as a textbook or reference guide. Organized by anatomic region, it is structured into five sections and sixty-six chapters to demonstrate proven successful surgical techniques. As a clear and concise text with excellent illustrations, it describes the history of each technique, its indications, and contraindications, as well as the surgical technique, technical alternatives, and pitfalls. In addition, it provides guidelines for rehabilitation and return to play recommendations. It also discusses outcomes and future directions, and it includes suggested readings, making this one of the most useful surgical techniques books available.

Surgical Techniques in Sports Medicine is an outstanding and unique contribution to the continuing development of orthopaedic sports medicine. I believe it will be an important and useful addition to sports medicine libraries everywhere.

James R. Andrews, M.D.
May 18, 2006

The field of sports medicine has evolved tremendously in the last few decades. Whereas the early emphasis was on non-operative management for many injuries, minimally invasive and arthroscopic surgery has revolutionized the field by allowing athletes to recover quickly and return to the playing field or the professional sports arena. In addition, we are seeing three other major evolving trends in our patient population. Our teenage athletes are suffering from injuries requiring surgical treatment, especially to the shoulder and elbow, previously seen primarily in their adult counterparts. The cause of this trend is in large part overuse and overexposure. While it is of paramount importance to identify these causes and educate the patient population to decrease this trend, it is also important to be able to effectively treat these young injured patients in order for them to pursue a desired activity or sport which may provide them with an education, livelihood, or simply enjoyment. Alternatively, we are caring for an adult population which is staying much more physically active later in life and sustaining injuries, such as tears of the ACL and rotator cuff which are being surgically managed as would be in younger patients. These people want to return to the activities and exercise which they enjoy and which are providing them a more healthy quality of life.

Newer, less invasive surgical techniques and rehabilitation are helping greatly in the endeavor. Lastly we are experiencing the increasing presentation of the athletically active arthritic patient. This is a very challenging group of patients to take care of, however, several of our contributors to this text are focusing a portion of their practice to treating the problems in these patients with promising results.

We have assembled a list of outstanding contributors who are well known and respected in their fields to describe their surgical techniques. While surgical techniques evolve quickly, these authors are among the "thought leaders" who will advance our science.

We are fortunate to be able to record their most recent and advance surgical procedures in this text. When applicable, both open and arthroscopic techniques are described to treat a given condition. This book is divided into upper and lower extremity techniques.

The chapters are written in a consistent fashion to allow the reader to easily find a section within various chapters. While clinical diagnosis and imaging are important for the evaluation of a problem, the emphasis of this book is on the surgical techniques. The surgical technique portion has detailed information including anesthesia, positioning, operating room set up, incisions/portal placement, superficial and deep dissection, and wound closure. Sections on post-operative rehabilitation will aid in the recovery of the patient. We hope that this book will adequately prepare the surgeon to perform even the more challenging sports medicine cases.

Neal S. Elattrache, M.D.
Christopher D. Harner, M.D.
Raffy Mirzayan, M.D.
Jon K. Sekiya, M.D.

GENERAL ACKNOWLEDGMENTS

We would like to acknowledge Jim Merritt, who initially began the project and believed that this would be a great addition to the orthopaedic sports medicine community. We would like to thank Acquisitions Editor, Bob Hurley, who also believed in us and green lighted the book, and thanks to his assistant, Eileen Wolfberg. We would like to especially thank Director of Marketing, Sharon Zinner, who has been helpful in navigating the publishing field. We also wanted to thank Managing Editors Michelle LaPlante and Jenny Koleth who were involved in various stages of the book's development.

We would like to especially thank the contributing authors who have made every effort to submit outstanding manuscripts which will aid in the understanding of performing the surgical procedures. This book would not have come to fruition without their hard work.

PERSONAL ACKNOWLEDGMENTS

I would like to acknowledge and thank my dedicated assistant and nurse, Teri Chavarria and Myrna Quirante, who take such outstanding care of my patients and me on a daily basis, and Karen Mohr who helps coordinate the Sports Medicine Fellowship and research. I would like to acknowledge all the hard work in producing this text book by my co-editors Raffy Mirzayan, M.D., John Sekiya, M.D., and my old friend and colleague Chris Harner, M.D. I would also like to acknowledge Frank W. Jobe, M.D., James E. Tibone, M.D., Bernie Morrey, M.D., James R. Andrews, M.D., and the late Robert K. Kerlan, M.D., who stand out among my mentors. I benefit from something each of them has taught me everyday.

—Neal S. ElAttrache

First and foremost, I would like to acknowledge the incredible work of my friend, old fellow, and new partner Jon Sekiya and his colleague Raffy Mirzayan. Without their dedication, this textbook would have never been completed. To my dear friend and colleague Neal ElAttrache, thank you

for this opportunity to bring East and West together on this monumental task. Finally, I would like to acknowledge Dr. Albert B. Ferguson, Jr, and Dr. Kenneth DeHaven, two old Dartmouth boys who taught me more than they will ever know.

—Christopher D. Harner

I would like to honor Frank W. Jobe, M.D., who has been a mentor and a driving force in my personal and professional endeavors in the field of sports medicine. Not only is he an outstanding surgeon and physician, he is a true gentleman.

I would like to thank all of the associates at the Kerlan-Jobe Orthopaedic Clinic, especially Neal ElAttrache, who have given me the education and experience in the field of sports medicine which has allowed me to flourish in my practice and provide the best care to my patients. I owe a great debt of gratitude to them.

I would like to thank Teri Chavarria and Myrna Quirante, Dr. ElAttrache's assistants, who were very helpful during the entire production process of this book. They always took my calls and made sure that the message was conveyed to Dr. ElAttrache.

Last, but definitely not least, I would like to thank my wife, Armena, for all the support and love she has given me through all of my life and my medical career.

—Raffy Mirzayan, M.D.

I would first like to thank Christopher Harner, my mentor and friend, who gave me the opportunity to be a part of this wonderful project and has been a role model for me in all aspects of my professional and personal life—thank you! I would like to thank my other co-editors Raffy Mirzayan and Neal ElAttrache for the wonderful collaboration in getting this book to completion—We did it! I would also like to thank my many other mentors and friends who have impacted my career in so many positive ways—Edward Wojtys, Freddie Fu, Jed Kuhn, Patrick McMahon, Richard Debski, Mark Miller, Jim Bradley, Mark Rodosky, Marc Philippon, Jim Carpenter, Wally Roeser, and Daniel Unger—You have helped me in so many ways and for this I will always be grateful!!!

—Jon K. Sekiya

1

SHOULDER

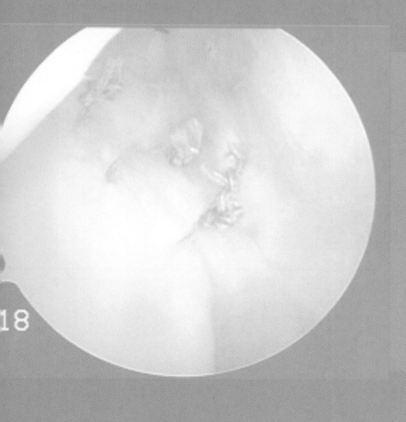
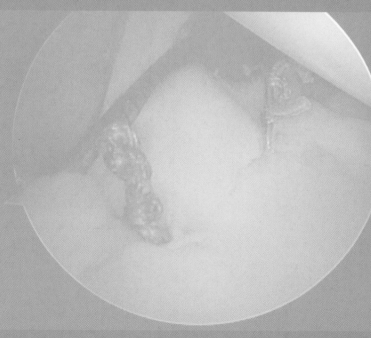

Part

A

INSTABILITY

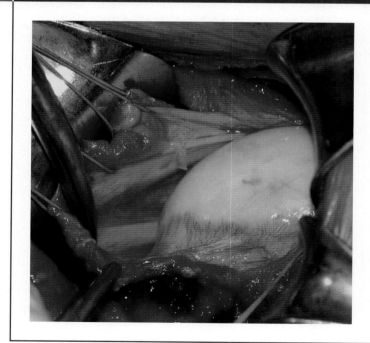

1

OPEN ANTERIOR INSTABILITY REPAIR

DAVID H. KIM, MD, FRANK W. JOBE, MD

■ HISTORY OF THE TECHNIQUE

Glenohumeral instability can present as a spectrum of disability, ranging from subtle anterior shoulder pain with apprehension to frank recurrent dislocations. Perthes[1] and Bankart[2] described that a separated labrum and capsule were the anatomic abnormalities responsible for anterior shoulder instability and reported on surgical techniques involving the reattachment of the avulsed labrum and capsule to the glenoid rim. Rowe et al.[3] reported on the long-term results of open Bankart repair. They noted 97% excellent or good results, with a 3.5% dislocation rate, but 31% of the patients had some degree of motion loss and only 33% of those patients involved in overhand athletics were able to return to their previous activity level. Other surgeons[4–12] have also reported overall successful outcomes with open Bankart repair with respect to stability, but have noted some overall loss of shoulder motion in their patients, especially loss of external rotation.

Moreover, patients with multidirectional instability due to capsular laxity have been treated with open surgical techniques. Neer and Foster[13] originally described the inferior capsular shift with a laterally based T-shaped capsular incision for treatment of patients with inferior and multidirectional instability. Other authors[14–18] have reported results of a modified open capsular shift technique with good clinical outcomes in terms of stability, but patients in these series also suffered from some degree of postoperative loss of external rotation. Specifically, overhead and throwing athletes had a difficult time returning to their prior competitive level.[15–18]

Overhead throwing athletes are particularly susceptible to shoulder problems and in particular, impingement of the rotator cuff on the posterosuperior glenoid rim and labrum. This phenomenon of "internal impingement" has been well described[19–27] and has been attributed to the loss of anterior glenohumeral stability leading to injury of the anterior capsulolabral complex, particularly during the late cocking phase of throwing with the shoulder in abduction and maximal external rotation.

Care for these patients led to the development of the anterior capsulolabral reconstruction (ACLR)[22,23,28–31] at the Kerlan-Jobe Orthopaedic Clinic. The goal was to design a procedure that would restore shoulder stability without compromising shoulder mobility postoperatively. The ACLR is a modification of the Bankart procedure in which a new capsulolabral complex is reconstructed by using suture anchors placed in the anterior glenoid rim and imbricating the capsule and inferior glenohumeral ligament with sutures. However, a capsular shift based on the glenoid side of the joint through a transversely oriented capsulotomy is utilized. Moreover, the native anatomy is preserved as much as possible—no muscle is detached, shortened, or transferred since the subscapularis muscle is split along the line of its muscle fibers.

■ INDICATIONS AND CONTRAINDICATIONS

A careful, detailed history will identify the majority of patients suffering from anterior glenohumeral instability. The apprehension and relocation tests are reliable clinical examination maneuvers to help confirm this diagnosis.[22] Initial management consisting of supervised therapy with a specific exercise program is often effective, especially in those patients with subtle glenohumeral instability. Operative intervention is reserved for those patients with persistent symptoms despite adequate conservative treatment. Successful surgery can be performed utilizing either an open or arthroscopic approach. The indications for open anterior stabilization surgery such as the ACLR are dependent on both patient and surgeon factors. For those patients in whom it is critical to maintain postoperative range of motion, such as overhead throwing athletes, the ACLR provides a reproducible technique to allow the restoration of stability without compromising mobility. Although this may be possible using arthroscopic techniques, currently there are no long-term reports in the literature supporting this practice. Furthermore, some studies have suggested that those patients involved in high-risk contact activities may be better served to have an open reconstruction.[32-35] In addition, those patients who require revision anterior instability surgery may also benefit from open techniques,[36-38] especially if the capsule is thinned or of poor quality. Finally, those patients in whom previous open reconstruction has been successful on one side may prefer to have an open procedure performed on their injured contralateral shoulder.

The skill and experience of the surgeon also play a role in determining whether open surgery is appropriate. Those surgeons whose arthroscopic experience may be limited and who do not feel confident in performing a consistent, reproducible reconstruction with arthroscopic techniques will provide a better service to their patients if open surgical techniques are utilized.

Contraindications to the ACLR procedure include the presence of significant anteroinferior glenoid bone loss and the occurrence of the engaging Hill-Sachs lesion of the posterior humeral head. In these cases, a modified Bristow procedure[39] or a glenoid reconstruction procedure using iliac crest bone graft is indicated. The ACLR procedure is also contraindicated when the pattern of instability is mainly posterior or if injury to the posterior labrum is the primary pathology.

■ SURGICAL TECHNIQUE

Anesthesia

Most patients are administered general anesthesia. An interscalene block with local anesthetic can also be used to supplement the general anesthetic and aid in pain management. It is recommended that this regional anesthesia be administered postoperatively after the patient awakes from general anesthesia, so that a careful neurologic evaluation can be performed reliably.

Positioning

The patient is placed supine on the edge of the operating room table with the affected arm supported by an arm board while two folded surgical towels are placed beneath the scapula for stabilization. The affected arm is draped free to allow for movement and control of shoulder and arm position during the procedure. The operating room table should be angled approximately 45 degrees with the feet turned away from the operative side to create extra working room

around the shoulder. It is also recommended that the operative lights be positioned prior to surgical prepping and draping with one light placed directly overhead and the second light placed over the surgeon's left shoulder if the procedure is being performed on the patient's right shoulder.

Surface Anatomy

The acromion, clavicle, acromioclavicular joint, and coracoid process should be readily identified. The proximal humerus, including the bicipital groove, should also be noted and this is facilitated with rotation of the arm. Finally, the axillary skin crease should be formed to run parallel to Langer skin lines so that the incision will heal in a more cosmetic fashion.

Skin Incision/Superficial Dissection

A standard axillary skin incision is made starting proximally from approximately 1 to 2 cm distal and lateral to the tip of the coracoid process and extending distally to the axillary crease. If preferred, the surgeon may use local anesthetic, such as 0.25% bupivacaine with diluted epinephrine (1:200,000 or 5 mcgm/mL), which can be infiltrated into the skin prior to incision to help with localized pain control and to reduce skin bleeding. The skin and subcutaneous tissue are undermined to visualize the deltopectoral interval **(Fig. 1-1)**. Occasionally, it can be difficult to find this interval, and dissection toward the coracoid process in a proximal and medial direction will often facilitate its identification. The cephalic vein is then identified and dissected to be retracted laterally with the deltoid muscle. The deltopectoral interval is then developed by undermining the deltoid muscle

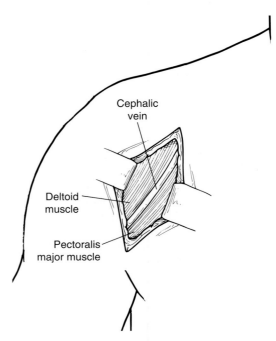

Cephalic vein

Deltoid muscle

Pectoralis major muscle

Fig. 1-1. Deltopectoral approach.

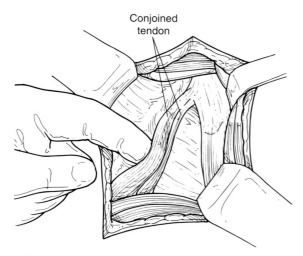

Fig. 1-2. Deep dissection lateral to conjoined tendon.

with a combination of blunt and sharp dissections and retracting it laterally with the cephalic vein, while the pectoralis major muscle is retracted medially. Retraction is performed with modified Goelet retractors to expose the underlying clavipectoral fascia and conjoined tendon.

Deeper Dissection

The clavipectoral fascia is incised along the lateral border of the conjoined tendon. It is important to start the dissection at the lateral border of the muscular portion of the coracobrachialis rather than the more medial tendinous part of the short head of the biceps muscle to ensure entering the correct dissection plane **(Fig. 1-2)**. Blunt dissection is carried out to

undermine the conjoined tendon, which is then retracted medially with a long narrow right angle retractor. Care should be taken to avoid overzealous medial retraction of the conjoined tendon to prevent injury to the underlying musculocutaneous nerve. The underlying subscapularis muscle is then visualized, and exposure can be improved with external rotation of the arm.

Subscapularis Division

The bicipital groove and lesser tuberosity of the proximal humerus are palpated, and the superior and inferior borders of the subscapularis muscle are identified. Inferiorly, the anterior humeral circumflex vessels can be readily identified, and if bleeding from these vessels occurs, they should be promptly cauterized or ligated to ensure hemostasis. The axillary nerve should also be easily palpable with a finger by sweeping medially and inferiorly at the inferior margin of the subscapularis muscle. The location of the axillary nerve should be carefully noted and it should be protected at all times. With a needle-point electrocautery device, the subscapularis tendon and muscle are then split horizontally along the course of its fibers between the upper two-thirds and lower one third of the muscle **(Fig. 1-3A,B)**. Care should be taken to divide just the subscapularis muscle and to preserve the underlying capsule. The tissue plane between the subscapularis and the capsule is developed with an elevator and is easier to identify if dissection is begun more medially within the muscular part of the subscapularis and continued laterally toward its tendinous portion **(Fig. 1-4)**. Once the overlying subscapularis is separated from the anterior capsule, a modified Gelpi self-retractor is used to keep the superior and inferior leaflets of the muscle apart and a three-pronged pitchfork is carefully placed on the

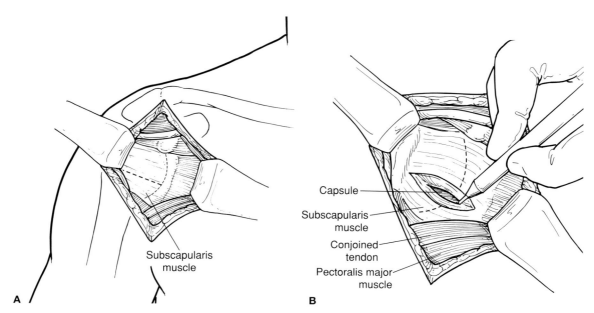

Fig. 1-3. A: Subscapularis muscle and tendon exposure and division between upper two thirds and lower one third. **B:** Transverse split of subscapularis muscle and tendon with electrocautery.

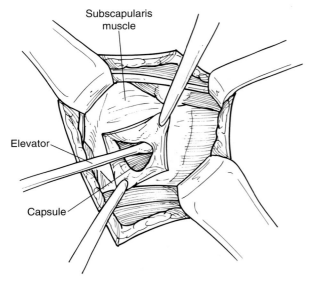

Fig. 1-4. Elevation of subscapularis from underlying capsule.

anterior glenoid neck to maintain retraction of the conjoined tendon and pectoralis muscle medially **(Fig. 1-5)**. The long narrow right angle retractor and the medial Goelet retractor can then be safely removed.

Anterior Capsule Division

The capsule, humeral head, and anterior glenoid are palpated, and a horizontal incision in the capsule is made with a long-handled no. 15 blade, starting from laterally and extending medially. Usually, this capsular incision parallels the split in the subscapularis muscle, but in cases where there is a large redundant capsule or in a revision surgery setting, care should be taken to identify the midanterior glenoid and the capsulotomy should be directed toward the 4 o'clock position of the glenoid of a right shoulder. Care should be

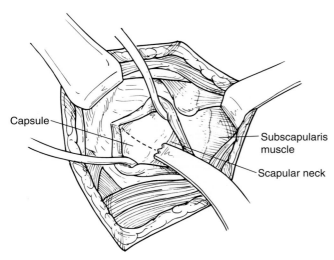

Fig. 1-5. Exposure of capsule to be split in line with subscapularis division.

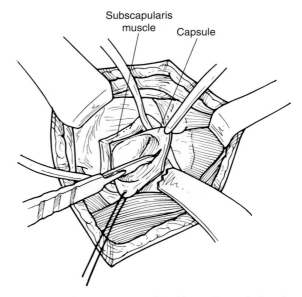

Fig. 1-6. Tagging sutures at glenoid margin and elevation of capsule from glenoid.

taken to preserve the anterior labrum as the incision is carried medially. Tag sutures with no. 2 braided suture are placed in the superior and inferior leaflets of the capsule, to the level of the glenoid margin in the medial and lateral directions **(Fig. 1-6)**. Exposure to the anterior glenoid and labrum is facilitated by placement of a single-prong (or double-prong) humeral head retractor between the humeral head and posterior rim of the glenoid to distract the joint. The glenoid articular surface, glenoid labrum, and capsule are then carefully inspected. The anterior glenoid labrum should be carefully probed to determine if a Bankart lesion is present. The capsule should also be inspected to assess tissue quality and the degree of laxity, and this information should be correlated with impressions from the examination under anesthesia and, if available, from findings of arthroscopic evaluation.

ACLR Reconstruction

If the anterior labrum is intact with no Bankart lesion but capsular laxity is noted, then the capsule is elevated subperiosteally from the anterior scapular neck with sharp dissection, taking care to preserve the anterior labrum. The inferior leaflet of the capsule will contain the important inferior glenohumeral ligament and should be dissected carefully down to the 6 o'clock position to allow for sufficient superior advancement. Extreme care should be taken to prevent injury to the nearby axillary nerve when mobilizing the inferior capsular flap. The superior leaflet should also be dissected from the anterior glenoid neck to allow for later mobilization inferiorly.

If a Bankart lesion is present, the anterior labrum should be sharply elevated from the face of the glenoid and dissected to expose the anterior glenoid neck. The glenoid rim and glenoid neck can then be abraded with a curette and power burr to promote a healing surface for the reattachment of the labrum. The detached labrum can then be incorporated with the capsular reconstruction as described below.

The anterior glenoid neck is debrided of any fibrous tissue, scar tissue, or remaining periosteum with a bone rongeur or curette. Next, three drill holes are placed 1 to 2 mm from the glenoid articular margin at the 2 o'clock, 4 o'clock, and 5:30 positions for the right shoulder **(Fig. 1-7)**. Suture anchors with nonabsorbable sutures are then sequentially placed into each drill hole. The inferior flap of the capsule will then be shifted proximally along the anterior glenoid margin while the superior flap will later be brought distally over the inferior flap and labrum. This technique not only tightens the capsule in a superior-inferior direction but also reinforces and augments the anterior labrum, while avoiding significant medial-lateral shortening of the capsule.

The humeral head retractor is removed and the glenohumeral joint irrigated to clear any loose debris. First, the most inferior sutures are brought through the inferior capsule in a horizontal mattress fashion, while pulling proximally on its tagging suture to shift this tissue superiorly **(Fig. 1-8)**. The sutures are then passed through capsular tissue under direct visualization, and care should be taken to stay medial to the tagging suture to avoid overtightening the capsule in a medial-lateral direction. Next, the middle sutures are passed in through the inferior capsule in a similar manner, followed by the most superior sutures. The position and placement of the sutures should be tested by pulling tightly on the sutures and noting the shift of the reconstructed capsule. The sutures are then tied in the standard fashion but are left uncut, to be used to anchor the superior flap of capsule.

Utilizing a similar technique, the superior flap of the capsule is pulled inferiorly with its tagging suture, and the most superior sutures are brought through the capsule in a horizontal mattress fashion, just medial to the tagging suture **(Fig. 1-9)**. Again, it is important to avoid moving the capsule

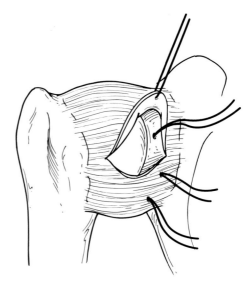

Fig. 1-8. Capsular reconstruction of inferior leaflet.

medially when the sutures passed through the capsule. Continuing inferiorly, the remaining sutures are passed through the superior capsule in a similar manner and are then tied securely. The sutures are then cut and the remainder of the capsule laterally is left overlapped but not closed with additional sutures **(Fig. 1-10)**. The patient's required range of motion during the postoperative period will dictate how much overlap and in which position this part of the lateral capsule will eventually heal.

The arm is then taken through a safe range of motion in which tension is placed on the repair. The patient may move within this safe zone without jeopardizing the reconstruction, and this allows for early range of motion postoperatively. The safe zone usually allows abduction above 90 degrees in the scapular plane and external rotation beyond 45 degrees before excessive tension is placed on the repair. If this safe zone cannot be achieved, then the reconstruction should be taken down and sutures replaced to allow for this

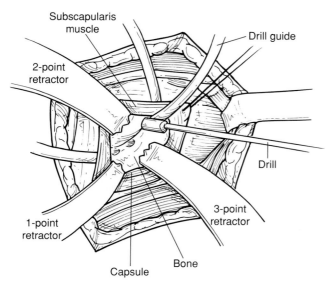

Fig. 1-7. Drill holes at glenoid margin for suture anchors.

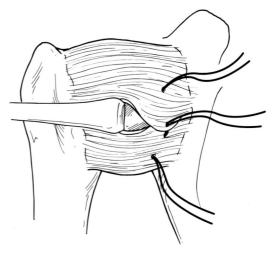

Fig. 1-9. Capsular reconstruction of superior leaflet.

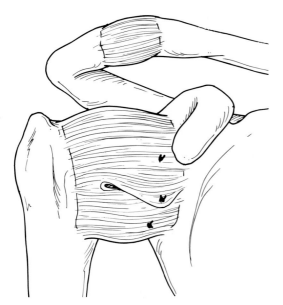

Fig. 1-10. Anterior capsulolabral reconstruction with transverse capsulotomy left unsutured.

motion. It is usually because the sutures have been placed too lateral within the capsular flaps and overtightening in a medial-lateral direction has occurred.

Closure Technique

The wound is irrigated profusely and the pitchfork retractor and modified Gelpi self-retractor are removed. The subscapularis muscle is reapproximated with interrupted no. 0 absorbable suture such as Vicryl (Ethicon, Inc, New Brunswick, NJ) **(Fig. 1-11)**. The deltopectoral interval typically does not require reapproximation, and the subcutaneous tissue is closed with interrupted 2–0 absorbable suture.

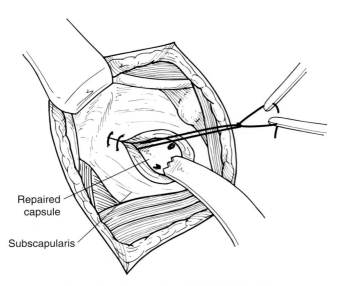

Repaired capsule

Subscapularis

Fig. 1-11. Closure of subscapularis tendon.

Finally, the skin is closed in a subcuticular fashion and reinforced with adhesive strips before a sterile dressing is applied and secured with foam tape. The arm is then placed in a sling with an abduction pillow orthosis, such as the UltraSling II (dj Orthopedics, Inc, Vista, CA)

■ TECHNICAL PITFALLS

It is critical to place the tagging sutures in the superior and inferior leaflets of the capsule at the level of the glenoid. These tagging sutures will guide you when placing the imbricating sutures from the bone anchors through capsular tissue. Placement of the tagging sutures too far lateral to the glenoid will lead to the imbricating sutures placed too far laterally and will cause overtightening of the capsule in the medial-lateral direction, which could contribute to loss of motion postoperatively.

The lateral capsule should be left open with no sutures placed in a "vests over pants" technique. Early in our experience, we were routinely closing the lateral capsule in this manner, and at times, this would lead to early motion loss and a longer recovery of external rotation. By leaving the lateral capsule overlapped but not closed with sutures, the patient could gain early full range of motion, and this dictated the amount of overlap and in which position the lateral capsule would eventually heal.

■ REHABILITATION/RETURN TO PLAY RECOMMENDATIONS

Immediately postoperatively, a sling and abduction pillow orthosis are worn full-time except during rehabilitative exercises. The patient is given ball-squeezing exercises and is encouraged to perform active elbow and wrist range of motion exercises the day of surgery. On the first postoperative day, passive and gentle active-assisted shoulder range of motion (ROM) exercises are begun with abduction, flexion, and external rotation in the scapular plane. Isometric shoulder strengthening exercises are also instituted as tolerated. Once the patient can actively abduct and forward flex the arm to 90 degrees, usually by 2 weeks, then the sling can be discontinued. At 2 weeks, active internal rotation and external rotation to neutral with the arm at the side with rubber tubing is begun. At 4 weeks, shoulder extension exercises, external rotation to tolerance, and active shoulder abduction to 90 degrees are allowed. At 6 to 8 weeks, strengthening exercises are continued with specific emphasis on the rotator cuff muscles and continued ROM exercises, especially concentrating on regaining full external rotation. Within 8 to 12 weeks, most patients will have achieved full forward flexion and abduction with some minor restriction in external rotation. As pain completely resolves and soft tissue healing is complete (usually by 3 months), a vigorous strengthening program is begun, continuing to refine the strength, power, and endurance of the rotator cuff muscles and also focusing on the scapular rotators and pectoralis and deltoid muscles. At 4 months, an isokinetic strength and endurance test can be performed as well as a careful evaluation of range of motion. Usually at least 80% strength of the contralateral shoulder is achieved and near full ROM is present by this time, and the patient may begin a progressive throwing (overhand) program. Most patients are then able to return to preinjury level activities and full overhand sports by 8 to 12 months postoperatively.

■ OUTCOMES AND FUTURE DIRECTIONS

This procedure has been performed on many skilled overhead-throwing athletes who have consistently been able to return to their previous level of competition[21,28,40] with excellent clinical results and minimal loss of motion. Similar successful results have been reported at other institutions in athletes with multidirectional instability.[41] In addition, a recent biomechanical study of cadaveric shoulders has demonstrated that the ACLR is comparable to an inferior capsular shift in terms of stability but resulted in less restriction of rotational range of motion.[42]

Initially, open surgery for anterior instability was felt to be superior compared to arthroscopic surgery.[9,35,43-45] However, recent advances in arthroscopic techniques and improvement in our understanding of the pathoanatomy of glenohumeral instability have led to several recent reports demonstrating similar successful results with arthroscopic repair compared with standard open techniques, both for Bankart repairs[10,46-52] and for capsular shifts.[46,53] However, to date, there have not yet been any long-term follow-up studies reporting the results of arthroscopic repair for anterior instability, especially in the overhand-throwing athlete.

■ SUGGESTED READINGS

Bankart ASB. Recurrent or habitual dislocation of the shoulder joint. Br Med J. 1923;2:1132–1133.

Cole BJ, L'Insalata J, Irrgang J, et al. Comparison of arthroscopic and open anterior shoulder stabilization: a two to six-year follow-up study. J Bone Joint Surg Am. 2000;82-A:1108–1114.

Gill TJ, Micheli LJ, Gebhard F, et al. Bankart repair for anterior instability of the shoulder: long-term outcome. J Bone Joint Surg Am. 1997;79:850–857.

Glousman RE, Jobe FW. Anterior and multidirectional glenohumeral instability. In: Jobe FW, ed. *Operative Techniques in Upper Extremity Sports Injuries*. St Louis: Mosby-Yearbook; 1996:191–210.

Itoi E, Watanabe W, Yamada S, et al. Range of motion after Bankart repair: vertical compared with horizontal capsulotomy. Am J Sports Med. 2001;29:441–445.

Jobe FW, Giangarra CE, Kvitne RS, et al. Anterior capsulolabral reconstruction of the shoulder in athletes in overhand sports. Am J Sports Med. 1991;19:428–434.

Jobe FW, Glousman RE. Anterior capsulolabral reconstruction. Tech Orthop. 1989;3:29–35.

Kvitne RS, Jobe FW. Anterior capsulolabral reconstruction for instability in the throwing athlete. In: Craig EV, ed. *Master Techniques in Orthopaedic Surgery: The Shoulder*. New York: Raven Press; 1995: 89–108.

Kvitne RS, Jobe FW, Jobe CM. Shoulder instability in the overhand or throwing athlete. Clin Sports Med. 1995;14:917–935.

Montgomery WH III, Jobe FW. Functional outcomes in athletes after modified anterior capsulolabral reconstruction. Am J Sports Med. 1994;22:352–358.

Perthes G. Uber operationen bei habitueller schulterluxation. Dtsch Z Chir. 1906;85:199–227.

Remia LF, Ravalin RV, Lemly KS, et al. Biomechanical evaluation of multidirectional glenohumeral instability and repair. Clin Orthop. 2003 Nov;(416):225–236.

Rowe CR, Patel D, Southmayd WW. The Bankart procedure: a long-term end-result study. J Bone Joint Surg Am. 1978;60:1–16.

■ REFERENCES

1. Perthes G. Uber operationen bei habitueller schulterluxation. Dtsch Z Chir. 1906;85:199–227.
2. Bankart ASB. Recurrent or habitual dislocation of the shoulder joint. Br Med J. 1923;2:1132–1133.
3. Rowe CR, Patel D, Southmayd WW. The Bankart procedure: a long-term end-result study. J Bone Joint Surg Am. 1978;60:1–16.
4. Gill TJ, Micheli LJ, Gebhard F, et al. Bankart repair for anterior instability of the shoulder: long-term outcome. J Bone Joint Surg Am. 1997;79:850–857.
5. Levine WN, Richmond JC, Donaldson WR. Use of the suture anchor in open Bankart reconstruction: a follow-up report. Am J Sports Med. 1994;22:723–726.
6. Rosenberg BN, Richmond JC, Levine WN. Long-term followup of Bankart reconstruction: incidence of late degenerative glenohumeral arthrosis. Am J Sports Med. 1995;23:538–544.
7. Potzl W, Witt KA, Hackenberg L, et al. Results of suture anchor repair of anteroinferior shoulder instability: a prospective clinical study of 85 shoulders. J Shoulder Elbow Surg. 2003;12:322–326.
8. Sperber A, Hamberg P, Karlsson J, et al. Comparison of an arthroscopic and an open procedure for posttraumatic instability of the shoulder: a prospective, randomized multicenter study. J Shoulder Elbow Surg. 2001;10:105–108.
9. Guanche CA, Quick DC, Sodergren KM, et al. Arthroscopic versus open reconstruction of the shoulder in patients with isolated Bankart lesions. Am J Sports Med. 1996;24:144–148.
10. Kim SH, Ha KI. Bankart repair in traumatic anterior shoulder instability: open versus arthroscopic technique. Arthroscopy. 2002;18:755–763.
11. Itoi E, Watanabe W, Yamada S, et al. Range of motion after Bankart repair. Vertical compared with horizontal capsulotomy. Am J Sports Med. 2001;29:441–445.
12. Thomas SC, Matsen FA III. An approach to the repair of avulsion of the glenohumeral ligaments in the management of traumatic anterior glenohumeral instability. J Bone Joint Surg Am. 1989;71: 506–513.
13. Neer CS II, Foster CR. Inferior capsular shift for involuntary inferior and multidirectional instability of the shoulder: a preliminary report. J Bone Joint Surg Am. 1980;62:897–908.
14. Wirth MA, Blatter G, Rockwood CA Jr. The capsular imbrication procedure for recurrent anterior instability of the shoulder. J Bone Joint Surg Am. 1996;78:246–259.
15. Altchek DW, Warren RF, Skyhar MJ, et al. T-plasty modification of the Bankart procedure for multidirectional instability of the anterior and inferior types. J Bone Joint Surg Am. 1991;73:105–112.

16. Cooper RA, Brems JJ. The inferior capsular-shift procedure for multidirectional instability of the shoulder. J Bone Joint Surg Am. 1992;74:1516–1521.

17. Bigliani LU, Kurzweil PR, Schwartzbach CC, et al. Inferior capsular shift procedure for anterior-inferior shoulder instability in athletes. Am J Sports Med. 1994;22:578–584.

18. Pollock RG, Owens JM, Flatow EL, et al. Operative results of the inferior capsular shift procedure for multidirectional instability of the shoulder. J Bone Joint Surg Am. 2000;82-A:919–928.

19. Kvitne RS, Jobe FW, Jobe CM. Shoulder instability in the overhand or throwing athlete. Clin Sports Med. 1995;14:917–935.

20. Davidson PA, Elattrache NS, Jobe CM, et al. Rotator cuff and posterior-superior glenoid labrum injury associated with increased glenohumeral motion: a new site of impingement. J Shoulder Elbow Surg. 1995;4:384–390.

21. Kvitne RS, Jobe FW. The diagnosis and treatment of anterior instability in the throwing athlete. Clin Orthop. 1993 Jun;(291):107–123.

22. Jobe FW, Kvitne RS, Giangarra CE. Shoulder pain in the overhand or throwing athlete: the relationship of anterior instability and rotator cuff impingement. Orthop Rev. 1989;18:963–975.

23. Jobe FW. Impingement problems in the athlete. Instr Course Lect. 1989;38:205–209.

24. Jobe CM. Posterior superior glenoid impingement: expanded spectrum. Arthroscopy. 1995;11:530–536.

25. Liu SH, Boynton E. Posterior superior impingement of the rotator cuff on the glenoid rim as a cause of shoulder pain in the overhead athlete. Arthroscopy. 1993;9:697–699.

26. Walch G, Liotard JP, Boileau P, et al. [Postero-superior glenoid impingement: another shoulder impingement]. Rev Chir Orthop Reparatrice Appar Mot. 1991;77:571–574. French.

27. Walch G, Boileau P, Noel E, et al. Impingement of the deep surface of the supraspinatus tendon on the posterosuperior glenoid rim: an arthroscopic study. J Shoulder Elbow Surg. 1992;1:238–245.

28. Jobe FW, Giangarra CE, Kvitne RS, et al. Anterior capsulolabral reconstruction of the shoulder in athletes in overhand sports. Am J Sports Med. 1991;19:428–434.

29. Jobe FW, Glousman RE. Anterior capsulolabral reconstruction. Tech Orthop. 1989;3:29–35.

30. Glousman RE, Jobe FW. Anterior and multidirectional glenohumeral instability. In: Jobe FW, ed. *Operative Techniques in Upper Extremity Sports Injuries*. St Louis: Mosby-Yearbook; 1996: 191–210.

31. Kvitne RS, Jobe FW. Anterior capsulolabral reconstruction for instability in the throwing athlete. In: Craig EV, ed. *Master Techniques in Orthopaedic Surgery: The Shoulder*. New York: Raven Press; 1995:89–108.

32. Roberts SN, Taylor DE, Brown JN, et al. Open and arthroscopic techniques for the treatment of traumatic anterior shoulder instability in Australian rules football players. J Shoulder Elbow Surg. 1999;8:403–409.

33. Uhorchak JM, Arciero RA, Huggard D, et al. Recurrent shoulder instability after open reconstruction in athletes involved in collision and contact sports. Am J Sports Med. 2000;28:794–799.

34. Hayashida K, Yoneda M, Nakagawa S, et al. Arthroscopic Bankart suture repair for traumatic anterior shoulder instability: analysis of the causes of a recurrence. Arthroscopy. 1998;14:295–301.

35. Grana WA, Buckley PD, Yates CK. Arthroscopic Bankart suture repair. Am J Sports Med. 1993;21:348–353.

36. Levine WN, Arroyo JS, Pollock RG, et al. Open revision stabilization surgery for recurrent anterior glenohumeral instability. Am J Sports Med. 2000;28:156–160.

37. Mologne TS, McBride MT, Lapoint JM. Assessment of failed arthroscopic anterior labral repairs: findings at open surgery. Am J Sports Med. 1997;25:813–817.

38. Zabinski SJ, Callaway GH, Cohen S, et al. Revision shoulder stabilization: 2- to 10-year results. J Shoulder Elbow Surg. 1999;8: 58–65.

39. Lombardo SJ, Kerlan RK, Jobe FW, et al. The modified Bristow procedure for recurrent dislocation of the shoulder. J Bone Joint Surg Am. 1976;58:256–261.

40. Montgomery WH III, Jobe FW. Functional outcomes in athletes after modified anterior capsulolabral reconstruction. Am J Sports Med. 1994;22:352–358.

41. Bak K, Spring BJ, Henderson JP. Inferior capsular shift procedure in athletes with multidirectional instability based on isolated capsular and ligamentous redundancy. Am J Sports Med. 2000;28: 466–471.

42. Remia LF, Ravalin RV, Lemly KS, et al. Biomechanical evaluation of multidirectional glenohumeral instability and repair. Clin Orthop. 2003 Nov;(416):225–236.

43. Geiger DF, Hurley JA, Tovey JA, et al. Results of arthroscopic versus open Bankart suture repair. Clin Orthop. 1997 Apr;(337):111–117.

44. Steinbeck J, Jerosch J. Arthroscopic transglenoid stabilization versus open anchor suturing in traumatic anterior instability of the shoulder. Am J Sports Med. 1998;26:373–378.

45. Koss S, Richmond JC, Woodward JS Jr. Two- to five-year followup of arthroscopic Bankart reconstruction using a suture anchor technique. Am J Sports Med. 1997;25:809–812.

46. Kim SH, Ha KI, Cho YB, et al. Arthroscopic anterior stabilization of the shoulder: two to six-year follow-up. J Bone Joint Surg Am. 2003;85-A:1511–1518.

47. Kim SH, Ha KI, Jung MW, et al. Accelerated rehabilitation after arthroscopic Bankart repair for selected cases: a prospective randomized clinical study. Arthroscopy. 2003;19:722–731.

48. Bottoni CR, Wilckens JH, DeBerardino TM, et al. A prospective, randomized evaluation of arthroscopic stabilization versus nonoperative treatment in patients with acute, traumatic, first-time shoulder dislocations. Am J Sports Med. 2002;30:576–580.

49. Cole BJ, L'Insalata J, Irrgang J, et al. Comparison of arthroscopic and open anterior shoulder stabilization. A two to six-year follow-up study. J Bone Joint Surg Am. 2000;82-A:1108–1114.

50. Gartsman GM, Roddey TS, Hammerman SM. Arthroscopic treatment of anterior-inferior glenohumeral instability: two to five-year follow-up. J Bone Joint Surg Am. 2000;82-A:991–1003.

51. O'Neill DB. Arthroscopic Bankart repair of anterior detachments of the glenoid labrum: a prospective study. J Bone Joint Surg Am. 1999;81:1357–1366.

52. Bacilla P, Field LD, Savoie FH III. Arthroscopic Bankart repair in a high demand patient population. Arthroscopy. 1997;13: 51–60.

53. Treacy SH, Savoie FH III, Field LD. Arthroscopic treatment of multidirectional instability. J Shoulder Elbow Surg. 1999;8:345–350.

ARTHROSCOPIC BANKART REPAIR

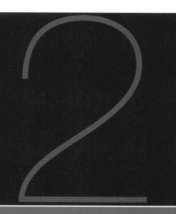

■ STEPHEN S. BURKHART, MD, JOHN R. KLEIN, MD

■ HISTORY OF THE TECHNIQUE

Arthroscopic Bankart repair results have traditionally been deemed as inferior to the results obtained through open repair. The first arthroscopic Bankart repairs were performed with transglenoid labral suturing, in which the labrum was often repaired in a medialized, nonanatomic position.[1–5] The development and the use of suture anchors in arthroscopic Bankart repair, along with the greater recognition of the need to repair the labrum to the glenoid rim or face, have allowed surgeons to achieve results that are comparable to open Bankart repair.[6–15]

The senior author (SSB) has previously reviewed his results of arthroscopic Bankart repair.[16] The redislocation rate in this series was 10.8%. However, the redislocation rate was only 4% for patients without significant bone defects. In patients with an engaging Hill-Sachs lesion or significant glenoid bone loss, the redislocation rate was 67%. In light of these results, it is our opinion that the failure of Bankart repairs, whether done arthroscopically or open, is not usually a failure of technique, but rather a failure to recognize and treat significant glenohumeral bone deficiency. Accordingly, we treat patients who have greater than 25% loss of the anterior glenoid or an engaging Hill-Sachs lesion with an open Latarjet procedure to restore the normal articular arc between the glenoid and the humerus.

■ INDICATIONS AND CONTRAINDICATIONS

In the contact or overhead athlete who dislocates his or her shoulder traumatically for the first time and has a documented Bankart lesion on magnetic resonance imaging (MRI) without significant bone loss, we recommend an arthroscopic Bankart repair since, in our clinical experience, the rate of redislocation without surgery in this group of athletes is quite high. For the older recreational athlete who dislocates his or her shoulder traumatically for the first time, we recommend nonoperative treatment. In all patients who have traumatically dislocated their shoulders more than once, we recommend an arthroscopic Bankart repair. Patients who have atraumatic shoulder instability and have evidence of ligamentous laxity on physical examination are initially treated nonoperatively with physical therapy.

In patients who have dislocated their shoulder multiple times and in patients who appear to have a bony Bankart lesion or a large Hill-Sachs lesion on radiographs, we obtain preoperative computed tomography (CT) scans with three-dimensional reconstructed images of the glenoid and humerus in order to assess the degree of glenohumeral bone loss. Typically, in patients who have a high degree of glenohumeral bone loss, we will perform an initial diagnostic shoulder arthroscopy in order to diagnose and arthroscopically repair any superior labral anterior to posterior (SLAP) lesion. We will also assess arthroscopically if there is an engaging Hill-Sachs lesion or quantify the degree of glenoid bone loss. If there is an engaging Hill-Sachs lesion and/or loss of greater than 25% of the anterior glenoid, we will reposition and reprep the patient and proceed to an open Latarjet procedure.

■ SURGICAL TECHNIQUE

After induction of general anesthesia, the patient is placed into the lateral decubitus position. Five to 10 pounds of balanced suspension are used with the arm in 20 to 30 degrees of abduction and 20 degrees of forward flexion (Star Sleeve Traction System; Arthrex, Inc, Naples, Fla). Glenohumeral arthroscopy is performed through the standard posterior portal with an arthroscopic pump maintaining a pressure of 60 mm Hg.

For anterior instability cases we use a standard anterior portal for suture placement and anchor placement. Often a lower anterior portal is needed for suture anchor placement in the 5 o'clock position of the glenoid.[17] While a posterior viewing portal is initially used, the anterosuperior portal gives the surgeon a better view of the anterior aspect of the glenoid. An unobstructed view is essential for glenoid bone preparation and correct suture anchor placement.

Anterior instability cases are often associated with SLAP lesions or posterior labral tears. It is, therefore, important to systematically examine both the superior labrum and posterior labrum to ensure that there are no concomitant injuries to these labral structures. While viewing through the posterior viewing portal, we take the arm out of traction and place it in external rotation and abduction to see if there is a peel-back lesion. As the arm is placed in abduction and external rotation, the superior labrum, if not well anchored, will shift medially over the corner of the glenoid onto the posterosuperior scapular neck.[18] A positive peel-back test confirms a posterosuperior SLAP lesion. It is also necessary to thoroughly probe the biceps root attachment since an isolated anterosuperior SLAP tear will have a negative peel-back test but will have a displaceable biceps root. Since swelling can obliterate the superior sulcus above the superior labrum, and an anterior capsulolabral repair can be a lengthy procedure, we initially prepare the bone of the superior glenoid neck, place anchors, and pass the sutures through the superior labrum. We do not, however, tie the sutures of the SLAP repair until the end of the procedure. The SLAP lesion produces some "pseudolaxity" within the glenohumeral joint, which improves the visualization and working space for anterior

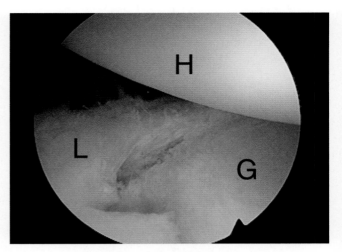

Fig. 2-1. Arthroscopic view from an anterosuperior portal demonstrating a Bankart lesion. L, anterior labrum; G, glenoid; H, humerus.

capsulolabral repair. Tying the sutures of the SLAP repair obliterates this laxity and makes anterior capsulolabral repair more difficult.

Once a Bankart lesion is identified **(Fig. 2-1)**, we use an arthroscopic elevator to mobilize the capsulolabral sleeve from the glenoid. During this step, the subscapularis muscle must be seen underneath the mobilized labral tissue **(Fig. 2-2A,B)**. This ensures that the anterior labrum has been sufficiently mobilized from the glenoid so that it may be later shifted back to its anatomic position on the glenoid. An arthroscopic shaver is then used to create a bleeding bone surface on the glenoid rim. During this step, the surgeon must be careful not to remove glenoid bone in order to avoid creating an iatrogenic glenoid bone deficiency. We also use an arthroscopic curette to remove a small portion of cartilage from the glenoid face **(Fig. 2-3)**. This will enable the surgeon

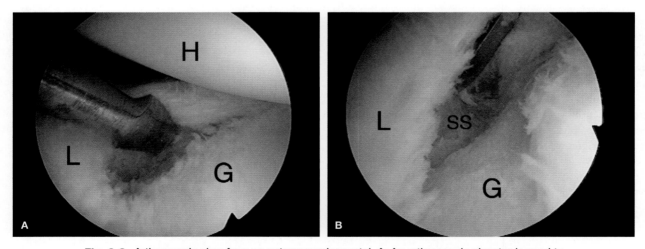

Fig. 2-2. Arthroscopic view from an anterosuperior portal. **A:** An arthroscopic elevator is used to mobilize the capsulolabral sleeve from the glenoid. **B:** Completed mobilization of the capsulolabral sleeve is confirmed with visualization of the underlying subscapularis muscle. L, anterior labrum; G, glenoid; H, humerus.

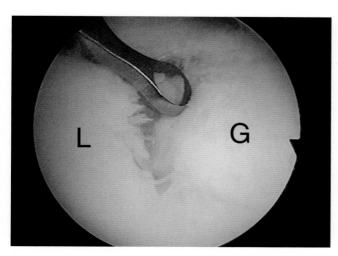

Fig. 2-3. Arthroscopic view from an anterosuperior portal demonstrating the use of an arthroscopic curette, which is used to remove a small portion of articular cartilage off the glenoid face. L, anterior labrum; G, glenoid.

to place the suture anchors onto the glenoid face and avoid having a medialized capsulolabral repair. After the glenoid is prepared, the suture anchors are placed. Usually three anchors are placed, beginning at the 5 o'clock position inferiorly (in a right shoulder) and then progressing superiorly.

In the vast majority of anterior instability cases, the angle of approach to place anchors in the lower anteroinferior quadrant is too oblique from a standard anterior portal. A lower anterior 5 o'clock portal is made for such cases. While viewing from an anterosuperior portal, we use a spinal needle to determine the proper location of this portal. Because only a small suture anchor delivery tube (Spear guide; Arthrex, Inc, Naples, Fla) is necessary for suture anchor

placement, only a small 3-mm skin incision is required **(Fig. 2-4A,B)**. We prefer to use 3.0 mm BioFastak suture anchors (Arthrex, Inc, Naples, Fla) loaded with no. 2 FiberWire (Arthrex, Inc, Naples, Fla). The BioFastak delivery cannula is the spear guide with a trocar, which is "walked" down the needle until its entry is visualized within the glenohumeral joint. We prefer to place the two lowest anchors through this percutaneous 5 o'clock portal **(Fig. 2-5A,B)**. The superiormost anchor is placed through the standard anterior portal.

Sutures are passed in a retrograde or antegrade fashion **(Fig. 2-6A,B,C)** from the standard anterior portal (45-degree Birdbeak suture passer, Sidewinder suture passer, Suturelasso, Viper suture passer; Arthrex, Inc, Naples, Fla). After all sutures have been passed through the labrum, the suture pairs are tied sequentially, from inferior to superior **(Fig. 2-7A,B)**. To ensure loop security (maintenance of a tight suture loop around the enclosed soft tissue) and knot security (resistance of the knot to failure by slippage) we use a double diameter knot pusher (Surgeon's Sixth Finger, Arthrex, Inc, Naples, Fla). Simple sutures are tied with stacked half hitches. We initially stack three half hitches followed by three half hitches on alternating posts. Switching posts can be easily performed without rethreading by flipping the half hitch through differential tensioning of the suture limbs.

■ TECHNICAL ALTERNATIVES AND PITFALLS

As noted earlier, the majority of our arthroscopic Bankart repair failures were due to the presence of glenohumeral bone defects. Accordingly, it is important to arthroscopically assess and quantify the amount of glenohumeral bone loss in each patient.

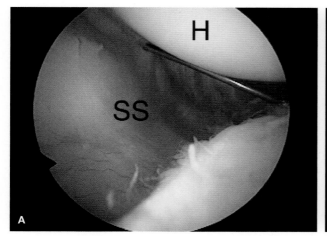
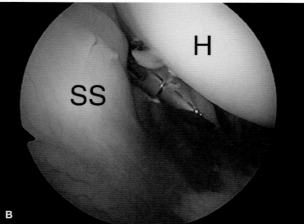

Fig. 2-4. Arthroscopic view from an anterosuperior portal demonstrating placement of the anterior 5 o'clock portal. **A:** A spinal needle is used to determine the correct angle of approach to place anchors in the lower anteroinferior quadrant of the glenoid. **B:** Through a percutaneous skin incision a Spear guide (Arthrex, Inc) is carefully passed alongside the spinal needle. SS, subscapularis; H, humerus.

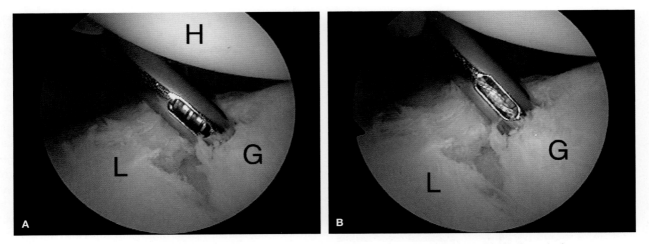

Fig. 2-5. Arthroscopic view from an anterosuperior portal. **A:** Using the Spear guide (Arthrex, Inc) a hole is tapped on the glenoid face. **B:** Placement of the 3.0 mm BioFastak suture anchor (Arthrex, Inc) through the Spear guide. L, anterior labrum; G, glenoid; H, humerus.

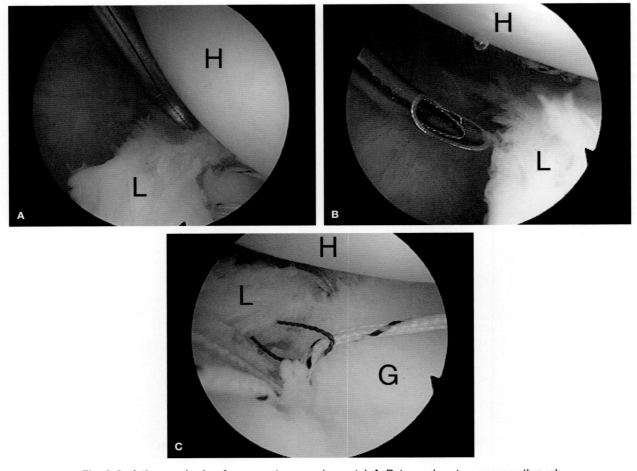

Fig. 2-6. Arthroscopic view from an anterosuperior portal. **A:** Retrograde suture passage through the capsulolabral sleeve can be accomplished with a Sidewinder suture passer (Arthrex, Inc). **B:** Alternatively the Suturelasso (Arthrex, Inc) can be used for retrograde suture passage. **C:** Successful suture passage through the capsulolabral sleeve using the Suturelasso. L, anterior labrum; G, glenoid; H, humerus.

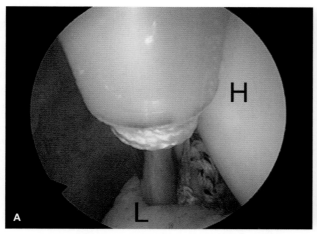 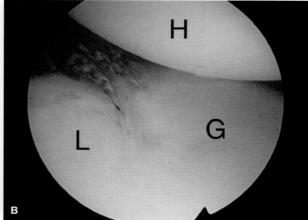

Fig. 2-7. Arthroscopic view from an anterosuperior portal. **A:** The use of the double diameter knot pusher (Surgeon's Sixth Finger, Arthrex, Inc) ensures loop security and knot security. **B:** Completed anatomic capsulolabral repair. L, anterior labrum; G, glenoid; H, humerus.

To identify an engaging Hill-Sachs lesion, the arm is taken out of traction and placed in a position of athletic function (a position defined as 90 degrees of abduction combined with external rotation of 90 degrees).[16,19] If the Hill-Sachs lesion engages the anterior rim of the glenoid with the arm in a functional (90-90) position this is classified as an engaging Hill-Sachs lesion. If a Hill-Sachs lesion engages the glenoid with the arm in a nonfunctional position of shoulder extension or of low shoulder abduction (<70 degrees), then this is defined as a nonengaging Hill-Sachs lesion. An engaging Hill-Sachs lesion is a relative contraindication to arthroscopic Bankart repair, since the Hill-Sachs lesion will continue to engage the anterior rim of the glenoid, giving the patient a continued sense of instability. Accordingly, in cases of engaging Hill-Sachs lesions, we recommend an open Latarjet procedure to extend the anterior glenoid arc by means of a coracoid bone graft so that the Hill-Sachs lesion cannot engage.

When viewing the glenoid from the anterosuperior portal, the glenoid normally has the shape of a pear—the inferior half of the glenoid is significantly wider than its superior half. If the patient has suffered significant inferior glenoid bone loss, the ratio is reversed and the superior half of the glenoid is wider than its inferior half.[20,21] Normally the bare spot of the glenoid represents the equidistant point between the anterior and posterior rims of the glenoid. Using a probe with calibrated laser marks, the amount of inferior bone loss can be quantified. An inverted pear glenoid is defined as bone loss of at least 25% of the inferior glenoid diameter. The presence of greater than 25% bone loss of the inferior glenoid diameter is a contraindication to arthroscopic Bankart repair.

■ REHABILITATION/RETURN TO PLAY RECOMMENDATIONS

Following surgery, the arm is placed in a sling with a small pillow. The sling is continuously worn for 4 weeks. Active flexion and extension of the elbow is encouraged. Passive external rotation is restricted to 0 degrees (straight ahead position). After 4 weeks, the sling is discontinued and patients are encouraged to perform passive overhead and internal rotation stretching with a rope and pulley. External rotation stretching is progressed with the goal of reaching 50% of the external rotation of the contralateral shoulder by 12 weeks. Isotonic strengthening of the rotator cuff, deltoid, and scapular stabilizers is not begun until 6 weeks after surgery. Progressive activities are allowed as strength increases. Unrestricted activities and return to play are not allowed until a minimum of 6 months after surgery.

■ OUTCOMES AND FUTURE DIRECTIONS

Recent reports of arthroscopic Bankart repair have demonstrated similar redislocation rates as open repairs. Unfortunately, newer techniques to augment arthroscopic Bankart repair, such as thermal shrinkage and capsular plication, continue to focus on the soft tissues. It is our belief that this attention is misdirected and that the real focus should be on the need to recognize and correctly treat the presence of glenohumeral bone deficiency, which, in our opinion, is the main cause of failure of arthroscopic Bankart repairs. Instead of overconstraining and overtightening these patients, we believe the treatment of choice is a bone grafting procedure (e.g., Latarjet procedure), which restores the normal articular arc of the glenohumeral joint.

■ SUGGESTED READINGS

Chow JCY, ed. *Advanced Arthroscopy*. New York: Springer-Verlag; 2001.

Codman EA. *The Shoulder*. Boston: Thomas Todd; 1934.

McGinty JB, Burkhart SS, Jackson RW, et al., eds. *Operative Arthroscopy*. Philadelphia: Lippincott Williams & Wilkins; 2003.

■ REFERENCES

1. Grana WA, Buckley PD, Yates CK. Arthroscopic Bankart suture repair. Am J Sports Med. 1993;21:348–353.
2. Green MR, Christensen KP. Arthroscopic Bankart procedure: two- to five-year followup with clinical correlation to severity of glenoid labral lesion. Am J Sports Med. 1995;23:276–281.
3. Kandziora F, Jager A, Bischof F, et al. Arthroscopic labrum refixation for post-traumatic anterior instability: suture anchor versus transglenoid fixation technique. Arthroscopy. 2000;16:359–366.
4. McIntyre LF, Caspari RB. The rationale and technique for arthroscopic reconstruction of anterior shoulder instability using multiple sutures. Orthop Clin North Am. 1993;24:55–58.
5. Morgan CD, Bodenstab AB. Arthroscopic Bankart suture repair: technique and early results. Arthroscopy. 1987;3:111–122.
6. Rowe CR, Patel D, Southmayd WW. The Bankart procedure. J Bone Joint Surg Am. 1978;60:1–16.
7. Thomas SC, Matsen FA. An approach to the repair of avulsion of the glenohumeral ligaments in the management of traumatic anterior glenohumeral instability. J Bone Joint Surg Am. 1989;71:506–513.
8. Abrams JS, Savoie FH, Tauro JC, et al. Recent advances in the evaluation and treatment of shoulder instability: anterior, posterior, and multidirectional. Arthroscopy. 2002;18(suppl):1–18.
9. Bacilla P, Field LD, Savoie FH. Arthroscopic Bankart repair in a high demand patient population. Arthroscopy. 1997;13:51–60.
10. Elrod BF. Arthroscopic reconstruction of traumatic anterior instability. Op Tech Sports Med. 1997;5:215–225.
11. Gartsman GM, Roddey TS, Hammerman SM. Arthroscopic treatment of anterior-inferior glenohumeral instability. J Bone Joint Surg Am. 2000;82:991–1003.
12. Kim SH, Ha KI, Kim YM. Arthroscopic revision Bankart repair: a prospective outcome study. Arthroscopy. 2002;18:469–482.
13. Kim SH, Ha KI, Kim SH. Bankart repair in traumatic anterior shoulder instability: open versus arthroscopic technique. Arthroscopy. 2002;18:755–763.
14. Ryu RK. Arthroscopic approach to traumatic anterior shoulder instability. Arthroscopy. 2003;19(suppl):94–101.
15. Wolf EM. Arthroscopic capsulolabral repair using suture anchors. Orthop Clin North Am. 1993;24:59–69.
16. Burkhart SS, DeBeer JF. Traumatic glenohumeral bone defects and their relationship to failure of arthroscopic Bankart repairs: significance of the inverted-pear glenoid and the humeral engaging Hill-Sachs lesion. Arthroscopy. 2000;16:677–694.
17. Davidson PA, Tibone JE. Anterior-inferior (5 o'clock) portal for shoulder arthroscopy. Arthroscopy. 1995;11:519–525.
18. Burkhart SS, Morgan CD, Kibler WB. The disabled shoulder: spectrum of pathology. Part I: Pathoanatomy and biomechanics. Arthroscopy. 2003;19:404–420.
19. Burkhart SS, Danaceau SM. Articular arc length mismatch as a cause of failed Bankart repair. Arthroscopy. 2000;16:740–744.
20. Burkhart SS, DeBeer JF, Tehrany AM, et al. Quantifying glenoid bone loss arthroscopically in shoulder instability. Arthroscopy. 2002;18:488–491.
21. Lo IK, Parten PM, Burkhart SS. The inverted pear glenoid: an indicator of significant glenoid bone loss. Arthroscopy. 2004;20:169–174.

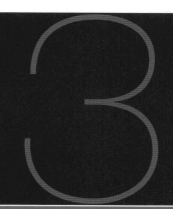

OPEN TREATMENT OF MULTIDIRECTIONAL SHOULDER INSTABILITY IN ATHLETES

■ ILYA VOLOSHIN, MD, KEVIN J. SETTER, MD, LOUIS U. BIGLIANI, MD

■ HISTORY OF THE TECHNIQUE

Multidirectional instability (MDI) of the shoulder was originally described by Neer and Foster[1] in 1980 as instability in more than one direction: anterior, posterior, or inferior. MDI is classically thought to have an atraumatic etiology; however, many patients, especially athletes, are subjected to microtrauma or even multiple frank traumatic episodes that attenuate their capsular restraints resulting in MDI. Bankart lesions and humeral head defects often associated with unidirectional traumatic instability may also be present, with less incidence, in patients with MDI.[2] From an operative standpoint, it is important to distinguish MDI from unidirectional instability for two reasons: (a) standard anterior reconstructions addressing Bankart lesions and the anterior capsule alone do not address the inferior and posterior components of instability in MDI,[1] (b) soft tissue imbalance created by tightening capsular structures on one side only have been shown to result in capsulorrhaphy arthropathy,[2-4] often at a young age, caused by fixed subluxation of the humeral head in the opposite direction.[4-6] Several reports in literature highlight the challenge of making the diagnosis of MDI.[7,8] Currently, there are no specific guidelines to define this group of patients. Since the original report by Neer and Foster in 1980,[1] reports of surgical treatment have utilized different criteria for assigning the diagnosis of MDI.[9-11] A recent report by McFarland et al.[12] demonstrated that the literature on this subject may be limited secondary to the variety of diagnostic criteria used to define MDI. Perhaps this has been the result of shoulder instability representing a spectrum of pathology often difficult to separate into two distinct entities—unidirectional and multidirectional. Although this distinction may be important in terms of reporting surgical results, from the surgical treatment standpoint there is a continuum of pathology that exists spanning both of these diagnostic entities.

A previously normal shoulder in an athlete can undergo adaptive capsular stretching due to sports participation (i.e., swimming or gymnastics) and subsequently undergo a traumatic episode resulting in instability in multiple directions. A study from our institution on material properties of inferior glenohumeral ligament, the main stabilizer of anterior translation of the humeral head,[13] demonstrated significant strain at the midsubstance of the ligament prior to its failure.[14] This is consistent with the findings in cadaveric specimens with isolated Bankart lesion, without capsular laxity, showing no increase in instability resulting in full dislocation.[15] We feel that using strict guidelines for MDI versus unidirectional instability in terms of operative intervention, especially in athletes who can exhibit an overlap caused by day-to-day microtrauma with a superimposed traumatic event, can lead to potentially missing important pathology that should be addressed. The senior author (LUB) favors the anterior-inferior capsular shift operation to address the continuum of capsular and labral pathology often present in athletes.

■ INDICATIONS AND CONTRAINDICATIONS

Athletes with MDI may present in a variety of ways. Neer[7] emphasized that the majority of his patients with this diagnosis were athletic, often exhibiting inherent ligamentous laxity who had been subjected to repetitive minor trauma or several major traumatic episodes. Participation in certain sports that expose the shoulder to repetitive microtrauma—swimming, weight lifting, gymnastics, and overhead activity sports, tends to predispose to MDI. Generalized joint laxity is also a contributing factor in MDI even without significant trauma.[1] Patients with MDI often present with shoulder and upper arm pain, fatigability, inability to carry heavy loads, and transitory numbness and weakness after activity. Often the clinical picture is not clear, however, and multiple encounters with the patient are needed to achieve the correct diagnosis.

A complete history of the symptoms is extremely important to determine the etiology and to elucidate the main direction of instability. Duration of symptoms, characterization of their severity, activity associated with their increase or decrease, presence or absence of the traumatic event, and history of systemic metabolic disorders resulting in generalized joint laxity should be actively sought. Instability must be separated into involuntary and voluntary. Voluntary dislocators must also be separated into patients who have positional instability and can dislocate on command and those with underlying psychiatric disorder—true voluntary instability. The patients who have positional instability and can voluntarily dislocate their shoulder when asked, but otherwise try to avoid dislocations, can have a successful result after surgical intervention after proper nonoperative management. Conversely, patients with true voluntary instability are poor surgical candidates and skillful neglect combined with nonoperative management and potentially psychiatric evaluation should be considered. The patient's motivation for improvement should also be assessed. Strict adherence to the postoperative rehabilitation program is extremely important for a successful outcome. More than one interview is usually necessary to sort through these important issues.

A thorough physical examination must be performed to detect potential other causes of pain. It is easy to make the wrong diagnosis in a loose shoulder with other lesions, such as acromioclavicular joint arthritis or cervical radiculitis, that are responsible for pain. Many athletes' shoulders exhibit laxity, which is normal, without the diagnosis of instability. This is a crucial point that must be remembered when examining a patient. Both shoulders as well as other joints (elbows, finger joints, and knees) must be examined for signs of generalized ligamentous laxity. Complete examination of the shoulder is crucial to determine the etiology of pain. Diagnostic injections with 1% lidocaine into the subacromial space or acromioclavicular joint are useful to differentiate subacromial pathology from glenohumeral lesions. Close inspection of scapulothoracic articulation must be performed. Any signs of muscular atrophy or scapular winging must be noted. Scapulothoracic instability may present with symptoms of vague pain and numbness and tingling similar to patients with microinstability of the glenohumeral joint. Specific tests on physical examination are useful to determine the direction of glenohumeral instability. Presence of pain during the performance of these tests is important and should be noted; however, apprehension, not pain, is a true positive result of these tests. Anterior apprehension test determines the presence of anterior instability.[16] This test is performed with the arm in abduction and external rotation

with the humerus being pushed forward. Posterior instability is tested with the arm flexed and internally rotated with the humerus pushed posteriorly.[16] Sulcus sign is important in making the diagnosis of MDI and is indicative of inferior laxity.[1] Downward pressure is applied to the adducted arm, creating an indentation of skin between the acromion and the humeral head. Inferior apprehension can be determined with the arm abducted and humerus pushed downward. Additional tests for glenohumeral instability, such as the fulcrum test, Fukuda test, relocation test, and push-pull stress test have been described and are helpful in making the diagnosis.[1,2] Often a patient cannot relax enough to adequately perform instability tests in the office. Exam under anesthesia in this type of patient is a very important part of operative treatment if a nonoperative approach fails.

Plain radiographs, anteroposterior view in internal, neutral, and external rotation, scapular-Y, and axillary views are obtained to evaluate for Hill-Sachs and glenoid bony defects as well as potential other pathologic conditions. Stress radiographs can demonstrate capsular laxity, but are not usually needed. Magnetic resonance imaging (MRI) is often helpful but not required to assess labral and capsular pathology. MRI with intra-articular contrast injection provides much more information about capsular redundancy and labral injuries.

An adequate course of nonoperative treatment is advised after establishing the diagnosis of MDI. Once other pathologic causes of the patient's symptoms have been eliminated (superior labrum anterior to posterior [SLAP] tears, tendonitis, acromioclavicular [AC] joint, etc.) and the diagnosis of MDI has been made, a mandatory period of rest is necessary to allow subsidence of pain and inflammation. Once the symptoms allow, the patient is started on a guided course of physiotherapy, including rotator cuff and periscapular muscle strengthening. Based on physical finding and patient symptoms, the therapy program should be individualized to the patient's specific needs. An adequate course of nonoperative treatment allows the surgeon to confirm the diagnosis and assess the motivation of the patient. Improper athletic technique can often be responsible for a patient's symptoms. Strict analysis and correction of the technique combined with biofeedback and muscle retraining can often alleviate symptoms.

An adequate course of nonoperative treatment includes a period of rest and avoidance of activity causing symptoms. A course of anti-inflammatory medications may facilitate a decrease in the inflammatory process that could be part of soft tissue injury. Exercises below shoulder level are instituted to strengthen the rotator cuff musculature and deltoid. Gradual progression of the intensity and duration of the exercises allows the muscles to retrain. This is followed by progression to sport-specific exercises and gradual return to competition. If the patient has prolonged symptoms (greater than 3 months of a well controlled nonoperative protocol) that have not responded to nonoperative treatment, is motivated, and does not have true voluntary instability, operative treatment is recommended.

■ SURGICAL TECHNIQUE

Pathologic instability is often a continuum between true traumatic unidirectional instability and MDI. Neer[7] indicated that one of the main reasons for failure of the surgical treatment of MDI, besides making the wrong diagnosis and operating on a voluntary dislocator, is an incomplete surgical correction of all elements responsible for the instability. For this reason, the senior author (LUB) has used the anterior-inferior capsular shift for MDI, which allows excellent inspection and the ability to correct any potential type of capsular and labral pathology found at surgery. This allows the surgeon to achieve proper balance and stabilization of the glenohumeral joint, without significant loss of range of motion. A recent study from our institution analyzed normal glenohumeral joint mechanics and the mechanics following an anterior tightening procedure versus an anterior-inferior capsular shift (presented at the ASES Closed Meeting, Dana Point, Calif, 2003). Anterior tightening adversely affected joint mechanics by decreasing joint stability (instability in posterior direction), limiting both external rotation and forward elevation, and increasing joint reaction forces. The anterior-inferior capsular shift improved joint stability while preserving external rotation with slight loss of maximum elevation. The anterior-inferior capsular shift more closely re-creates normal joint mechanics when compared to isolated anterior tightening. This operation allows the surgeon to precisely titrate the reduction of the capsular volume on all sides of the glenohumeral joint by proper tensioning, overlapping, and plicating the capsule in the areas that are redundant. This can be accomplished from the anterior approach even in patients with posterior instability as a primary component of MDI.

Examination under Anesthesia

Muscle guarding can prevent adequate instability testing in the unanesthetized patient. A thorough examination under anesthesia is critical. True laxity of the shoulder can be determined at this time. This exam can either confirm the previous findings in the office or pinpoint an additional direction of laxity. Usually the directions of instability have been determined preoperatively after complete workup. Some axial pressure should be applied to the humerus to appreciate translations of the humeral head over the glenoid rim. Experience and practice is important in this technique to understand the position of the humeral head relative to the glenoid during testing.

Positioning

Interscalene block is administered and supplemented with local subcutaneous tissue injection of Marcaine in the medial axillary region. The patient is placed in a beach chair position and all the bony prominences and neurovascular structures are well padded. The patient's head is secured to prevent hyperflexion, hyperextension, or lateral bending of the neck.

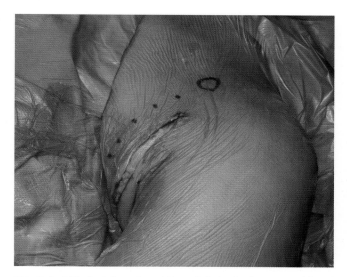

Fig. 3-1. Skin incision placed 3 cm inferior to the coracoid and extending inferiorly 7 cm into the axillary crease.

The patient's upper extremity is prepped and draped from the sternum, neck, and the medial border of the scapula. Prophylactic intravenous antibiotics are administered prior to incision.

Incision

A concealed axillary incision beginning approximately 3 cm inferior to the coracoid and extending inferiorly 7 cm into the axillary crease is used **(Fig. 3-1)**. Full thickness subcutaneous skin flaps are developed allowing exposure to the clavicle. The deltopectoral interval is identified **(Fig. 3-2)**. Blunt dissection and electrocautery are used to separate the clavicular portion of the pectoralis major and the deltoid muscles. Most often, the cephalic vein is retracted laterally with the deltoid, as it has less contributories from the medial side. Although not routine, if warranted for lack of exposure, the upper 0.5 to 1 cm of the pectoralis major may be released from the humeral insertion while protecting the biceps tendon, which

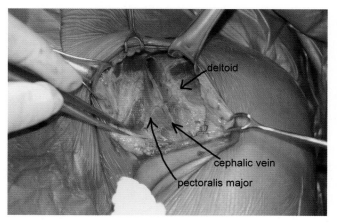

Fig. 3-2. Identification of the deltopectoral interval.

lies deep to the pectoralis tendon. This is tagged and anatomically repaired at the end of the procedure.

Dissection

The clavipectoral fascia is then incised lateral to the conjoint tendon. It is important to recognize that distally, the muscle belly of the short head of the bicep is more lateral than the tendon. Care should be taken not to enter this plane when dissecting lateral to the conjoint tendon. A medium Richardson retractor can then be used to retract the conjoint tendon medially **(Fig. 3-3)**. Care is taken to prevent injury to the musculocutaneous nerve, normally passing about 5.6 cm inferior to the coracoid; this distance can be as short as 3.5 cm.[17] The coracoid and the coracoacromial ligament are then identified. The leading edge of the coracoacromial (CA) ligament is then resected, improving superior visualization of the rotator interval **(Fig. 3-4)**. A complete anterior bursectomy is then performed, allowing excellent exposure and clear identification of the subscapularis. The upper border of the subscapularis is identified by finding the rotator interval. The lower border is heralded by the anterior circumflex artery and its two venae comitantes. These vessels are then coagulated using the needle tipped Bovie or tied, depending on their girth. The incision on the subscapularis is started 1 cm medial to the tendinous insertion on the lesser tuberosity **(Fig. 3-5)**. This ensures a stout cuff of subscapularis to repair back to at the conclusion of the procedure. Great care is taken to avoid violation of the

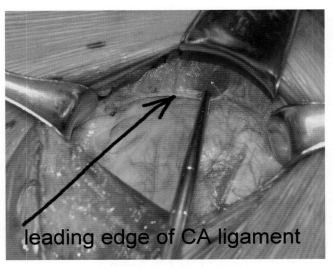

Fig. 3-4. The leading edge of the coracoacromial (CA) ligament is excised granting superior exposure to the rotator interval.

underlying capsule. Separating the subscapularis and the anterior glenohumeral capsule can be very challenging. The upper portion of the subscapularis is confluent with the capsule; however, inferiorly the capsule and subscapularis muscle are not confluent **(Fig. 3-6)**.[18] Blunt dissection at the inferior aspect of the subscapularis muscle facilitates identification of the plane between the capsule and the subscapularis. Once the plane has been clearly identified inferiorly, an elevator or Mayo scissors can then be used to tease the "confluent" portion of the subscapularis off the anterior capsule **(Fig. 3-7)**.

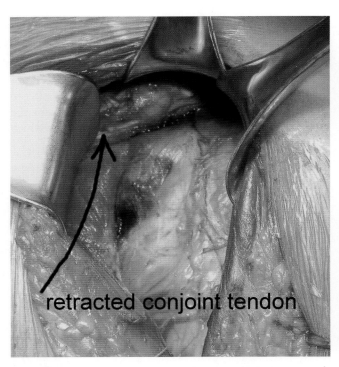

Fig. 3-3. Conjoint tendon retracted medially, exposing the bursal layer covering the subscapularis.

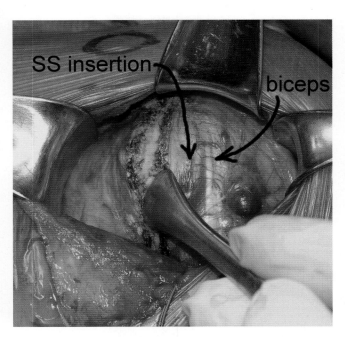

Fig. 3-5. The subscapularis (SS) is incised leaving a stout cuff of tissue laterally to facilitate later repair.

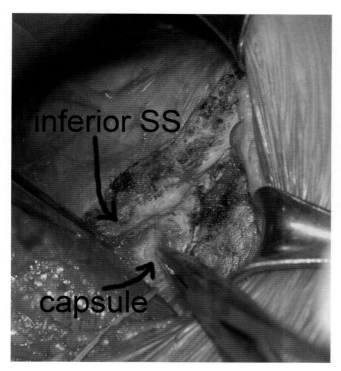

Fig. 3-6. The interval between the inferior subscapularis (SS) muscle and the anterior capsule.

Tag stitches can be placed to help keep traction on the subscapularis during the separation.

Inferiorly, extreme care should be exercised to avoid injury to the axillary nerve coursing around the inferior border of the subscapularis on its way to the quadrangular space. The "tug test" may be helpful in identifying the nerve,

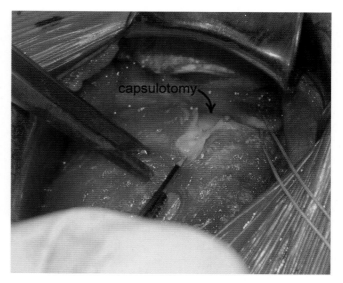

Fig. 3-8. Separation of the confluent upper portion of the subscapularis (SS) and the anterior capsule.

but the vast majority of times the nerve can be visualized.[19] Once the subscapularis has been completely released, the capsule is incised, approximately 0.5 cm medial to the subscapularis, once again leaving an adequate cuff of tissue for the subsequent repair (Fig. 3-8). Some have utilized suture anchors on the humeral side for capsular repair, but we have found this unnecessary if an adequate cuff of tissue is left behind. The capsular incision is initiated superiorly at the rotator interval and continued inferiorly with traction sutures placed in the free edge (Fig. 3-9). It is important to externally rotate and adduct the humerus during the inferior capsular release to protect the axillary nerve. The plane of

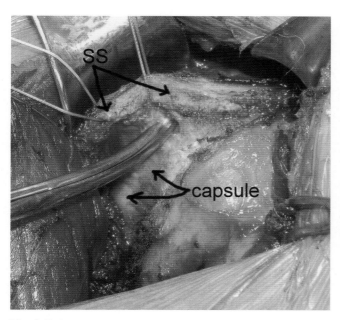

Fig. 3-7. Separation of the subscapularis (SS) from anterior capsule with Mayo scissors.

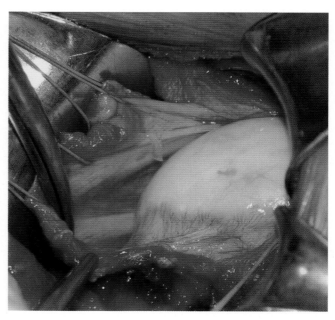

Fig. 3-9. Traction sutures are placed in the lateral edge of the anterior capsule.

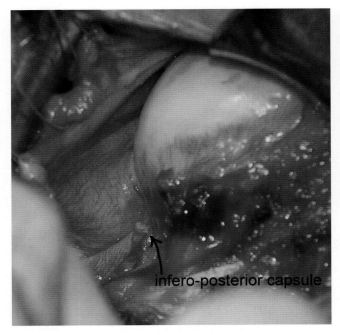

Fig. 3-10. Capsular release is extended as far posteriorly as necessary to eliminate inferior and posterior capsular redundancy.

dissection moves away from the nerve with the external rotation of the arm.

The inferior capsule is detached sharply with a scalpel. The amount of capsule incised from the neck of the humerus, and therefore the amount available to be shifted, is determined by the amount of instability and degree of capsular redundancy. This amount can be titrated depending on the specific pathology of the capsule. Placement of a finger in the inferior pouch and posteriorly around the neck of the humerus can assist in determining how much redundant capsule needs to be released prior to shifting. The release of the inferior capsule can be extended as far posteriorly as necessary to eliminate the redundancy in

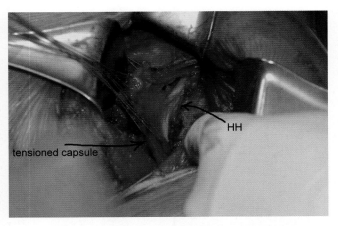

Fig. 3-12. Humeral head (HH) is reduced concentrically after posterior and inferior capsule is tensioned as part of the capsular shift.

posterior capsule **(Fig. 3-10)**. Posterior laxity can be reduced with an extensive shift of the posteroinferior capsule. As can be seen in **Figure 3-11**, without tension on the capsule the head is easily displaced posteriorly. However, when the shift is simulated with tension applied to the tag stitches, the posterior instability is greatly reduced **(Fig. 3-12)**. Proper mobilization has been achieved if pulling up on the tag sutures pushes the finger out from the posterior and inferior pouch, eliminating capsular redundancy **(Figs. 3-13, 3-14)**.

An important anatomic point should be made regarding the inferior attachment of the capsule. It has been shown that most often the inferior aspect of the capsule splits and has a dual attachment to the inferior humeral neck **(Fig. 3-15)**.[19a] In order to perform an adequate shift of the capsule and tension the posterior part of the capsule, both layers need to be released from the neck of the humerus to prevent the tethering of the capsule. After both inner and outer layers of the capsule have been released inferiorly and posteriorly around

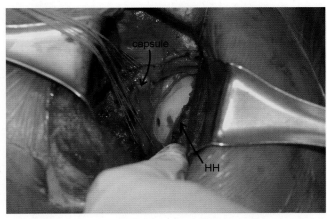

Fig. 3-11. Slight posteriorly directed force on the humeral head (HH) creates posterior subluxation secondary to the redundant posterior capsule.

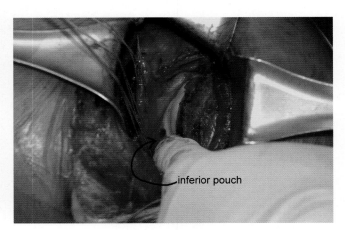

Fig. 3-13. Inferior redundancy is assessed by placing the index finger into the inferior capsular pouch.

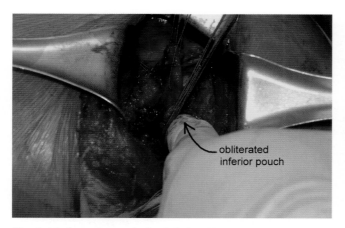

Fig. 3-14. Capsular tensioning is judged based on the elimination of the inferior redundancy with the finger pushed out of the inferior capsular pouch.

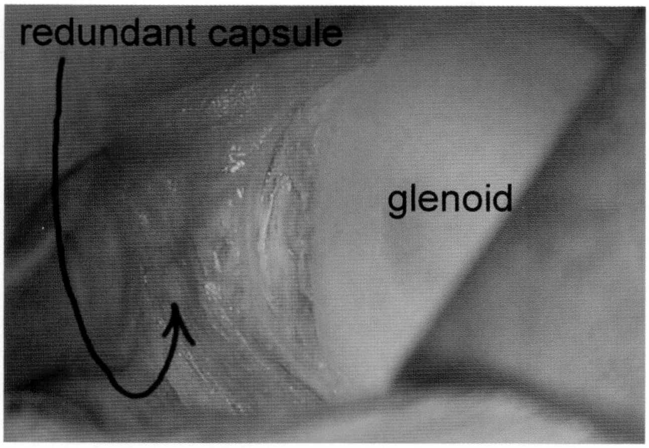

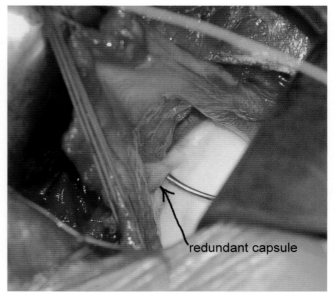

Fig. 3-16. Anteromedial capsular redundancy is often present in multidirectional instability (MDI).

the neck of the humerus, the posterior and inferior redundancy can be eliminated with superior traction. It is also critical to pull the capsule laterally and look at the superficial surface of the capsule. Often there are residual attachments from the subscapularis that need to be released to allow a complete shift of the capsule.

A Fukuda retractor is hooked behind the posterior glenoid rim to retract the humerus posteriorly. The joint is inspected for bony or labral pathology. Glenohumeral ligament and labral avulsion from bone are repaired anatomically prior to the capsular shift. The anterior inferior glenoid rim is prepared with a curette to bleeding bone. Suture anchors are placed at the articular cartilage-scapular neck margin and used for fixation. Medial placement of the suture anchors has been implicated in a few failures in one

series.[20] Often a Bankart lesion is not identified, but anteromedial capsular redundancy is present (Fig. 3-16). In these situations an anterior crimping (barrel) stitch is placed.[21] The stitch is started on the superficial side of the capsule at the capsule-labral junction. It is passed through the capsule and then back out in a mattress fashion (Fig. 3-17). Once tied the anterior medial redundancy is obliterated and an anterior inferior bumper is created (Fig. 3-18). The capsule should be palpated to check if the desired tension was achieved. If the capsule is still felt to be loose anteriorly, an additional crimping stitch can be placed.

One of the most useful attributes of removing the capsule from the humeral side is the ability to titrate the amount of capsular shift to the pathology identified intraoperatively. For MDI patients who have a less posterior

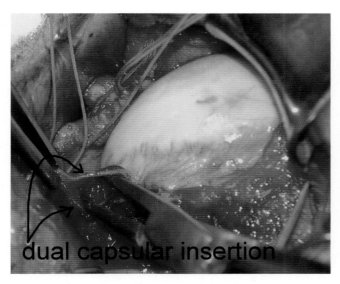

Fig. 3-15. The dual insertion of the inferior capsule on the humeral neck. Both insertions need to be released for an adequate shift of the posterior and inferior capsule.

Fig. 3-17. Placement of the "barrel stitch."

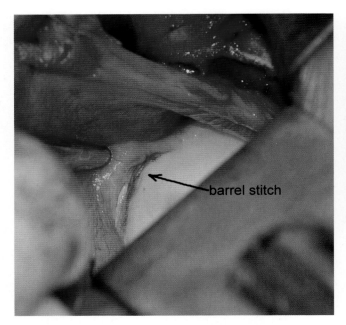

Fig. 3-18. Obliteration of the anteromedial capsular redundancy with the "barrel stitch."

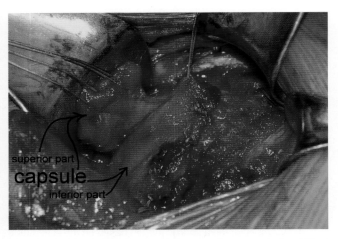

Fig. 3-20. The inferior part of the anterior capsule is shifted superolaterally and repaired to the remaining capsular tissue on the humeral neck.

component of instability and capsular redundancy, only the anterior and inferior capsules are mobilized. However, many of these patients have instability in all directions with the large and patulous capsule circumferentially. In these cases, the posterior and inferior capsules are released off the humerus, as described above, and mobilized superolaterally, eliminating the global capsular redundancy and creating equilibrium in capsular tension circumferentially. The anterior capsule can be split horizontally between the inferior and middle glenohumeral ligaments when necessary. The incision is carried medially, along this plane, to but not through the labrum (Fig. 3-19).

The arm is positioned between 20 degrees to 30 degrees of abduction and 20 degrees to 30 degrees of external rota-

tion in preparation for the capsular shift. More abduction and external rotation is used in overhead athletes. Less abduction and external rotation is used in patients with large Hill-Sachs lesions or anterior glenoid bone deficiency. The inferior aspect of the capsule is advanced superiorly and held under tension using the tag sutures while it is reattached to the remnant of capsular tissue left behind (Fig. 3-20). If the horizontal "T" has been made it is repaired with a pants-over-vest technique over the lower portion of the capsule (Fig. 3-21). The rotator interval is closed only laterally if there is a substantial preoperative sulcus sign or widening identified intraoperatively. Overtightening should be avoided as this may lead to loss of external rotation. This is prevented by frequent reevaluation of capsular tension while repairing the capsule back to the humeral neck.

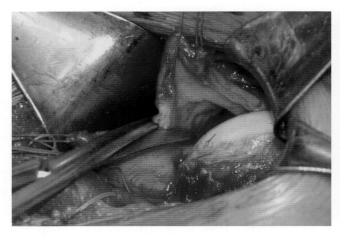

Fig. 3-19. Horizontal capsulotomy in the redundant anterior capsule.

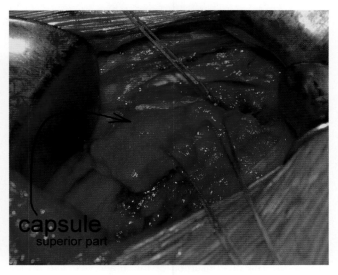

Fig. 3-21. The superior part of the anterior capsule is repaired over the inferior part in the pants-over-vest fashion.

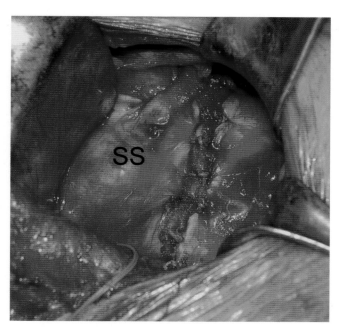

Fig. 3-22. The subscapularis (SS) is repaired anatomically to its insertion on the humerus.

The subscapularis is then closed anatomically and a layered closure performed **(Fig. 3-22)**. Drains are not routinely used.

■ REHABILITATION

In patients whose posterior component of instability was not significant, a sling is used for 6 weeks postoperatively to protect the repair. However, exercises are initiated at 10 days within a protected range of motion. This range is determined intraoperatively based on the repair. In general, however, isometrics, elevation to 90 degrees, and external rotation to 20 degrees to 30 degrees are begun from 10 days to 2 weeks. From 2 to 4 weeks, elevation to 140 degrees and external rotation to 30 degrees to 40 degrees are allowed. From 4 to 6 weeks, elevation is increased to 160 degrees and external rotation to 40 degrees to 50 degrees. Resistive exercises are also begun at this stage. After 6 weeks external rotation is increased further and terminal elevation stretching is allowed. The goal is to achieve full motion over several months and avoid too rapid progression that may lead to recurrent instability. Close monitoring of these patients will help to identify those who may be progressing too rapidly and those who may need more aggressive therapy. Return to contact sports is not generally allowed until a minimum of 6 months has elapsed.

In patients who have had a significant release of the posterior capsule a brace holding the arm in neutral rotation for 6 weeks is used. Subsequently, range-of-motion exercises are started gradually. At 12 weeks postoperatively progressive strengthening is initiated and progressed on an individual basis.

■ OUTCOMES/RESULTS

The success of earlier reports on open reconstructive procedures for shoulder instability was measured only by elimination of dislocations.[22-28] In the past several decades attention has turned more to maintenance of motion and function, especially with regard to overhead athletes. Many of these earlier procedures were "nonanatomic" and did not address the specific pathoanatomy of MDI patients—the capsular redundancy and instability in multiple directions. In the past decade, however, the focus has shifted to "anatomic" repairs, which restore the normal glenohumeral anatomy and repair the capsular pathology. Labral repairs combined with proper capsulorrhaphy procedures address all potential sites of pathology in MDI (detached labrum and capsular redundancy). The capsulorrhaphy can be performed using a lateral approach to the joint[1] or a medial approach.[29-31] Care is taken to preserve the length of the subscapularis to prevent the loss of external rotation and overtightening, which can lead to degenerative changes in the glenoid.[3]

Altchek et al.[29] reported on a T-plasty modification of the Bankart procedure performed on 42 shoulders of mostly young male athletes. Patients were satisfied with 40 shoulders (95%). Throwing athletes, however, found that they were unable to throw a ball with as much speed as before the operation.

Rubinstein et al.[32] reported on a large series of 76 athletes treated with anterior capsulolabral reconstruction through a longitudinal subscapularis split with a medial-based capsular shift. Most of the patients returned to previous sports with the majority having subtle instability and activity related pain. Seven had a history of a dislocating event.

We prefer anterior-inferior capsular shift (AICS) with a lateral approach to the joint. This operation is well suited for athletes with the common clinical picture of MDI. The AICS eliminates laxity in the rotator interval, anterosuperior capsule, anteroinferior capsule, posteroinferior capsule, and far posterior capsule with re-creation of equal tension on all sides. Infrequent, but described, capsular avulsion of the humerus can easily be addressed with this operation. The versatility of the AICS is its major advantage, especially important in athletes who can reveal a variety of intraoperative pathology related to microtrauma to the shoulder. Neer and Foster's[1] initial report on inferior capsular shift on 36 patients with MDI revealed only one unsatisfactory result. One decade later, Neer[7] reported on more than 100 additional anterior-inferior capsular shifts with similar results. The senior author (LUB) reported on 68 anterior-inferior capsular shifts performed in 63 young athletes.[9] Ninety-two percent returned to their sport and 75% maintained their level of competitiveness. Seven patients (10.3%) reported a single episode of probable subluxation that was not followed by recurrent instability and did not affect the final result, whereas two patients (2.7%) dislocated postoperatively. Both of these cases were associated with traumatic episode. The average loss of external rotation was 7 degrees. Cooper and Brems[33] reported on the AICS in

38 patients (43 shoulders) with MDI. Thirty-nine shoulders (91%) functioned well with no instability. Sixteen of 43 shoulders (37%) were stable enough to return to the same sport, some to a lower level. The failures occurred in the early postoperative period less than 2 years postsurgery. These reports demonstrate that the results held up to a 6-year follow-up.

■ CONCLUSION

MDI is not uncommon in athletes. A high degree of suspicion and awareness is needed to make the correct diagnosis. Etiological factors include repetitive microtrauma, inherent joint laxity, and multiple traumatic events. Standard operations simply addressing only one direction of instability are doomed for failure and create fixed joint subluxation in the opposite direction with subsequent development of capsulorrhaphy arthropathy at a young age. Careful patient selection for operative intervention is important to maximize successful results. The operations addressing not only labral lesion but also capsular redundancy have shown to provide similar successful results. Experience with anterior-inferior capsular shift has been very satisfying with results withstanding the test of time.

■ SUGGESTED READINGS

Altchek DW, Wakren RF, Skyhar MJ, et al. T-plasty modification of the Bankart procedure for multidirectional instability of the anterior and inferior types. J Bone Joint Surg Am. 1991;73(1):105–112.

Bigliani LU, Kurzweil PR, Schwartzbach CC, et al. Inferior capsular shift procedure for anterior-inferior shoulder instability in athletes. Am J Sports Med. 1994;22(5):578–584.

Bigliani LU, Pollock RG, Soslowsky LJ, et al. Tensile properties of the inferior glenohumeral ligament. J Orthop Res. 1992;10(2):187–197.

Hawkins RJ, Angelo RL. Glenohumeral osteoarthrosis. A late complication of the Putti-Platt repair. J Bone Joint Surg Am. 1990;72(8):1193–1197.

Jobe FW, Guingarra CE, Kvitne RS, et al. Anterior capsulolabral reconstruction of the shoulder in athletes in overhand sports. Am J Sports Med. 1991;19(5):428–434.

Neer CS II, Foster CR. Inferior capsular shift for involuntary inferior and multidirectional instability of the shoulder: a preliminary report. J Bone Joint Surg Am. 1980;62(6):897–908.

Neer CS I. Involuntary inferior and multidirectional instability of the shoulder: etiology, recognition, and treatment. Instr Course Lect. 1985;34:232–238.

O'Brien SJ, Neves MC, Arnockzky SP, et al. The anatomy and histology of the inferior glenohumeral ligament complex of the shoulder. Am J Sports Med. 1990;18:449–456.

Rowe CR, Zarins B, Ciullo JV. Recurrent anterior dislocation of the shoulder after surgical repair: apparent causes of failure and treatment. J Bone Joint Surg Am. 1984;66(2):159–168.

■ REFERENCES

1. Neer CS II, Foster CR. Inferior capsular shift for involuntary inferior and multidirectional instability of the shoulder: a preliminary report. J Bone Joint Surg Am. 1980;62(6):897–908.
2. Neer CS I. *Shoulder Reconstruction*. ed. N.C. II. Philadelph6ia: WB Saunders; 1990:273–341.
3. Hawkins RJ, Angelo RL. Glenohumeral osteoarthrosis: a late complication of the Putti-Platt repair. J Bone Joint Surg Am. 1990;72(8):1193–1197.
4. Young DC, Rockwood CA Jr. Complications of a failed Bristow procedure and their management. J Bone Joint Surg Am. 1991;73(7):969–981.
5. Hawkins RH, Hawkins RJ. Failed anterior reconstruction for shoulder instability. J Bone Joint Surg Br. 1985;67(5):709–714.
6. Rowe CR, Zarins B, Ciullo JV. Recurrent anterior dislocation of the shoulder after surgical repair: apparent causes of failure and treatment. J Bone Joint Surg Am. 1984;66(2):159–168.
7. Neer CS I. Involuntary inferior and multidirectional instability of the shoulder: etiology, recognition, and treatment. Instr Course Lect. 1985;34:232–238.
8. Yamaguchi K, Flatow EL. Management of multidirectional instability. Clin Sports Med. 1995;14(4):885–902.
9. Bigliani LU, Kurzweil PR, Schwartzbach CC, et al. Inferior capsular shift procedure for anterior-inferior shoulder instability in athletes. Am J Sports Med. 1994;22(5):578–584.
10. Emery RJ, Mullaji AB. Glenohumeral joint instability in normal adolescents: incidence and significance. J Bone Joint Surg Br. 1991;73(3):406–408.
11. McFarland EG, Campbell G, McDowell J. Posterior shoulder laxity in asymptomatic athletes. Am J Sports Med. 1996;24(4):468–471.
12. McFarland EG, Kim TK, Park HB, et al. The effect of variation in definition on the diagnosis of multidirectional instability of the shoulder. J Bone Joint Surg Am. 2003;85-A(11):2138–2144.
13. O'Brien SJ, Neves MC, Arnockzky SP, et al. The anatomy and histology of the inferior glenohumeral ligament complex of the shoulder. Am J Sports Med. 1990;18:449–456.
14. Bigliani LU, Pollock RG, Soslowsky LJ, et al. Tensile properties of the inferior glenohumeral ligament. J Orthop Res. 1992;10(2):187–197.
15. Speer KP, Deng X, Borrero S, et al. Biomechanical evaluation of a simulated Bankart lesion. J Bone Joint Surg Am. 1994;76:1819–1826.
16. Gerber C, Ganz R. Clinical assessment of instability of the shoulder: with special reference to anterior and posterior drawer tests. J Bone Joint Surg Br. 1984;66(4):551–556.
17. Flatow EL, Bigliani LU, April EW. An anatomic study of the musculocutaneous nerve and its relationship to the coracoid process. Clin Orthop. 1989;244:166–171.
18. Sugalski MT, Wiater JM, Levine WN, et al. The confluence of the subscapularis insertion and the glenohumeral joint capsule. Paper presented at: OREF New York Resident Research Competition and Symposium; 2003; New York.
19. Flatow EL, Bigliani LU. Locating and protecting the axillary nerve in shoulder surgery: the tug test. Orthop Rev. 1992;21:503–505.
19a. Sugalski MT, Levine WN, Bigliani LU. J Shoulder Elbow Surg. 2005;14(1):91–95.
20. Levine WN, Richmond JC, Donaldson WR. Use of the suture anchor in open Bankart reconstruction: a follow-up report. Am J Sports Med. 1994;22(5):723–736.
21. Ahmad CS, Freehill MQ, Blaine TA, et al. Anteromedial capsular redundancy and labral deficiency in shoulder instability. Am J Sports Med. 2003;31(2):247–252.
22. Bankart A. Recurrent or habitual dislocation of the shoulder joint. Brit Med J. 1923;2:1132–1133.
23. DePalma A. Factors influencing the choice of a modified Magnuson procedure for recurrent anterior dislocation of the shoulder with a note on technique. Surg Clin North Am. 1963;43:1647–1649.
24. Barry TP, Lombardo SJ, Kerlan RK, et al. The coracoid transfer for recurrent anterior instability of the shoulder in adolescents. J Bone Joint Surg Am. 1985;67(3):383–387.

25. Braly WG, Tullos HS. A modification of the Bristow procedure for recurrent anterior shoulder dislocation and subluxation. Am J Sports Med. 1985;13(2):81–86.
26. Hill JA, Lombardo SJ, Kerlan RK, et al. The modification Bristow-Helfet procedure for recurrent anterior shoulder subluxations and dislocations. Am J Sports Med. 1981;9(5):283–287.
27. Hovelius LK, Sandstrom BC, Rosmark DL, et al. Long-term results with the Bankart and Bristow-Latarjet procedures: recurrent shoulder instability and arthropathy. J Shoulder Elbow Surg. 2001;10(5):445–452.
28. Lombardo SJ, Kerlan RK, Jobe FW, et al. The modified Bristow procedure for recurrent dislocation of the shoulder. J Bone Joint Surg Am. 1976;58(2):256–261.
29. Altchek DW, Warren RF, Skyhar MJ, et al. T-plasty modification of the Bankart procedure for multidirectional instability of the anterior and inferior types. J Bone Joint Surg Am. 1991;73(1):105–112.
30. Jobe FW, Giangarra CE, Kvitne RS, et al. Anterior capsulolabral reconstruction of the shoulder in athletes in overhand sports. Am J Sports Med. 1991;19(5):428–434.
31. Pollock RB, Bigliani LU. Glenohumeral instability: evaluation and treatment. J Am Acad Orthop Surg. 1993;1:24–32.
32. Rubenstein DL, JF, Glousman RE, et al. Anterior capsulolabral reconstruction of the shoulder in athletes. J Shoulder Elbow Surg. 1992;1:229–237.
33. Cooper RA, Brems JJ. The inferior capsular-shift procedure for multidirectional instability of the shoulder. J Bone Joint Surg Am. 1992;74(10):1516–1521.

ARTHROSCOPIC SUTURE PLICATION FOR MULTIDIRECTIONAL INSTABILITY OF THE SHOULDER

4

■ JOSEPH P. BURNS, MD, STEVEN J. SNYDER, MD

■ HISTORY OF THE TECHNIQUE

Multidirectional instability (MDI) of the shoulder can be a very difficult problem to effectively diagnose and treat. Patients with complaints of shoulder instability often present with a mixed bag of pathology, having complex histories and variable physical findings. As the understanding of the spectrum of instability has improved, surgical treatment techniques have likewise evolved, becoming more specialized to the various types of pathology that can be present. Early stabilization procedures such as the Putti-Platt, Magnuson-Stack, or Bristow were designed to prevent unidirectional anteroinferior instability, but were poor options for MDI as they did not address the excessive capsular redundancy present in MDI patients, nor could they effectively treat components of posterior instability. These procedures were predicated upon significantly altering normal anterior shoulder anatomy, such as the subscapularis or conjoint tendon, to compensate for dysfunctional capsulolabral structures within the joint. In 1980, Neer and Foster[1] popularized the open capsular shift for MDI patients. This procedure effectively reduced capsular volume and proved successful in preventing recurrent instability in anterior, inferior, and posterior directions. While the open capsular shift did not disrupt normal anatomy to the extent of other procedures, it still involved the neurovascular risks of a large surgical dissection, caused considerable scar formation and iatrogenic damage to the shoulder, and required a fairly substantial postoperative recuperation.

In more recent years, the advent of the arthroscope has lead to significant advancements in both the understanding and treatment of MDI. An organized diagnostic examination now allows all relevant anatomy to be fully evaluated in all areas of the shoulder joint. In the past, open procedures did not allow such close inspection of shoulder anatomy and as a result many of the more subtle or posterior pathologic conditions would go unseen and untreated.

In cases of MDI, the arthroscope has also significantly advanced the understanding of shoulder stability and its dependence upon capsular volume. Arthroscopists began noticing that MDI patients had intact structures but increased capsular redundancy. Pathologic instability was often associated with a "drive-through sign" where, owing to excessive ligamentous laxity and redundancy, the arthroscope could be passed across the entirety of the glenohumeral joint without significant resistance. In an effort to spare the normal extra-articular structures and treat only the pathologic anatomy in MDI patients, orthopedists began investigating ways of using the arthroscope to manage the redundant capsule from within the glenohumeral joint.

Early arthroscopic efforts in treating shoulder instability involved transglenoid drilling to stabilize the ligaments to bone.[2-4] Although effective in reducing capsular redundancy and stabilizing the shoulder, the technique required a posterior dissection for knot-tying, involved risk to both the glenoid and the suprascapular nerve, and was more effective for traumatic, unidirectional anteroinferior instability than for the pancapsular involvement of MDI.

Arthroscopic tack devices have also been used in an effort to keep the stabilization procedure "all inside" and avoid any extra-articular dissection. Created from both permanent and biodegradable materials, these tack devices have had suboptimal long-term results and have been associated with excessive morbidity related to tack breakage, tack migration, articular surface damage, and long-term synovitis.[5-9]

Several years ago, arthroscopists began using thermal shrinkage as a means to tighten lax shoulder capsules.[10-12] Although the immediate and short-term reports from the early users seemed promising, the longer-term results have been disappointing and inferior to those of the more traditional open techniques.[13] Anecdotal reports of irreparable capsular necrosis, serious nerve injuries, and articular cartilage damage combined with thermal capsulorrhaphy's digression from an anatomic reconstruction have made surgeons increasingly wary of the technique.

At the Southern California Orthopedic Institute (SCOI), an all-inside, all-arthroscopic technique was developed in 1992. Named arthroscopic pancapsular plication (APCP), this technique minimizes morbidity and risk to the patient, allows close evaluation of the entire glenohumeral joint, and enables precise reconstruction of the pathologic anatomy while sparing what is normal. Capsular stitches used in APCP, with or without suture anchors, allow the surgeon to selectively tighten lax ligaments, re-create and widen the labral "bumper," and complete the operation with minimal morbidity or surgical scarring.

■ INDICATIONS AND CONTRAINDICATIONS

MDI of the shoulder has been defined as symptomatic shoulder laxity in more than one direction (anterior, posterior, and/or inferior), but it can be a difficult diagnosis to confirm.[14,15] Symptoms can vary from subtle painful subluxations to recurrent frank dislocations. Patients with MDI often have symptoms resulting from relatively little or no trauma and usually have normal radiographs. However, a traumatic episode and the presence of a Bankart labral injury or Hill-Sachs fracture do not exclude the potential for MDI as a diagnosis. A thorough history is necessary to establish the activity or position of the upper extremity that reproduces symptoms. An office physical exam as well as an exam under anesthesia are both critical in assessing laxity and planning surgery.

In patients with MDI, some degree of generalized ligamentous laxity is the norm, and it should always be tested and documented. Patients may also have varying degrees of ability to voluntarily sublux or dislocate their shoulders. Physical examination may reveal either obvious or subtle findings such as excessive anterior and posterior glide, a positive sulcus sign, or the ability to voluntarily sublux the shoulder upon request. A positive early warning sign (EWS) is the ability of a patient to easily and willingly dislocate or sublux his or her shoulder, usually with the arm held comfortably at the side. Surgical stabilization of such patients is prone to failure, as these "muscular" subluxators will often stretch out any repair, arthroscopic or open. Other "positional" subluxators are still able to voluntarily sublux their shoulders, but need to bring the arm into a flexed, adducted, and internally rotated position to do so. These patients are more hesitant to sublux their shoulders upon request, as the subluxation is uncomfortable or painful. Positional subluxators are felt to be somewhat better surgical candidates than purely muscular subluxators. A third group, those patients who cannot and will not voluntarily sublux their shoulders at all, makes up the best candidates for surgery. A careful history and office physical exam should differentiate these patient groups.

Once the diagnosis of MDI has been made, many patients will improve with conservative therapy. With a combined program that includes patient education, activity modification, and physical therapy, some patients will avoid surgical intervention. Therapy should be focused on rotator cuff strengthening, periscapular muscular strengthening, maximizing humero–scapulo–thoracic dynamics, and plyometrics. Surgical intervention is indicated when a comprehensive therapy program fails to provide acceptable relief.

■ SURGICAL TECHNIQUE

Anesthesia and Positioning

The patient is given general anesthesia and positioned in the lateral decubitus position. A bean bag is used to maintain proper position and an axillary roll is placed under the dependent thorax to relieve pressure on the dependent shoulder and neurovascular structures. The thorax is allowed to tilt posteriorly 20 degrees, as per standard arthroscopy protocol.

Exam Under Anesthesia

Prior to prepping and draping the positioned patient, examination of the shoulder is performed to thoroughly document the degree and direction of laxity. At our center, this examination is video recorded. Anterior laxity is assessed with the shoulder abducted in a neutral and externally rotated position. Using the weight of the arm to slightly compress the joint, the proximal humerus is gently glided anteriorly and posteriorly, taking note as to whether the humeral head reaches the glenoid edge, goes beyond the edge, or frankly dislocates. Anterior laxity and instability is corrected with anterior capsular plication. Posterior laxity is assessed by positioning the shoulder in a forward flexed, adducted, and internally rotated position. While stabilizing the scapular spine, the examiner gives a gentle posteriorly directed force through the humeral shaft and slowly extends the arm back into an abducted position. With a posterior force applied, a shoulder with posterior laxity will sublux in the adducted position, and the examiner will feel a reduction as the arm is moved into the abducted position. Posterior laxity and instability are corrected with posterior capsular plication and closure of the posterior portal. Inferior laxity is evaluated by the subacromial sulcus test. With the arm at the side, the examiner exerts a downward pull on the arm in both neutral and external rotation. With a competent rotator interval, the amount of displacement inferiorly should decrease with the arm in an externally rotated position. If the rotator interval is incompetent, the inferior displacement of the humerus is similar in both positions. Inferior laxity and instability is corrected by plicating the rotator interval.

The information gained under anesthesia must be compared to that obtained during the office physical exam and to the exam of the contralateral arm. Laxity, a function of the soft tissues, and instability, a subjective feeling of the joint disassociating, are not synonomous and should be evaluated independently. The examiner must use all information available to determine which areas of the joint need surgical plication and which do not. In true MDI, a patient will be lax and unstable in multiple directions and the following pancapsular plication will be carried out.

Procedure

After surgical skin preparation, the arm is placed in a padded traction sleeve with approximately 10 lb of one point inline traction holding it in standard 70 degrees of abduction and 10 degrees forward flexion. Weight can be altered for larger or smaller limbs. The pertinent acromial and clavicular borders are marked on the skin with a sterile marker. The glenohumeral joint is entered using a standard posterior portal created approximately 2 cm inferior and 1 cm medial to the posterolateral acromial angle.

Once the arthroscope is inside the joint and the joint is distended with fluid, an anterosuperior portal (ASP) is created using an outside-in technique. A spinal needle is used to ensure proper placement prior to making a skin incision. Ideal portal placement is 1 cm anterior to the anterolateral acromial angle, angled toward the axilla within Langer lines, entering the joint in the superior aspect of the rotator interval, just anterior and superior to the biceps tendon. This position anticipates the placement of a second portal, the anterior midglenoid portal (AMGP), which will be placed later in the procedure. Of note, the rotator interval tissue is often very robust tissue and difficult to penetrate with a working cannula. It often needs to be dilated with a smaller obturator prior to placement of the cannula. At SCOI, a 5.75 mm clear cannula is used in the ASP (Crystal Cannula, Arthrex, Inc, Naples, Fla).

Once the posterior and anterosuperior portals are established, a comprehensive 15-point arthroscopic glenohumeral examination is performed.[16] A bursal arthroscopic examination can be performed when indicated. While examining the glenohumeral joint, special attention should be paid to several areas. The amount of overall volume is noted. A patulous posterior capsule will often allow a very broad view of the posterior joint, termed a "skybox view" **(Fig. 4-1)**. The status of the biceps anchor and anteroinferior labrum will always be noted, but the humeral attachment of the glenohumeral ligaments, both anteriorly and posteriorly, must be inspected as well. When ruptured anteriorly, this is termed a humeral avulsion of the glenohumeral ligaments (HAGL) lesion and is best viewed with the arthroscope in the anterior superior portal, anterior to the humeral head, with the lens looking up laterally at the humeral capsular insertion. When the ligaments are ruptured posteriorly, it is termed a reverse HAGL (RHAGL). A RHAGL is best

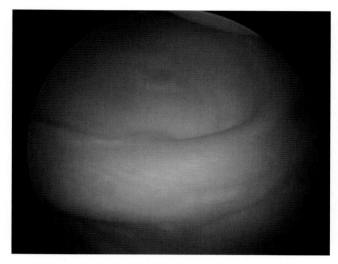

Fig. 4-1. The "skybox view" of the posterior glenohumeral joint in a patient with excessive capsular volume.

identified with the arthroscope in the anterior superior portal, posterior to the humeral head, with the lens looking up lateral at the humeral capsular insertion. It is important to rule out such capsular tears prior to performing an arthroscopic pancapsular plication **(Fig. 4-2)**.

After completing a standard arthroscopic examination and ruling out capsulolabral tears, the AMGP is created using outside-in technique. A spinal needle ensures proper spacing and placement both exteriorly as well as within the joint. Typically the incision is made approximately 2 cm distal and 1 cm lateral to the ASP, entering the joint at the

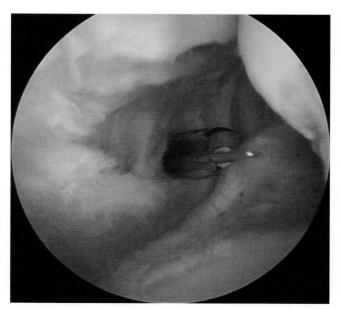

Fig. 4-2. Reverse HAGL ligamentous injury as seen from the ASP. The ligamentous structures have been avulsed from the humerus *(upper right)* and have retracted toward the glenoid *(lower right)*. The posterior cannula is seen in the center.

superior edge of the subscapularis tendon such that the two anterior portals share the rotator interval, maximizing the distance between the two portals. This AMGP cannula will be the anterior working portal and ideally should angle somewhat inferiorly within the joint. As the procedure begins with suturing posteriorly, a 5.75-mm smooth clear cannula (Crystal Cannula, Arthrex, Inc, Naples, Fla) is used in this AMGP until later in the case.

After placement of the two anterior cannulas, the arthroscope is placed in the ASP. Using a small diameter arthroscope, the scope may fit through the ASP cannula itself. A clear flexible 6.5-mm cannula (Clearflex or Dry Doc, Linvatec, Inc, Largo, Fla) is placed in the posterior portal using a switching stick technique. This cannula is used as the "working cannula" for plication as its diameter and flexibility allow passage of all necessary instruments including the curved stitching needles (Spectrum Suture Hook, Linvatec, Inc, Largo, Fla).

The capsular plication usually begins in the posterior inferior quadrant. With the arthroscope in the anterosuperior portal, a manual synovial rasp is used to lightly abrade the synovium overlying the posterior and inferior capsule, especially along the capsular aspect of the glenoid labrum **(Fig. 4-3)**. Care is taken not to violate the integrity of the capsule. Synovial capillary bleeding is encouraged to promote healing of the plicated capsular surfaces. Briefly turning off the saline flow allows confirmation of capsular bleeding **(Fig. 4-4)**.

After rasping the capsule and labral edge, the capsule is ready to be plicated. Prior to stitching, an atraumatic grasper may be used to assess the degree and ease of plication that the capsule will allow. For posterior stitching, a 45-degree curved suture hook is used (Spectrum Suture Hook, Linvatec, Inc, Largo, Fla), although 60-degree instruments are available as well. Posteriorly, use a curve-to-the-right suture hook in left shoulders and a curve-to-the-left in right shoulders. The suture hook should be preloaded with a Suture Shuttle Relay (Linvatec, Inc, Largo, Fla).

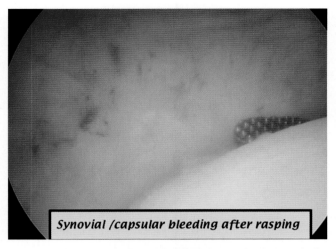

Fig. 4-4. After turning off fluid flow and decreasing intra-articular pressure, bleeding from the abraded synovium can be confirmed.

A "pinch-tuck" stitch is used to suture whenever possible. This technique ensures that the needle does not capture the axillary nerve and that the desired amount of tissue can be folded up against the labrum edge. Beginning as far inferior as possible, usually around the 6 to 7 o'clock area, the first pinch-tuck stitch is performed by passing the needle perpendicularly through the capsule 1 to 1.5 cm from the labral border, depending on the degree of capsular redundancy. A palpable "pop" should be felt as the tip pierces the capsule. The curved needle is rotated 180 degrees and advanced back through the capsule into the joint to create a 4 to 5 mm "pinch" of the capsular tissue **(Fig. 4-5)**. The corkscrew design of the suture hook tends to advance distally with rotation; therefore, effort should be made to slightly pull the hook back to prevent overadvancement as the pinch is made.

In the next part of the pinch-tuck, the needle, with the pinch of abraded capsule, is then advanced up to just below

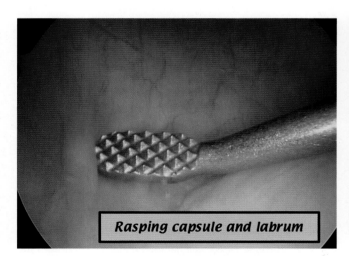

Fig. 4-3. A specialized rasp is used to abrade the entire synovium and labrum in efforts to stimulate a maximal healing response.

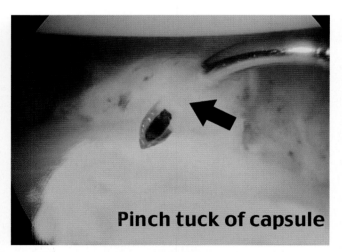

Fig. 4-5. A capsular "pinch" with the 45-degree "curve-to-the-left" suture hook (Spectrum Suture Hook, Linvatec, Inc, Largo, Fla). After advancing this capsular tissue, the needle will next be passed under the labrum to complete the pinch-tuck.

16. Snyder SJ. Diagnostic arthroscopy of the shoulder: normal anatomy and variations. In: Snyder SJ, ed. *Shoulder Arthroscopy*, 2nd ed. New York: McGraw-Hill; 2003:22–38.

17. Millett PJ, Clavert P, Warner JJP. Arthroscopic management of anterior, posterior, and multidirectional shoulder instability: pearls and pitfalls. Arthroscopy. 2003;19:86–93.

18. Price MR, Tillett ED, Acland RD, et al. Determining the relationship of the axillary nerve to the shoulder joint capsule from an arthroscopic perspective. J Bone Joint Surg Am. 2004;86A: 2135–2142.

19. Schamblin ML, Snyder SJ. Arthroscopic capsular plication techniques. Tech Shoulder Elbow Surg. 2004;5:193–199.

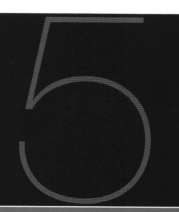

POSTERIOR SHOULDER INSTABILITY REPAIR

JAMES C. DREESE, MD, JAMES P. BRADLEY, MD

■ HISTORY OF ARTHROSCOPIC TREATMENT

In comparison to anterior shoulder instability, posterior instability is a relatively rare entity. Most authors agree that posterior shoulder instability represents only 5% to 10% of shoulder instability cases.[1-3] It encompasses a broad spectrum of pathology ranging from the more common recurrent posterior subluxation (RPS) to the less common locked posterior dislocation (LPD). Consequently, posterior instability may present in a variety of patient populations and clinical scenarios. As a result, confusion has traditionally existed in attempting to diagnose and treat this ill-defined, uncommon entity. Initial attempts in clarifying the distinctions of posterior instability were made in 1962 when McLaughlin[1] recognized that differences exist between "fixed and recurrent subluxations of the shoulder," suggesting that the etiology and treatment of the two are distinctly different. Since that time additional knowledge has been gained in the differences between unidirectional versus multidirectional (MDI), traumatic versus atraumatic, acute versus chronic, and voluntary versus involuntary posterior instability. In many respects each of these may represent a distinct form of posterior instability with its own underlying predispositions, anatomical abnormalities, and treatment algorithms.[4-9] Our collective understanding of posterior shoulder instability continues to be an evolving process.

Recent advances in our understanding of the spectrum of posterior instability have been gained through the study of shoulder injuries in athletes, patients with generalized ligamentous laxity, and patients with posttraumatic injuries.[4-8,10-12] Acute posterior dislocations typically occur as a result of a direct blow to the anterior shoulder or indirect forces that couple shoulder flexion, internal rotation, and adduction.[6] The most common indirect causes are accidental electric shock and convulsive seizures. Chronic LPD presents with the humeral head locked over the posterior glenoid rim. As a result of incomplete radiographic studies and a failure to recognize the posterior shoulder prominence and mechanical block to external rotation, 60% to 80% of LPD cases are overlooked by the treating physician. These patients are often given a diagnosis of "frozen shoulder" but fail to improve their external rotation with physical therapy. Patients with both acute posterior dislocations and LPD may suffer a significant osseous defect to the anteromedial humeral head,[2] that is often referred to as the reverse Hill-Sachs lesion (**Fig. 5-1**). In addition, a minority of patients with posterior dislocations will also suffer a posterior capsulolabral detachment, often referred to as a reverse Bankart tear (**Fig. 5-2**). Failure to recognize a posterior shoulder dislocation in the acute period complicates treatment and leads to a predictably poorer prognosis.

In contrast to posterior shoulder dislocations, RPS is often the result of chronic repetitive microtrauma to the posterior capsule without a single traumatic antecedent event. Gradually the patient develops insidious pain with laxity of the posterior capsule and fatigue of the static and dynamic stabilizers.[6] RPS may also result from a traumatic reverse Bankart lesion or as a component of MDI.[6,7] The capsulolabral avulsion is seen less commonly in posterior instability than it is in anterior instability.[13,14] Other proposed mechanisms of RPS include excessive retroversion of the humeral head, an engaging Hill-Sachs lesion, excessive retroversion of the glenoid, and hypoplasia of the glenoid.[2,6,15,16]

Many patients with RPS can be managed successfully without surgery. Numerous authors have proposed a period of no less than 6 months of physical therapy prior to considering surgical treatment.[7,8,17] Effective rehabilitation includes avoidance of aggravating activities, restoration of a full range of motion, and shoulder strengthening.

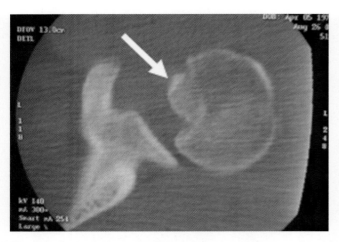

Fig. 5-1. Computed tomography scan demonstrating an osseous impression defect, also known as a reverse Hill-Sachs lesion *(arrow)*, in a patient following reduction of a posterior shoulder dislocation.

Strengthening of the rotator cuff, posterior deltoid, and periscapular musculature are critical. The premise of such directed physical therapy is to enable dynamic muscular stabilizers to offset the deficient static capsulolabral restraints. Response to physical therapy is dependent upon the type of RPS present. While patients with atraumatic MDI have enjoyed encouraging success rates with physical therapy alone, the results have not been as optimistic in patients with recurrent traumatic posterior instability.[7,17] Restated, patients with a history of macrotrauma initiating the RPS have poorer success rates with rehabilitation alone than patients with recurrent microtrauma or generalized

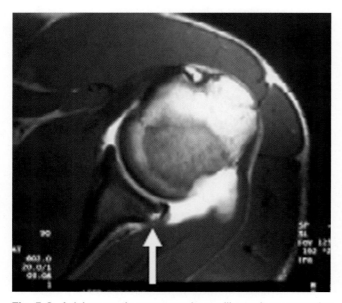

Fig. 5-2. Axial magnetic resonance image illustrating a posterior labral detachment, also known as a reverse Bankart tear, with some posterior capsular stripping from the glenoid rim *(arrow)* in a patient with recurrent traumatic posterior instability.

ligamentous laxity. Subjectively, nearly 70% of patients will improve following an appropriate rehabilitation protocol. Objectively, the recurrent subluxation is generally not eliminated, but the functional disability is diminished enough that it does not prevent activities.[18,19] If the disability fails to improve with an extended 6-month period of directed rehabilitation, or in select cases of posterior instability resulting from a macrotraumatic event, surgical intervention should be considered.

The surgical treatment of posterior instability has historically included posterior capsular tightening procedures, osseous reconstructions, and combinations of both. In contrast to the surgical treatment of anterior shoulder instability, surgical results of posterior shoulder instability have in general been less consistent. The laterally based posterior capsular shift, as described by Neer and Foster,[20] remains the gold standard in the treatment of RPS. Preliminary results of the capsular shift in 25 patients revealed good to excellent results in nearly 90% of patients[21] and longer follow-up studies in 38 patients revealed satisfactory results in 80%.[22] Similarly, results of a medially based capsular shift have yielded success rates near 90%.[7] However, Tibone and Bradley[6] reported 40% failure rates in a group of 40 high-performance athletes after undergoing a medially based capsulorrhaphy. The high rate of failures was attributed to an incomplete correction of ligament laxity and unrecognized MDI. Additional soft tissue tightening procedures have included McGlaughlin's[1] description of subscapularis tendon insertion transposition from the lesser tuberosity to fill the reverse Hill-Sachs lesion, Severin's[23] account of the reverse Putti-Platt procedure to divide and advance the infraspinatus laterally over a capsular plication, Boyd and Sisk's[2] report of rerouting the long head of the biceps to the posterior glenoid rim to function as a sling around the posterolateral humeral head, and the report from Tibone et al.[24] on repair of a posterior labral tear with a staple. Osseous reconstructions have included a posterior opening wedge glenoid osteotomy, rotational osteotomy of the proximal humerus, and augmentation of the posterior glenoid with a bone block.[25–28] Because each of these procedures has comparatively proven to be either less effective, less safe, or more technically demanding, the posterior capsular shift remains the gold standard in the treatment of posterior shoulder instability.

In the 1990s preliminary results of arthroscopic techniques in the treatment of RPS began to surface. In 1995, Papendick and Savoie[13] reported 95% overall satisfactory results in a group of athletes treated by one of four arthroscopic stabilization procedures. In a follow-up study Savoie and Field[11] reported 90% success rates at an average follow-up of 34 months. In 1996, Wolf[29] described the use of an arthroscopic suture anchor technique in a series of 17 patients, with successful results in 88%. McIntyre et al.[12] reported 25% failure rates following an arthroscopic posterior capsular shift with suture capsulorrhaphies in 20 patients with RPS at a mean follow-up of 31 months.

Further investigation suggested that four of the five failures occurred in patients with a voluntary component to their instability. Antoniou et al.[30] reported 85% success rates following arthroscopic suture capsulorrhaphy in a series of 41 patients at an average of 28 months follow-up. Ten patients in this series of Antoniou et al. exhibited MDI and also underwent rotator interval closure at the time of surgery. Wolf and Eakin[31] reported a group of 14 patients with unidirectional posterior shoulder instability. Patients with RPS as a result of isolated capsular redundancy were treated with suture capsulorrhaphy alone, and patients with labral detachments were treated with arthroscopic suture anchors. At 33 months average follow-up 12 of 14 patients (86%) had good or excellent results and 9 of 10 patients participating in competitive athletics returned to full activity. Studies by Mair et al.[14] and Williams et al.[32] have reported minimum 2-year follow-up success rates greater than 90% following use of a bioabsorbable tack to repair a traumatic posterior Bankart lesion. Although these published reports present preliminary results, arthroscopic capsulorrhaphy and labral repair techniques have thus far proven to be effective in the treatment of posterior shoulder instability.

Thermal capsulorrhaphy techniques have also been proposed in the treatment of posterior shoulder instability. The technique utilizes either laser or radiofrequency energy to induce thermal damage to the tissue of the redundant posterior capsule.[9,33–35] The degree of the capsular response has proven to be both time and temperature dependent.

An inflammatory reaction results in response to thermal energy, leading to shortening and denaturation of collagen fibrils. Over a period of at least 3 to 4 months a process of remodeling occurs whereby collagen fibroplasia and capsular thickening lead to reduction of the capsular volume. However, there are limits to the degree that capsular tissue can be shortened before the collagen is significantly weakened and its biomechanical properties are irreparably affected. The thermal energy induces a variable response on the part of the patient. Some patients form abundant scar tissue and exhibit significant reduction in capsular volume, while other patients do not respond to such a favorable extent. In addition, the long-term properties of the thermally modified tissue are unknown. Initial short-term results of thermal capsulorrhaphy in shoulder instability were encouraging with success rates near 90%.[36–38] More recent studies have not been as encouraging, with failure rates near 40%.[39,40] In particular, patients with MDI have shown particularly high failure rates.[39–41] Consequently, many surgeons have abandoned the use of thermal capsulorrhaphy in the treatment of shoulder instability.

■ INDICATIONS AND CONTRAINDICATIONS

Patients failing extensive physical therapy protocols should receive surgical consideration. The application of arthroscopic techniques to the treatment of shoulder instability is rapidly expanding. The development of arthroscopic techniques with the use of suture anchors has obviated the need for transglenoid drilling. Interval plication and suture capsulorrhaphy techniques have improved arthroscopic results, making them comparable to open procedures.[11,12,14,29,30,32] Advantages of arthroscopic techniques over traditional open techniques include less disruption of normal shoulder anatomy, better visualization of intra-articular landmarks, the ability to perform concomitant anterior and posterior stabilization procedures, and complete visualization of both the intra-articular and subacromial spaces. The surgeon's transition from open to arthroscopic techniques can be difficult. Arthroscopic techniques require the surgeon be familiar with anchor placement, suture management, and arthroscopic knot tying. A thorough understanding of arthroscopic anatomy is vital to the success of arthroscopic stabilization procedures.

Traditional open techniques have proven valuable in the treatment of posterior shoulder instability. As mentioned previously success rates near 80% to 90% have been achieved.[7,22] Contrary to arthroscopic techniques, open techniques require larger incisions, a deltoid-splitting approach, and splitting either the bipennate infraspinatus muscle or developing the interval between the infraspinatus and the teres minor. On the other hand, open techniques allow complete visualization of the posterior capsule and offer the opportunity to perform a reliable capsular shift or posterior labral repair. As a result open capsular shift techniques serve as reliable reconstruction methods in the surgical treatment of posterior shoulder instability. Indications for an open posterior shift include recurrent posterior shoulder instability in patients who have failed a reasonable rehabilitation program but continue to have functional impairment or pain with activity, a surgeon's preference over arthroscopic techniques, posterior instability in a contact athlete, the presence of a large reverse bony Bankart lesion, and instability in the setting of a large engaging reverse Hill-Sachs lesion. Relative indications include active patients with an acute antecedent macrotraumatic injury. Contraindications include patients who have not undergone appropriate conservative treatment, patients with muscular voluntary instability and psychogenic disorders, and patients unable or unwilling to comply with postoperative limitations.

Arthroscopic techniques have also shown promise in the treatment of posterior shoulder instability. As mentioned previously, success rates near 90% have been reported following arthroscopic procedures.[3,30,32] These results include patients with isolated posterior labral tears, unidirectional posterior instability, and MDI with a primary posterior component. The technique for each is distinctly different, but early results have been similarly successful. The senior author (JPB) has in review a prospective series of 66 patients with posterior unidirectional instability in 72 shoulders. At an average of 17.5 months follow-up (range 3 to 39 months) 91% good to excellent results were achieved by ASES criteria.

The patient population is largely comprised of high school, college, and professional athletes ranging in age from 14 to 58 years. Two failures in the study group have occurred to date, both of which were recurrent posterior subluxations resulting from macrotraumatic events.

Indications for arthroscopic posterior stabilization include patients with continued disabling isolated RPS following a rehabilitation program, RPS with a posterior labral tear, MDI with a primary posterior component, and voluntary positional posterior instability. Relative indications include patients with an antecedent macrotraumatic injury. Contraindications include patients not having completed a reasonable rehabilitation program, a surgeon's preference for traditional open techniques, a large engaging reverse Hill-Sachs lesion requiring subscapularis transfer or an osteochondral allograft, a large reverse bony Bankart lesion, patients with muscular voluntary instability and underlying psychogenic disorders, and patients unable or unwilling to comply with postoperative limitations. Relative contraindications may include chronic instability resulting in compromised capsulolabral tissue, patients who have undergone previous open surgery, and posterior instability in a contact athlete. However, successful results have been achieved following arthroscopic treatment of posterior labral tears in contact athletes.[14,32] As arthroscopic techniques continue to evolve the surgical indications will likely broaden.

■ SURGICAL TECHNIQUES

Arthroscopic Technique

The procedure can be performed under interscalene block or general endotracheal anesthesia with an interscalene block for postoperative pain control. The examination under anesthesia (EUA) is performed on a firm surface with the scapula relatively fixed and the humeral head free to rotate. Passive range of motion is documented, with differences between the affected and unaffected shoulders noted. We prefer to first examine the opposite shoulder, followed by examination of the affected side. A load and shift maneuver, as described by Murrell and Warren,[5] is performed with the patient supine. The arm is held in 90 degrees of abduction and neutral rotation while a posterior force is applied in an attempt to translate the humeral head over the posterior glenoid **(Fig. 5-3)**. Translation is graded 0 if the humeral head does not translate to the glenoid rim, 1+ if the humeral head translates to the glenoid rim and is increased compared to the uninvolved shoulder, 2+ if the humeral head translates over the glenoid rim but spontaneously reduces, and 3+ if the humeral head translates over the glenoid rim and does not spontaneously reduce. A sulcus sign is performed with the arm adducted and in neutral rotation to assess whether the instability has an inferior component. The sulcus sign is a measure of the distance between the undersurface of the acromion and the humeral head. Translation is graded as 1+ if the distance is

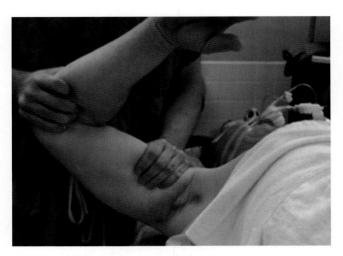

Fig. 5-3. Clinical photograph of the posterior load and shift maneuver performed at 90 degrees abduction and neutral rotation.

less than 1 cm, 2+ if the distance is between 1 and 2 cm, and 3+ if the distance is greater than 2 cm. A 3+ sulcus sign that remains 2+ or greater in external rotation is considered pathopneumonic for MDI. Testing is completed on both the affected and unaffected shoulders, and differences between the two are documented.

The patient is also examined for signs of generalized ligamentous laxity as described by Beighton et al.[42] in 1973. Patients are assessed one point for the presence of the following criteria in each extremity: greater than 10 degrees elbow hyperextension, greater than 10 degrees knee hyperextension, the ability to perform a thumb-to-forearm maneuver, greater than 90 degrees extension at the small finger metacarpophalangeal joint, and the ability to place the hands flat on the floor with the knee straight. A maximum score of nine points can be generated with this scoring system. Although some disagreement exists, a Beighton score of five or greater is generally considered to be diagnostic of generalized ligamentous laxity. Patients with RPS have been shown to have increased laxity scores when compared to age- and sex-matched controls without instability.[7]

The patient is then placed in the lateral decubitus position with the affected shoulder positioned superior. An inflatable bean bag and kidney rests hold the patient in position. Foam cushions are placed to protect the peroneal nerve at the neck of the fibula on the down leg. An axillary roll is placed in the axilla. The operating table is placed in a slight reverse Trendelenburg position. The full upper extremity is prepped to the level of the sternum anteriorly and the medial border of the scapula posteriorly. The operative shoulder is placed in 10 lb of traction and is positioned in 45 degrees of abduction and 20 degrees of forward flexion **(Fig. 5-4)**. The bony landmarks, including the acromion, distal clavicle, and coracoid process, are demarcated with a marking pen **(Fig. 5-5)**.

Following prepping and draping, the glenohumeral joint is injected with 20 cc of sterile saline through an 18-gauge spinal needle to inflate the joint. A standard posterior portal to the anterior portal to allow improved visualization of the posterior capsule and labrum. A switching stick can then be utilized in replacing the posterior cannula with an 8.25-mm distally threaded clear cannula (Arthrex, Inc, Naples, Fla), thus allowing passage of an arthroscopic probe through the clear cannula to explore the posterior labrum for evidence of tears.

Posterior Labral Tear

In situations where the posterior labrum is detached suture anchors are employed in performing the repair. The posterior labrum is visualized from both the posterior **(Fig. 5-6)** and anterior portals to appreciate the full extent of the tear. The arthroscope then remains in the anterior portal and the posterior portal serves as the working portal for the repair. An arthroscopic rasp or chisel is used to mobilize the torn labrum from the glenoid rim. A motorized synovial shaver is used to debride and decorticate the glenoid rim to achieve a bleeding surface **(Fig. 5-7)**. An arthroscopic rasp or motorized synovial shaver can then be utilized in abrading the capsule adjacent to the labral tear. Care must be taken in the use of the motorized shaver for this purpose because the posterior capsule is thin and can be easily penetrated with an aggressive technique.

An arthroscopic awl is then employed to penetrate the bare area of the humerus, under the infraspinatus tendon, in an effort to achieve some punctuate bleeding to augment the healing response. Suture anchors are then placed at the articular margin of the glenoid rim, rather than down on the glenoid neck, to perform the labral repair **(Fig. 5-8)**. The number of suture anchors depends on the size of the labral tear. A posterior labral tear extending from 6 o'clock to 9 o'clock is typically repaired with suture anchors at the 6:30, 7:30, and 8:30 positions. We prefer the 3.0-mm BioFastak suture anchor (Arthrex, Inc, Naples, Fla) but a number of other

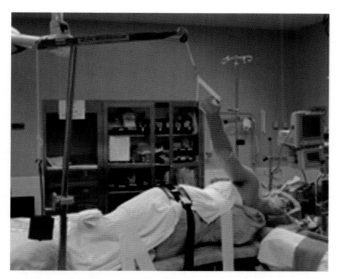

Fig. 5-4. Lateral decubitus positioning for shoulder arthroscopy.

is established. An anterior portal is then established high in the rotator interval via an inside-to-outside technique with a switching stick. Alternatively, it can also be established via an outside-to-inside technique with the assistance of a spinal needle. Typically, only anterior and posterior portals are required to perform the procedure. Sometimes an accessory 7 o'clock portal may be needed. A diagnostic arthroscopy of the glenohumeral joint is then undertaken. The labrum, capsule, biceps tendon, subscapularis, rotator interval, rotator cuff, and articular surfaces are visualized in systematic fashion. This ensures that no associated lesions will be overlooked by poorly directed tunnel vision. Lesions typically seen in posterior instability include a patulous posterior capsule, posterior labral tears, labral fraying and splitting, widening of the rotator interval, and undersurface partial-thickness rotator cuff tears. After viewing the glenohumeral joint from the posterior portal, the arthroscope is switched

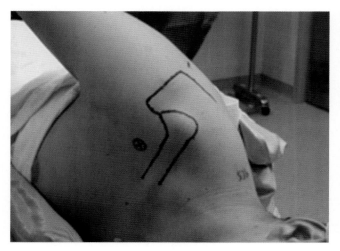

Fig. 5-5. Skin markings of the bony landmarks in preparation for arthroscopy.

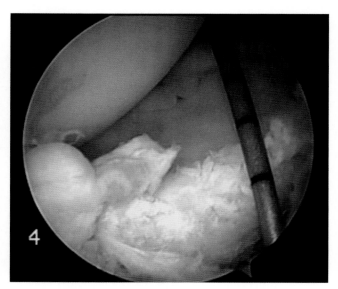

Fig. 5-6. Arthroscopic view from the posterior portal demonstrating a displaced posterior labral tear.

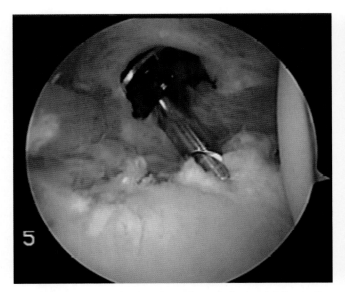

Fig. 5-7. Arthroscopic view from the anterior portal illustrating debridement of the glenoid rim with a motorized synovial shaver adjacent to a posterior labral tear.

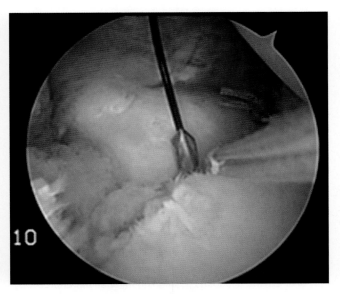

Fig. 5-9. Arthroscopic view from the anterior portal showing advancement of the no. 0 PDS from behind the torn posterior labrum to the glenoid articular margin.

commercially available anchors are also adequate. The suture anchor is placed with the sutures oriented perpendicular to the glenoid rim to facilitate passage of the most posterior suture limb through the torn labrum. During placement of the suture anchor care must be taken to avoid inadvertent injury to the articular cartilage.

Following placement of the suture anchors a 45-degree Spectrum suture hook (Linvatec Corp, Largo, Fla) is then loaded with a no. 0 polydiaxanone sulphate (PDS) suture (Ethicon, Somerville, NJ). Alternatively, there are other commercially available suture passers and suture relays that

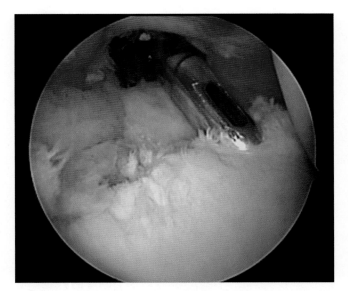

Fig. 5-8. Arthroscopic view from the anterior portal showing placement of a suture anchor at the articular margin of the glenoid rim.

will also suffice. The suture passer is delivered through the torn labrum and advanced superiorly, reentering the joint at the edge of the glenoid articular cartilage **(Fig. 5-9)**. Advancing the suture passer in this fashion reintroduces tension into the posterior band of the inferior glenohumeral ligament (IGHL). This tension must be restored to reestablish posterior stability. Patients with acute injuries and less evidence of capsular stretching do not require the same degree of capsular advancement as those with more chronic instability or MDI. In the case of an acute labral tear without significant capsular laxity the 6 o'clock position on the labral tear is advanced to the 6:30 suture anchor. In the setting of a labral tear with some capsular laxity, the suture passer is advanced through the posterior capsule approximately 1 cm lateral to the edge of the labral tear and then is advanced as described previously, underneath the labral tear, to the edge of the articular cartilage. The PDS is then fed into the glenohumeral joint and the suture passer is withdrawn through the posterior clear cannula. While withdrawing the suture passer from the posterior clear cannula, additional suture is advanced into the joint to prevent inadvertently pulling the suture through the torn edge of the labrum. An arthroscopic suture grasper is used to withdraw both the most posterior suture in the suture anchor and the end of the PDS suture that has been advanced through the torn labrum **(Fig. 5-10)**. This step detangles the sutures inside the cannula. The PDS is then fashioned into a single loop and tightly tied over the end of the braided suture. It is important not to tie the braided suture over the end of the PDS suture as this construct will unravel while pulling through the labrum and capsule. The most lateral PDS suture, which has not been tied to the braided suture, is then pulled through the clear cannula. This advances the most

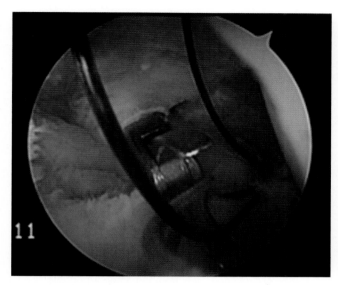

Fig. 5-10. Arthroscopic view from the anterior portal demonstrating use of a suture grasper to capture the most posterior suture from the suture anchor and the anterior limb of the PDS suture.

posterior suture in the suture anchor behind the labral tear **(Fig. 5-11)**. Additional sutures are then placed in similar fashion to complete the labral repair. The labral tear at the 7 o'clock position is advanced to the 7:30 suture anchor and the 8 o'clock labral tear position is advanced to the 8:30 suture anchor. If the capsule requires further advancement suture capsulorrhaphies, as described later in this section, these can be performed in the intervals between the suture anchors directly to the newly secured labrum. Knots are tied following passage of each suture. This allows continued assessment of the repair and the degree of the capsular shift

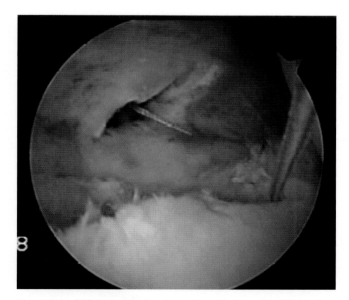

Fig. 5-11. Arthroscopic view from the anterior portal illustrating the completed passage of the posterior suture from the suture anchor behind the posterior labral tear.

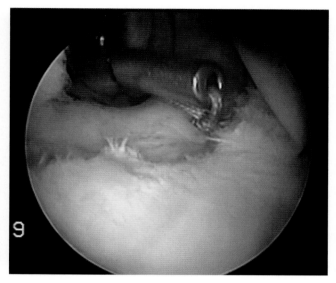

Fig. 5-12. Arthroscopic view from the anterior portal demonstrating the past point technique.

achieved by each suture. Care must be taken with the sharp Spectrum suture passer tip to avoid cutting or placing undue tension on previously tied sutures.

When tying the sutures we prefer the sliding, locking Westin knot, but there are a number of arthroscopic knot-tying techniques that work well. What is most important is that the surgeon be familiar with the knot utilized and be skilled in its use. The posterior braided suture exiting through the capsule is threaded through a knot pusher and the end is secured with a hemostat. This suture serves as the post, which in effect will advance the capsule and labrum to the glenoid rim when the knot is tightened. Regardless of the knot-tying technique utilized each half hitch must be completely seated before the next half hitch is thrown. Placing tension on the nonpost suture and advancing the knot pusher "past point" will lock the Westin knot **(Fig. 5-12)**. In order to prevent the knots from unraveling each half hitch must be secured square to the preceding hitch. A total of three half hitches are placed to secure the Westin knot. The posterior capsular portal incision is then closed by passage of a PDS suture through the crescent Spectrum suture passer **(Fig. 5-13)** and retrieving the suture with an arthroscopic penetrator **(Fig. 5-14)**. The PDS is then tied in the subacromial space, closing the posterior capsular incision **(Fig. 5-15)**.

Posterior Capsulorrhaphy

Most patients with unidirectional posterior instability and primary posterior MDI do not have a posterior labral tear.[13,14] If the EUA exhibits unidirectional posterior instability but the diagnostic arthroscopy, as described earlier, does not reveal a posterior labral tear, a posterior suture capsulorrhaphy is performed. Posterior labral fraying and splitting without a discrete displaced tear are common in these

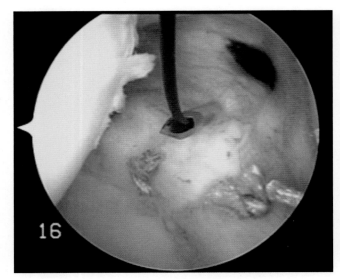

Fig. 5-13. Arthroscopic view from the anterior portal showing advancement of the Spectrum crescent suture passer through one side of the posterior capsular portal incision.

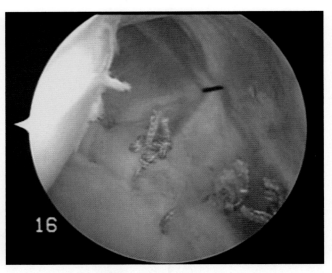

Fig. 5-15. Arthroscopic view from the anterior portal following closure of the posterior capsular portal incision.

situations. These patients will typically display significant capsular laxity at arthroscopy **(Fig. 5-16)**.

The capsule from the 7 o'clock position to 10 o'clock position is abraded with an arthroscopic rasp or a motorized synovial shaver. Care must be taken in the use of a motorized shaver on the posterior capsule as it is thin and easily penetrated by aggressive application of the shaver. An arthroscopic awl is used to create some punctate bleeding by penetrating the subchondral bone along the bare area of the humerus. Suture capsulorrhaphies are placed from inferior (6 o'clock) to superior (10 o'clock). Advancement from 1 cm

lateral to the capsulolabral junction to the glenoid rim has proven to be safe.[43] A 45-degree Spectrum suture passer pierces the capsule 1 cm lateral to the labrum at the 6:30 position on the glenoid. The capsule is then lifted and advanced superiorly and medially, with the suture passer reentering the joint at the junction of the annular labral fibers and the glenoid articular cartilage rim. Depending on the degree of capsular laxity present, the 6:30 capsular suture is typically advanced to the 7:30 position on the glenoid. A no. 0 PDS suture is then fed through the suture passer into the joint **(Fig. 5-17)**. The ends are retrieved with a suture grasper. One end of the PDS is tied over the end of a braided no. 2 suture and the opposite end of the PDS is advanced out of the clear cannula, pulling the braided suture

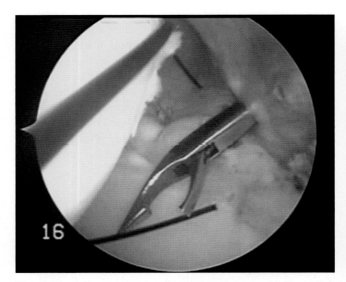

Fig. 5-14. Arthroscopic view from the anterior portal illustrating passage of an arthroscopic penetrator through the opposite side of the posterior capsular portal incision to capture the PDS suture.

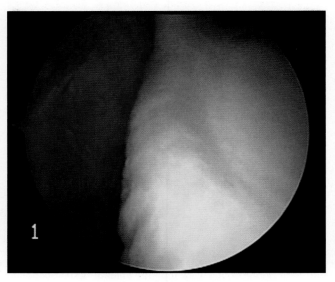

Fig. 5-16. Arthroscopic view from the posterior portal demonstrating a capacious posterior capsule.

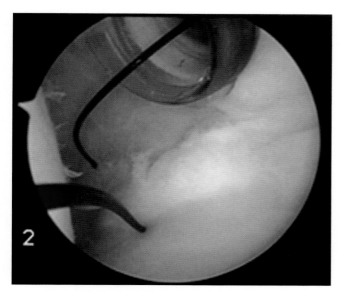

Fig. 5-17. Arthroscopic view from the anterior portal showing passage of a PDS suture in preparation for a 1-cm advancement of the capsule from the 6:30 position to the 7:30 position on the glenoid.

into position. This suture is tied, as described previously, and the reduction in capsular volume is assessed. Restoring adequate tension in the posterior band of the IGHL is critical to the success of the reconstruction. If adequate, a second 1 cm capsulorrhaphy suture is placed at the 7:30 position on the capsule that advances to the 8:30 position on the glenoid. Additional sutures are then placed at the 8:30 and 9:30 positions on the capsule, advancing to the 9:30 and 10:30 positions on the glenoid **(Fig. 5-18)**. Sutures are tied after each is passed rather than waiting until the end to tie all of them at the same time. If the initial 6:30 capsular

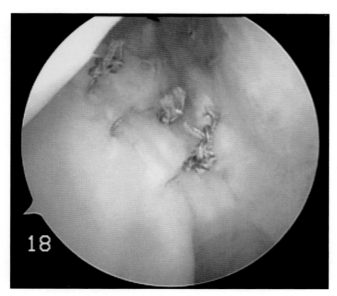

Fig. 5-18. Arthroscopic view from the anterior portal following multiple posteroinferior suture capsulorrhaphies.

suture is deemed to not have been advanced far enough superior on the glenoid, it can be removed and only that one suture need be replaced. On the other hand, if the sutures are not tied until the end one errant suture may necessitate removal of all other sutures to achieve correction. The posterior capsular portal incision is then closed as previously described (Figs. 5-13, 5-14, 5-15).

In the setting of MDI with a primary posterior component, the rotator interval requires closure for reasons discussed in the next section. The rotator interval is viewed in the glenohumeral joint with the arthroscope in the posterior portal. A crescent suture passer is advanced from the anterior portal through the anterior capsule just above the superior border of the subscapularis tendon. As the suture passer is visualized entering the glenohumeral joint, it is then passed through the middle glenohumeral ligament (MGHL) at the inferior border of the rotator interval. A no. 0 PDS suture is then fed into the joint, and the suture passer is withdrawn from the joint as additional suture is advanced. An arthroscopic penetrator is then passed through the anterior portal, through the anterior capsule in the superior aspect of the rotator interval, and through the superior glenohumeral ligament (SGHL). The penetrator is then advanced to capture the PDS that has been passed through the MGHL. The penetrator and PDS suture are then withdrawn from the anterior cannula. The PDS suture is then visualized in the subacromial space and is tied as previously discussed. In cases of significant rotator interval widening, additional sutures placed in similar fashion may be necessary to achieve the necessary plication.

■ TECHNICAL ALTERNATIVES AND PITFALLS

There is open debate regarding whether the lateral decubitus or beach chair position better facilitates shoulder arthroscopy. We prefer the lateral position because we feel it allows better access to both the anterior and posterior aspects of the shoulder. Placing the shoulder in 10 lb traction in the position of 45 degrees abduction and 20 degrees of forward flexion in effect displaces the humeral head anteriorly and inferiorly, bringing the posterior labrum into clear view. We have not been able to achieve such an unimpeded approach to the posteroinferior shoulder capsule in the beach chair position without imparting injury to the articular cartilage of the humeral head in the process.

We prefer to inject the glenohumeral joint with 20 to 30 cc of sterile saline prior to placement of the cannula into the glenohumeral joint. It inflates the joint to allow safer insertion of the cannula, limiting risk to the articular cartilage of the humeral head and glenoid.

After a determination of posterior labral pathology or capsular laxity is made, a posterior working portal must be established. Placement of an 8.25-mm distally threaded clear cannula (Arthrex, Inc, Naples, Fla) over a switching stick into the posterior portal will allow passage of both the crescent and 45-degree suture hooks. Smaller cannulas will not accommodate the 45-degree suture hook.

Difficulty in the placement of suture anchors can be encountered if the posterior portal is located too far superior or medial in the posterior capsule. The conventional posterior portal is located near 10 o'clock on the glenoid, which makes approach to the posteroinferior glenoid difficult for the placement of suture anchors. We therefore place the posterior portal approximately 1 cm inferior and 1 cm lateral to the standard posterior portal in patients with demonstrable posterior instability on EUA. When the posterior portal has been made too far superior, an auxiliary posterior portal can then be made inferior and lateral to the existing posterior portal. A spinal needle can be utilized in positioning the auxiliary portal at 7 o'clock on the glenoid and approximately 1 cm lateral to the glenoid rim on the posterior capsule for approach to the posteroinferior glenoid at a 30- to 45-degree angle in the sagittal plane. Cadaveric studies by Davidson and Rivenburgh[44] have shown the 7 o'clock portal to be located a safe distance from the axillary nerve and posterior humeral circumflex artery (39 ± 4 mm), and the suprascapular nerve and artery (29 ± 3 mm). The use of blunt trocars in the placement of the portal further decreases the risk of neurovascular injury.

We do not routinely close the rotator interval in patients with unidirectional posterior instability. This practice is supported by several other studies in the literature.[14,29–31] Harryman et al.[45] sectioned the rotator interval and found that in a position of 60 degrees flexion and 60 degrees abduction a significant increase in posterior translation occurred. However, in posterior instability's provocative position of 60 degrees flexion and 90 degrees internal rotation, no significant increase in posterior translation occurred following sectioning of the rotator interval. Furthermore, although imbrication of the rotator interval significantly decreased posterior translation at a position of 60 degrees flexion and 60 degrees abduction, it did not have a similar effect in the provocative position. A sectioned rotator interval did lead to a significant increase in inferior translation, which was corrected by imbrication of the rotator interval tissue. Therefore, we do perform rotator interval closure in patients with an inferior component to their instability, as defined by a 2+ or greater sulcus sign that does not improve in external rotation.

■ ALTERNATIVE SURGICAL TECHNIQUES: OPEN POSTERIOR CAPSULORRHAPHY

The patient is placed supine on the operating table and a thorough EUA is performed. Following completion of the EUA the patient is positioned on a bean bag in the lateral decubitus position as previously described. The bony landmarks of the shoulder are demarcated with a marking pen (Fig. 5-5).

A diagnostic shoulder arthroscopy utilizing anterior and posterior portals technique is performed to evaluate the articular surfaces of the glenoid and humeral head, labrum, capsule, rotator cuff, rotator interval, and glenohumeral ligaments. After the diagnosis is confirmed by EUA and diagnostic arthroscopy, the arthroscopic procedure is terminated.

The approach for open capsulorrhaphy extends from just posterior to the acromioclavicular joint to the axillary fold **(Fig. 5-19)**. The incision generally measures nearly 10 cm in length. The deltoid muscle is split in line with its fibers from the scapular spine, beginning 2 to 3 cm medial to the posterolateral corner of the acromion and extending distally approximately 5 to 6 cm **(Fig. 5-20A)**. Care must be taken to avoid splitting the deltoid muscle inferior to the teres minor and subsequently injuring the axillary nerve, which enters the deltoid muscle at the inferior border of the teres minor. The deltoid typically does not require reflection from the spine of the scapula, except occasionally in muscular individuals. It is essential to place the split in the deltoid medial to the posterolateral border of the acromion to ensure proper visualization of the glenohumeral joint.

Beneath the deltoid lies the external rotators of the shoulders, including the bipennate infraspinatus and the teres minor (Fig. 5-20B). The interval between the muscles may be indistinct, but the raphe separating the two heads of the bipennate infraspinatus is typically unmistakable. This raphe lies above the equator of the humeral head and should not be confused with the interval between the infraspinatus and teres minor muscles, which is usually located below the equator of the humeral head. The interval between the bipennate heads of the infraspinatus is bluntly developed to expose the posterior

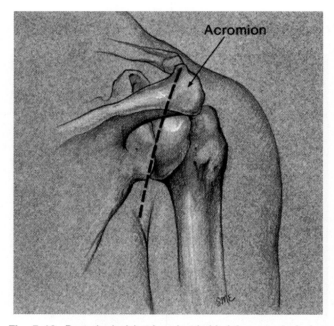

Fig. 5-19. Posterior incision from just behind the acromioclavicular joint toward the posterior axillary fold. (From Garrett WE Jr, Speer KP, Kirkendall DT, eds. **Principles and Practice of Orthopaedic Sports Medicine.** Philadelphia: Lippincott Williams & Wilkins.)

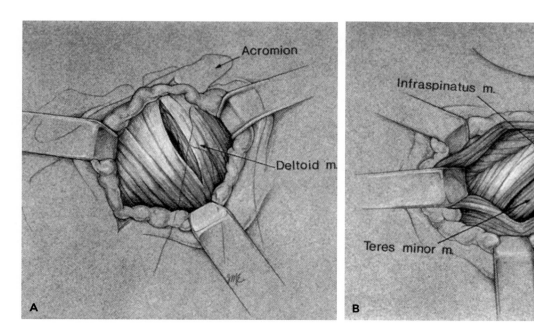

Fig. 5-20. A: The deltoid is split in line with its fibers beginning approximately 2 to 3 cm medial to the posterolateral corner of the acromion. **B:** The underlying infraspinatus and teres minor muscles are exposed. (From Garrett WE Jr, Speer KP, Kirkendall DT, eds. *Principles and Practice of Orthopaedic Sports Medicine*. Philadelphia: Lippincott Williams & Wilkins.)

capsule over the equator of the glenoid. Care must be taken to avoid splitting the infraspinatus more than 1.5 cm medial to the glenoid rim to protect the suprascapular nerve. Narrow deep Richardson retractors work well as blunt retractors in this setting. The capsule is closely associated with the tendons laterally, necessitating sharp dissection to develop this interval. Medially the capsule is more readily freed from the overlying muscle belly with the assistance of a periosteal elevator.

Following complete exposure of the posterior capsule a transverse arthrotomy is made in a medial to lateral direction. Medially the arthrotomy is continued to the lateral edge, but not through, the labrum **(Fig. 5-21)**. The vertical limb of the capsulotomy is then carried out just lateral to the labrum. The superior and inferior capsular flaps are then developed **(Fig. 5-22)**. Tagging sutures are placed in the superior and inferior limbs of the capsule. Care must be taken in

Fig. 5-21. The T-shaped capsular incision is marked to the lateral edge, but not through, the labrum. (From Garrett WE Jr, Speer KP, Kirkendall DT, eds. *Principles and Practice of Orthopaedic Sports Medicine*. Philadelphia: Lippincott Williams & Wilkins.)

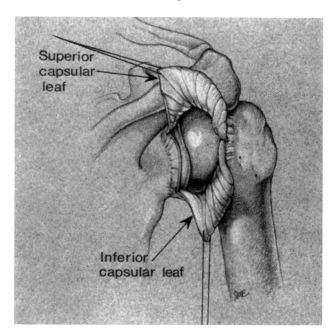

Fig. 5-22. The capsular incision has been made. The superior and inferior capsular flaps are mobilized. (From Garrett WE Jr, Speer KP, Kirkendall DT, eds. *Principles and Practice of Orthopaedic Sports Medicine*. Philadelphia: Lippincott Williams & Wilkins.)

developing the inferior capsular flap because of the close proximity of the axillary nerve.

Treatment at this point is directed at the pathology present. In the setting of a posterior labral tear, or reverse Bankart tear, the labrum must be reflected to permit access to the glenoid rim to allow placement of suture anchors. If the labrum is intact the sutures that anchor the capsulorrhaphy are placed through the labrum. The capsulorrhaphy is initiated by advancing the inferior flap in the superior and medial direction. The degree of advancement of the inferior flap is dependent upon the direction and degree of the instability. While a patient suffering from unidirectional posterior instability can be effectively treated by a primarily medial capsular shift, a patient with MDI will also require a superior advancement of the inferior capsular flap to correct the inferior component of the instability. Determination of the appropriate advancement and capsular tension is made with the arm in a relaxed, neutral position. The capsular flap is secured to the labrum with no. 1 nonabsorbable sutures **(Fig. 5-23)**. The superior flap is then advanced over the inferior flap in the inferior and medial directions **(Fig. 5-24)**. The remaining gap in the capsule is then closed with interrupted mattress sutures. Drains are generally not necessary. The interval between the bipennate heads of the infraspinatus, or between the infraspinatus and teres minor, typically reapproximates nicely without need for sutures. The superficial deltoid fascia is then repaired with interrupted no. 0 absorbable sutures. The subcutaneous tissue is reapproximated with no. 2-0 absorbable suture. The incision is closed with a subcuticular suture to improve cosmesis.

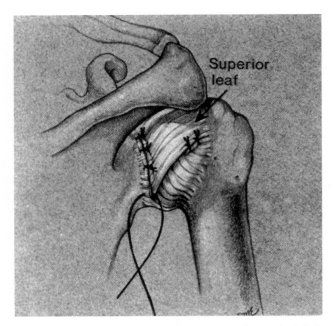

Fig. 5-24. The superior capsular flap is sutured over the inferior capsular flap following medial and inferior advancement. (From Garrett WE Jr, Speer KP, Kirkendall DT, eds. Principles and Practice of Orthopaedic Sports Medicine. Philadelphia: Lippincott Williams & Wilkins.)

■ REHABILITATION/RETURN TO PLAY RECOMMENDATIONS

The physical therapy rehabilitation program following RPS/posterior dislocation surgical repair varies in length of time depending on several underlying patient characteristics: the absence or presence of generalized ligamentous laxity, unidirectional posterior instability versus MDI with a primary posterior component, traumatic versus atraumatic etiologies, acute versus chronic conditions, and the absence or presence of a patient predisposition to form abundant scar tissue. Patients with traumatic injuries, acute conditions, a predisposition to form abundant scar tissue, and no evidence of generalized ligamentous laxity are typically immobilized in an UltraSling (DonJoy, Carlsbad, Calif) for 4 weeks postoperatively. Conversely, patients with atraumatic etiologies, chronic conditions, absence of a predisposition to form abundant scar tissue formation, and evidence of generalized ligamentous laxity are typically immobilized in the UltraSling for 6 weeks postoperatively. Patients in the latter group are continually evaluated for development of increasing stiffness, at which time the sling is discontinued and the patient progressed to the second stage of the rehabilitation program.

The rehabilitation program consists of a series of phases. Initially, the posterior capsule must be protected by avoiding extremes of internal rotation. The UltraSling achieves this by abducting the shoulder approximately 30 degrees. Cryotherapy is employed for edema control. Immobilization is removed for gentle passive range of motion exercises. Progression of passive motion is limited based on the above

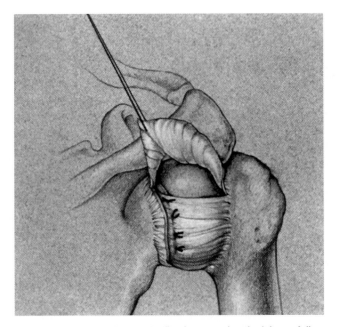

Fig. 5-23. The inferior capsular flap is sutured to the labrum following medial and superior advancement. (From Garrett WE Jr, Speer KP, Kirkendall DT, eds. Principles and Practice of Orthopaedic Sports Medicine. Philadelphia: Lippincott Williams & Wilkins.)

criteria, but in general we allow 90 degrees forward flexion and external rotation to 0 degrees by 4 weeks postsurgery. Once again, internal rotation is avoided to protect the posterior capsule. Passive motion should be within pain-free limits of the patient. Active elbow, wrist, and hand exercises are encouraged.

As mentioned previously the UltraSling is discontinued at 4 to 6 weeks postsurgery. Gentle passive range of motion exercises are progressed and pain-free gentle internal rotation is instituted. Extremes of internal rotation are avoided. Active-assisted range of motion exercises, such as wand exercises, begin at this time as well. Periscapular strengthening begins with shoulder shrug exercises. Isometric internal and external rotation with the arm at the side and the elbow flexed 90 degrees is begun according to the patient's tolerance. Active horizontal abduction in the prone position with movement restricted from 45 degrees of horizontal adduction to full horizontal abduction is allowed. Cryotherapy for edema control continues.

At 6 to 8 weeks postsurgery passive and active-assisted range of motion are advanced. Active external rotation with surgical tubing begins. Passive internal rotation continues, followed by active internal rotation in the supine position with the arm at the side and the elbow flexed 90 degrees. Active shoulder flexion as tolerated and shoulder abduction to 90 degrees are allowed.

At 2 to 3 months postsurgery, range of motion and mobilization is progressed to achieve full passive and active motion. Stretching exercises for the anterior and posterior capsule are instituted. Isotonic strengthening continues with emphasis on the rotator cuff and posterior deltoid. Active internal rotation with surgical tubing begins. Horizontal abduction may be increased to include beginning from a starting position at 90 degrees of horizontal adduction. Proprioceptive neuromuscular facilitation of upper extremity patterns is added.

By 4 months postsurgery the shoulder should be pain free and have no significant amount of swelling. Resisted strengthening with free weights continues, with a concentration on eccentric rotator cuff strengthening. Isokinetic strengthening and endurance exercises for shoulder internal and external rotation, with the arm at the side, and horizontal abduction are added. At 5 months postsurgery isotonic and isokinetic exercises are advanced. Continued eccentric rotator cuff strengthening and total body conditioning, with an emphasis on strength and endurance, are encouraged.

At 6 months postsurgery throwing athletes undergo isokinetic testing. When patients are able to achieve at least 80% strength and endurance compared to the uninvolved side an integrated throwing protocol is instituted. Progression to the next stage in the throwing program is dependent on the ability to perform the prior stage in a pain-free fashion. Throwers begin an easy-tossing program at a distance of 20 ft without a windup. Stretching and the application of heat to increase circulation prior to throwing sessions are critical.

By 7 months light throwing with an easy windup to 30 ft is allowed 2 to 3 days per week for 10 minutes per session. The distance and frequency are gradually increased. By 9 months postsurgery long, easy throws from the midoutfield (150 to 200 feet) are allowed. The ball should reach home plate on five or six bounces. The throwing frequency is increased to a schedule of 15 minutes of throwing on 2 consecutive days followed by a day of rest. By 10 months stronger throws from the outfield are allowed, reaching home plate on only one or two bounces. At 11 months pitchers are allowed to throw one-half to three-quarter speed from the mound with emphasis on technique and accuracy. A schedule of 30 minutes of throwing on 2 consecutive days, followed by a day of rest, continues to be followed. By 12 months postsurgery throwers are allowed to throw from their position at three-quarter to full speed. When able to perform full-speed throwing for 2 consecutive weeks, the throwing athlete is permitted to return to full competition.

Nonthrowing athletes and nonathletes are managed by different criteria than throwing athletes. At 6 months postsurgery isokinetic testing is performed. When patients are able to achieve at least 80% strength and endurance compared to the uninvolved side, nonthrowing athletes begin a sport-specific program. Return to full competition is permitted with successful completion of a sport-specific program. In general, power athletes and contact athletes, such as weight lifters and football players, can return to full competition by 9 to 12 months postsurgery. Noncontact athletes such as golfers, basketball players, swimmers, and cheerleaders can generally return to full competition by 8 to 12 months. Athletes must achieve a full, pain-free range of motion, full strength and endurance, and return of proprioceptive function prior to return to full competition. Nonathletes are allowed to return to full recreational activity with restoration of a full, pain-free range of motion and full strength. This can generally be achieved by 6 to 8 months postsurgery.

■ SUMMARY

Posterior shoulder instability is a broad entity ranging from RPS to LPD. It is much less common than anterior shoulder instability, but probably occurs more frequently than suggested in the literature. Traditionally confusion existed in the distinction between the different forms of posterior instability, but a much greater understanding has been gained more recently. Good success rates can be gained by a prolonged course of physical therapy with avoidance of activities in the provocative position. Patients with RPS resulting from chronic, repetitive microtrauma or generalized ligamentous laxity tend to respond best to a rehabilitation program. Patients failing conservative measures should be considered for surgical reconstruction. Traditional open techniques have proven to be 80% to 90% effective at long-term follow-up.

Open reconstructive methods are both reliable and reproducible. Arthroscopic techniques have shown encouraging preliminary results. Although long-term results do not yet exist, short-term results suggest that success rates near 90% can be achieved by arthroscopic reconstructive procedures. Furthermore, arthroscopic methods afford the ability to perform simultaneous anterior and posterior reconstructions, avoid splitting the deltoid and rotator cuff, and offer excellent visualization of both the glenohumeral joint and subacromial space. A directed physical therapy program postsurgery is vital to a successful outcome. Throwing athletes and power athletes are generally able to return to full competition within 9 to 12 months postsurgery. Nonathletes are generally able to return to full activity within 6 to 9 months postsurgery.

■ SUGGESTED READINGS

Antoniou J, Duckworth DT, Harryman DT II. Capsulolabral augmentation for the management of posteroinferior instability of the shoulder. J Bone Joint Surg Am. 2000;82(9):1220.

Boyd HB, Sisk TD. Recurrent posterior dislocation of the shoulder. J Bone Joint Surg Am. 1972;54A:779.

D'Alessandro DF, Bradley JP, Fleischli JE, et al. Prospective evaluation of thermal capsulorrhaphy for shoulder instability. Am J Sports Med. 2004;32:21–33.

Eakin CL, Dvirnak P, Miller CM, et al. The relationship of the axillary nerve to arthroscopically placed capsulolabral sutures. Am J Sports Med. 1998;26:505–509.

Fronek J, Warren RF, Bowen M. Posterior subluxation of the glenohumeral joint. J Bone Joint Surg Am. 1989;71A:205.

Harryman DT, Sidles JA, Harris SL, et al. The role of the rotator interval capsule in passive motion and stability of the shoulder. J Bone Joint Surg Am. 1992;74:53–66.

Mair SD, Zarzour RH, Speer KP. Posterior labral injury in contact athletes. Am J Sports Med. 1998;26:753.

McIntyre LF, Caspari RB, Savoie FH III. The arthroscopic treatment of posterior shoulder instability: two-year results of a multiple suture technique. Arthroscopy. 1997;13:426.

McLaughlin HL. Posterior dislocation of the shoulder. J Bone Joint Surg Am. 1952;34A:584.

Murrell GA, Warren RF. The surgical treatment of posterior shoulder instability. Clin Sports Med. 1995;14:903.

Neer CS II, Foster CR. Inferior capsular shift for involuntary inferior and multidirectional instability of the shoulder. J Bone Joint Surg Am. 1980;62A:897.

Tibone JE, Bradley JP. The treatment of posterior subluxation in athletes. Clin Orthop. 1993;291:124.

Wolf EM, Eakin CL. Arthroscopic capsular plication for posterior shoulder instability. Arthroscopy. 1998;14:153–163.

■ REFERENCES

1. McLaughlin HL. Posterior dislocation of the shoulder. J Bone Joint Surg Am. 1952;34A:584.
2. Boyd HB, Sisk TD. Recurrent posterior dislocation of the shoulder. J Bone Joint Surg Am. 1972;54A:779.
3. Hayashi K, Markel MD, Thabit G III, et al. The effect of nonablative laser energy on joint capsule properties: an in vitro mechanical study using a rabbit model. Am J Sports Med. 1995;25:482–487.
4. Pollock RG, Bigliani LU. Recurrent posterior shoulder instability. Clin Orthop. 1993;291:85.
5. Murrell GA, Warren RF. The surgical treatment of posterior shoulder instability. Clin Sports Med. 1995;14:903.
6. Tibone JE, Bradley JP. The treatment of posterior subluxation in athletes. Clin Orthop. 1993;291:124–137.
7. Fronek J, Warren RF, Bowen M. Posterior subluxation of the glenohumeral joint. J Bone Joint Surg Am. 1989;71A:205.
8. Hawkins RJ, Koppert G, Johnston G. Recurrent posterior instability (subluxation) of the shoulder. J Bone Joint Surg Am. 1984;66A:169.
9. Hayashi K, Thabit G III, Bogdanske JJ, et al. The effect of nonablative laser energy on the ultrastructure of joint capsular collagen. Arthroscopy. 1996;12:474–481.
10. Tibone JE, Ting A. Capsulorrhaphy with a staple for recurrent posterior subluxation of the shoulder. J Bone Joint Surg Am. 1990;12A:999.
11. Savoie FH, Field LD. Arthroscopic management of posterior shoulder instability. Oper Tech Sports Med. 1997;5:226.
12. McIntyre LF, Caspari RB, Savoie FH III. The arthroscopic treatment of posterior shoulder instability: two-year results of a multiple suture technique. Arthroscopy. 1997;13:426.
13. Papendick LW, Savoie FH III. Anatomy-specific repair techniques for posterior shoulder instability. J South Orthop Assoc. 1995; 4:169.
14. Mair SD, Zarzour RH, Speer KP. Posterior labral injury in contact athletes. Am J Sports Med. 1998;26:753.
15. Rowe CR, Zarins B. Recurrent transient subluxation of the shoulder. J Bone Joint Surg Am. 1981;63A:863–872.
16. Surin V, Blader S, Markhede G, et al. Rotational osteotomy of the humerus for posterior instability of the shoulder. J Bone Joint Surg Am. 1990;72A:181–186.
17. Burkhead WZ Jr, Rockwood CA Jr. Treatment of instability of the shoulder with an exercise program. J Bone Joint Surg Am. 1992;74A:890–896.
18. Hurley JA, Anderson TE, Dear W, et al. Posterior shoulder instability: surgical versus conservative results with evaluation of glenoid version. Am J Sports Med. 1992;20:396–400.
19. Hindenach JCR. Recurrent posterior dislocation of the shoulder. J Bone Joint Surg Am. 1947;29A:582.
20. Neer CS II, Foster CR. Inferior capsular shift for involuntary inferior and multidirectional instability of the shoulder. J Bone Joint Surg Am. 1980;62A:897.
21. Bigliani LU, Endrizzi DP, McIlveon SJ. Operative management of posterior shoulder instability. Orthop Trans. 1989;13:232.
22. Bigliani LU, Pollock RG, Endrizzi DP, et al. Surgical repair of posterior instability of the shoulder: long term results. Paper presented at: Ninth Combined Meeting of the Orthopaedic Associations of the English-Speaking World; June 1992; Toronto.
23. Severin E. Anterior and posterior recurrent dislocation of the shoulder: the Putti-Platt operation. Acta Orthop Scand. 1953;23:14.
24. Tibone JE, Prietto C, Jobe FW, et al. Staple capsulorrhaphy for recurrent posterior shoulder dislocation. Am J Sports Med. 1981;4:135.
25. Scott DJ Jr. Treatment of recurrent posterior dislocations of the shoulder by glenoplasty. J Bone Joint Surg. 1967;49A:471.
26. Chaudhuri GK, Sengupta A, Saha AK. Rotation osteotomy of the shaft of the humerus for recurrent dislocation of the shoulder: anterior and posterior. Acta Orthop Scand. 1974;45:193.
27. McLaughlin HL. Follow-up notes on article previously published in the journal posterior dislocation of the shoulder. J Bone Joint Surg Am. 1962, 44A:1477.
28. Jones V. Recurrent posterior dislocation of the shoulder: report of a case treated by posterior bone block. J Bone Joint Surg Br. 1958;40B:203.
29. Wolf EM. Arthroscopic shoulder stabilization using suture anchors: technique and results. Paper presented at: AANA Annual Meeting, April 1996; Washington D.C.

30. Antoniou J, Duckworth DT, Harryman DT II. Capsulolabral augmentation for the management of posteroinferior instability of the shoulder. J Bone Joint Surg Am. 2000;82(9):1220.

31. Wolf EM, Eakin CL. Arthroscopic capsular plication for posterior shoulder instability. Arthroscopy. 1998;14:153–163.

32. Williams RJ III, Strickland S, Cohen M, et al. Arthroscopic repair for traumatic posterior shoulder instability. Am J Sports Med. 2003:31(2):203.

33. Hayashi K, Thabit G III, Massa KL, et al. The effect of thermal heating on the length and histologic properties of the glenohumeral joint capsule. Am J Sports Med. 1997;25:107–112.

34. Lopez MJ, Hayashi K, Fanton GS, et al. The effect of radiofrequency energy on the ultrastructure of joint capsular collagen. Arthroscopy. 1998;14:495–501.

35. Naseef GS III, Foster TE, Trauner K, et al. The thermal properties of bovine joint capsule: the basic science of laser- and radiofrequency-induced capsular shrinkage. Am J Sports Med. 1997;25: 670–674.

36. Thabit G III. The arthroscopically assisted holmium YAG laser surgery in the shoulder. Op Tech Sports Med. 1998;6:131–138.

37. Khan AM, Fanton GS. Arthroscopic capsulorrhaphy for recurrent instability in the athlete. Sports Med Arthrosc Rev. 2000;8:239–250.

38. Levitz CL, Dugas J, Andrews JR. The use of arthroscopic thermal capsulorrhaphy to treat internal impingement in baseball players. Arthroscopy. 2001;17(6):573–577.

39. D'Alessandro DF, Bradley JP, Fleischli JE, et al. Prospective evaluation of thermal capsulorrhaphy for shoulder instability. Am J Sports Med. 2004;32:21–33.

40. Miniaci A, McBirnie J. Thermal capsular shrinkage for treatment of multidirectional instability of the shoulder. J Bone Joint Surg Am. 2003;85:2283–2287.

41. Noonan TJ, Tokish JM, Briggs KK, et al. Laser-assisted thermal capsulorrhaphy. Arthroscopy. 2003;19(8):815–819.

42. Beighton P, Solomon L, Soskolne CL. Articular mobility in an African population. Ann Rheum Dis. 1973;32:413–418.

43. Eakin CL, Dvirnak P, Miller CM, et al. The relationship of the axillary nerve to arthroscopically placed capsulolabral sutures. Am J Sports Med 1998;26:505–509.

44. Davidson PA, Rivenburgh DW. The 7-o'clock posteroinferior portal for shoulder arthroscopy. Am J Sports Med. 2002;30: 693–696.

45. Harryman DT, Sidles JA, Harris SL, et al. The role of the rotator interval capsule in passive motion and stability of the shoulder. J Bone Joint Surg Am. 1992;74:53–66.

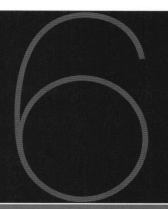

INTERNAL IMPINGEMENT OF THE GLENOHUMERAL JOINT

■ CHRISTOPHER M. JOBE, MD

SURGERY IS THE TREATMENT OF THE ACUTE, FOCAL AND TRAUMATIC.
—*Francis D. Moore, MD[1]*

The orthopedic surgeon might add "the dynamic" to Moore's definition of surgery. In orthopedics, as in other fields of surgery, mechanical problems are frequently related to an anatomic structure or a structural abnormality, but in the shoulder, mechanical problems are frequently related to a dynamic event. The shoulder patient often has an exaggeration of an event in the shoulder that is normal. These exaggerations are in magnitude or in frequency of a normal activity, necessitating different terms in discussing the normal and abnormal. For example, the normal shoulder has a certain amount of laxity, while an abnormal and symptomatic laxity is termed instability. In the subacromial space we see contact between the rotator cuff and the undersurface of the coracoacromial arch, termed "buffering" by Flatow and Soslowsky.[2] In the pathologic or symptomatic setting, this is called subacromial (or external) impingement. In like fashion, internal impingement of the glenohumeral joint is an exaggeration of a normally occurring event that becomes abnormal or symptomatic when it is performed with increased force or increased frequency.[3]

In medical texts we usually begin with a description of the pathogenesis of diseases and proceed to their clinical picture. Because there are rival pathomechanical explanations, we should begin with the known portion of the clinical picture and then proceed to the possible pathomechanics and a more detailed clinical description.

The groups of patients with similar pathology described in the literature thus far include: overhead-throwing athletes, nonathletes with interior impingement on a repetitive or traumatic basis or anterior-internal impingement, and athletes with loss of internal rotation.

The most studied patient is the overhead-throwing athlete.[4-8] The patient best known to the sports medicine physician and trainer is the thrower. The most frequent presenting complaint is a posterior pain in the shoulder at the initiation of the acceleration phase of throwing **(Fig. 6-1)**. The most common physical finding is a positive relocation test with 90 degrees abduction and maximum external rotation and horizontal abduction producing the pain. In the second phase of the relocation test posterior pressure on the humerus relieves the pain **(Figs. 6-2A,B and 6-3A,B)**.

The majority of overhead-throwing athletes can be treated by removing them from throwing for a period of time during which there would be strengthening of the muscles, total conditioning of the body, and finally correction of kinematic rhythm. Most importantly, because of the high energies involved, correction of the body mechanics or "style" **(Fig. 6-4)** is needed. A minority of throwers will develop recurrent symptoms on return to throwing and will be found to have a surgical (i.e., structural) lesion **(Table 6-1)**.

Further study by professional trainers has shown that there is a prodromal phase before the thrower becomes truly symptomatic. During that phase the athlete complains of some stiffness and slowness to warmup. By resting and correcting mechanics in this earlier phase, the time away from play can be cut in half.

Any pathomechanical explanation would therefore include: features of the athletes or other patients' anatomy and function, a dynamic event that can be aggravated by factors local or remote to the shoulder, correction by training, and later a surgical lesion or lesions beyond the reach of physical therapy.

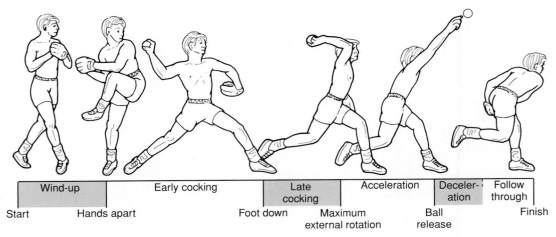

Fig. 6-1. Phases of the baseball pitch.

■ PATHOMECHANICS OF THE OVERHEAD ATHLETE

The rival explanations for this condition involve one of two common features of overhead sports: the first is the extreme angulation of the joint achieved at the initiation of acceleration and the second is the tendency for overhead athletes to develop a tight posterior capsule.

Superimposed on one or both of these mechanisms is the transfer of enormous energy in overhead activities. Most of these activities consist of a controlled fall. The thrower or racquet player falls toward a target, turning his body into a large body rotating over his ipsilateral foot. He stops the fall with the contralateral foot and guides the retained kinetic energy into his torso. In like fashion the energy is guided into smaller and therefore more rapidly moving segments of the body. The large transfer we are discussing here occurs at the initiation of acceleration (Fig. 6-1). After releasing the ball or striking it with a racquet the athlete must dissipate the energy retained within his or her body in order to prevent injury. This is most safely done by a follow-through motion that converts the athlete back to a large forward moving object, this time rotating over the contralateral foot.

As he or she is now a large object moving more slowly, there is more time in which to dissipate the retained energy with the large muscles of the pelvis and lower limbs.

■ PATHOMECHANICS OF INTERNAL IMPINGEMENT

There are several limitations on the normal range of motion of the glenohumeral joint. The bony dimensions of the glenoid limit the spinning motion of the humeral head. It is one of the unfortunate but mathematical ironies of geometry that small decreases in the bony limits on humeral motion result in large decreases in the bony stability of the joint calculated as area of coverage is a geometric function.

The capsule also limits motion of the humeral head in rotation. For most positions of the shoulder the capsule is lax and only becomes taut in end-range positions. For instance, in the abduction-external rotation (ABER) position the anterior-inferior capsule tightens toward the end of the range, resulting in a slight posterior translation of the humeral head. For most positions of the glenohumeral joint, alignment and stability are provided by muscle, mainly the

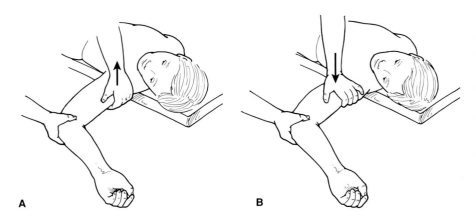

A   **B**

Fig. 6-2. Relocation test: The patient is supine with the arm off the table at 90 degrees abduction and maximum external rotation. **A:** The examiner grasps the humeral head posteriorly and pushes anteriorly. Sometimes the examiner feels sliding (subluxation) of the humeral head, and this sliding typically elicits pain located at the posterior joint line. **B:** The examiner grasps the humeral head anteriorly and pushes posteriorly to relocate the head and lift the rotator cuff off the posterior labrum. If the patient feels pain in the first half of the test (A), it is usually relieved in the second half of the test.

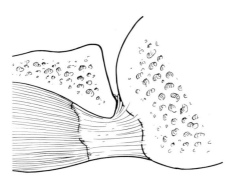

Fig. 6-3. Impingement of the rotator cuff on the posterosuperior glenoid labrum during humeral abduction and maximum external rotation. Cross-section from a cadaver.

rotator cuff. The rotator cuff in a dynamic fashion functions to protect the capsule from stretch in the end-range positions.

The superior part of the glenohumeral joint is where the glenohumeral structures can make contact in elevation. The two positions where this contact may occur are ABER and forward flexion-internal rotation. In the ABER position the greater tuberosity approaches the posterior-superior glenoid. The structures between these two bones, the labrum and the internal fibers of the rotator cuff, are compressed between these two bones.[9,10] An additional structure at risk is the anterior-inferior capsule that is stretched in this position (Table 6-1). Full forward flexion produces a similar compression of the superior labrum.[11]

In the forward flexion-internal rotation position it is the lesser tuberosity that approaches the anterior-superior glenoid. The fibers of the rotator cuff, in this case the subscapularis tendon, are pushed against the anterior-superior labrum **(Table 6-2)**.[12–15] The superior glenohumeral ligament and the biceps pulley can be damaged as well. The contact is against subscapularis below 90 degrees of elevation, and against the biceps tendon and pulley above 90 degrees.

It has been shown in arthroscopy that the vast majority of patients without symptoms in these areas achieve these internal contacts easily. The presence of damage to structures at risk and the accompanying symptoms point to these contacts being made with an increased load or increased frequency.

The structures at risk in the ABER position are the internal fibers of the rotator cuff and the opposing labrum.[8] The adjacent bones are less frequently injured. Supraspinatus and infraspinatus are vulnerable in the ABER position and the subscapularis in the forward flexion-internal rotation position. The area of labrum that makes contact with these portions of the rotator cuff is also at risk for developing a superior labral anterior to posterior (SLAP) lesion.[4] The underlying bone, either tuberosity or glenoid, is less frequently injured but also affected or thickened.[16–18] Finally, stretching of the capsule with resulting subluxation of the shoulder can occur. The combined injury may include one or more of the above-mentioned five structures **(Fig. 6-5)**.

■ PATIENT AT RISK

Although this injury can occur in an acute fashion, it is most often seen as a result of a repetitive motion and is therefore more common in the athlete. Mechanical predisposition to this occurs from several possible sources: (a) weak cuff, (b) a malpositioned scapula, (c) weak trunk and thigh muscles, (d) errors of technique and kinematics, and (e) repetitive positioning **(Table 6-3)**.

Weak rotator cuff muscles can result in angular forces at the shoulder that are unopposed by a protective rotator cuff. This would occur in the position of initiation of the acceleration phase. A professional level thrower at this point has precariously balanced his humeral head on his glenoid and at the initiation of acceleration exerts a very strong contraction of his subscapularis. This serves the double purpose of accelerating the arm and protecting the anterior capsule. A thrower who is poorly conditioned would be at increased risk at late stages of a game because of subscapularis fatigue.

The scapula can be pathologically rotated forward in the sagittal and transverse planes by tight protractors or weakness in retractors and upward rotators. This position of relative protraction leads to increased angulation of the glenohumeral joint at the initiation of acceleration.

Weak trunk muscles can affect a thrower's position, resulting in the need for the shoulder to make similar compensatory adjustments. The kinematics of the shoulder during

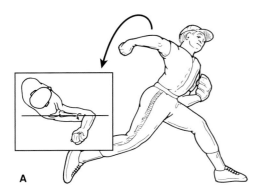

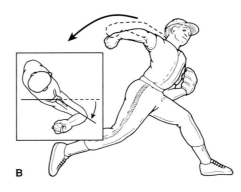

Fig. 6-4. Pitching mechanics. **A:** Normal pitching mechanics from a side view and an overhead view. **B:** Pathologic pitching mechanics from a side view and an overhead view.

TABLE 6-1	Posterior Glenoid Impingement	
	Early	**Later**
Structure	**Reversible lesion**	**Structural lesion**
Rotator cuff	Fraying or irritation	Partial or full thickness tear
Labrum	Irritation Fraying	SLAP
Glenoid	Sclerosis Hypertrophy	Fatigue fracture Osteophyte
Greater tuberosity	Cyst Sclerosis	Fracture
Anterior capsule	Traction	Instability

this very important transition time are thrown off. This scapulohumeral malposition may also result from weak muscles of the lower limb, for example, weakness of the ipsilateral quadriceps.

Finally, for the athlete, there are errors in technique. An example of this is what is called by pitching coaches "opening up too soon." This can result from an error in contralateral foot placement at the end of the early phase of cocking. If the contralateral lower limb is too far externally rotated, this will rotate the pelvis toward the target too early. Then the torso will rotate forward too early, leaving the arm trailing behind. The anterior muscles of the shoulder have to pull the arm forward, leading to both earlier muscle fatigue and increased angulation in the joint with resultant repetitive contact in the posterior-superior rotator cuff and posterior labrum. Eventually there may be stretching of the anterior-inferior capsule.

Some occupations can cause chronic ABER positioning of the shoulder. An example would be someone who drives a forklift **(Fig. 6-6)**. Although the steering mechanism of a forklift resembles that of an automobile, the technique with which it is driven does not. Because the loads in front obscure his view, the driver spends most of his day driving backward. This leaves the shoulder of the hand on the wheel in the ABER position. The glenohumeral angulation becomes greater as the scapular positioner's fatigue.

TABLE 6-2	Anterior Glenoid Impingement	
Structure	**Reversible**	**Structural**
Subscapularis tendon	Fraying	Tear
Anterior superior labrum	Fraying	SLAP
SGHL, CHL	Fraying	Biceps subluxation
Biceps pulley		Anterior superior GH subluxation

SGHL, superior glenohumeral ligament; CHL, coracohumeral ligament;
GH, glenohumeral.

■ ALTERNATIVE PATHOMECHANICS IN THE TIGHT POSTERIOR CAPSULE

An alternative etiologic theory for this combination of SLAP lesions with partial rotator cuff tears has been proposed but has some clinical features with the internal impingement theory.[19] It has been noted that there is a very high incidence of tight posterior capsule in throwing and other overhead athletes.[6,7,20] A tight posterior capsule has been shown to produce an upward force on the humeral head in the initiation of the acceleration phase of throwing.[20] In addition, at that same instant, the tight posterior capsule is producing a downward shear force on the labrum.[18] As with glenoid impingement, this is a load on the posterior-superior labrum for which it was not designed. This results in the development of a "peel-back mechanism" that leads to a SLAP lesion. A SLAP lesion may affect ligament insertions especially in the superior and middle glenohumeral ligaments and lead to an additional secondary instability. It has been noted that correction of a SLAP lesion alone in these patients often corrects the patient's problem. As with glenoid impingement there are reversible

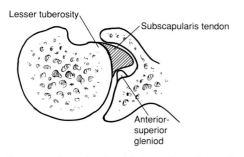

Fig. 6-5. Cross-section of a shoulder specimen frozen in forward flexion and internal rotation as would occur in the active compression test. The lesser tuberosity is brought against the anterior-superior glenoid. The anterior-superior labrum and the upper fibers of the subscapularis are compressed between the two bones.

TABLE 6-3	Causes of Internal Impingement

1. Weak rotator cuff resulting in early fatigue and reliance upon boney and ligamentous restraints on glenohumeral motion
2. Weak scapular rotators and lack of scapular mobility resulting in the need for more extreme glenohumeral positions
3. Weak torso and lower limb muscles resulting in disruption of the smooth flow of kinetic energy and scapular malposition
4. Errors in technique (sports)
5. Repetitive positioning (i.e., ABER) on the job

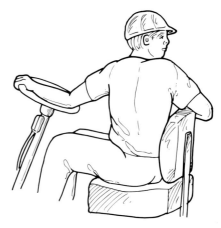

Fig. 6-6. To drive safely, forklift drivers must drive in reverse, putting at least one shoulder into the abducted externally rotated position. Fatigue of the upward rotators of the scapula would cause the driver to rest the glenohumeral joint in the impinged position. Some drivers place the opposite arm, the right arm in this illustration, into abduction-external rotation. They do this so they can use the right hand on the frame to assist with rotating the torso. This second position would place both shoulders at risk.

aspects to this mechanism. In many athletes, the posterior capsule can be stretched. Even after SLAP repair, rehabilitation emphasizes reconditioning of the entire body and restoration of proper mechanics.

■ CLINICAL SIGNS AND SYMPTOMS

Internal impingement in overhead athletes has been divided into three clinical phases by the physicians and trainers who most often treat the patients **(Table 6-4)**. In the first stage the patient complains of stiffness and slowness to warmup. There is no actual pain in this prodromal phase, so there is a negative relocation test. During this phase a knowledgeable trainer will diagnose the athlete, take him or her off of their athletic event for 2 weeks, strengthen the rotator cuff and the scapular rotators and any other affected muscles of the limb, torso, and legs, and correct any kinematic problems. The athlete is then returned to the coach for style correction and then to the lineup.

Stage II is the first phase in which there is actually pain. The pain is usually posterior in the shoulder, early in the acceleration phase. On physical examination, the patient has a positive relocation test, which is a re-creation of the glenohumeral position at the initiation of acceleration. The pain is thought to be created by the posterior superior-internal impingement of the shoulder, and the pain relief sign is

assumed to be produced by the decrease in angulation and decreased contact of the posterior shoulder. Because of the pain, the athlete is felt to be more severely affected than in stage I and is pulled from the lineup for a 1-month period during which time corrections in flexibility and muscle strength are made by the trainer. Corrections in kinematics are instituted, and then corrections in performance style are made.[21]

Stage III looks clinically very similar to stage II except the patient now has the additional clinical finding of failing to respond to a careful rehabilitation program as outlined above. Failure to respond to rehabilitation is felt to indicate one or more structural lesions that can require surgery.[22] Further studies are done in these athletes such as magnetic resonance (MR) arthrogram to elucidate the problems. In addition, arthroscopy could be undertaken to look for subluxation as

TABLE 6-4	Posterior Internal Impingement	
Stage	**Description**	**Treatment**
I	Sensation of stiffness Slowness to warmup	Brief withdrawal from lineup Strengthening Correct kinematics Correct style
II	Posterior pain at initiation of acceleration Positive relocation at 90 degrees	Longer respite from throwing Similar conditioning as for stage I
III	Clinically the same as stage II Failure of nonoperative treatment Findings pointing to one or more surgical lesions	Workup for surgical lesions Arthroscopy Surgical correction (see appropriate chapter)

TABLE 6-5	Workup of the Patient

HISTORY:
  Location of the pain
  Timing
  Associated factors
PHYSICAL EXAM:
  Range of motion (internal rotation deficit)
  Illiciting maneuvers
  Impingement: Relocation test, Neer and Hawkins
  SLAP: Active compression test
  Relocation at 120 degrees abduction
  Speed test
  Subluxation
  Scapula position and flexibility
  Scapulohumeral kinematics
  Torso strength and flexibility
  Lower limb and pelvic strength
ASSESSMENT OF ACTIVITY PERFORMANCE:
  Imaging:
    X-ray: boney sclerosis, and unusual structure
    MR arthrogram: SLAP and nondisplaced fracture, partial
      cuff tear, cysts
    Diagnostic arthroscopy

well as to treat any SLAP lesions or partial rotator cuff tears. Following surgical correction the patient is put through a rehabilitation program appropriate for whatever surgery he or she has had. In addition the rehabilitation program aims to correct whatever mechanical predisposition the athlete had to glenoid impingement.

■ WORKUP OF THE PATIENT

The workup of the patient is a summary of what this chapter has covered **(Table 6-5)**. The patient's complaints indicate a glenohumeral problem and the workup begins there. The exam looks for dynamic problems by applying the relocation test and by looking for an internal rotation deficiency. We look for structural problems such as: SLAP, partial cuff tears, sclerosis along the glenoid, tuberosity damage, and instability.

We then move back down the kinetic chain looking for etiologic factors. Malpositioning of the scapula, the base of the glenohumeral joint, can be seen at rest or kinematically. Weakness or decreased range of the torso can affect the base that positions the scapula. Weakness or poor positioning of the lower limb can affect the position of the torso. Some of the analysis may require the help of an expert coach or trainer who can spot foot malposition that might cause the shoulder injury.

■ TREATMENT

The treatment of the specific structural lesions is covered in other chapters in this text. There is, however, an additional

caveat to be gained from the unifying concepts of internal impingement and internal rotation deficiency. That concept is what appears to be instability and may be a result of one of the other lesions. This is understandable, as these lesions, especially the SLAP, affect capsular attachments. Among the glenohumeral internal rotation deficit (GIRD) patients, Morgan and Burkhart found that repairing the SLAP often corrected the instability.[7] Among the anterior-internal impingement patients, correction of labrum or pulley damage had a similar effect on correcting the anterior-superior subluxation occurring in that group of patients. To summarize, it seems best to correct the other lesions first before deciding that the shoulder has a separate instability problem.

■ AREAS FOR FUTURE RESEARCH

The controversy between internal impingement and GIRD as explanations and the addition of anterior-internal impingement points out that we are just starting to understand this group of injuries. Certainly, these three mechanisms do not rule out the addition of as yet undescribed mechanisms. This will remain an area of future research.

In addition, more work needs to be done on the groups of patients already mentioned. The overhead athlete is the best studied for both posterior-internal impingement and GIRD. Industrial exposure has only been mentioned and is as yet unstudied. Anterior-internal impingement has been studied a little more in terms of mechanism, but is essentially an open field for exploration.

And finally, it has yet to be determined how much these pathways contribute to a final common pathway of larger rotator cuff tears.

■ REFERENCES

1. Sabiston DC, ed. *Davis-Christopher Textbook of Surgery: The Biological Basis of Modern Surgical Practice.* 10th ed. Philadelphia: WB Saunders; 1972:19.
2. Flatow EL, Soslowsky LJ. Excursion of the rotator cuff under the acromion: patterns of subacromial contact. Am J Sports Med. 1994;22:779–788.
3. McFarland EG, Hsu CY, Neira C, et al. Internal impingement of the shoulder: a clinical and arthroscopic analysis. J Shoulder Elbow Surg. 1999;8:458–460.
4. Jazrawi LM, McCluskey GM III, Andrews JR. Superior labral anterior and posterior lesions and internal impingement in the overhead athlete. Instr Course Lect. 2003;52:43–63.
5. Halbrecht JL, Tirman P, Atkin D. Internal impingement of the shoulder: comparison of findings between the throwing and non-throwing shoulders of college baseball players. Arthroscopy. 1999; 15:253–258.
6. Burkhart SS, Morgan CD. The disabled throwing shoulder: spectrum of pathology Part I: pathoanatomy and biomechanics. Arthroscopy. 2003;19:404–420.
7. Burkhart SS, Morgan CD. The disabled throwing shoulder: spectrum of pathology Part II: evaluation and treatment of SLAP lesions in throwers. Arthroscopy. 2003;19:531–539.

8. Paley KJ, Jobe FW, Pink MM, et al. Arthroscopic findings in the overhand throwing athlete: evidence for posterior internal impingement of the rotator cuff. Arthroscopy. 2000;16:35–40.

9. Jobe CM. Posterior superior glenoid impingement: expanded spectrum. Arthroscopy. 1995;11:530–536.

10. Walch G, Liotard JP, Boileau P, et al. Postero-superior glenoid impingement: another shoulder impingement. Rev Chir Orthop Reparatrice Appar Mot. 1991;77:571–574.

11. Kim TK, McFarland EG. Internal impingement of the shoulder in flexion. Clin Orthop Relat Res. 2004;421:112–119.

12. Gerber C, Sebesta A. Impingement of the deep surface of the subscapularis tendon and the reflection pulley on the anterosuperior glenoid rim: a preliminary report. J Shoulder Elbow Surg. 2000;9:483–490.

13. Habermeyer P, Magosch P, Pritsch M, et al. Anterosuperior impingement of the shoulder as a result of pulley lesions: a prospective arthroscopic study. J Shoulder Elbow Surg. 2004;13:5–12.

14. Parentis MA, Jobe CM, Pink MM, et al. An anatomic evaluation of the active compression test. J Shoulder Elbow Surg. 2004;13:410–416.

15. Struhl S. Anterior internal impingement: an arthroscopic observation. Arthroscopy. 2002;18:2–7.

16. Edelson G, Teitz C. Internal impingement in the shoulder. J Shoulder Elbow Surg. 2000;9:308–315.

17. Meister K, Buckley B, Batts J, et al. The posterior impingement sign: diagnosis of rotator cuff and posterior labral tears secondary to internal impingement in overhand athletes. Am J Orthop. 2004;33:412–415.

18. Pearce CE, Burkhart SS. The pitcher's mound: a late sequela of posterior type II SLAP lesions. Arthroscopy. 2000;16:214–216.

19. Morgan CD, Burkhart SS, Palmeri M, et al. Type II SLAP lesions: three subtypes and their relationships to superior instability and rotator cuff tears. Arthroscopy. 1998;14:553–565.

20. Tyler TF, Nicholas SJ, Roy T, et al. Quantification of posterior capsule tightness and motion loss in patients with shoulder impingement. Am J Sports Med. 2000;28:668–673.

21. McClure PW, Bialker J, Neff N, et al. Shoulder function and 3-dimensional kinematics in people with shoulder impingement syndrome before and after a 6-week exercise program. Phys Ther. 2004;84:832–848.

22. Kaplan LD, McMahon PJ. Internal impingement: findings on magnetic resonance imaging and arthroscopic evaluation. Arthroscopy. 2004;20:701–704.

Part

B

ROTATOR CUFF

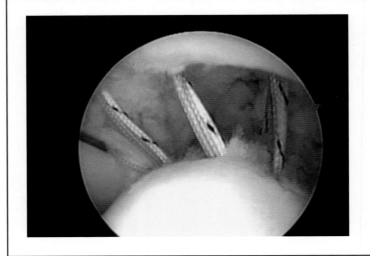

7

ARTHROSCOPIC SUBACROMIAL DECOMPRESSION, DISTAL CLAVICLE RESECTION, AND CORACOPLASTY

STEVEN B. SINGLETON, MD, JAMES M. BOTHWELL, MD, JOHN E. CONWAY, MD

■ ARTHROSCOPIC SUBACROMIAL DECOMPRESSION

History of the Technique

Subacromial decompression as a treatment for impingement syndrome was first described by Neer in 1972.[1–4] The goal of the procedure was to reduce extrinsic compression on the rotator cuff musculature by increasing the volume of the subacromial space. The original description entailed the open exposure of the anterior acromion and subacromial space to resect the coracoacromial ligament, the anterior lip of the acromion, and the subacromial bursa. Over the past 30 years, multiple investigators have noted satisfactory results with this procedure when performed in the proper setting.[3–5]

The advent of shoulder arthroscopy has furthered the evolution of the subacromial decompression. Neer's description of the open technique has been the gold standard by which arthroscopic techniques have been measured. Many, including Ellman,[6] have proposed various techniques for arthroscopic subacromial decompression that differ slightly in their means, but have the very same end point: that is, to increase the volume of the subacromial space. The main advantage of arthroscopic subacromial decompression is sparing of the deltoid muscle origin and, therefore, an expedited recovery. In general, most authors report good to excellent results in the majority (73% to 88%) of their patients.[3–10]

Indications and Contraindications

The main indications for arthroscopic subacromial decompression include the following: (a) Symptomatic subacromial impingement refractory to a comprehensive rehabilitation program usually lasting 6 to 12 months, where the impingement is either classical extrinsic or chronic secondary with adaptive changes; (b) when rotator cuff repair is performed.

The contraindications for arthroscopic subacromial decompression include the following: (a) Shoulder stiffness, (b) massive or irreparable rotator cuff tear, (c) inaccurate diagnosis: be aware of instability.

Preoperatively, consider the amount of anterior acromion to be resected. The supraspinatus outlet view enables one to determine the acromial morphology and may prove helpful in determining the appropriate volume of bone removal for adequate acromioplasty. Similarly, postoperative radiographic evaluation utilizing the supraspinatus outlet view to evaluate the decompression may be useful, especially for those learning the arthroscopic technique.

Surgical Technique

Anesthesia and patient positioning are the same for the three procedures described in this chapter. General anesthetic or interscalene regional block is used. Hypotensive anesthesia maintaining systolic blood pressure at or below 95 mm Hg will assist visualization by minimizing intraoperative bleeding. Our preference in performing arthroscopic shoulder procedures is the lateral decubitus position. The arm is suspended with 10 to 12 lb of arm traction in 30 degrees of abduction, and in 20 degrees to 30 degrees of forward flexion. The spine of the scapula, lateral acromion, and anterior and posterior borders of the clavicle are marked on the skin. When indicated, the location and angle of obliquity of the acromioclavicular (AC) joint is also noted on the skin **(Fig. 7-1)**.

Procedure

A 30-degree arthroscope is placed in the standard posterior portal. This portal is located approximately 2 cm inferior

65

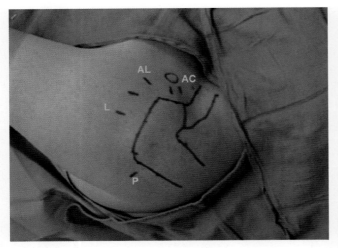

Fig. 7-1. Anterior view of shoulder with portal locations noted. Note location of AC joint portal *(AC)* for distal clavicle excision and of anterolateral portal *(AL)* for coracoplasty. P, posterior portal; L, lateral portal.

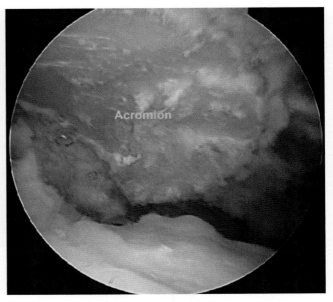

Fig. 7-2. Thirty-degree arthroscope location: Posterior portal. Undersurface of acromion during arthroscopic acromioplasty.

and 1.5 cm medial to the posterior angle of the acromion in the "soft spot." An anterior portal is established approximately 1 cm anterior to the anterior edge of the acromion. If this procedure is done in conjunction with an arthroscopic distal clavicle excision, an AC joint portal, as described below, can be utilized. A thorough diagnostic examination of the glenohumeral joint is performed. Any indicated intraarticular procedures may be accomplished. In the same posterior portal, the arthroscope is removed from the glenohumeral joint and reintroduced into the subacromial space. The anterior cannula is redirected into the subacromial space and is utilized primarily as an inflow portal. A midlateral portal (working portal) is established approximately 4.0 cm lateral to the midportion of the lateral acromion, in line with the posterior border of the clavicle. A complete bursectomy of the subacromial space is performed using an arthroscopic shaver. Cautery or a radiofrequency device is used for hemostasis. This is an essential step because visualization of the complete undersurface of the acromion is necessary for this procedure. After completion of the subacromial bursectomy, the cautery or radiofrequency device is used to outline the anterior and lateral aspects of the acromion. The coracoacromial ligament is detached in its entirety from the anterior aspect of the acromion. Care should be taken to coagulate the acromial branch of the thoracoacromial artery because this can be a significant source of bleeding as the ligament is detached. The ligament should be further resected until the anterior deltoid fascia is visualized. The undersurface of the acromion should be visualized in its entirety from its posterior border to its anterior border such that its morphology is visualized and confirmed based on preoperative radiographs **(Fig. 7-2).** An arthroscopic burr is inserted via the midlateral working portal and used to remove the appropriate amount of anterior acromion to produce a flat undersurface from its

lateral to medial borders. Caution should be exercised to not violate the capsule of the acromioclavicular joint or to excessively detach the deltoid fascia from the acromion. The anterior border of the acromion should be resected to be coplanar with the anterior edge of the clavicle (usually a resection of 5 to 8 mm from the anterior border). It is essential for adequate decompression that the resection of the acromion be flat from its lateral to medial borders, including the acromioclavicular joint **(Fig. 7-3A)**. An arthroscopic rasp may be utilized to smooth the resection of the undersurface of the acromion. Final evaluation and visualization of the acromion after resection is performed by tilting the angle of the lens parallel to acromion (medial or lateral) (Fig. 7-3B). Also, one may visualize the undersurface of the acromion from the midlateral portal and place a switching stick from the posterior border to the anterior border of the acromion to confirm that the decompression is adequate. A last option is to use digital palpation to evaluate the acromial undersurface. Portals are reapproximated and dressings applied. The patient's extremity is placed in an immobilizer for comfort; however, passive motion is begun immediately and full range of motion is the short-term immediate goal, followed by strengthening once full range of motion is encountered.

Pitfalls of the Technique

There are several potential complications to be aware of and to avoid. It is important to choose a burr for the resection that is able to smoothly resect the appropriate amount of bone from the undersurface without being too aggressive. Our personal choice is a 12-fluted barrel burr that is able to

Approximately 2 mm of the medial acromial facet may also be debrided. As the joint space opens, a larger 4-mm burr may be inserted. This will hasten the bony debridement; however, it may also obscure visualization by leading to bleeding or fluid control problems. The arthroscope is then switched to the posterior superior portal to allow burr access to the more anterior portions of the distal clavicle and the acromion. This portion of the bony debridement is addressed in a similar fashion as that which began in the posterior portion of the joint. Care is taken to ensure that an adequate bony debridement of the most posterior and anterior portions of the joint is performed. The remaining AC interval should measure approximately 10 to 12 mm. Appropriately done, the inferior AC joint capsule/ligaments are not disrupted. The AC interval is thoroughly irrigated with saline; then, closure is performed with simple nylon sutures or a simple absorbable subcuticular stitch of the surgeon's choice. Sterile dressings are placed. The postoperative care and rehabilitation will proceed in a fashion identical to that of the arthroscopy indirect approach.

Rehabilitation

As noted previously, rehabilitation begins immediately with passive and active assisted range of motion. Active range of motion begins by postop day 7 to 10. We place an emphasis on regaining full active range of motion prior to instituting any strengthening activity. The rehabilitation program should focus on scapula stabilization and control of the trunk. As the patient progresses, return to full activity and sports may occur as early as 6 weeks. However, in a throwing athlete, a more reasonable time frame for return may be as long as 3 to 4 months. Keep in mind that when resection of the distal clavicle is performed in conjunction with a subacromial decompression or other intra-articular procedure, the latter may provide constraints to the rehabilitation program, and the patient's return to sports will be slower.

■ SUBCORACOID IMPINGEMENT

History of the Technique

Subcoracoid, or coracoid, impingement is an increasingly recognized cause of persistent anterior shoulder pain. Subcoracoid impingement is defined as the mechanical contact between the coracoid and the lesser tuberosity of the humerus.[23] Patients note pain and tenderness in the anterior shoulder that is exacerbated with increasing degrees of flexion, adduction, and internal rotation. The origin of the pain presumably occurs because of impingement of the subscapularis tendon between the coracoid process and the lesser tuberosity.

Several investigators have noted that many factors may decrease the coracohumeral space, thus leading to subcoracoid stenosis and possibly impingement.[24-26] A strong association has been noted recently between subcoracoid stenosis and anterior superior rotator cuff tears.[27-30] Controversy exists as to whether this coracohumeral narrowing leads to the development of these rotator cuff tears, or if the subcoracoid impingement develops secondary to the anterosuperior translation of the humeral head that may be present in patients with large rotator cuff tears. Further, it is postulated that contracture of the posterior glenohumeral joint capsule may play a role in the development of subcoracoid impingement.

The coracohumeral space in asymptomatic shoulders has been reported to be between 8.7 and 11 mm. Gerber et al.,[24] Dines et al.,[25] Karnaugh et al.,[26] Dumontier et al.,[27] and Burkhart et al.[28-30] have demonstrated different means by which to assess the subcoracoid space using preoperative imaging and intraoperative observation. These investigators have also proposed different techniques for surgical decompression of the subcoracoid space for patients with persistent subcoracoid impingement that is unresponsive to nonoperative management. These techniques include osteotomy of the neck of the coracoid process, resection of the tip of the coracoid, or resection of most all of the coracoid process. The technique we now favor, and that currently proposed by Burkhart, is to perform an arthroscopic coracoplasty. In the arthroscopic coracoplasty, the coracohumeral space is increased by resecting the posterolateral aspect of the coracoid in line with the subscapularis tendon.

Indications

The indications for arthroscopic coracoplasty are evolving. At this time, the indications for this procedure include the following: Recalcitrant anterior shoulder pain in patients whose clinical findings, preoperative imaging, and intraoperative examination confirm the presence of subcoracoid stenosis and subcoracoid impingement, isolated subscapularis tendon tears with associated subcoracoid stenosis and subcoracoid impingement, anterior superior rotator cuff tears and rotator interval lesions associated with subcoracoid stenosis and subcoracoid impingement.

It is recognized that both subacromial impingement and subcoracoid impingement may occur in patients with combined subscapularis, supraspinatus, and infraspinatus tendon tears.

Procedure

During arthroscopic coracoplasty, a 70-degree arthroscope may be helpful by providing an "aerial" view of the coracoid and the subscapularis tendon. A standard posterior portal is used typically for visualization of the coracoid. In cases where the rotator interval tissue obstructs visualization and the proper angle of approach, the portion of the rotator interval directly over the coracoid is resected using a radiofrequency and shaver device. Although it may be visualized through the subacromial space, the coracoid is more easily seen and coracoplasty more easily performed through a small window in the rotator interval. The anterolateral portal is used for approaching the coracoid and the sub-scapularis tendon. This portal is located 2 to 3 mm anterior to the biceps and 2 to 4 cm from the anterolateral corner of the acromion. Proper placement of this portal to allow adequate access to the posterolateral coracoid and access to the subscapularis tendon for repair is essential. Localization initially with an 18-gauge spinal needle is helpful **(Fig. 7-10)**. After completing a thorough intra-articular glenohumeral joint examination, a shaver or radiofrequency device is introduced through an anterolateral portal. The coracoid is identifiable by palpating through the rotator interval tissue just above the superior edge of the subscapularis tendon. A window in the rotator interval tissue is created in this location directly adjacent to the coracoid tip. Via the anterolateral portal, all soft tissue is resected from the posterior aspect of the coracoid tip. Care is taken to avoid dissection medial to the coracoid. A 4-mm burr (Stonecutter 7205330, Dyonics, Smith & Nephew, Memphis, Tenn) is then introduced into the anterolateral portal, and the coracoid is resected in line with the subscapularis tendon. The goal is to resect the posterolateral aspect of the coracoid space and prevent impingement of the coracoid against the subscapularis tendon and lesser tuberosity **(Fig. 7-11)**. Manipulating the arm into forward flexion and internal rotation with the traction removed helps assess the adequacy of the coracoplasty. The humerus may be pushed posteriorly by an assistant while burring the posterolateral tip of the coracoid to improve access to this space. The 4-mm burr or an arthroscopic probe with a known tip length may be used as a reference tool to estimate

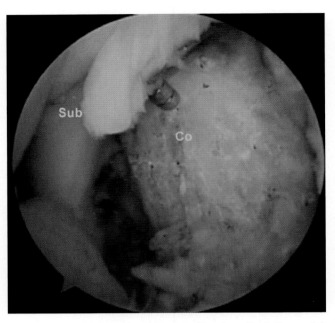

Fig. 7-11. Thirty-degree arthroscope location: Posterior portal. Note impingement of subscapularis tendon onto coracoid tip with the upper extremity moved into a position of forward flexion, adduction, and internal rotation.

the distance between the remaining coracoid and subscapularis tendon. The end point for the resection is to obtain 7 mm of clearance between the remaining coracoid and subscapularis tendon **(Fig. 7-12)**. After subcoracoid decompression, any remaining pathology may be addressed. This may include isolated subscapularis tendon repair, repair of larger

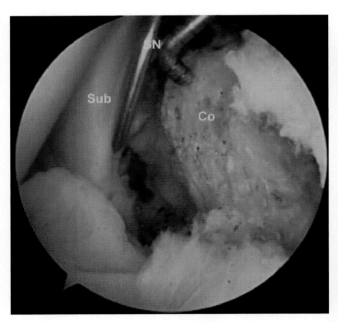

Fig. 7-10. Thirty-degree arthroscope location: Posterior portal. Note coracoid *(Co)* in this view through a window in the rotator interval just superior to the superior border of the subscapularis tendon *(Sub)*. Spinal needle *(SN)* enters the coracohumeral space via the anterolateral portal. The probe touches the posterolateral tip of the coracoid.

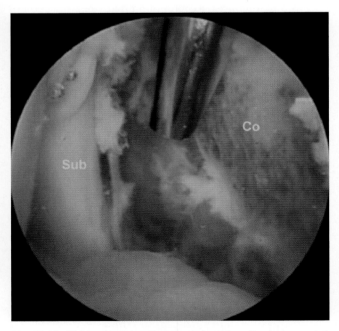

Fig. 7-12. Thirty-degree arthroscope location: Posterior portal. Referencing the coracoplasty *(Co)* after resection of the posterolateral coracoid using a 4-mm burr as a reference tool.

tears that involve portions of the subscapularis, supraspinatus, and infraspinatus tendons, or repair of rotator interval and proximal biceps tendon lesions.

Rehabilitation

Following isolated coracoplasty, patients may begin a program of rehabilitation that is similar to that for patients who have had subacromial decompressions. The arm position of forward flexion, adduction, and internal rotation is avoided for 4 to 6 weeks in the immediate postoperative period. For patients who have other intra-articular pathology addressed, the rehabilitation program should be modified based on any limitations necessitated by the other procedures.

Technical Alternatives/Pitfalls of the Technique

The most important aspect of this procedure is appropriate anterolateral portal placement. This will allow the surgeon access to the coracoid tip and to the leading edge of the subscapularis tendon. Using a spinal needle to assist in placement of this portal is essential. Care must be taken to avoid dissection medial to the coracoid tip to avoid neurologic injury. To that end, only the posterolateral portion of the coracoid need be resected. The goal is to increase the coracohumeral distance. This is done by resecting the posterolateral portion of the tip of the coracoid just anterior to the superior border of the subscapularis tendon.

Visualization of the coracoid through the subacromial space is possible but difficult because of the large amount of fibro-fatty bursal tissue that surrounds the coracoid. The coracoid is much more easily approached intra-articularly through a small window in the rotator interval for three reasons: (a) It avoids the large amount of subacromial bursal tissue surrounding the coracoid, which provides for better visualization, (b) it allows for a direct assessment of the coracohumeral space both before and after coracoplasty, which will help to ensure that the coracoid decompression is adequate, and (3) it facilitates surgeon evaluation of the subscapularis tendon.

■ REFERENCES

1. Neer CS II. Anterior acromioplasty for the chronic impingement syndrome in the shoulder: a preliminary report. J Bone Joint Surg. 1972;54A:41–50.
2. Neer CS II. Impingement lesions. Clin Orthop. 1983;173:70–77.
3. Altchek DW, Carson EW. Arthroscopic acromioplasty: current status. Orthop Clin North Am. April 1997;28(2):157–168.
4. Altchek DW, Carson EW. Arthroscopic acromioplasty: indications and technique. Instr Course Lect. 1998;47:21–28.
5. Spangehl MJ, Hawkins RH, McCormack RG, et al. Arthroscopic versus open acromioplasty: a prospective, randomized, blinded study. J Shoulder Elbow Surg. March–April 2002;11(2):101–107.
6. Ellman H. Arthroscopic subacromial decompression: an analysis of one to three year results. Arthroscopy. 1987;3:173.
7. Esch JC. Arthroscopic subacromial decompression and postoperative management. Orthop Clin North Am. January 1993;24(1):161–171.
8. Hawkins RJ, Plancher KD, Saddemi SR, et al. Arthroscopic subacromial decompression. J Shoulder Elbow Surg. May–June 2001; 10(3):225–230.
9. Stephens SR, Warren RF, Payne LZ, et al. Arthroscopic acromioplasty: a 6- to 10-year follow-up. Arthroscopy. 1998;14(4):382–388.
10. Kolowich PA. Arthroscopic decompression of the shoulder in athletes. Clin Sports Med. October 1996;15(4):701–713.
11. Hunt JL, Moore RJ, Krishnan J. The fate of the coracoacromial ligament in arthroscopic acromioplasty: an anatomical study. J Shoulder Elbow Surg. November–December 2000;9(6):491–494.
12. Levy O, Copeland SA. Regeneration of the coracoacromial ligament after acromioplasty and arthroscopic subacromial decompression. J Shoulder Elbow Surg. July–August 2001;10(4):317–320.
13. Ogilvie-Harris DJ, Wiley AM, Sattarian J. Failed acromioplasty for impingement syndrome. J Bone Joint Surg. 1990;72:1070–1072.
14. Connor PM, Yamaguchi K, Pollock RG, et al. Comparison of arthroscopic and open revision decompression for failed anterior acromioplasty. Orthopedics. June 2000;23(6):549–554.
15. Mumford EB. Acromioclavicular dislocation. J Bone Joint Surg Am. 1941;23:799–802.
16. Gurd FB. The treatment of complete dislocation of the outer end of the clavicle: a hitherto undescribed operation. Ann Surg. 1941;113:1094–1098.
17. Matthews LS, Parks BG, Pavlovich LJ Jr, et al. Arthroscopic versus open distal clavicle resection: a biomechanical analysis on a cadaveric model. Arthroscopy. 1999;15:240–247.
18. Johnson LL. Diagnostic and Surgical Arthroscopy, the Knee and Other Joints. St. Louis: CV Mosby; 1981.
19. Flatow EL, Cordasco FA, Bigliani LU. Arthroscopic resection of the outer end of the clavicle from a superior approach: a critical, quantitative, radiographic assessment of bone removal. Arthroscopy. August 1992;8:55–64.
20. Bigliani LU, Nicholson GP, Flatow EL. Arthroscopic resection of the distal clavicle. Orthop Clin North Am. 1993;24:133–141.
21. Levine WN, Barron OA, Yamaguchi K, et al. Arthroscopic distal clavicle resection from a bursal approach. Arthroscopy. 1998;14:52–56.
22. Eskola A, Santavirta S, Jiljakka HT, et al. The results of operative resection of the lateral end of the clavicle. J Bone Joint Surg Am. 1997;78:584–587.
23. Gerber C, Terrier F, Ganz R. The role of the coracoid process in the chronic impingement syndrome. J Bone Joint Surg Br. 1985; 67:703–708.
24. Gerber C, Terrier F, Zehnder R, et al. The subcoracoid space: an anatomic study. Clin Orthop. 1987;215:132–138.
25. Dines DM, Warren RF, Inglis AE, et al. The coracoid impingement syndrome. J Bone Joint Surg Br. 1990;72:314–316.
26. Karnaugh RD, Sperling JW, Warren RF. Arthroscopic treatment of coracoid impingement. Arthroscopy. 2001;17:784–787.
27. Dumontier C, Sautet A, Gagey O, et al. Rotator interval lesions and their relation to coracoid impingement syndrome. J Shoulder Elbow Surg. 2001;10:37–46.
28. Burkhart SS, Tehrany AM. Arthroscopic subscapularis repair: technique and preliminary result. Arthroscopy. 2002;18:454–463.
29. Lo IK, Burkhart SS. Combined subcoracoid and subacromial impingement in association with anterosuperior rotator cuff tears: an arthroscopic approach. Arthroscopy. December 2003;15(10): 1068–1078.
30. Lo IK, Burkhart SS. Current concepts in rotator cuff repair. J Sports Med. 2003;31(2):308–324.

LATISSIMUS DORSI
TENDON TRANSFER

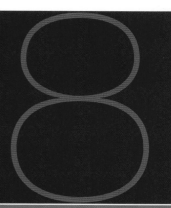

JOHN G. COSTOUROS, MD, CHRISTIAN GERBER, MD,
JON J. P. WARNER, MD

Irreparable tendon tears of the rotator cuff are found in a small proportion of patients with rotator cuff tears as approximately 95% of all tears are reparable by conventional methods at the time of surgery.[1] Although the prevalence of irreparable tendon tears is quite low, they profoundly impact the functional capacity of patients and can be associated with significant levels of pain. Tendon transfer techniques, including the latissimus dorsi tendon transfer, have been developed in order to improve pain and function in selected patients with massive, irreparable rotator cuff tears.

Massive, irreparable tears are defined as tears involving at least two rotator cuff tendons with retraction that is not amenable to mobilization and repair to the anatomical footprint with the arm in less than 60 degrees of abduction.[2] Recent advances have enabled the surgeon to preoperatively determine whether or not a large rotator cuff tear is amenable to primary repair or, if it is technically reparable, whether or not it will be associated with a good functional outcome.[3] This is based on both clinical and radiographic findings that are made prior to surgery.

Posterosuperior rotator cuff tears are the most common type of configuration of massive rotator cuff tendon tears. These involve the supraspinatus, infraspinatus, and, less commonly, the teres minor. The latissimus dorsi transfer offers a reasonable solution to patients with significant pain and dysfunction associated with a massive, irreparable posterosuperior rotator cuff tears.

HISTORY OF THE TECHNIQUE

Latissimus dorsi tendon transfer was first described in 1988 by Christian Gerber for the management of irreparable, massive, posterosuperior rotator cuff tendon tears.[2] The use of the latissimus dorsi has been well described in the treatment of brachial plexus birth palsy, in which patients display a similar functional deficit[4–7] **(Fig. 8-1A,B)**. Active external rotation of the adducted and abducted arm is lost, which severely impairs the ability of the patient to position the arm in space. Thus, the glenohumeral joint must compensate by generating much more flexion and abduction to reach the same height.[2]

In the treatment of brachial plexus birth palsy, variations in technique have shared the same goal of converting the teres major and latissimus dorsi to external rotators of the shoulder.[4–7] Since 1934, when L'Episcopo[5] first described his surgical procedure, this has proven to be an effective form of treatment. For this reason, it was seen that massive rotator cuff tears constituted an analogous problem of the adult that might be amenable to a similar treatment. Latissimus dorsi transfer was conceived as a method to provide containment of the humeral head in the setting of a massive, irreparable rotator cuff tear with the additional benefit of external rotation force. In this way, a fixed fulcrum of rotation would increase the efficiency of the remaining rotator cuff muscles and the deltoid in order to generate improved motion.[2,8,9]

INDICATIONS AND CONTRAINDICATIONS

The indications for tendon transfer have been established based on a number of clinical studies and observations[2,9,10] **(Table 8-1)**. In general, this procedure is indicated in individuals who have refractory pain, weakness, and dysfunction of the shoulder in the setting of an irreparable posterosuperior rotator cuff tear. Good subscapularis and deltoid function as well as minimal evidence of osteoarthritis are prerequisites prior to considering this procedure **(Figs. 8-2A,B,C,D,E,F, 8-3)**.

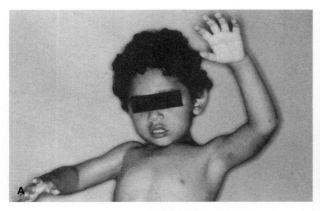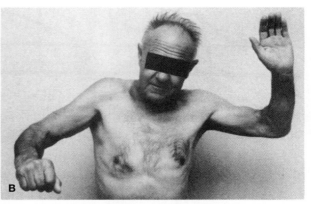

Fig. 8-1. Residual functional deficit is similar in patients with **(A)** brachial plexus birth palsy as well as **(B)** massive posterosuperior rotator cuff tears. In both cases, loss of abduction and external rotation limits the efficiency of arm motion in flexion and abduction. (Reprinted with permission from Gerber C, Vinh TS, Hertel R, et al. Latissimus dorsi transfer for the treatment of massive tears of the rotator cuff: a preliminary report. Clin Orthop Rel Res. 1988;51–61.)

Patients with an irreparable posterosuperior tear will have a lag between passive and active external rotation. In these cases, the patient's arm will fall into internal rotation when the examiner releases it from maximal passive external rotation **(Fig. 8-4A,B)**. When the arm is at the side in adduction, this degree of lag is consistent with an irreparable tear of the infraspinatus **(Fig. 8-5A,B)**. When the patient's arm is abducted and held in maximal passive external rotation position, the patient may be able to actively maintain this position if the teres minor is intact.

The degree of weakness is important in the clinical decision making and in determining whether this tendon transfer is an appropriate method of treatment. If the patient has mild to moderate weakness, then a latissimus transfer can be expected to give sufficient force to elevate the arm against gravity above shoulder level. We determine this by assisting the patient in raising the arm. If the degree of assistance required to raise the arm overhead is minimal, then a latissimus transfer is indicated. If, however, the patient requires a great deal of assistance to raise the arm and when the exam-iner releases the arm the patient cannot maintain it overhead, then a latissimus transfer is not likely to effectively restore the patient's ability to raise the arm overhead. We describe this patient as having a pseudoparalysis **(Fig. 8-6A,B)**.

Contraindications to latissimus dorsi tendon transfer include associated anterosuperior tears that involve the subscapularis, cases of static anterior or posterior subluxation, advanced arthritis, axillary nerve injury, or infection. Of course, all considerations for treatment must be catered to an individual patient's disability and expectations for pain relief and functional recovery. Comorbid conditions including diabetes, cardiovascular disease, pulmonary disease, uncontrolled seizure disorder, or immunosuppression may have a negative impact on the patient's potential for recovery and ability to adhere to a rigorous postoperative rehabilitation regimen.

Weakness of the subscapularis and deltoid are clinically assessed by the lift-off and extension lag signs, respectively[11,12] **(Fig. 8-7A,B,C,D)**. Dynamic anterosuperior subluxation can be elicited by asking the patient to actively abduct the arm and indicates deficiency of the subscapularis **(Fig. 8-8A,B)**. If these clinical signs are present, latissimus dorsi tendon transfer should not be performed.

Radiographic evaluation in all patients consists of a true anteroposterior plain radiograph with the arm in neutral rotation. This enables the assessment of the acromiohumeral distance **(Fig. 8-9A,B)**. An acromiohumeral distance of 5 mm or less is a relative contraindication to performing the latissimus transfer. Cranial migration of the humerus perpetuates subacromial impingement and reduces the efficiency of the deltoid muscle as an abductor. The axillary lateral radiograph allows one to determine the presence of static anterior and posterior subluxation and the stage of glenohumeral arthritis (Fig. 8-9A,B). Further imaging includes either a computed tomography (CT) or magnetic resonance imaging (MRI) with intra-articular contrast. MRI is the currently preferred

TABLE 8-1	Surgical Indications for Latissimus Dorsi Transfer in Posterosuperior Defects

- Chronic supraspinatus/infraspinatus and/or teres minor tear or failed prior repair with retraction that is not amenable to surgical mobilization.
- Isolated supraspinatus/infraspinatus and/or teres minor tear that is mobile but has a high likelihood of failure (fatty degeneration III or IV, acromiohumeral distance <5 mm on true AP).
- No evidence of static anterior or posterior subluxation on the axillary lateral radiograph.
- Fatty degeneration of the supraspinatus or infraspinatus muscles of grade III or IV on MRI or CT scan.

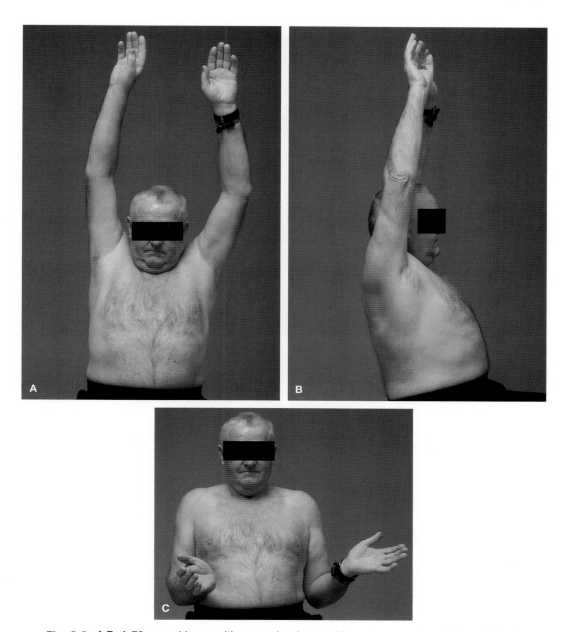

Fig. 8-2. A,B: A 72-year-old man with a massive, irreparable posterosuperior rotator cuff tear is able to maintain good flexion due to maintenance of a good anterior-posterior force couple and a well-functioning deltoid. **C:** However, he displays a significant loss of active external rotation.

method for assessment of tear quality and size, degree of retraction, and degree of fatty degeneration and muscle atrophy[13,14] **(Fig. 8-10A,B)**. Massive tears of Goutallier stage III or greater suggest an irreparable tear with poor-quality tissue likely to be encountered at the time of surgery.[3]

■ SURGICAL TECHNIQUES

Dr. Gerber's Technique in Beach Chair

Surgery is performed under general anesthesia combined with patient-controlled interscalene analgesia (PCIA),

which facilitates early passive mobilization postoperatively. The patient is placed in a beach-chair position in such a manner that sufficient access to the entire scapula and latissimus dorsi muscle belly is possible using a full-length bean bag. A mechanical arm holder is not used during the operation.

The bony landmarks of the shoulder are palpated and outlined, including the acromion, acromioclavicular joint, coracoid process, and clavicle. An anterosuperior approach to the rotator cuff is performed through a 12-cm incision parallel to the Langer lines over the lateral one third of the acromion **(Fig. 8-11A)**. In general, this incision begins at the posterolateral edge of the acromion and ends anteriorly 2 to

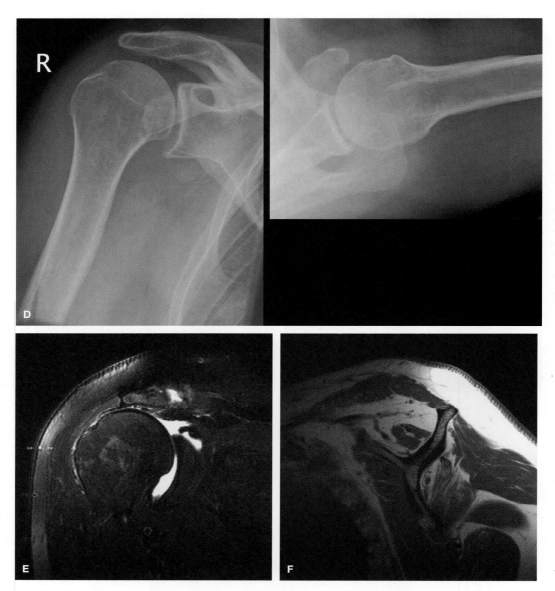

Fig. 8-2. (*Continued*) **D:** Plain radiographs that include a true AP of the glenohumeral joint and axillary lateral display superior subluxation and good maintenance of joint space consistent with mild to moderate osteoarthritis. **E:** Coronal MRI demonstrates a complete tear of the supraspinatus with retraction. **F:** Oblique sagittal plane MRI demonstrates severe fatty degeneration of the supraspinatus and infraspinatus muscles.

3 cm lateral to the coracoid process. The anterolateral deltoid is detached from its origin with a thin wafer of bone using a flexible half-inch osteotome in order to allow for preferential bone-to-bone healing following repair of the deltoid at the completion of the procedure (Fig. 8-11B,C,D). The deltoid is split no more than 5 cm from its origin at the junction of the anterior and middle raphe in order to avoid possible injury to the axillary nerve.

The subacromial bursa is resected sharply, and minimal anterior acromioplasty is performed as well as distal clavicle resection if needed. A subacromial retractor (Sulzer Medica, Winterthur, Switzerland) **(Fig. 8-12)** is placed in order to allow visualization of the entire rotator cuff, from the teres minor to the subscapularis. The long head of the biceps is routinely tenodesed into the bicipital groove using a nonabsorbable anchor, as there is frequently degeneration in the setting of a massive tear and may persist as a significant pain generator following surgery.

Mobilization of the supraspinatus and infraspinatus tendons is then performed, beginning on the bursal surface and proceeding to the articular surface, followed by placement of traction sutures using nonabsorbable, braided suture (no. 2 Ethibond, Ethicon, Johnson & Johnson, Westwood, Mass) in a modified Mason-Allen configuration **(Fig. 8-13)**. Mobilization may include release of the coracohumeral ligament, interval slide, and circumferential capsulotomy.

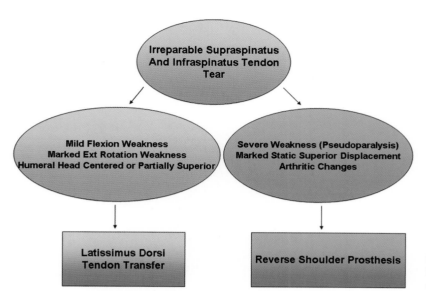

Fig. 8-3. Treatment algorithm for patients with irreparable tears of the posterosuperior rotator cuff.

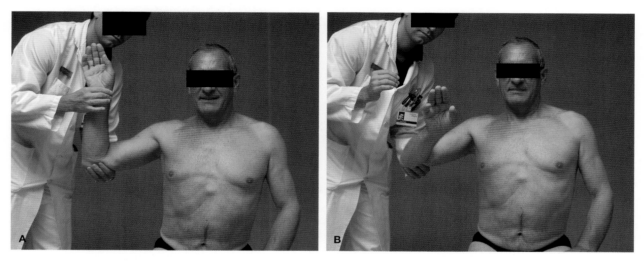

Fig. 8-4. A 59-year-old man with a chronic, massive tear of the posterosuperior rotator cuff. Demonstration of the external rotation lag sign **(A,B)** with the arm at 90 degrees of abduction, which indicates disruption of the infraspinatus and teres minor.

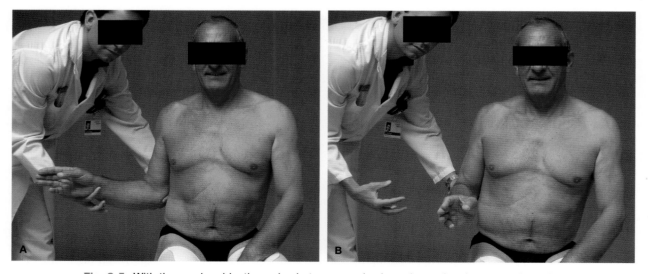

Fig. 8-5. With the arm in adduction, a lag between maximal passive and active external rotation **(A,B)** is pathognomonic of a tear of the infraspinatus.

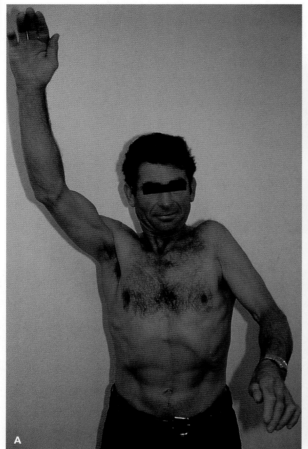
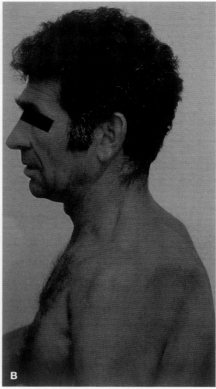

Fig. 8-6. A 52-year-old mason with a traumatic posterosuperior rotator cuff injury. At examination, he showed **(A)** the inability to raise the arm against gravity, or pseudoparalysis, with **(B)** clinical evidence of severe atrophy of the supraspinatus and infraspinatus muscles. (Reprinted with permission from Gerber C. Massive rotator cuff tears. In: Iannotti JP, Williams GR, eds. *Disorders of the Shoulder: Diagnosis and Management.* Philadelphia: Lippincott Williams & Wilkins; 1999:60.)

Release of the articular side of the posterosuperior cuff does not extend beyond 1.5 cm medial to the glenoid rim in order to avoid inadvertent injury to the suprascapular nerve.[15]

Attention is then directed to harvesting the latissimus dorsi tendon. With the arm fully elevated, adducted, and internally rotated, with the help of a second assistant, the anterior border of the latissimus dorsi muscle is palpated. An approximately 25-cm incision is made from the anterior border of the latissimus dorsi muscle, which curves to the posterolateral upper humerus about 4 cm distally and does not traverse the axilla **(Fig. 8-14A)**. Sharp dissection is used to raise subcutaneous flaps just superficial to the underlying fascia over the posterior deltoid, long head of the triceps, teres major, and latissimus dorsi. The anterior latissimus is dissected off the chest wall fascia, beginning at the level of the muscle belly and proceeding proximally toward the insertion of the tendon on the proximal humerus (Fig. 8-14B). The radial nerve crosses over the humerus immediately distal to the insertion of the latissimus tendon on the

humerus, while the circumflex vessels and axillary nerve are located just proximal to the tendon.

The interval between the superior border of the latissimus and the inferior border of the teres major is often difficult to distinguish, but can be more easily identified at the more proximal portion of either muscles. The latissimus tendon is released from its insertion using a long-handled no. 15 scalpel and tagged with two no. 3 Ethibond sutures in a Krakow configuration (Fig. 8-14C,D,E). As traction is applied on the muscle, dissection can continue distally in order to achieve sufficient excursion of the musculotendinous unit and in order to reach the superolateral aspect of the greater tuberosity (Fig. 8-14F). The thoracodorsal neurovascular pedicle does not necessarily need to be identified, but can be found as it enters the muscle approximately 10 cm distal to the musculotendinous junction.

The interval between the inferior border of the posterior deltoid and underlying teres minor is identified and developed using a combination of sharp and blunt dissection. A curved Mayo clamp is passed from the previous anterosupe-

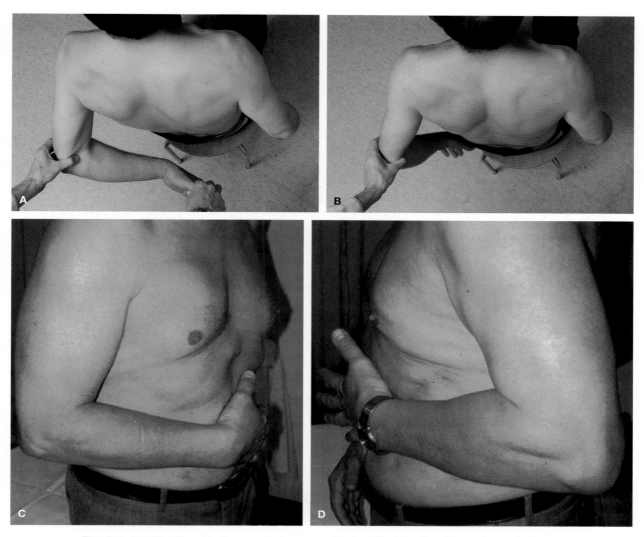

Fig. 8-7. The lift-off and belly press tests are used to test the integrity of the subscapularis tendon. In the lift-off test, the patient is asked to lift his or her hand off the lower back. It has been found to be more sensitive and specific if there is the presence of an internal rotation lag sign after the clinician releases the hand from maximal internal rotation with the arm off the back **(A,B)**. In the belly press sign **(C,D)**, the patient exerts an internal rotation force on the belly, with the elbow forward and anterior to the midline of the trunk. If the subscapularis is ruptured, the patient is unable to keep his or her hand on the stomach with resisted internal rotation, and the elbow will fall back posteriorly. (Reprinted with permission from Gerber A, Clavert P, Millett PJ, et al. Split pectoralis major transfer and teres major tendon transfers for reconstruction of irreparable tears of the subscapularis. Tech Shoulder Elbow Surg. 2004;5:5–12.)

rior exposure into this interval (Fig. 8-14F). It is extremely important to adequately develop this potential space in order to allow for free and unrestricted excursion of the tendon transfer with the proximal humerus. The latissimus dorsi tendon is then transferred to the superolateral humerus (Fig. 8-14G,H).

The tagged end of the latissimus is sutured to the superior border of the subscapularis through bone tunnels passing through the lesser tuberosity (Fig. 8-14I). The previously mobilized supraspinatus and infraspinatus tendons are either repaired to a bony trough at their anatomic insertion through bone tunnels (if sufficient mobilization is possible) prior to

transfer of the latissimus or, more often, repaired to the medial border of the tendon transfer. The lateral border of the tendon transfer is repaired through bone tunnels passing through the greater tuberosity and exiting laterally over a titanium cortical bone augmentation device that prevents cutting of the sutures through the bone (Stratec/Synthes, Paoli, Penn) **(Fig. 8-15)**.

Suction drains are routinely placed in both the inferior and anterosuperior wounds deep into the fascia. The deltoid split is reapproximated with a running 0 polydiaxanone suture (PDS) monofilament suture (Ethicon, Johnson & Johnson, Westwood, Mass). The osteotomy of the anterolateral middle deltoid is repaired with no. 2 FiberWire (Arthrex, Inc, Naples,

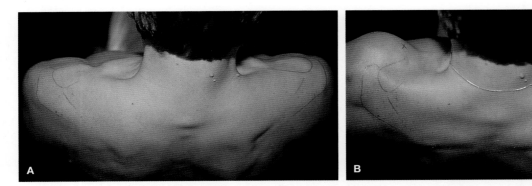

Fig. 8-8. Dynamic anterosuperior subluxation indicates major injury to the supraspinatus and subscapularis. The clinical diagnosis is made if **(A)** the patient has normal contour of both shoulders at rest and **(B)** subluxates his or her shoulder anterosuperiorly while resisting abduction. The condition of anterosuperior subluxation can be precipitated by open or arthroscopic subacromial decompression, with release of the coracoacromial ligament. If anterosuperior subluxation becomes static, clinically or radiographically, successful restoration of overhead elevation by direct surgical repair is exceedingly rare, and subacromial decompression is detrimental. (Reprinted with permission from Gerber C. Massive rotator cuff tears. In: Iannotti JP, Williams GR, eds. *Disorders of the Shoulder: Diagnosis and Management*. Philadelphia: Lippincott Williams & Wilkins; 1999:69.)

Fla) passed through drill holes in the lateral acromion. The superficial fascia of the deltoid split is reinforced with a running monofilament suture (2-0 PDS, Ethicon, Johnson & Johnson, Westwood, Mass).

Watertight sterile dressings are applied to enable early aqua therapy postoperatively. Prior to transfer off the table, the patient is placed into an abduction brace (SOBER Abductor, Pharmap, Crolles, France) at 45 degrees of

abduction and 45 degrees of external rotation, which is worn continuously for 6 weeks following surgery **(Fig. 8-16)**.

■ REHABILITATION

A range of passive motion exercises with the arm maintained in 45 degrees of external rotation and isometric contraction

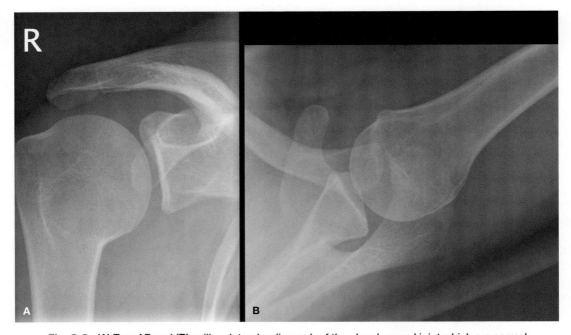

Fig. 8-9. **(A)** True AP and **(B)** axillary lateral radiograph of the glenohumeral joint which are normal in this case. The true AP view of the glenohumeral joint allows for assessment of the acromiohumeral distance (ACHD) and static superior subluxation, whereas the axillary lateral view is used to assess for static anterior or posterior subluxation.

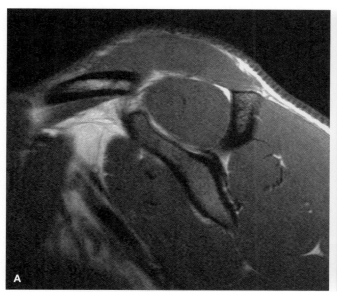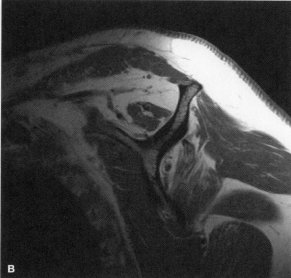

Fig. 8-10. Magnetic resonance images parallel to the glenoid plane through the base of the cora-coid. **A:** The subscapularis, supraspinatus, infraspinatus, and teres minor are homogeneous, convex, and voluminous in a normal rotator cuff. **B:** In a massive posterosuperior tear, the subscapularis exhibits normal signal characteristics and volume, but the supra- and infraspinatus show fatty infiltration and atrophy. If a line drawn from the top of the scapular spine to the highest point on the coracoid does not pass through the substance of the muscle belly, it indicates significant atrophy of the supraspinatus muscle.

of the deltoid are initiated on postoperative day 1. Passive motion is important not only with respect to tendon healing, but also to maintain glenohumeral motion and prevent adhesion of the tendon transfer to surrounding soft tissues.[16] Aqua therapy is also initiated at this time on a routine basis. The splint is discontinued after 6 weeks at which time active external rotation and abduction are initiated as well as passive internal rotation. The patient is allowed to begin performing gentle activities of daily living at this time. Strengthening exercises are not allowed until 3 months following surgery and are continued for 6 to 9 months. It may take up to 12 months for complete retraining of the transferred latissimus dorsi to occur.

Dr. Warner's Technique in Lateral Decubitus

The patient is placed into a lateral decubitus position on a long bean bag that is contoured around the patient. An articulated hydraulic arm holder (Spider Arm Positioner, Tenet Medical Engineering, Calgary, Alberta, Canada) is used on the contralateral side of the operative table, and this permits placement of the arm in the proper position for tendon harvesting as well as for setting the tension of the tendon transfer during fixation. This positioning allows the surgeon to perform the procedure with one assistant, provided the arm holder is available **(Fig. 8-17)**.

An anterosuperior approach is utilized and the deltoid is split directly off the lateral acromion. The deltoid is then

elevated using electrocautery in the subperiosteal plane off the anterior and posterior acromion so that this sleeve is in continuity with the deltoid and trapezius fascia. By making this vertical split directly laterally, we are able to expose the humerus from the teres minor to the subscapularis **(Fig. 8-18)**. Furthermore, the dissection is performed parallel to the muscle fibers of the deltoid, which we believe protects the deltoid from disruption when it is repaired.

If the coracoacromial ligament has not been disrupted by prior surgery, we are careful to define it and avoid its detachment as it is an important restraint to superior displacement of the humeral head in patients with a massive rotator cuff tear. More often than not, however, an acromioplasty and resection of the coracoacromial ligament have already been performed. In cases where there has been no acromioplasty, we perform a modified acromioplasty using a small saw and remove only the undersurface of the acromion from lateral to anterior, being careful not to detach the origin of the coracoacromial ligament.

Adhesions often exist between the acromion and the rotator cuff as well as between the rotator cuff and the deltoid. Internal rotation of the arm will expose the posterior rotator cuff while external rotation will expose the anterior rotator cuff. Adhesions are sharply released in this interval.

If the supraspinatus and infraspinatus tendon remnants are discernible, they are mobilized as much as possible, and sutures are placed through them to be used to secure the latissimus dorsi along its medial edge following the transfer.

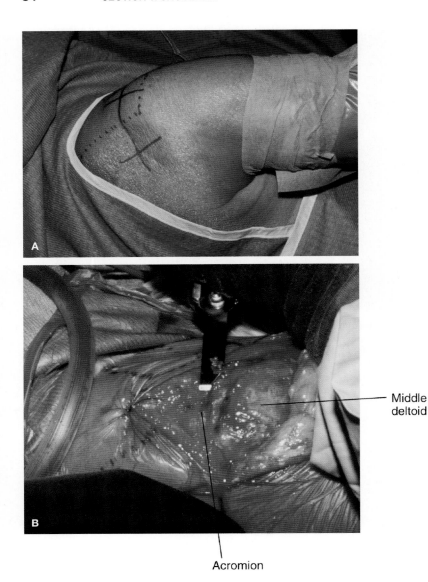

Middle
deltoid

Acromion

Fig. 8-11. Anterosuperior exposure. **A:** The incision is parallel to the Langer lines over the lateral one third of the acromion beginning at the posterolateral edge of the acromion and extending anteriorly to 2 to 3 cm lateral to the coracoid process. **B:** Deltoid exposure with middle deltoid detachment using half-inch straight osteotome from anterolateral acromion.

Once it is defined, the remnant of the infraspinatus or teres minor is secured with several sutures of nonabsorbable, braided material (no. 2 Ethibond, Ethicon, Johnson & Johnson, Westwood, Mass). The upper insertion of the subscapularis is also defined and sutures are placed through it as well.

The biceps, if present, is usually degenerated in these individuals and, in such cases, it is tenodesed within the bicipital groove using a bone anchor (TwinFix, Smith & Nephew Endoscopy, Andover, Mass).

Next, the greater tuberosity is debrided clear of soft tissue and the remnant of the stump of the torn tendon. A rongeur is used to abrade the bone, but a bone trough is not created. We prefer to use suture anchors to fix the tendon transfer as these can be placed at points along the greater tuberosity to secure the latissimus tendon directly into the "footprint" of the supraspinatus and infraspinatus. Usually, 3 or 4 screw-in anchors appropriate for tuberosity fixation are placed into the greater tuberosity.

The latissimus dorsi is harvested only after all of the above preparatory steps have been performed. Exposure of the latissimus dorsi is facilitated by placing the patient's arm into flexion, adduction, and internal rotation. The articulated hydraulic arm holder can maintain the arm in this position during tendon dissection. It is helpful at this stage of the procedure for the assistant to stand on the side opposite the surgeon as this facilitates retraction and exposure of the tendon insertion during the dissection.

An L-shaped incision is made along the anterior belly of the latissimus muscle and then along the posterior axillary line. Curving the incision laterally at its proximal portion will make exposure of the tendon insertion easier **(Fig. 8-19A)**. During the dissection, the muscles of the latissimus (most anterior muscle on the chest wall), teres major, long head of the triceps, and posterior deltoid are defined. The latissimus is dissected first from its attachments to the anterior chest wall, followed by identification of the interval between it and the teres major (Fig. 8-19B). This interval can be variable

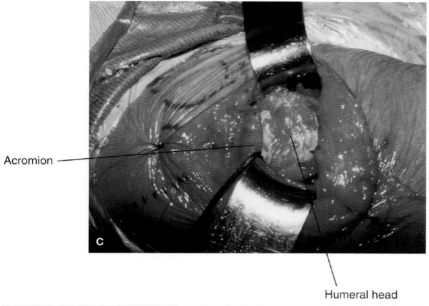

Acromion

Humeral head

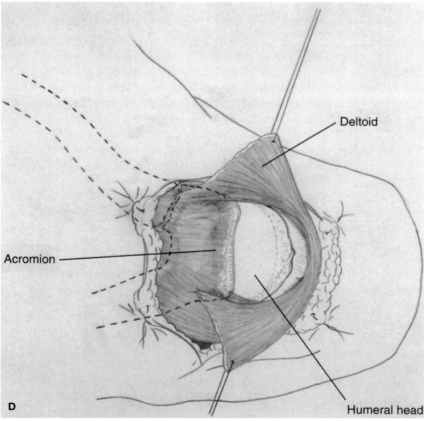

Deltoid

Acromion

Humeral head

Fig. 8-11. (*Continued*) **C,D:** Middle deltoid detachment enables exposure underlying humeral head and rotator cuff. (Reprinted with permission from Holovacs TF, Espinosa N, Gerber C. Latissimus dorsi transfers in rotator cuff reconstruction. In: Craig EV, Thompson, RC eds. *Master Techniques in Orthopaedic Surgery: The Shoulder*. Philadelphia: Lippincott Williams & Wilkins; 2004:366–368.)

and difficult to define; in some patients, the two muscles may seem to be conjoined. However, careful dissection and retraction that places each under tension will allow clear dissection of the latissimus muscle from the teres major.

As the dissection proceeds toward the insertion of the latissimus dorsi tendon, several fascial bands may be encountered that course anteriorly. If the surgeon palpates

the insertion of the tendon on the humerus, the correct plane of dissection can be clarified. Maintenance of the arm in internal rotation will make this step easier.

The tendon insertion is then isolated and the latissimus is sharply detached from the humerus. A traction suture in a whipstitch configuration facilitates dissection of the muscle toward its origin until the thoracodorsal neurovascular pedicle

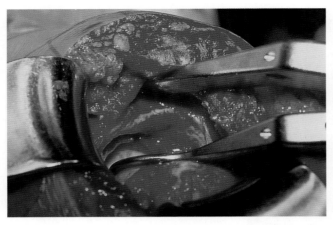

Fig. 8-12. Subacromial retractor used during anterosuperior exposure (Sulzer Medica, Winterthur, Switzerland). This device has a ring that is used to retract the humeral head inferiorly and a straight limb analogous to a lamina spreader that distracts the acromion superiorly to enlarge the subacromial space. This greatly facilitates identification and mobilization of a retracted rotator cuff tendon. (Reprinted with permission from Gerber C. Massive rotator cuff tears. In: Iannotti JP, Williams GR, eds. *Disorders of the Shoulder: Diagnosis and Management*. Philadelphia: Lippincott Williams & Wilkins; 1999:70.)

is identified (Fig. 8-19C). This structure courses on the chest wall and can be clearly defined if tension is maintained on the tendon by an assistant. We place sutures on either edge of the tendon in order to facilitate this step (Fig. 8-19D).

The extent of tendon release and mobilization of the musculotendinous unit is determined by the surgeon intraoperatively such that it can be pulled to the level of the posterior acromion. This will ensure sufficient length for the transfer over the greater tuberosity. We usually release the tendon from attachments to the chest wall all the way to the inferior edge of the scapula. Although the neurovascular pedicle is identified, its dissection and release is never necessary to gain mobility for the transfer.

Before transferring the tendon, we prefer to augment it with fascia lata from the ipsilateral thigh. Based on our initial experience, the tendon in many patients is quite diminutive

and some patients had late rupture of the transfer. For this reason, we started to use the fascia lata to augment the tendon (Fig. 8-19E). A strip of fascia lata is typically 2 to 3 cm wide by 6 to 8 cm long. The defect in the fascia is then closed.

The fascia lata is secured to the latissimus tendon from the musculotendinous junction to the end of the tendon. Although the length of the tendon is almost never a problem, it is possible to lengthen the tendon with the graft. We use braided nonabsorbable suture (no. 2 Ethibond, Ethicon, Westwood, Mass) along the length of the tendon and the graft.

The interval underneath the deltoid and superficial to the teres minor is then dissected from the posterior, and a curved clamp is placed underneath the acromion so that it comes into this interval (Fig. 8-19F,G). This interval is then sharply and bluntly dissected to ensure that free and unrestricted excursion of the tendon transfer is possible.

A clamp is then passed from the anterosuperior incision beneath the acromion and deltoid in order to grasp the sutures in the latissimus tendon for the transfer. The arm is then placed in a position to tension the tendon transfer. This is approximately 45 degrees of abduction and 45 degrees of external rotation. The tendon is then fixed to the posterior rotator cuff and over the greater tuberosity using the previously placed bone anchors. Finally, it is fixed to the subscapularis, and the sutures in the remnants of the supraspinatus and infraspinatus are sewn into the medial edge of the tendon (Fig. 8-19H). The deltoid is then repaired to the acromion with transosseous sutures and the deltoid split is closed in a side-to-side fashion. After placing a sterile dressing, the shoulder is placed into a prefabricated abduction orthosis to maintain arm position and to protect the graft from excessive tension (SOBER Abductor, Pharmap, Crolles, France) (Fig. 8-16).

■ REHABILITATION

Phase I (first 6 weeks) consists of continuous wearing of the brace and passive motion by the therapist, bringing the arm into abduction and external rotation. Adduction and internal

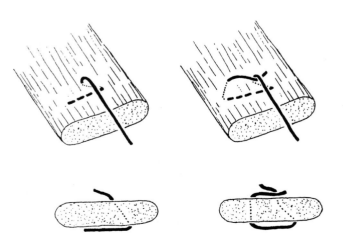
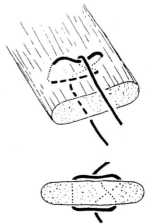

Fig. 8-13. A modified Mason-Allen tendon-grasping technique increases the pullout strength of the suture by a factor greater than two when compared with a simple stitch or with a mattress-type suture. (Reprinted with permission from Gerber C. Massive rotator cuff tears. In: Iannotti JP, Williams GR, eds. *Disorders of the Shoulder: Diagnosis and Management*. Philadelphia: Lippincott Williams & Wilkins; 1999:70.)

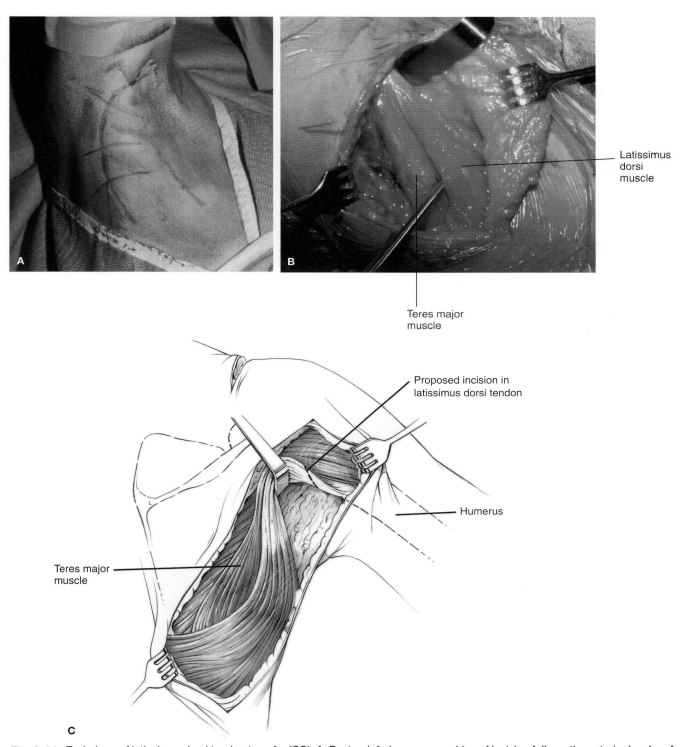

Fig. 8-14. Technique of latissimus dorsi tendon transfer (CG). A: Posteroinferior exposure. Line of incision follows the anterior border of the latissimus dorsi muscle belly and curves 4 cm proximal to the axillary fold ending at the inner one third of the proximal humerus. B: Latissimus dorsi exposure with identification of the posterior deltoid and teres major superiorly. C: Identification of insertion of latissimus muscle on proximal humerus and release with Metzenbaum scissors or no. 15 scalpel blade.

rotation are not permitted. This ensures that the tendon moves in its new soft-tissue tunnel and will not become tethered while it heals.

Phase II (second 6 weeks) consists of removal of the brace and then active-assisted range of motion as well as continued

passive range of motion exercises. The patient is permitted to use the arm for daily living activities, and water therapy may be commenced to facilitate return of passive motion arcs.

Phase III (12 to 16 weeks) consists of ongoing active-assisted motion and initiation of biofeedback program. A

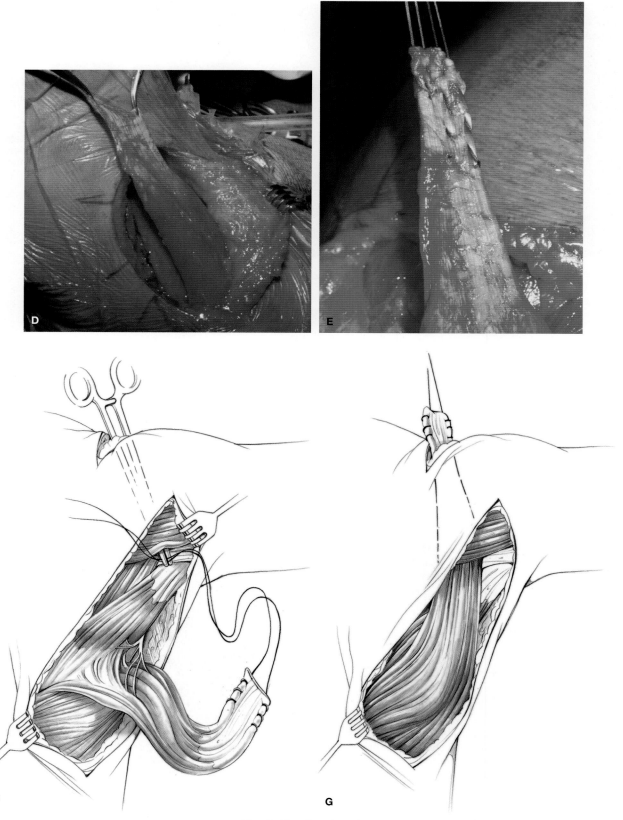

Fig. 8-14. (*Continued*)

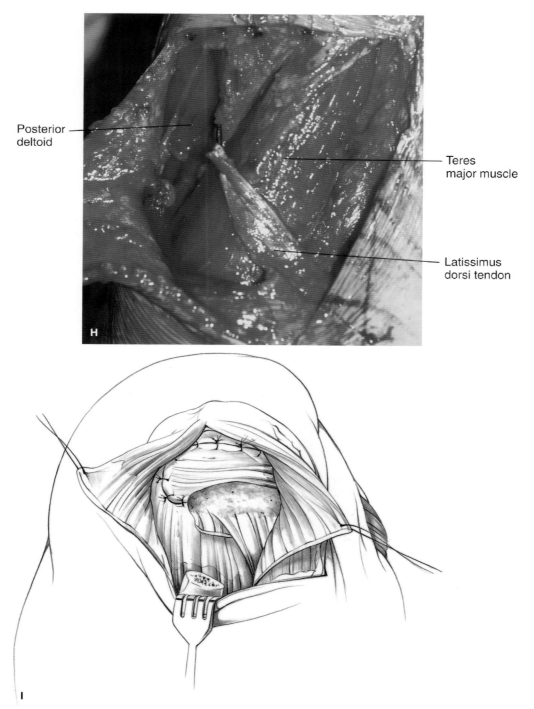

Posterior deltoid

Teres major muscle

Latissimus dorsi tendon

Fig. 8-14. (*Continued*) **D:** Fully released tendon. **E:** Traction sutures are placed in a Krakow configuration. **F:** The muscle is dissected until the pedicle is identified, a clamp is passed between the deltoid and external rotators, and the tendon is **(G,H)** pulled superiorly into the subacromial space. The tendon is sutured to the tip of the greater tuberosity and the remaining stump of the supraspinatus and infraspinatus are sutured end-to-side to the latissimus tendon **(I)**. (C,F,G,I. Reprinted with permission from Gerber C. Massive rotator cuff tears. In: Iannotti JP, Williams GR, eds. *Disorders of the Shoulder: Diagnosis and Management*, Philadelphia: Lippincott Williams & Wilkins; 1999:80–81.) (A,B,D,E,H: Reprinted with permission from Holovacs TF, Espinosa N, Gerber C. Latissimus dorsi transfers in rotator cuff reconstruction. In: Craig EV, Thompson RC, eds. *Master Techniques in Orthopaedic Surgery: The Shoulder*. Philadelphia: Lippincott Williams & Wilkins; 2004:366, 370, 81, 373.)

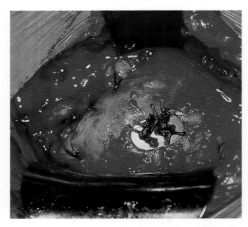

Fig. 8-15. Direct repair of the lateral border of the tendon transfer is achieved with transosseous sutures that are augmented using a titanium cortical bone augmentation device (Stratec/Synthes, Paoli, Penn). (Reprinted with permission from Gerber C. Massive rotator cuff tears. In: Iannotti JP, Williams GR, eds. *Disorders of the Shoulder: Diagnosis and Management.* Philadelphia: Lippincott Williams & Wilkins; 1999:72.)

cutaneous biofeedback device is used by the patient (Myotrac, Thought Technology, Ltd, Montreal, Quebec, Canada). The patient is then instructed by the therapist on the methods of training the latissimus transfer to become an active elevator and external rotator of the shoulder. The biofeedback unit is applied over the latissimus muscle. The first maneuver that the patient is instructed to perform is the J-maneuver. The patient's shoulder is placed in approximately 90 degrees of flexion and the patient is instructed to pull downward and across the body. This will cause the latissimus to contract while the biofeedback unit gives the patient audiovisual feedback. During sustained contraction of the latissimus muscle, the

patient then attempts to raise the arm into flexion, so as to trace the letter "J" with his or her hand. This maneuver sustains contraction of the latissimus muscle during elevation of the arm **(Fig. 8-20A,B)**.

Once the patient is able to initiate and maintain contraction of the latissimus with the J-maneuver, he or she is instructed to attempt contraction of the latissimus with external rotation. This can be facilitated by having the patient lie on his or her opposite side while pulling downward followed by active external rotation.

During phase IV (16 weeks), biofeedback continues as long as necessary, and it may take up to 1 year for patients to successfully train the tendon transfer to actively assist in arm elevation and external rotation. Strengthening is begun when the patient achieves latissimus contraction during elevation, and we try to limit this to elastic bands rather than free weights.

■ TECHNICAL ALTERNATIVES AND PITFALLS

Although the latissimus dorsi transfer provides, in our opinion, the optimal solution for massive, irreparable posterosuperior rotator cuff tendon tears, other options have been described and may offer a viable alternative to patients.

The supraspinatus advancement, first described by Debeyre et al.[17] is a technique that is more of a muscle "slide" rather than a transfer **(Fig. 8-21A,B,C,D,E,F,G,H,I,J)**. Nonetheless, it has been deemed effective in the treatment of isolated, irreparable tears of the supraspinatus. It is performed by releasing the muscle belly of the supraspinatus in order to allow lateral advancement of the tendon, being cognizant not to injure the suprascapular neurovascular pedicle. Despite the success of Debeyre et al., this technique remains largely historical as others have not been able to validate its usefulness.

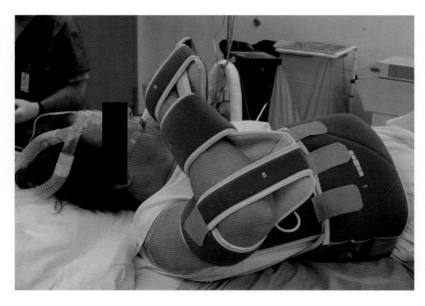

Fig. 8-16. Abduction brace for postoperative protection of tendon transfer. (SOBER Abductor, Pharmap, Crolles, France.)

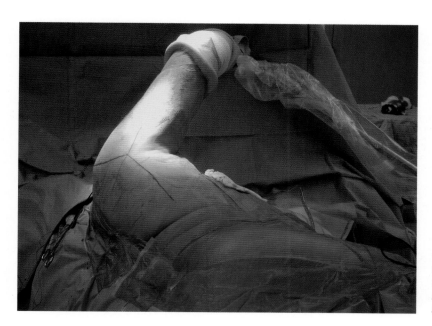

Fig. 8-17. Patient positioning in the lateral decubitus position for latissimus dorsi tendon transfer using an articulated pneumatic arm holder. (Spider Arm Positioner, Tenet Medical Engineering, Calgary, Alberta, Canada.)

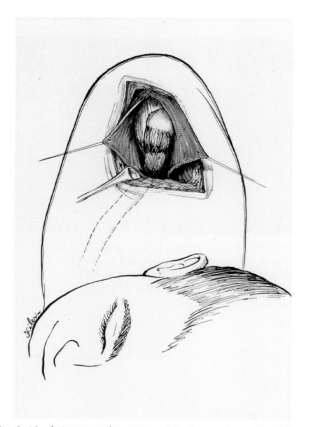

Fig. 8-18. Anterosuperior approach to the rotator cuff utilizing a deltoid split directly off the lateral acromion. The deltoid is elevated using electrocautery in the subperiosteal plane off the anterior and posterior acromion so that this sleeve is in continuity with the deltoid and trapezius fascia.

Cofield[18] has described a partial subscapularis transfer that utilizes the superior two thirds of the tendon to replace an irreparable supraspinatus tear. This rotational flap has been effective in his hands for medium-sized tears, but, unfortunately, much less effective in the treatment of massive tears.[19] Karas and Giachello[19] have shown that patients who undergo transfer of the subscapularis for an irreparable supraspinatus tear actually had worse function after the procedure.

Takagishi[20] has described the trapezius transfer for isolated irreparable tears of the supraspinatus. The technique involves transfer of the acromial portion of the tendon to the greater tuberosity.

Apoil and Augereau[21] have recommended the lateral deltoid transfer based on the original description by Takagishi[20] **(Fig. 8-22A,B,C)**. This technique involves release of an approximately 2.5-cm-wide strip of the anterolateral deltoid from the acromion, which is transferred to the supraspinatus stump or the superior aspect of the glenoid. Despite the research of Takagishi and others, our concern is that the critical importance of a functional deltoid, especially if further treatment of rotator cuff arthropathy is undertaken using the reverse shoulder prosthesis, obviates the perceived advantage of a deltoid transfer.

Finally, Malkani et al.[22] have recently reported on the transfer of the long head of the triceps in the treatment of irreparable tears of the supraspinatus and infraspinatus. In a review of 19 shoulders in 18 patients who underwent this surgical procedure at minimum 2 years follow-up, 100% of patients were satisfied in their outcome, with average overall improvement in their UCLA scores.

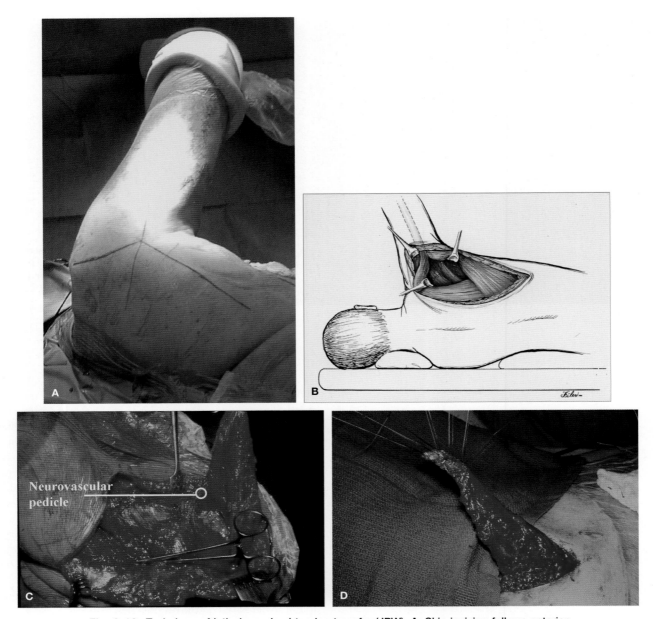

Fig. 8-19. Technique of latissimus dorsi tendon transfer (JPW). **A:** Skin incision follows anterior border of latissimus and curves along posterior axillary line. **B:** Identification of teres major (superior)—latissimus dorsi (inferior) interval. **C:** Thoracodorsal neurovascular pedicle. **D:** During mobilization of musculotendinous unit, the tendon is tagged with a nonabsorbable suture in a Krakow configuration to facilitate traction and later transfer.

The main pitfalls are associated with this procedure may be divided into intraoperative and postoperative complications. Intraoperative complications can include axillary nerve injury during passage of the graft or during graft harvest from the proximal humerus, inadequate tendon length due to anatomic variations, poor technique, or poor mobilization of the muscle belly prior to transfer, and injury to the thoracodorsal neurovascular pedicle during harvest. Postoperative complications may include rupture of the tendon transfer, infection, nerve injury, deltoid detachment, and persistent pain.

■ OUTCOMES

Gerber et al. were the first to report on the outcome of latissimus dorsi transfer in 1988.[2] They noted that these patients gained an average of 50 degrees of active elevation and 13

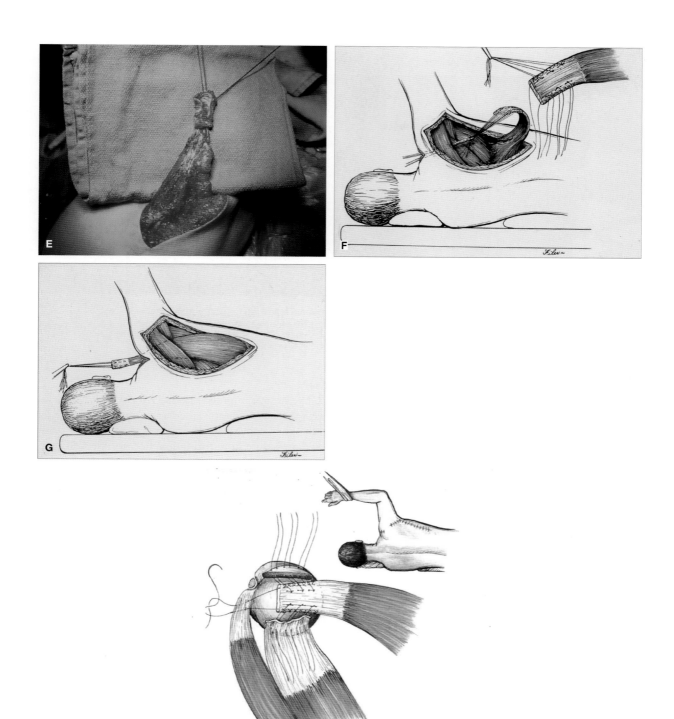

Fig. 8-19. (*Continued*) **E:** Fascia lata augmentation of latissimus tendon. **F,G:** Transfer of tendon through interval defined by inferior border of posterior head of deltoid and teres minor into subacromial space. **H:** Definitive fixation of tendon transfer using bone anchors or transosseous tunnels.

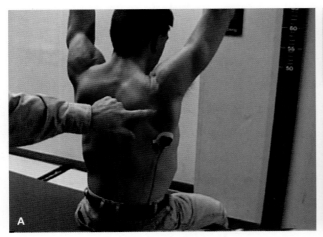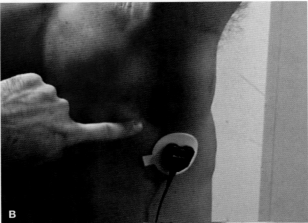

Fig. 8-20. A,B: Biofeedback training of latissimus muscle following tendon transfer involves use of a biofeedback unit (Myotrac, Thought Technology, Ltd, Montreal, Quebec, Canada) and the J-maneuver.

degrees of active external rotation following this procedure. They demonstrated that a pre-existing injury of the subscapularis and inability to repair that tendon were associated with poor recovery of function.[3,9]

More recently, Gerber et al.[23] have reviewed the mid- to long-term clinical and radiographic outcome of patients who underwent latissimus dorsi transfer at an average follow-up of 53 months (range 24 to 126 months). Thirteen of these patients had a deficient subscapularis. The age and gender-matched Constant score improved from 55% to 73%, with significant improvements in pain, flexion, external rotation, and strength in abduction. It was again noted that patients with a dysfunctional subscapularis did significantly worse in all parameters tested.

One explanation for inferior results in the setting of combined anterosuperior defects has been proposed by Burkhart,[24,25] who emphasized the importance of a balanced force couple and fulcrum in the shoulder. Others have confirmed this concept in biomechanical studies.[26,27]

The effectiveness of latissimus dorsi transfer has also been compared in primary versus revision settings. Warner and Parsons[28] found significant functional differences postoperatively in salvage settings compared to primary settings. At a mean follow-up of 19 months, patients who underwent latissimus dorsi transfer as a salvage procedure had a higher rate of rupture of the transfer (44% versus 17%) as well as significantly worse Constant scores (55% versus 70%).

Aoki et al.[29] reported on 12 cases of latissimus dorsi transfer for irreparable rotator cuff tears at an average follow-up of 3 years. They noted excellent results in 4 out of 12, good results in 4 out of 12, and poor results in 3 out of 12, and were able to correlate electromyogram (EMG) activity of the muscle during active motion in 9 out of 12 cases.

Active flexion improved from 99 to 135 degrees on average with associated improvements in strength in external rotation. They concluded this technique to be an effective salvage procedure in restoring function and decreasing pain in irreparable tears.

Irlenbusch et al.[30] performed a latissimus dorsi transfer in 22 patients, 7 of which were for failed prior open rotator cuff repair surgeries at an average 9-month follow-up. Average Constant scores improved from 43 to 67 versus 33 to 62 in revision cases. Poor results were associated with concomitant rupture of the subscapularis or deltoid insufficiency. Pain improved significantly in all patients.

■ FUTURE DIRECTIONS

The indications and techniques for latissimus dorsi tendon transfer continue to evolve. An increased understanding of the natural history of irreparable massive rotator cuff tears as well as the underlying biochemical mechanisms that instigate fatty infiltration, muscle atrophy, and tendon degeneration will help guide treatment decisions in the future and improve outcomes. The role of latissimus transfer combined with reverse shoulder arthroplasty is currently under investigation and may prove to be superior in the treatment of rotator cuff arthropathy in the setting of a significant impairment to external rotation **(Fig. 8-23A,B,C,D)**. The use of growth factors and gene therapy may improve tendon to bone healing and allow for earlier mobilization and perhaps greater range of motion and strength following surgery. Finally, improvements in rehabilitation, including advances in biofeedback training, may optimize clinical outcomes.

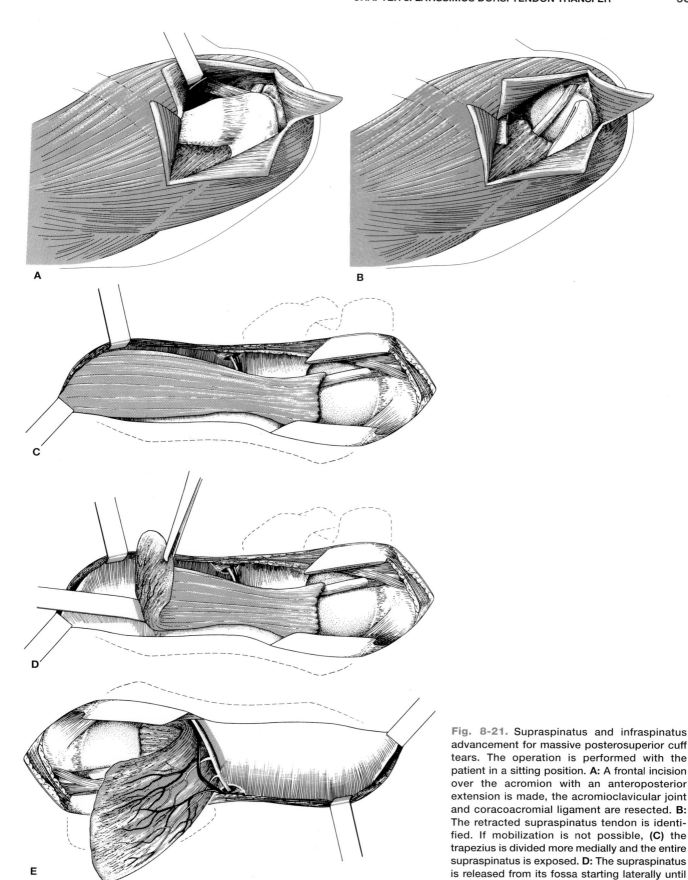

Fig. 8-21. Supraspinatus and infraspinatus advancement for massive posterosuperior cuff tears. The operation is performed with the patient in a sitting position. **A:** A frontal incision over the acromion with an anteroposterior extension is made, the acromioclavicular joint and coracoacromial ligament are resected. **B:** The retracted supraspinatus tendon is identified. If mobilization is not possible, **(C)** the trapezius is divided more medially and the entire supraspinatus is exposed. **D:** The supraspinatus is released from its fossa starting laterally until **(E)** the neurovascular pedicle is fully exposed.

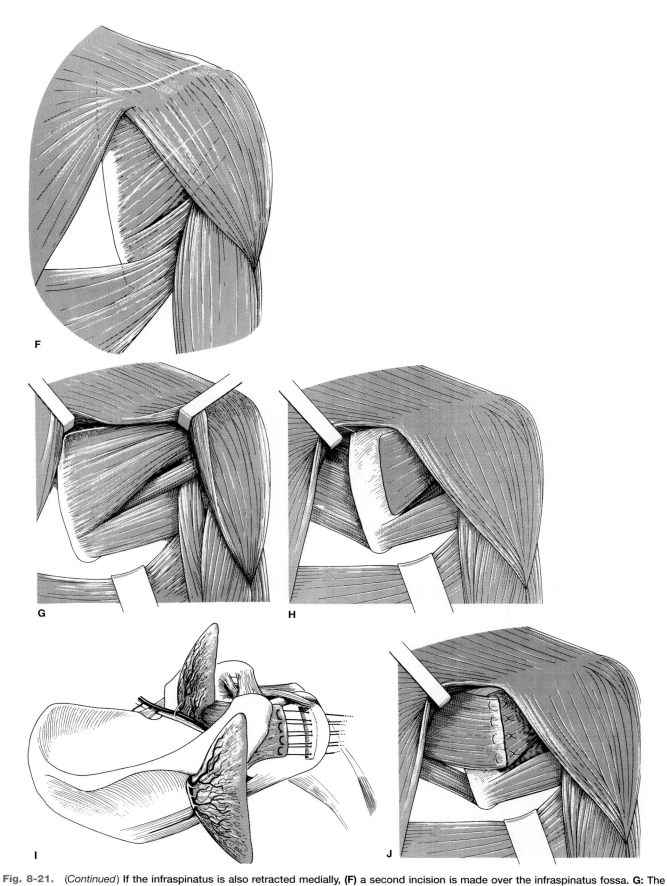

Fig. 8-21. (*Continued*) If the infraspinatus is also retracted medially, **(F)** a second incision is made over the infraspinatus fossa. **G:** The infraspinatus is released from the infraspinatus fossa. **H:** The insertion of the rhomboids at the medial border of the scapula is then released. **I:** Both musculotendinous units are then advanced and the tendon stumps are sutured to a bony trough at the greater tuberosity. **J:** The rhomboids are then sutured to the infraspinatus in the hope of augmenting the dynamic effect of the musculotendinous unit and protecting the infraspinatus from sliding too laterally. (Reprinted with permission from Gerber C. Massive rotator cuff tears. In: Iannotti JP, Williams GR, eds. *Disorders of the Shoulder: Diagnosis and Management*. Philadelphia: Lippincott Williams & Wilkins; 1999:77–78.)

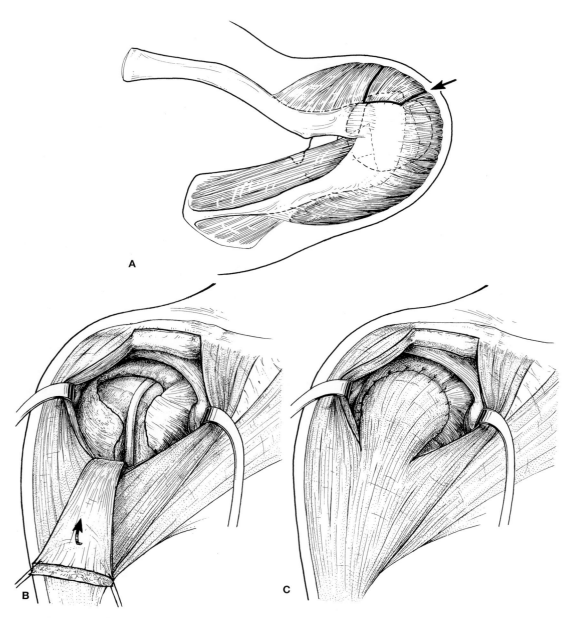

Fig. 8-22. Deltoid flap technique. **A:** An anterolateral strip of approximately 2.5 cm is tailored through a superolateral approach. **B:** The tear is identified and debrided. **C:** The deltoid flap is sutured to the stump of the supraspinatus, infraspinatus, subscapularis, or superior labrum depending on the pathology that is present. (Reprinted with permission from Gerber C. Massive rotator cuff tears. In: Iannotti JP, Williams GR, eds. *Disorders of the Shoulder: Diagnosis and Management*. Philadelphia: Lippincott Williams & Wilkins; 1999:79.)

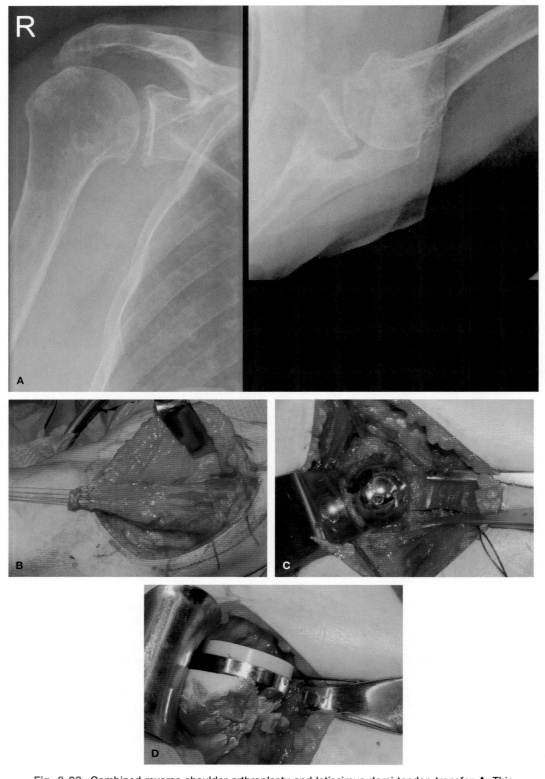

Fig. 8-23. Combined reverse shoulder arthroplasty and latissimus dorsi tendon transfer. **A:** This 67-year-old patient with glenohumeral arthritis had irreparable tears of the supraspinatus and infraspinatus tendons with evidence of mild static posterosuperior subluxation. On clinical examination, the patient displayed a 40-degree lag in external rotation with the arm in adduction. **B:** Isolation of latissimus dorsi tendon for subsequent transfer through a separate posteroinferior incision. **C:** Placement of glenosphere. **D:** Transosseous sutures are used to secure the tendon transfer just inferior to the humeral prosthesis.

■ REFERENCES

 1. Warner JJ, Gerber C. Treatment of massive rotator cuff tears: posterior-superior and anterior-superior. In: Iannotti JP, ed. *The Rotator Cuff: Current Concepts and Complex Problems.* Rosemont: American Academy of Orthopaedic Surgeons; 1998;232:59–94.
 2. Gerber C, Vinh TS, Hertel R, et al. Latissimus dorsi transfer for the treatment of massive tears of the rotator cuff: a preliminary report. Clin Orthop Rel Res. 1988;51–61.
 3. Gerber C, Fuchs B, Hodler J. The results of repair of massive tears of the rotator cuff. J Bone Joint Surg Am. 2000;82:505–515.
 4. Hoffer MM, Wickenden R, Roper B. Brachial plexus birth palsies: results of tendon transfers to the rotator cuff. J Bone Joint Surg Am. 1978;60:691–695.
 5. L'Episcopo JB. Tendon transfer in obstetrical paralysis. Am J Surg. 1934;25:122–125.
 6. Wickstrom J, Haslam ET, Hutchinson RH. The surgical management of residual deformities of the shoulder following birth injuries of the brachial plexus. J Bone Joint Surg Am. 1955;37A:27–36.
 7. Zachary RB. Transplantation of teres major and latissimus dorsi for loss of external rotation of the shoulder. Lancet. 1947;2:757–760.
 8. Burkhart SS. Biomechanics of rotator cuff repair: converting the ritual to a science. Instr Course Lect. 1998;47:43–50.
 9. Gerber C. Latissimus dorsi transfer for the treatment of irreparable tears of the rotator cuff. Clin Orthop Rel Res. 1992;275:152–160.
10. Miniaci A, MacLeod M. Transfer of the latissimus dorsi muscle after failed repair of a massive tear of the rotator cuff: a two- to five-year review. J Bone Joint Surg Am. 1999;81:1120–1127.
11. Gerber C, Krushell RJ. Isolated rupture of the tendon of the subscapularis muscle: clinical features in 16 cases. J Bone Joint Surg Br. 1991;73:389–394.
12. Hertel R, Ballmer FT, Lombert SM, et al. Lag signs in the diagnosis of rotator cuff rupture. J Shoulder Elbow Surg. 1996;5:307–513.
13. Fuchs B, Weishaupt D, Zanetti M, et al. Fatty degeneration of the muscles of the rotator cuff: assessment by computed tomography versus magnetic resonance imaging. J Shoulder Elbow Surg. 1999;8:599–605.
14. Goutallier D, Postel JM, Bernageau J, et al. Fatty muscle degeneration in cuff ruptures: pre- and postoperative evaluation by CT scan. Clin Orthop Rel Res. 1994;304:78–83.
15. Warner JP, Krushell RJ, Masquelet A, et al. Anatomy and relationships of the suprascapular nerve: anatomical constraints to mobilization of the supraspinatus and infraspinatus muscles in the management of massive rotator-cuff tears. J Bone Joint Surg Am. 1992;74:36–45.
16. Silva MJ, Boyer MI, Gelberman RH: Recent progress in flexor tendon healing. J Orthop Sci. 2002;7:508–514.
17. Debeyre J, Patie D, Elmelik E. Repair of ruptures of the rotator cuff of the shoulder. J Bone Joint Surg Br. 1965;47:36–42.
18. Cofield RH. Subscapular muscle transposition for repair of chronic rotator cuff tears. Surg Gynecol Obstet. 1982;154:667–672.
19. Karas SE, Giachello TL. Subscapularis transfer for reconstruction of massive tears of the rotator cuff. J Bone Joint Surg Am. 1996;78:239–245.
20. Takagishi N. The new operation for the massive rotator cuff rupture. J Jpn Orthop Assoc. 1978;52:775–780.
21. Apoil A, Augereau B. [Deltoid flap repair of large losses of substance of the shoulder rotator cuff]. Chirurgie. 1985;111:287–290.
22. Malkani AL, Sundine MJ, Tillett ED, et al. Transfer of the long head of the triceps tendon for irreparable rotator cuff tears. Clin Orthop Rel Res. 2004;428:228–236.
23. Gerber C, Maquieira G, Espinosa N. Latissimus dorsi transfer for the treatment of irreparable rotator cuff tears. J Bone Joint Surg Am. 2006;88:113–120.
24. Burkhart SS. Arthroscopic treatment of massive rotator cuff tears: clinical results and biomechanical rationale. Clin Orthop Rel Res. 1991;267:45–56.
25. Burkhart SS. Fluoroscopic comparison of kinematic patterns in massive rotator cuff tears: a suspension bridge model. Clin Orthop Rel Res. 1992;284:144–152.
26. Loehr JF, Helmig P, Sojbjerg JO, et al. Shoulder instability caused by rotator cuff lesions: an in vitro study. Clin Orthop Rel Res. 1994;304:84–90.
27. Thompson WO, Debski RE, Boardman ND III, et al. A biomechanical analysis of rotator cuff deficiency in a cadaveric model. Am J Sports Med. 1996;24:286–292.
28. Warner JJ, Parsons IM. Latissimus dorsi tendon transfer: a comparative analysis of primary and salvage reconstruction of massive, irreparable rotator cuff tears. J Shoulder Elbow Surg. 2001;10:514–521.
29. Aoki M, Okamura K, Fukushima S, et al. Transfer of latissimus dorsi for irreparable rotator-cuff tears. J Bone Joint Surg Br. 1996;78:761–766.
30. Irlenbusch U, Bensdorf M, Gansen HK, et al. [Latissimus dorsi transfer in case of irreparable rotator cuff tear—a comparative analysis of primary and failed rotator cuff surgery, in dependence of deficiency grade and additional lesions]. Z Orthop Ihre Grenzgeb. 2003;141:650–656.

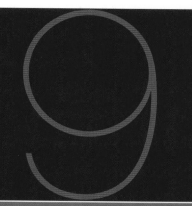

ROTATOR CUFF REPAIR
PART I. ARTHROSCOPIC APPROACH

■ CARLOS A. GUANCHE, MD

■ HISTORY OF THE TECHNIQUE

The treatment of rotator cuff tears has certainly improved over the past few years as a result of an increased understanding of the mechanics and anatomy of the involved tissues. However, the quantum leap has occurred as a result of the increasing use of the arthroscope in the management of these injuries. Initially, the use of the tool was confined to the diagnosis and occasionally management of subacromial bone spurs. The thinking has now shifted to an all-arthroscopic treatment. This is reminiscent of the history of the treatment of meniscal tears, chronic anterior cruciate ligament (ACL) insufficiency, shoulder impingement, and shoulder instability. Over time, clinical practice favors the arthroscopic treatment despite initial skepticism and lack of scientific evidence to support the procedures.

All-arthroscopic cuff repair is probably the most technically challenging of the commonly performed procedures done in the shoulder. It constitutes a natural extension of the arthroscopic-assisted mini-open repair. The latter has many of the advantages of an all-arthroscopic repair with less of the technical demands pertaining to the mobilization and securing of the rotator cuff to the greater tuberosity. No matter which repair technique is chosen, some fundamental principles of cuff repair should be applied.[1] These include preservation (or meticulous repair) of the deltoid, adequate subacromial decompression, surgical release to produce a freely mobile muscle-tendon unit, secure fixation of the tendon to the greater tuberosity, and closely supervised rehabilitation.

There clearly is no best technique. The most important factor is the individual surgeon's experience and comfort level. A good open repair will always be superior to a badly performed arthroscopic one. There are also technical considerations related to size of tear, quality of tissue, available equipment, and patient expectations. Preoperative imaging can assist with planning and discussion of options with the patient. A surgeon wishing to make the transition to arthroscopic repair should do so in a stepwise and careful fashion, first perfecting arthroscopic acromioplasty and the mini-open technique followed by progression to all-arthroscopic techniques.

The history of arthroscopic rotator cuff repairs can be traced back to the pioneers of shoulder arthroscopy such as Lanny Johnson who began repairing rotator cuff tears with a removable staple. Following that, Eugene Wolf pioneered the use of suture anchors in the subacromial space. This was closely followed by Steven Snyder,[2] who has written and presented extensively on the suture anchor technique dating back to the 1980s. More recently, Stephen Burkhart[3] has further advanced the surgery with the use of a variety of tools designed to expedite the surgical procedure.

■ INDICATIONS AND CONTRAINDICATIONS

There are two common reasons for surgical intervention in rotator cuff tears. They are pain and weakness. The two are commonly inseparable when it comes to the treatment of the entity. In general, as has been discussed above, the type of procedure should not matter as much as the ability to provide an adequate repair by whatever means are used. However, the use of minimally invasive procedures clearly impacts the patient's decision on whether or not to proceed with the intervention.[1]

Historically, open repair has been espoused as reproducibly improving strength as well as reducing pain. Recently, the ability to reproducibly improve function has also been shown with arthroscopic techniques. The outcomes appear to be as good with open, mini-open, or arthroscopic techniques, the only caveat being that the surgeon must be proficient in the chosen technique.[4]

The indication for repair of a tear (either complete or partial) is that it remains symptomatic despite a supervised course of physical therapy with or without the judicious use of subacromial cortisone injection(s). Although complete tears have historically been the only types to undergo repair, there is a growing body of knowledge that appears to support the repair of partial thickness tears in higher-level throwing athletes and laborers that continue to be symptomatic despite conservative measures. Initially, arthroscopic repair was described for tears measuring less than 2 cm. With the growing armamentarium of surgical tools and techniques, such as margin convergence, side-to-side repair, and transtendon repair, the size of the tear has become irrelevant to many surgeons.[2,3]

In addition to the above considerations, it is important to acknowledge that there are typically several other areas that need to be addressed at the time of rotator cuff repair. These most commonly include the need to perform a subacromial decompression (and possibly a distal clavicle resection), but often also the management of labral and biceps pathologies. The critical factor in this consideration is the time available for a successful arthroscopic procedure. The allotted time for surgical repair of the cuff is limited by fluid extravasation. Typically, the surgeon must accomplish any associated procedures in a minimal amount of time in order to accomplish the more daunting task of rotator cuff repair before fluid extravasation precludes successful repair.

Contraindications to arthroscopic repair include all of the usual parameters commonly employed in open and mini-open techniques. These include the attempt to repair obviously degenerative cuff tears showing not only intraoperative degenerative changes but also fatty infiltration and muscle atrophy on imaging studies. In addition, the quality of the bony bed available for the repair must be such that anchors can be successfully implanted and maintain their purchase. Finally, as discussed above, the techniques of all-arthroscopic repair can be difficult in inexperienced hands. The physician should be proficient with the techniques and should also be ready to convert to either an open or mini-open technique should the complexity of the procedure preclude a good outcome.

■ SURGICAL TECHNIQUE

The options for positioning during arthroscopic rotator cuff repair include the beach chair and lateral positions. The literature is replete with good outcomes in either position. This chapter will assume that the patient is in the lateral decubitus position with traction applied across the upper extremity in standard fashion. The basic setup for lateral decubitus arthroscopic surgical intervention in the shoulder has been well described by multiple authors and will not be discussed in detail here.[5]

The procedure can be performed under either general or regional anesthesia, depending on the experience of both the surgeon and the anesthetist involved in the procedure. The use of hypotensive anesthesia is helpful in most cases, especially with surgeons who are beginning the technique. This is obviously accomplished with a general anesthetic. The systolic pressure should be ideally maintained at 90 mm Hg. In addition, the use of preemptive analgesia is highly desirable. Typically, prior to sterile prep and drape of the patient, the subacromial space is infiltrated with 30 cc of 0.5% Marcaine with 1:100,000 epinephrine. This allows for both postoperative comfort for the patient and also simplifies anesthetic management.[6] An interscalene block is also effective for intraoperative and postoperative pain control and allows for easier blood pressure control intraoperatively.

Standard anterior and posterior glenohumeral portals are established with the arthroscope being inserted in the posterior portal. The procedure begins with the intra-articular visualization of the entire glenohumeral joint and management of any additional pathology that may be present. The articular surfaces of the glenoid and humerus should be carefully evaluated for concomitant damage. Similarly, the labral structures should be assessed and any pathology that is found should be addressed first before turning to the rotator cuff.

Following completion of any work in the glenohumeral joint, the rotator cuff is now addressed. The important factors of size of the tear (in the anterior to posterior and medial to lateral directions) should be delineated. In addition, full-thickness tears must be assessed for the pattern of tearing.[7] This is important to decide the order of repair, including considerations for side-to-side suturing ("margin convergence"), prior to suture anchor implantation. In addition, whether or not the tear is repairable must also be addressed. The factors employed in this consideration include whether the tear is immediately repairable or if significant soft tissue releases must be undertaken. This is, perhaps, the critical junction in the decision-making process for most surgeons. If extensive mobilization and complex suturing patterns will be required, then the surgeon must decide whether these techniques fit within their proficiency. If there is any doubt, then the arthroscopic procedure should be abandoned and traditional techniques employed.

Partial thickness tears are increasingly documented and newer techniques allow transtendon repair. The partial thickness tear may be equally symptomatic to a complete tear in those with excessive physical demands. The average thickness of a rotator cuff insertion is approximately 15 mm.[8] It is, therefore, important to document the thickness of tearing involved in any area. Once this is documented, the patient's size, activity level, and degree of clinical weakness are taken into account in order to decide whether to debride or repair a partial tear. The traditional indication for repair of a partial thickness cuff tear has been one greater than 50% of the thickness of the tendon. However, this is weighed against the patient's age, activity level, and physical demands.

A 30% tear in an elderly and relative sedentary individual is clearly different than the same tear in a professional baseball player. The general recommendation is that a greater than 50% partial tear should be repaired either with a transtendon technique or by completing the tear and repairing it through whatever means the surgeon decides. Those tears involving less than 50% of the thickness should be treated with debridement of the torn portion as well as consideration of other anatomic factors, including labral and subacromial pathology.

In cases where there is a clear intra-articular partial tear, yet the depth is not completely known, it is useful to insert a suture through the area of partial tearing as a marker suture.[2] This is accomplished with the use of a spinal needle that is placed near the anterolateral corner of the acromion through the area of partial tearing and visualized in the joint. Once this is visualized, a large diameter suture is placed through the needle and visualized in the joint. Several centimeters of suture are advanced into the joint and the needle is withdrawn. The suture is now a useful landmark to visualize the subacromial portion of the partial inner surface tear **(Fig. 9-1)**. Any tearing visualized in this portion of the cuff should then be taken into account when deciding on the overall size of the partial tear.

Once the intra-articular visualization is completed, the subacromial space is entered through the posterior portal. The arthroscopic sheath is placed immediately adjacent to the acromion and swept in a medial to lateral direction in order to release any subacromial adhesions that may be present. Palpating the coracoacromial ligament with the trocar delineates the most anterior portion of the subacromial space. Once oriented, the trocar is withdrawn and the arthroscope is placed in the sheath. A lateral portal is now established using direct visualization. In general, the ideal location for the portal is about 2 cm below the lateral acromion at about the midportion of the bone. The most common error in placing the portal is superior placement. This becomes a

critical factor once it is necessary to reach further medially with grasping tools and suture passers. In general, it is much better to err on the side of being too low rather than too high since this will not preclude access to the medial structures.

The use of arthroscopic cannulas in all of the portals is encouraged for entering the subacromial space, thus limiting the trauma to the soft tissues and increasing distension of the space. The cannulas that are employed are 7-mm clear devices (Crystal Cannula; Arthrex, Inc, Naples, Fla) that allow visualization of instruments and sutures within the sheath of the device as they are advanced. These are maintained throughout the rest of the procedure. If the arthroscope is placed in a particular portal, it is simply inserted through the cannula in many cases.

Once the lateral portal is established, a shaver is employed to perform a thorough bursectomy. In addition, it is useful to have a cautery device available for control of any bleeding that may arise during the debridement. This may be either a standard electrocautery instrument or a newer bipolar or monopolar radiofrequency device. It is safe to start debriding white tissue laterally and avoiding yellowish tissue medially. The yellowish, fatty tissue is well vascularized and can lead to bleeding. Regardless of the method chosen, it is important to perform a complete bursectomy at the beginning of the procedure. Not only does this allow for complete visualization of the subacromial space, but it also prevents impaired visualization later in the procedure when fluid is absorbed by many of the periarticular structures.

Following a thorough exposure of the cuff tendons, any suture markers that were previously placed are assessed for bursal-sided pathology. This should be taken into consideration when the decision is made to debride or repair a partial thickness tear. The area of tearing is now definitively assessed for dimensions, shape, and repairability.

In addition, the anterior acromion and the distal clavicle are now addressed, if necessary. An acromioplasty is often done in conjunction with a rotator cuff repair. The procedure is certainly indicated in cases where there is a prominent anterior and often lateral spur that abuts the rotator cuff. The coracoacromial ligament is released without a formal resection of the soft tissue. In any case, the acromioplasty must be carried out swiftly and decisively since the surgical steps involved in the arthroscopic cuff repair will take a considerable amount of time. A good rule of thumb is to complete the ancillary procedures of acromioplasty (and distal clavicle excision, if indicated) in 20 to 30 minutes so that there is ample time to complete the other tasks.

In most situations, once the cuff pattern is deciphered, no significant soft tissue release is indicated. In those cases where there is significant retraction of the cuff, a mobilization of the tissues needs to be undertaken. The first step is to release the adhesions in the subacromial space. If that does not suffice, then a rotator interval slide is completed. This typically includes release of the coracohumeral ligament. This is accomplished by visualizing from the posterior portal, while pulling traction from the lateral portal. The release is

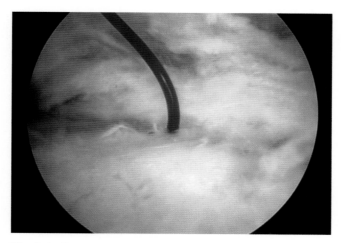

Fig. 9-1. Suture marker in the subacromial space. Note the normal bursal tissue.

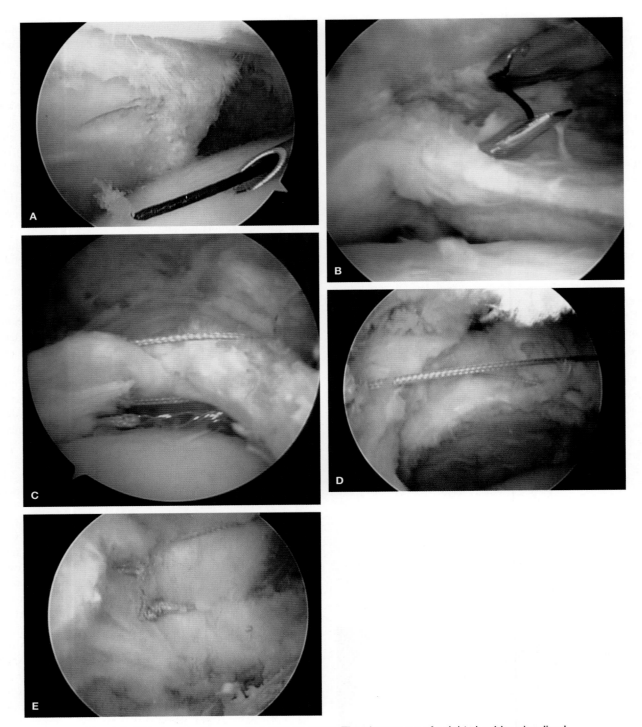

Fig. 9-2. Side-to-side closure using suture Lassos. The pictures are of a right shoulder, visualized from the lateral portal. **A:** Lasso in position with shuttle visualized. **B:** Shuttle being grasped from opposite portal. **C:** Suture being shuttled across defect. **D:** Final suture position prior to knot tying. **E:** Final closure obtained with two sutures.

then accomplished by using an electrocautery device via the anterior portal. The release is complete when the lateral coracoid process is visualized.

In cases where there is still significant retraction, consideration should be given to releasing the cuff intra-articularly at the junction of the cuff and the capsule. Visualizing from the posterior portal, elevating the cuff from the lateral portal, and then using either mechanical shavers or blunt arthroscopic elevators to release the interval between the cuff and glenoid accomplish the process. The release should not extend more than 1.5 cm medial to the glenoid face for fear of damaging the suprascapular nerve as it crosses the spinoglenoid notch.

Following mobilization, the greater tuberosity is cleared of soft tissue to create a bony bleeding bed. Any remnant of cuff and any adherent tissue should be removed first with a shaver blade and, if necessary, with a small burr. In cases of good bone quality, a gentle burring of the area of the tuberosity is indicated in order to stimulate a healing response. However, it is critical not to violate the cortical layer of the tuberosity for fear of compromising the strength of the suture anchor fixation that is required for solid cuff approximation. If there is any doubt as to the quality of the bone, then a shaver should only be used.

A side-to-side repair, if necessary, should be done prior to any suture anchor insertion. In cases of large tears, this is often the only repair undertaken. A simple approximation can change the moment arm of the functioning cuff to effect good movement and clinical results.[7] The procedure for side-to-side closure can be undertaken with a variety of instruments. My technique of choice is the use of Lasso devices (Arthrex, Inc, Naples, Fla) that allow the passage of sutures through one side of the rotator cuff tissue and retrieved from the opposite portal by first piercing the tissue from the bursal side, delivering the suture across the tear, and then repeating the process from the other side **(Fig. 9-2A,B,C,D,E)**. In general, one suture should be used for every 5 mm of cuff tear that requires approximation. The repair is undertaken from medial to lateral. Tying of the sutures is delayed until all of the side-to-side stitches are placed. This makes sequential suture passing much simpler. Permanent suture is employed in the side to side since absorbable sutures tend to be variably absorbed in some situations and can also give significantly when tension is applied. The security obtained with permanent suture, in my opinion, outweighs any benefit of the absorbable materials. The knot employed for side-to-side repairs is a reverse half hitch with alternating posts. As will be discussed later, using a sliding knot to approximate two layers of tissue could cause the suture to saw through the tissue and fail.

Following completion of any side-to-side repair, attention is then placed on the lateral portion of the cuff. In terms of suture anchor fixation, the critical point in planning involves the determination of how many anchors will be employed and in what location to place them. In general, the rule of thumb is to use one anchor per 1 cm of tearing in the anterior to posterior direction.

The choice of anchor is also a decision that is highly debated. Several anchors are available that allow solid bony fixation and are reproducible with respect to their technique of insertion. The anchors vary in size and in the material from which they are made. The surgeon must first decide whether to employ a permanent anchor or one that is bioabsorbable. My preference is the use of Corkscrew anchors (Arthrex, Inc, Naples, Fla), which are manufactured either of titanium metal or a polylactic acid material (pl-DLA)

that is bioabsorbable. They are manufactured in two sizes, 5.0 mm and 6.5 mm, with the larger anchors reserved for softer bone. Currently, there are no true indications for one type of anchor over another, despite the theoretical concerns of metal interference with subsequent MRI studies. In general, most of the metal anchors are manufactured with non-ferrous materials that create minimal artifact.

Following the thorough preparation of the tuberosity, anchor placement is now performed. The ideal position for visualization of the location of all the anchors is from the lateral portal. In this position, one has a bird's-eye view of the location without distortion from the arthroscope. The area for placement of each anchor is now chosen. Anchor insertion is performed via an accessory portal (5 mm in size) that is first located with the use of a spinal needle to ensure accurate placement and a good working angle. The usual location is proximal to the lateral portal and anterior, although this may vary with the configuration of the cuff tear **(Fig. 9-3)**.

The steps in the insertion of the anchor vary depending on the product employed. However, a few general principles apply. The angle of insertion is critical. The device should be placed in the subchondral bone immediately under the articular margin. The reason for this position is to maximize the quality of available bone and also to allow pulling of the sutures around the corner, rather than directly. This serves to increase the strength of fixation.[7] Generally, the anchors are inserted at a 45-degree angle to the bone (dead man's angle), which provides the highest pullout strength.

Anchors are typically placed followed by suture passing, then subsequent insertion of additional anchors and so on until the entire tear is addressed. It is generally a good idea not to insert multiple anchors prior to suture passing since that can create problems with suture management. In general, an anterior anchor is placed first, the sutures passed through the cuff, followed by a more posterior anchor placement. This is important in cases where the scope is maintained in the posterior portal as it will not block the view of the scope.

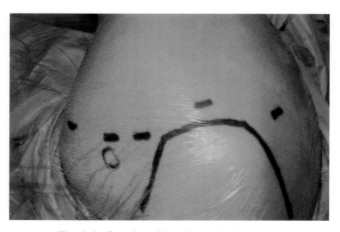

Fig. 9-3. Portal position for anchor insertion.

Once the first anchor is placed, there are a variety of techniques available for suture passing. My technique of choice is the use of the suture Lassos (Arthrex, Inc, Naples, Fla). These devices are available in a variety of angles that allow access to any type of cuff tear **(Fig. 9-4)**. Employing a Lasso for passage, the two limbs of a suture are separated into different portals with the limb that is closest to the cuff being prepared for passage through the cuff. Typically, the first anchor is placed anteriorly and the cuff is sutured from the posterior portal. With this in mind, the medial suture is now brought out the anterior portal. From the posterior portal, a suture Lasso device is inserted. The straight devices are certainly easier to maneuver; however, in some situations, the use of a curved device allows access to the cuff in a more medial position for ideal suture placement. The position for suture placement is now chosen and it is typically about 1 cm medial to the edge of the tendon. The Lasso device is then employed to pierce the tendon and deliver a loop of suture that is to be used for passing the anchor's suture. The suture loop is grasped from the anterior portal. The medial suture is now passed back through the cuff in a retrograde fashion using the suture loop. The two limbs of the suture are now in the posterior portal.

A device that simplifies the complexity of suture management is the Suture Saver (Linvatec, Inc, Largo, Fla). These are thin, color-coded sleeves that can be used to keep a pair of sutures together and also to keep them from becoming entangled with multiple other sutures that are often used in larger repairs. The process for employing these is as follows: Once the two limbs of a suture are delivered out of the portal, a switching stick is placed in the arthroscopic cannula, the cannula is withdrawn, the two loops of suture are pulled out of the cannula, and a Suture Saver is placed around the limbs. The cannula is then reinserted into the portal and the Suture Saver is advanced along the same channel as the cannula **(Fig. 9-5)**. The device can then be used to advance the

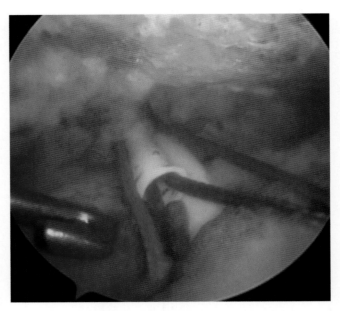

Fig. 9-5. Suture Savers viewed in place in subacromial space. Note separation of multiple suture limbs with these devices.

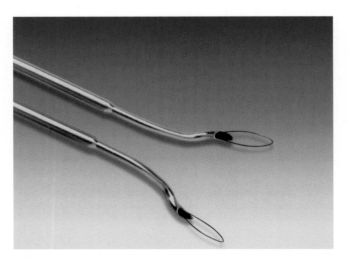

Fig. 9-4. Corkscrew Lasso devices. Note the shuttle device within the end of the needle.

cuff somewhat, allowing for planning of subsequent suture passes. The procedure is now repeated as many times as necessary for closure of the defect. Simple sutures are employed for most situations where a single row of anchors is placed. In most tears, two anchors are typically inserted since this distributes the stresses better.

An alternative technique, termed the mattress double anchor (MDA), employs a double row of anchors. In this technique, the first limb is passed as previously discussed. A second anchor is then placed about 1 cm lateral to the first anchor. This anchor is first prepared for this technique by unloading the sutures within the anchor and reloading them such that they are looped around each other **(Fig. 9-6A)**. It is important to ensure that the anchor's eyelet allow this maneuver. For this reason, I typically use the BioCorkscrew (Arthrex, Naples, FL) device since it has a suture eyelet that allows several loops of suture to pass through without damage to the others. The second anchor is then placed into the greater tuberosity. The loops of suture are then visualized and the loop that would pull a suture from medial to lateral into the anchor's eyelet is then identified. This loop is then delivered out of the subacromial space and loaded with the previously passed single loop of suture that is through the rotator cuff (Fig. 9-6B). Once this suture limb is passed through the second anchor's eyelet, it is now through the cuff and through the second anchor. When this loop is tied, it will serve to seat the cuff tissue down to the tuberosity and help to re-create the footprint of the rotator cuff in a more anatomical pattern (Fig. 6C). This construct has been tested in laboratory studies and appears to be superior to traditional single-pass techniques, both with respect to pullout and deformation.[9]

Following successful anchor insertion and suture passing, the next step is knot tying. A few words with respect to the

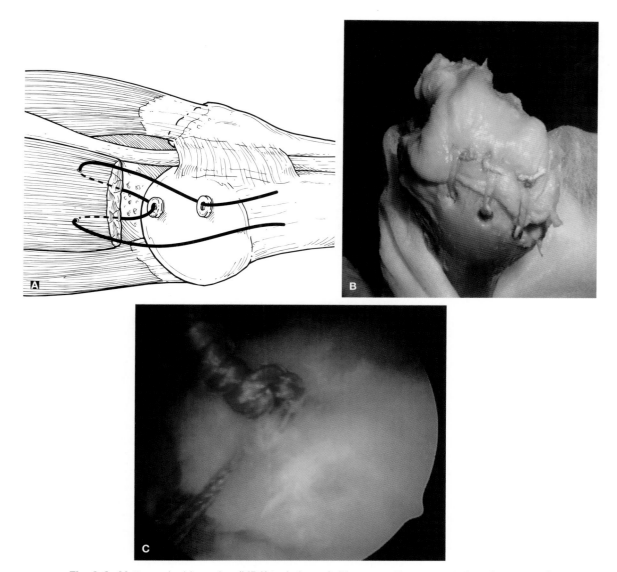

Fig. 9-6. Mattress double anchor (MDA) technique. **A:** Diagrammatic representation of concept of interlocking two anchors. **B:** Cadaveric example of approximation of cuff obtained with technique. **C:** Arthroscopic view of MDA technique in a right shoulder viewed from the lateral portal.

perceived difficulties in knot tying are in order. First, the technique is not more difficult than any other arthroscopic step. The important principle to keep in mind is that the technique of knot tying takes practice. One needs to be proficient with the technical steps involved in the process for any particular knot. The practice needs to take place well before the surgical procedure is attempted. In addition, it is important to ensure that there are no twists or tangles between the limbs. This is ensured by running the knot pusher down each suture limb immediately after delivering them to the lateral portal and before the knot-tying process begins.

It is also important to be familiar with two different techniques. One should be a sliding knot configuration, such as the Samsung Medical Center (SMC, Weston, Tenn) Slider, or any of a number of these techniques that have become

commonplace in arthroscopic shoulder surgery. The other technique is reverse half hitches with alternating posts. This technique is employed either when the sutures do not slide within the anchor or when one is tying a side-to-side repair. In these situations, having the suture slide from one side to the other may cause trauma to the soft tissues and may inadvertently cut through one side of the tissue, thus disrupting the repair. Although the topic of knot tying is of great importance, this chapter will not cover it in detail; the reader is referred to any of a number of articles that discuss these knots in greater detail.[10–12]

Once the knot to be employed has been decided upon, it is time to complete the repair by tying all of the sutures. It does not matter whether the knot tying occurs from anterior to posterior or vice versa. The important principle is to tie the knots in order so that the cuff is brought back to an anatomic or near anatomic location as each limb is secured. In general, the best angle for knot tying is obtained from the lateral portal. In most cases, the arthroscope is placed in the posterior portal, the suture limbs are brought out in pairs into the lateral portal, then tied one at a time. There should be only one pair of sutures within the working portal during knot tying and advancement of the sutures. Multiple sutures within the working portal tend to become entangled and often compromise several limbs of suture beyond salvage. In some cases, a separate portal may be created away from the lateral portal in order to "park" the sutures prior to tying.

The final configuration is now visualized from multiple angles. It is important to look from both the posterior and lateral portals to ensure that the closure is complete. In addition, the glenohumeral joint can be re-entered in order to ensure that the closure is complete and that some semblance of a footprint has been re-created.

Skin closure is performed with absorbable sutures placed subcutaneously, followed by a sterile dressing. An UltraSling (DJ Ortho, Vista, Calif) is applied in most cases and the patient is instructed to maintain the device in place for a period of 4 weeks. The sling maintains a small amount of abduction in the shoulder that relieves some tension at the repair site. The design of the sling (or the use of a larger abduction orthosis) should not be understood as a necessary device to maintain the cuff in place. The cuff should rest comfortably at the repaired position without undue tension before being placed in any device.

Physical therapy is instituted immediately (within 48 hours), with the sling being removed several times per day for pendulum exercises as well as passive range of motion, including supine and upright motion with passive assistive devices as tolerated by the patient. The positions to avoid include horizontal extension and external rotation when the shoulder is abducted. In most cases, passive motion is allowed to 90 degrees of abduction and forward flexion immediately post-op and for the first 6 weeks. Elbow range of motion and grip strengthening are also encouraged in the early stages. This is predicated on good tissue quality and an anatomic reconstruction of the cuff. In those cases where a suboptimal repair has been performed or tissue quality is poor, the institution of physical therapy and any motion may be delayed by up to 6 weeks.

Active exercises begin at 6 weeks, and range of motion is also progressed as tolerated at this point. A general strengthening program is now instituted with attention to the lower extremities, trunk, and scapula, especially in throwing athletes. Unrestricted activities such as contact sports are allowed at 4 months. In throwing athletes, a functional program is instituted at about 4 months, with unrestricted throwing being allowed only when the program has been completed, but certainly not before 6 months postoperative. The criteria that should be met before instituting the throwing program include full shoulder motion; trunk, scapula, and rotator cuff muscle endurance, balance, and strength

have been restored; and there is no pain with activity or during examination.[13]

■ PITFALLS OF THE TECHNIQUE

The most common problem observed is the failure to recognize, treat, or convert to open repair in the face of poor cuff mobility by those surgeons without extensive experience in arthroscopic management. This is especially important in tears greater than 3 cm.

Overdebridement of the tuberosity is also a factor that contributes to poor repair. This is especially important in osteoporotic patients with whom fixation is ordinarily an issue. The use of motorized burrs should be avoided in these patients. Simply using a standard shaver and being slightly aggressive will accomplish a thorough soft tissue debridement.

Other general factors that come into play center about surgical "exposure." The most important is the use of a fluid inflow pump. These devices allow the surgeon to increase visualization by increasing the pressure within the subacromial space or glenohumeral joint. This serves to distend the space and to tamponade any acute bleeding that may impair visualization. If a pump is not used, two inflow cannulas should be used to maintain an adequate pressure to prevent bleeding. Concurrently, an electrocautery device should be readily available to deal with occasional excessive bleeding that occurs during the procedure. Through a combination of increasing fluid pressure, electrocautery control of bleeders, and maintaining the systolic blood pressure at 90 mm Hg, visualization can be maintained throughout the procedure, allowing effective arthroscopic repairs.

Finally, and probably most important, is suture management. This is a critical part of the procedure, since often one suture limb that becomes entangled or frayed can compromise the entire repair. The key steps in the process include stepwise anchor insertion and suture passing, "storing" of sutures away from the area where other sutures are being passed or manipulated, and ensuring that each suture limb is free of twists and soft tissue entrapment prior to knot tying.

■ RESULTS

The literature on arthroscopic cuff repair contains many retrospective studies that generally have favorable results. The limitations of these studies are as follows: they are retrospective and nonrandomized, they are relatively short term with only 2- to 3-year follow-up in most cases, and there is clearly a general lack of documentation of the integrity of the repair. Multiple studies have shown a significant improvement in satisfaction, function, and pain with the use of arthroscopic techniques. The level of success has certainly been comparable to that documented with the use of the mini-open technique. Of note, several authors have recently shown their outcomes to be comparable to the traditional open cuff repairs with respect to all measured parameters when dealing with small and medium tears.[14–16]

In experienced hands, the application of arthroscopic techniques in essentially all tears has been espoused. In one study, nine patients with massive cuff tears were treated with arthroscopic double interval slides, side-to-side fixation, and suture anchor placement. At a mean follow-up time of 17.9 months, eight of nine patients were satisfied with the procedure. The mean UCLA score increased from 10.0 preoperatively to 28.3 postoperatively, and all patients showed some improvement in active motion, strength, or function. Active forward flexion improved significantly, from a preoperative mean of 108 degrees to a postoperative mean of 146.1 degrees.[14]

■ SUMMARY

The all-arthroscopic management of any rotator cuff tear is certainly a viable option in most cases where the surgeon has studied and practiced the procedure in the laboratory setting. It does, however, require a major commitment to thoroughly understanding the techniques and to having the necessary equipment available for all possible scenarios that may be encountered.

It is also a certainty that the surgeon must be ready to switch to alternative open and mini-open techniques should the arthroscopic procedure not allow a solid repair. As discussed earlier, the reasons that this occurs are many and the surgeon should be able to recognize them.

In conjunction with the cuff pathology, it is not uncommon to encounter other problems that need surgical intervention. This is especially true in young throwers. A typical scenario may include a concomitant labral repair and acromioplasty along with a rotator cuff repair. Time management is critical in these cases, and surgeons must be honest about their abilities.

Lastly, the historically daunting tasks of suture management and knot tying have to be met head on with practice and understanding of the principles. Education is key in this regard, and surgeons are encouraged to seek continuing medical education employing cadaveric tissue as well as surgical simulators such as the Alex surgical simulator (Pacific Research, Vashon, Wash). The critical factor in increasing the ability of surgeons to perform these procedures comfortably, after all, has been education.

■ REFERENCES

1. Yamaguchi K, Levine WN, Marra G, et al. Transitioning to arthroscopic rotator cuff repair: the pros and cons. J Bone Joint Surg. 2003;85-A:144–155.
2. Snyder SJ. Basic techniques for arthroscopic shoulder reconstruction. In: Snyder SJ, ed. *Shoulder Arthroscopy*. Philadelphia: Lippincott Williams & Wilkins; 2003:46–65.
3. Burkart S. Arthroscopic repair of massive rotator cuff tear: concept of margin convergence. Tech Shoulder Elbow Surg. 2000;1:232–239.
4. Gartsman GM, Khan M, Hammerman SM. Arthroscopic repair of full-thickness tears of the rotator cuff. J Bone Joint Surg. 1998;80(A):832–840.
5. Snyder SJ. Operating room setup for shoulder arthroscopy. In: Snyder SJ, ed. *Shoulder Arthroscopy*. Philadelphia: Lippincott Williams & Wilkins; 2003:14–22.
6. Tetzloff JE, Brems JJ, Dilger J. Intra-articular morphine and bupivacaine reduces postoperative pain after rotator cuff repair. Reg Anesth. 2000;25:611–614.
7. Lo IK, Burkhart SS. Current concepts in arthroscopic rotator cuff repair. Am J Sports Med. 2003;31(2):308–324.
8. Dugas JR, Campbell DA, Warren RF, et al. Anatomy and dimensions of rotator cuff insertions. J Should Elbow Surg. 2002;11(5):498–503.
9. Mazzocca AG, Millett PJ, Santangelo SA, et al. Arthroscopic single versus double row suture anchor rotator cuff repair. Paper presented at: American Orthopaedic Society for Sports Medicine Annual Meeting, June 27, 2004; Quebec City, Quebec.
10. Kim SH, Ha KI. The SMC knot—a new slip knot with locking mechanism. Arthroscopy. 2000;16:563–565.
11. Snyder SJ. Technique of arthroscopic rotator cuff repair using implantable 4-mm Revo suture anchors, suture Shuttle relays, and no. 2 nonabsorbable mattress sutures. Orthop Clin North Am. 1997;28:267–275.
12. Weston PV. A new cinch knot. Obstet Gynecol. 1991;78:144–147.
13. Conway JE. The management of partial thickness rotator cuff tears in throwers. Op Tech Sports Med. 2002;10(2):75–85.
14. Lo IK, Burkhart SS. Arthroscopic repair of massive, contracted, immobile rotator cuff tears using single and double interval slides: technique and preliminary results. Arthroscopy. 2004;20(1):22–33.
15. Gartsman GM, Brinker M, Khan M. Early effectiveness of arthroscopic repair for full-thickness tears of the rotator cuff: an outcome analysis. J Bone Joint Surg. 1998;80A:33–40.
16. Weber S. Comparison of all arthroscopic and mini-open rotator cuff repairs. Paper presented at Annual Meeting of the Arthroscopy Association of North America, April 20, 2001; Seattle, Wash.

ROTATOR CUFF REPAIR
PART II. TRANSOSSEOUS-EQUIVALENT
ROTATOR CUFF REPAIR

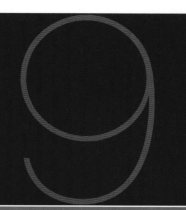

■ NEAL S. ELATTRACHE, MD, MAXWELL C. PARK, MD

■ TRANSOSSEOUS-EQUIVALENT ROTATOR CUFF REPAIR

The authors' preferred method depends on several factors when considering arthroscopic rotator cuff repair, particularly of the supraspinatus: (a) patient age, (b) size of tear, (c) degree of retraction, (d) chronicity of tear, and (e) tissue quality.[17,18] Other factors contribute to healing potential over a repaired rotator cuff footprint. For example, increasing the contact area and pressure distribution between tendon and tuberosity may help to optimize healing potential; in addition, repair strength may influence healing, particularly in the immediate postoperative period. Such parameters can be influenced by technique.[17,19–23] Park et al.[22] have found that a transosseous-equivalent repair using suture-bridges **(Fig. 9-7)** can improve pressurized contact area **(Fig. 9-8)** and overall pressure at a repaired rotator cuff insertion.

Park et al.[23] have also demonstrated that a transosseous-equivalent repair utilizing four-suture-bridges has an ultimate failure strength significantly stronger than a double-row repair; the gap formation was found to be similar to the double-row repair. Kim et al.[20] have also shown that a double-row repair can be significantly stronger than a single-row repair, with suture anchors that are double-loaded for the lateral row. Notably, the maximum force that can be generated by the adult supraspinatus is 302 N[3]. The yield failure load for all repairs has exceeded this number, except for the single-row repair with double-loaded suture anchors, which on average showed a yield failure load of 265 N[7]; this would be sufficient for a 50% tear (maximal supraspinatus force estimated to be 151 N).

Given the above considerations, our approach to arthroscopic rotator cuff repair is guided by the size of tear in the anterior-posterior direction. Given the adult rotator cuff footprint is roughly 24 mm in the anterior-posterior direction,[24,25] we simplify the approach by dividing tear size into fourths: 6 mm, 12 mm, 18 mm, and 24 mm; the estimated footprint dimension in the medial-lateral direction is 12 mm.[24,25]

For a <6-mm tear, we advocate a single-anchor repair. Theoretically this leaves 75% of the footprint intact; the additional anchor should provide sufficient strength and would restore a large majority of the footprint. If the chronicity of tear reveals a retracted tendon, a side-to-side repair may be necessary to facilitate tendon closure.[26]

For a <12-mm tear, a single-row or double-row repair is preferred. If the patient is young and the tissue quality is satisfactory, a single-row may be sufficient. If the tissue (tendon or bone) is compromised, an additional row may be necessary to provide adequate strength. A transosseous-equivalent repair is considered when the far lateral tissue is compromised and the tear approaches 12 mm in size; usually only two-suture-bridges are necessary, which restores up to 62.3% of the entire footprint[22] and would be more than adequate in a <12-mm tear. Care should be taken to assess any partial thickness undersurface tears, which may mean that less than 50% of the footprint is intact. A suture-bridge technique may be the best option, as this has been shown to restore the most area at a repaired insertion compared to a double-row technique.[22] If retracted, care is taken to mobilize the tendon and maximize medialization of the suture anchors in order to reduce "tension mismatch"[27]; side-to-side repairs are used as necessary.

For a <18-mm tear, which may involve overlapping infraspinatus tendon posteriorly,[24] a double-row or suture-bridge technique is preferred. The majority of the footprint is bare in this situation, and restoration of footprint dimensions is sought to help maximize the potential for healing. If the tear is readily mobilized and the tissue quality is not questionable, a double-row repair would be adequate. Again, however, if the far lateral tissue is compromised, as is often

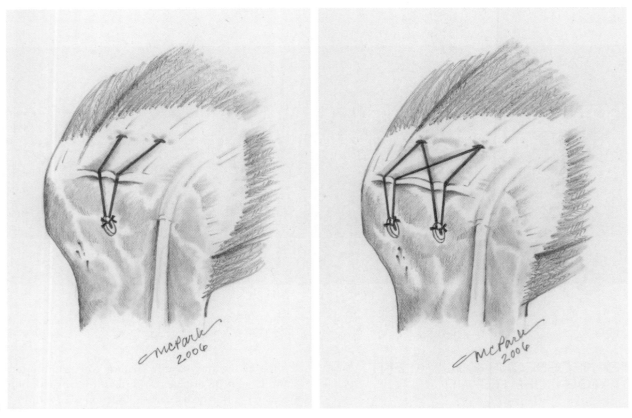

Fig. 9-7. Transosseous-equivalent repair using suture-bridges. **A:** Two-suture-bridge. **B:** Four-suture-bridge.

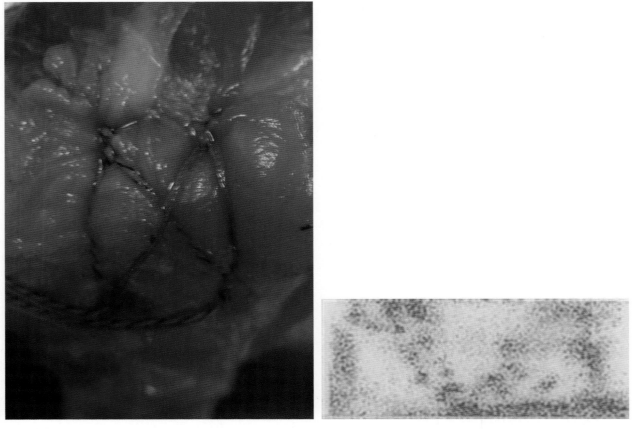

Fig. 9-8. A: Cadaveric specimen demonstrating a four-suture-bridge repair technique. **B:** Pressure-sensitive film demonstrating improved pressurized contact area.

the case in elderly patients or with chronic tears, the suture-bridge technique is preferred as this method does not rely on the lateral edge of torn tendon for fixation.[23] Tendon mobilization techniques are used for retracted tears, such as slides.[26] Re-creating the anterior and posterior "force couple" is a goal with tears that cannot be fully mobilized.[26]

For tears ≤24 mm (up to a complete tear of the supraspinatus, also involving the anterior portion of infraspinatus),[24] a suture-bridge technique is used. Four-suture-bridges are used to restore up to 77.6% of the footprint.[22] When the repair can be fully mobilized, the strength is significantly greater than a double-row technique, and gap formation is satisfactorily low.[23] However, when the goal is re-creating the force-couple, a transossesous-equivalent repair using only two-suture-bridges may be sufficient; if retraction is persistent, medialized single- or double-row techniques may be the best and only options.

Postoperatively, we immobilize the shoulder in 30 degrees of abduction, as this has been shown to reduce tension on the rotator cuff repair.[28,29] Passive range of motion is dictated by limits assessed intraoperatively. Supervised passive range of motion may begin at 0 to 6 weeks. Active exercises are initiated at 6 to 12 weeks depending on the patient's clinical progress. Progressive strengthening begins at roughly 12 weeks.

■ REFERENCES

17. Boileau P, Brassart N, Watkinson DJ, et al. Arthroscopic repair of full-thickness tears of the supraspinatus: does the tendon really heal? J Bone Joint Surg. 2005;87A(6):1229–1240.

18. Cofleld RH. Parvizi J, Hoffmeyer PJ, et al. Surgical repair of chronic rotator cuff tears; a prospective long-term study. J Bone Joint Surg. 2001;83A(1):71–77.

19. Apreleva M, Ozbaydar M, Fitzgibbons PG, et al. Rotator cuff tears: the effect of the reconstruction method on three-dimensional repair site area. Arthroscopy. 2002;18(5):519–526.

20. Kim DH, ElAttrache NS, Tibone JE, et al. A biomechanical analysis of a suture anchor rotator cuff footprint repair technique. Am J Sports Med. 2006 Mar;34(3):407–414.

21. Park MC. Cadet ER, Levine WN, et al. Tendon-to-bone pressure distributions at a repaired rotator cuff footprint using transosseous suture and suture anchor fixation techniques. Am J Sports Med. 2005;33(8):1154–1159.

22. Park MC, ElAttrache NS, Tibone JE, et al. Part I: Footprint contact characteristics for an arthroscopic transosseous-equivalent rotator cuff repair technique. 2005. Accepted Journal of Shoulder and Elbow Surgery.

23. Park MC, Tibone JE, ElAttrache NS, et al. Part II: Biomechanical assessment for a footprint-restoring arthroscopic transosseous-equivalent rotator cuff repair technique compared to a double-row technique. 2005. Accepted Journal of Shoulder and Elbow Surgery.

24. Minagawa H, Itoi E, Konno N, et al. Humeral attachment of the supraspinatus and infraspinatus tendons: an anatomic study. Arthroscopy. 1998;14(3):302–306.

25. Ruotolo C, Fow JE, Nottage WM. The supraspinatus footprint: an anatomic study of the supraspinatus insertion. Arthroscopy. 2004;20(3):246–249.

26. Lo IKY, Burkhart SS. Current concepts in arthroscopic rotator cuff repair. Am J Sports Med. 2003;31(2):308–324.

27. Burkhart SS, Johnson TC, Wirth MA, et al. Cyclic loading of transosseous rotator cuff repairs: tension overload as a possible cause of failure. Arthroscopy. 1997;13(2):172–176.

28. Hatakeyama Y, Itoi E, Pradhan RL, et al. Effect of arm elevation and rotation on the strain in the repaired rotator cuff tendon. Am J Sports Med. 2001;29(6):788–794.

29. Reilly P, Bull AMJ, Amis AA, et al. Passive tension and gap formation of rotator cuff repairs. J Shoulder Elbow Surg. 2004;13(6):664–647.

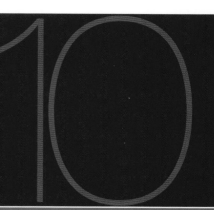

REPAIR OF PARTIAL-THICKNESS ARTICULAR-SURFACE ROTATOR CUFF TEARS

JOHN E. CONWAY, MD

■ HISTORY OF THE TECHNIQUE

In 1934, Ernest Amory Codman described partial-thickness, articular-surface rotator cuff tears involving the supraspinatus tendon as "rim rents" and expressed his confidence that "these rim rents account for the great majority of sore shoulders." He also accurately predicted that "these lesions never heal."[1,2] Stephen Snyder later called these defects partial-thickness articular-surface supraspinatus tendon avulsions and coined the term PASTA lesion **(Fig. 10-1)**. Since their original description, considerable attention has been placed on recognizing, understanding, and treating incomplete thickness rotator cuff tears. However, much controversy still exists and simply put, these tears vary widely in presentation. Although the significance of pattern and pathomechanics are now well recognized, the best methods for diagnosis and treatment are yet to be determined.

Several useful classifications for these tears are available. Ellman classified incomplete rotator cuff tears, based on location, as articular surface, bursal surface, or intratendinous and graded these lesions with measurements of both the depth and the area of the defect[3] **(Table 10-1)**. The grade classification was later revised to consider the depth of the tear as a percentage of the tendon.[4] Snyder proposed a similar classification that assigned a letter for each location and a number for grade in an effort to simplify the description of the lesion. In this system, the grade principally reflects the width of the defect, but also considers the presence of intratendinous delamination ("flap formation") and retraction.[5,6] Unfortunately, these classification systems are best suited to describe tears isolated to the supraspinatus tendon and consider neither the pathomechanics involved nor the significance of anterior/posterior location of the tear as important elements. Several pathomechanisms have been recently proposed for anteriorly located partial thickness tears that involve the upper subscapularis tendon[7,8] and Habermeyer et al.[7] have proposed a classification system that considers associated pathology. Similarly, the relatively posterior and intratendinous tear pattern commonly reported in young overhead throwing athletes has been recently graded for severity based on depth, width, and delamination in an attempt to provide prognosis and direction for treatment.[9]

A complete discussion of the pathomechanics of rotator cuff disease would exceed the scope of this article; however, there are several factors contributing to the articular-surface location of some incomplete tears that warrant description.[8,10–18] The articular surface of the rotator cuff has fewer arterioles and overall less vascularity than the bursa surface. The articular surface has a higher modulus of elasticity and therefore greater stiffness than the bursa surface. Eccentric forces tend to be concentrated more in the articular surface. Bursal surface contact of the rotator cuff against the margin of the acromion may produce tensile undersurface fiber failure. And finally, the articular surface has a less favorable stress strain curve than the bursal surface. The pathomechanics explaining associated intratendinous tears are less clear but probably involve shear within the five-layered architecture of the rotator cuff tendon.[15–17,19–23]

■ INDICATIONS AND CONTRAINDICATIONS

Débridement of the torn rotator cuff tendon has been recommended in order to stimulate a healing response,[24] and some authors have suggested that acromioplasty without tendon repair would provide good surgical outcomes.[6,25,26] However, Weber[27] reported that, on second-look arthroscopy

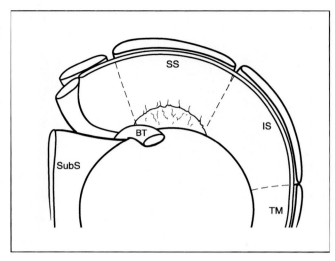

Fig. 10-1. Diagram demonstrating the common tear location for partial-thickness articular-surface supraspinatus tendon avulsion injuries (PASTA lesion). SubS, subscapularis tendon; BT, biceps tendon; SS, supraspinatus tendon; IS, infraspinatus tendon; TM, teres minor tendon. (Modified and reprinted with permission from Conway JE. The management of partial thickness rotator cuff tears in throwers. Oper Tech Sport Med. 2002;10(2):75–85.)

following arthroscopic rotator cuff tear débridement, "healing . . . was never observed." Fukuda et al.[21] also reported that "apparent evidence of spontaneous repair" of joint sided partial rotator cuff tears "was absent." It is probable that the continued separation of the torn tendon edges, the poor vascularity of the involved tissues,[3,28] and the formation of a synovial covering, both on the visibly exposed segment of the tear and within the intratendinous segment of the tear,[23,28,29] precludes any potential for spontaneous healing or healing following simple arthroscopic débridement.[23,27]

Progression of both the depth of the articular-surface tear and the extent of the intratendinous tear is of considerable concern, and rotator cuff repair may be advisable for the long-term function of the shoulder in some patients.[5,27,29–35] However, the percentage of depth, width, and delamination of the tear that calls for repair, using either open or arthroscopic methods, is controversial.[25,27,29,33,36] Because of the

risk for both tear progression and less satisfactory surgical outcomes, some authors have suggested that partial thickness rotator cuff tears >50% of the thickness of the tendon should be repaired.[3,25,27,30,37,38] Conversely, others have argued that in some patients, particularly overhead athletes, repair potentially increases the morbidity of the procedure and that 75% was a more reasonable depth mitigating for repair.[9,39] Finally, while many have suggested that tear completion and bursal side repair are reasonable for small full thickness tears, controversy still exists regarding the efficacy of such treatment for incomplete tears.

With such variable presentation, there is certainly no "most appropriate" method to surgically manage all partial thickness articular surface rotator cuff tears, and, of course, articular side repair methods will differ greatly from bursal side repair methods. Many factors affect the treatment decision process, and some of these include the tear size, location, depth, delamination, retraction, and chronicity as well as the tissue quality, bone density, and associated shoulder conditions. The patient's age, medical condition, smoking history, occupation, avocation, and expectations are also important. Finally, the surgeon's interest, training, experience, and skill in arthroscopic rotator cuff repair methods must be considered. This article will simply present a modification of a previously described articular side method for the arthroscopic repair of a deep partial thickness articular surface rotator cuff tear involving the supraspinatus tendon.[5,9–11]

■ SURGICAL TECHNIQUE

The patient is positioned in the 30-degree posterior-lateral decubitus position with 20 degrees Fowler's tilt and the arm is suspended with 10 pounds traction through a shoulder traction device that allows for manual application of shoulder abduction. Following routine shoulder prep, landmarks and portal sites are outlined (**Fig. 10-2**). During creation of the posterior portal, penetrate the posterior capsule parallel to the glenoid and along the middle of the glenoid rim. A superior or medial portal position may limit visualization during rotator cuff repair. On arthroscopic examination of the glenohumeral joint, observe any

TABLE 10-1	Ellman Classification for Partial Thickness Rotator Cuff Tears		
Location	**Grade**	**Revised grade**	**Area of defect**
A: Articular surface	1: <3 mm deep	1: Fraying	Base of tear (mm) ×
B: Bursal surface	2: 3–6 mm deep	2: <50% depth	Max retraction (mm) =
C: Interstitial	3: >6 mm deep	3: >50% depth	Area in mm²

Sources: Ellman H. Diagnosis and treatment of incomplete rotator cuff tears. Clin Orthop. 1990;254:64–74; Ellman H, Gartsman GM, Hengst TC, eds. *Arthroscopic Shoulder Surgery and Related Procedures*. Philadelphia: Lea and Febiger Publishers; 1993.

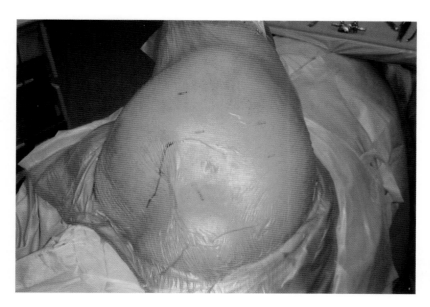

Fig. 10-2. Photograph of a patient in the lateral decubitus position with the shoulder prepped for arthroscopy. Landmarks and proposed arthroscopic portals are outlined.

apparent articular surface "draping" or "pillowing" of either the supraspinatus or infraspinatus tendon, as this may represent occult intratendinous delamination. A probe may be used to define the extent of the intratendinous tear. Also be aware that reduction of the articular surface margin to the tuberosity may increase the relative depth of a small intratendinous tear, creating a need for transtendinous mattress sutures following tendon-to-bone repair.

With the shoulder suspended in the typical lateral decubitus traction position, both visualization of and access to the torn tendon margins and the greater tuberosity are limited. However, increasing glenohumeral abduction will separate the torn edge of the rotator cuff tendon away from the humerus and provide better exposure of both the tendon and the tuberosity **(Fig. 10-3)**. Unfortunately, even the improved access gained by glenohumeral abduction may be insufficient to allow complete access to these structures. Since suture anchor placement will require a lateral transtendinous portal, this same portal may be used to provide the necessary access to the tendon and tuberosity **(Fig. 10-4A,B)**. An 18-gauge spinal needle placed in a transcutaneous manner through the deepest segment of the tear will identify the site along the lateral margin of the acromion for portal placement. The fibers of both the deltoid and the tendon are then split using a no.11 blade on a no. 7 blade handle producing a 5 to 6 mm portal through the tendon. This step appears to minimize the trauma to the remaining intact fibers of the cuff tendon and a cannula is rarely necessary. By placing an anchor adjacent to the tendon portal and appropriately passing the anchor sutures, the portal will be closed when sutures are tied in the subacromial space.

Limit the extent of tendon débridement to preserve tissue for repair, but remove obviously diseased and poor quality tissue. Optimally, the articular margin of the tear should be directly repaired to the articular margin to the tuberosity and adequate mobility of the tendon edge may be confirmed using an arthroscopic soft tissue grasping instrument placed through the transtendinous portal. However, as there may be considerable loss of the articular surface tendon fibers following débridement, reasonable expectations must be preserved during suture placement. When required, mobility of the supraspinatus tendon is improved by release of both the tendon and the coracohumeral ligament from the base of the coracoid using a combination of biting instruments, shavers, and ablators. Remember to remain aware of the location and vulnerability

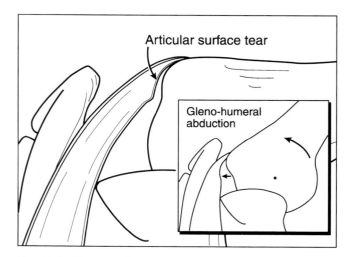

Fig. 10-3. Diagram of a coronal view of an articular surface tear in the supraspinatus tendon with the glenohumeral joint positioned in both adduction and abduction (*inset*) demonstrating the improved visualization of the rotator cuff tendon tear and the greater tuberosity with abduction. (Modified and reprinted with permission from Conway JE. The management of partial thickness rotator cuff tears in throwers. Oper Tech Sport Med. 2002; 10(2):75–85.)

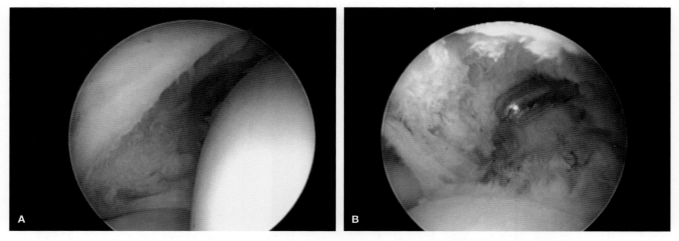

Fig. 10-4. Arthroscopic photographs of an articular surface tear in the supraspinatus tendon with the glenohumeral joint positioned in both adduction **(A)** and abduction **(B)** demonstrating the improved visualization of the rotator cuff tendon tear and the greater tuberosity with abduction. A transtendinous portal has been created in the lateral segment of the tear allowing introduction of a mechanical shaver for debridement of the tuberosity.

of the suprascapular nerve. When significant intratendinous delamination is recognized, the rotator cuff repair will need to be accomplished in two segments, performing tendon-to-bone repair first. A simple method for intratendinous repair has been previously described.[5,37]

Subacromial impingement is widely considered to be a common cause for articular surface rotator cuff tears. As such, many patients requiring PASTA lesion repair will have either moderate or marked hypertrophy of the subacromial and subdeltoid bursa. Since the repair method described here requires that sutures are passed blindly through the subacromial space and since these same sutures must be safely identified and protected within the subacromial space, it is well advised that the surgeon complete the bursectomy before beginning suture anchor placement. Acromioplasty may be delayed until after tendon repair is completed when hemostasis within the subacromial space is a concern.

Next, the need for either one or two rows of suture anchors is determined, and appropriate suture anchor sites are identified. My preference has been to use two rows of suture anchors when the depth of the tear exceeds 75% **(Fig. 10-5)**. Typically the PASTA lesion tear pattern will be wider along the articular margin, thus requiring a greater number of anchors in the medial row than in the lateral low. However, the lateral anchors should be introduced first as this will allow for the manipulation of sutures without loss of visualization of the tuberosity. As noted above, glenohumeral abduction facilitates visualization of and access to the supraspinatus tendon insertion site onto the greater tuberosity, and this position is certainly useful during both abrasion of the tuberosity and capture of the tendon-to-bone sutures. However, because of the angle to the humeral head and the potential for

subchondral penetration, insertion of the suture anchors should be done with minimal glenohumeral abduction (Fig. 10-5).

Select the suture anchor type based on bone quality, site location, and surgeon preference. Bioabsorbable anchors are often preferred in this setting and have several potential advantages over metal anchors, including improved postoperative magnetic resonance imaging (MRI). Test the security of the anchor fixation with longitudinal traction on the

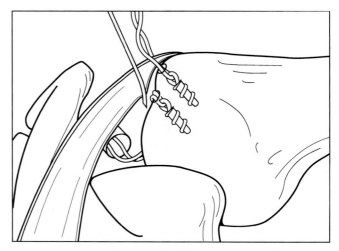

Fig. 10-5. Diagram showing two suture anchors inserted using a trans-tendinous method as described in the text. The lateral row sutures have been passed through the tendon while the medial row sutures exit an anterior cannula. Either straight or curved hollow needles are used to retrieve the sutures through the tendon. (Modified and reprinted with permission from Conway JE. The management of partial thickness rotator cuff tears in throwers. Oper Tech Sport Med. 2002;10(2):75–85.)

sutures and confirm that the suture anchor islet remains well beneath the surface of the bone. When the bone is less dense, metal anchors may be more appropriate. Following anchor placement, both limbs of the paired sutures are passed into the glenohumeral joint using a suture retriever through the transtendinous portal and then withdrawn into the anterior cannula. The suture pairs are divided for exposure and capture.

The sutures are then captured and placed through the tendon using a modification of a transcutaneous method previously described by Snyder[5] for the repair of Snyder classification type A4 anterior articular-surface flap tears. Although many instruments are available for this purpose, I have been most satisfied using one of two hollow needle options. The first option makes use of straight and curved Meniscal Mender II (Instrument Makar, Inc, Okemos, MI) needles and a Shuttle Relay (Linvatec, Inc, Largo, FL). The second option makes use of straight and curved Arthrex MiniLasso Suture Retrievers (Arthrex, Inc, Naples, FL).

The tendon is reduced to the greater tuberosity with a soft tissue grasper, and appropriate suture placement is determined. A hollow suture-passing needle is then passed though both the skin and the tendon into the joint space. The sutures are captured and withdrawn through the tendon using the suture-retrieving loop **(Fig. 10-6A,B)**. Although the individual suture limbs may be passed together or separately, my preference is to pass the sutures through the tendon together in pairs directly above the suture anchor tunnel in an effort to ensure that both the sutures will slide in the anchor islet during suture tying. This option may potentially produce tighter loops.

When the lateral row anchors have been introduced and the paired sets of suture have been passed through the tendon, the steps are repeated for the medial row. The anterior anchors are implanted first in order to more easily manage the suture pairs within the joint. Remember to observe the suture anchor entry angle as subchondral penetration risk is greater for the medial row anchors. For this row, an effort is made to place the suture-passing needles through thick healthy appearing tissue at the margins of the articular surface tear. The suture pairs are separated approximately 1 cm apart across the tendon fibers directly over the suture anchor tunnel and then drawn through the tendon utilizing the method described for the lateral suture row **(Fig. 10-7A,B)**. A soft tissue grasper may be employed to mobilize the tendon to the tuberosity while identifying proper suture placement. After the last sutures are placed, the tendon defect should appear filled with crossing suture pairs **(Fig. 10-8)**. Be aware that it is easy to underestimate the extent of retraction in the posterior margin of the tear, resulting in sutures placed too anterior for anatomic tendon repair. Finally, be certain that reduction of the tendon edge has not created an intratendinous defect that will require concomitant repair.

Externally, the suture pairs exit the skin surrounding the transtendinous portal site and should be separated approximately 1 cm apart **(Fig. 10-9)**. Within the subacromial space, the suture pairs exit the bursal side of the tendon where they are easily identified and separated for tying. My preference has been to tie the lateral suture pairs first.

Tight suture loops and secure knots are paramount to tendon repair success. Although many factors are important, mobilization of the tendon from the scapula, reduction of the torn tendon edge to the tuberosity, accurate alignment of the suture pairs over the suture anchor tunnel, and capture of healthy tendon tissue are essential. In addition, the suture must slide easily through the tendon and the anchor eyelet. To that end, the anchor eyelet must be aligned with the

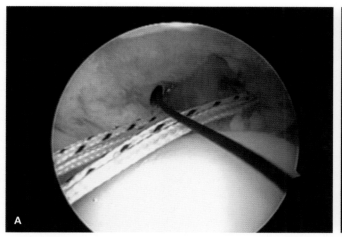 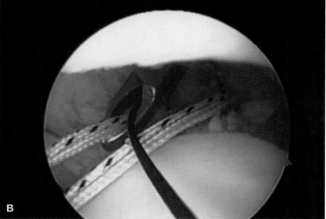

Fig. 10-6. Arthroscopic photographs demonstrating initial suture placement for the lateral suture anchor. A hollow needle placed through the tendon allows introduction of a suture retrieving loop **(A)**. Limbs of both suture pairs and the suture-retrieving loop are captured together with a suture retriever **(B)** and the sutures are passed through the tendon.

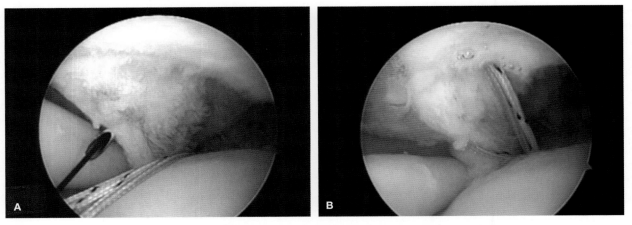

Fig. 10-7. Arthroscopic photographs demonstrating appropriate positioning of a suture passing needle **(A)** and paired sutures **(B)** for the first of two medial row suture anchors.

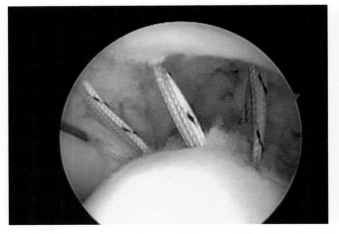

Fig. 10-8. Arthroscopic photograph demonstrating the apparent filling of the rotator cuff tendon defect with suture pairs using the method described in the text. One anchor was place laterally and two were placed medially positioning six sutures for tendon-to-bone repair.

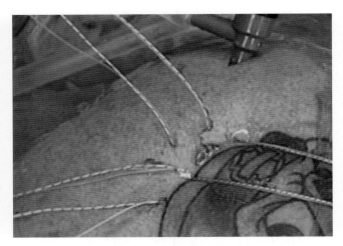

Fig. 10-9. Photograph of six sutures surrounding an arthroscopic portal along the lateral margin of the acromion.

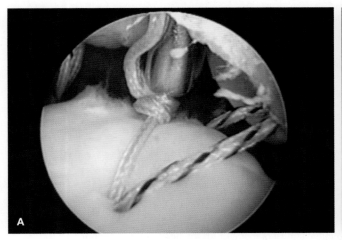

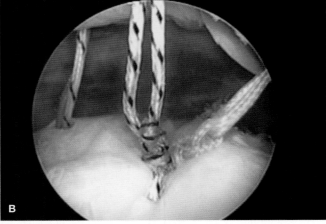

Fig. 10-10. Arthroscopic photographs demonstrating the reduction of the tendon and the sutures over the respective suture anchor tunnel using lateral traction on one suture pair while tying the second suture pair **(A)**. The sutures are exchanged and the second suture pair is similarly tied **(B)**.

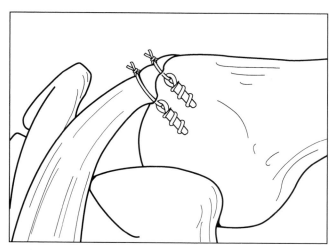

Fig. 10-11. Diagram of a coronal view of a repaired articular-surface tear in the supraspinatus tendon using two rows of suture anchors. (Modified and reprinted with permission from Conway JE. The management of partial thickness rotator cuff tears in throwers. Oper Tech Sport Med. 2002;10(2):75–85.)

direction of the suture passing through the tendon; the suture must pass through the tendon, through the eyelet, and back through the tendon without twisting or crossing; and the suture knot must be tied through the same portal through which the respective anchor was inserted. When two sutures must slide in the same islet, tension must be maintained on the second suture pair to prevent entanglement in the soft tissue or the other suture. Finally, a knot pusher must be used to tighten the loop before locking the knot, and, of course, the surgeon must be able to reliably tie secure arthroscopic knots.

A simple technique to achieve these elements in the repair process is as follows. Using the method described above, for each suture anchor there are two suture pairs passing together through the tendon. Forcefully retracting both

limbs of one suture pair, "the traction suture," in the far lateral portal, optimally positions the torn tendon for direct reduction to the tuberosity and aligns the suture set to be tied, "the tying suture," over the respective suture anchor tunnel. The tying suture is then drawn through the transtendinous lateral portal with a suture retriever, which positions this tying suture in line with the suture anchor tunnel. The tying suture is then tied using any reliable method. The suture sets are exchanged in the portals, and the second suture is tied **(Fig. 10-10A,B)**. Both sutures are cut and attention is turned to the next suture pair.

After all sutures have been tied, the repair is tested with humeral rotation and glenohumeral abduction **(Fig. 10-11)**. Secure attachment of the tendon to the greater tuberosity should be observed. Finally, return the arthroscope to the glenohumeral joint and similarly observe the repair while rotating the shoulder. The margin of the tear should appear stable and well seated against the tuberosity **(Fig. 12A,B)**. When intratendinous delamination extends medially <2 to 3 cm, transtendinous mattress sutures placed with arthroscopic methods will probably provide adequate fixation for tissue healing.

Supraspinatus outlet impingement symptoms are commonly reported in patients with articular surface rotator cuff tears, and subacromial decompression should be considered in selected cases. Be aware that controversy remains regarding the need for and extent of acromial resection.[39–46] Furthermore, outlet impingement is common but rarely the primary cause of shoulder pain in young overhead athletes,[40,41] and published treatment methods that included acromioplasty failed to yield good results.[39–41,46] In some patients, subacromial decompression may be accomplished by simply thinning a hypertrophic coracoacromial ligament with an ablator. However, relative indications for an acromioplasty include the following: coracoacromial ligament abrasion, bursal-surface rotator cuff tear, anterior location of the articular-surface tear, near full-thickness articular-

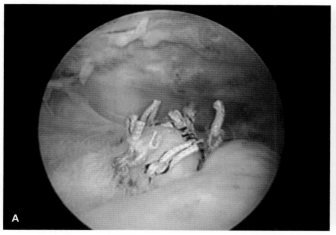
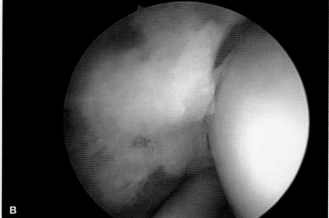

Fig. 10-12. Arthroscopic photographs of the completed repair as view from the bursal surface **(A)** and the articular surface **(B)**.

surface tear, extensive intratendinous tear, sagittal-oblique MRI demonstrating a prominent anterior edge of the acromion, positive subacromial impingement signs, and age >30 years.

■ REHABILITATION

An UltraSling shoulder immobilizer (dj Orthopedics, LLC, Vista, CA) is applied in the operating room and worn for 3 weeks. The immobilizer is removed several times a day for gentle passive motion exercises, avoiding horizontal extension and external rotation while the shoulder is abducted. Range of motion is evaluated frequently in the office or in therapy during the first 2 weeks. Early joint stiffness and motion loss are treated by a physical therapist with gentle stretching exercises. No shoulder rotation above 60 degrees of glenohumeral abduction is allowed until 3 weeks following surgery. Glenohumeral abduction in the scapular plane and glenohumeral external rotation without abduction are considered the two most important planes of motion to recover during the first week following surgery.

Lower extremity, trunk, and scapula exercises are begun immediately. At 3 to 4 weeks, passive motion is usually recovered, and a supervised strengthening program for the shoulder begins and continues under the direction of a physical therapist. Progress is made toward recovering internal and external rotation strength with the glenohumeral joint adducted before active abduction exercises begin.

■ FUTURE DIRECTIONS

MRI studies and arthroscopic methods may continue to improve, allowing earlier detection and repair of partial thickness rotator cuff tears that exceed 50% depth. Better understanding of the tear morphology and pathomechanisms that lead to tear progression will guide future decisions regarding treatment options.

■ REFERENCES

1. Codman EA. *The Shoulder*. Boston: Thomas Todd Publishers; 1934.
2. Codman EA, Akerson ID. The pathology associated with rupture of the supraspinatus tendon. Ann Surg. 1931;93:348.
3. Ellman H. Diagnosis and treatment of incomplete rotator cuff tears. Clin Orthop. 1990;254:64–74.
4. Ellman H, Gartsman GM, Hengst TC, eds. *Arthroscopic Shoulder Surgery and Related Procedures*. Philadelphia: Lea and Febiger Publishers; 1993.
5. Snyder SJ. Arthroscopic evaluation and treatment of the rotator cuff. In: *Shoulder Arthroscopy*. New York: McGraw-Hill; 1994: 133–168.
6. Snyder SJ, Pachelli AF, Del Pizzo W, et al. Partial thickness rotator cuff tears: results of arthroscopic treatment. Arthroscopy. 1991;7:1–7.
7. Habermeyer P, Magosch P, Pritsch M, et al. Anterosuperior impingement of the shoulder as a result of pulley lesions: a prospective arthroscopic study. J Shoulder Elbow Surg. 2004;13:5–12.
8. Lo IKY, Burkhart SS. Combined subcoracoid and subacromial impingement in association with anterior superior rotator cuff tears: An arthroscopic approach. Arthroscopy, 2003;19(10):1142–1150.
9. Conway JE, Singleton SB. Posterior articular-surface intratendinous rotator cuff tears in throwers. In: Krishnan S, Hawkins R, Warren R, eds. *The Shoulder and the Overhead Athlete*. Philadelphia: Lippincott Williams and Wilkins; 2004:135–145.
10. Conway JE. Arthroscopic repair of partial-thickness rotator cuff tears and SLAP lesions in professional baseball players. Oper Tech Sport Med. 2000;8:281–292.
11. Conway JE. The management of partial thickness rotator cuff tears in throwers. Oper Tech Sport Med. 2002;10(2):75–85.
12. Lehman RC, Perry CR. Arthroscopic surgery for partial rotator cuff tears. Arthroscopy. 2003;19:1–4.
13. Snyder SJ. Technique of arthroscopic rotator cuff repair using implantable 4 mm Revo suture anchors, suture shuttle relays, and no. 2 nonabsorbable mattress sutures. Orthop Clin North Amer. 1997;28(2):267–275.
14. Walch G. Posterosuperior glenoid impingement. In: Burkhead WZ Jr, ed. *Rotator Cuff Disorders*. Baltimore: Williams and Wilkins; 1996:193–198.
15. Jobe CM. Current concepts: superior glenoid impingement. Clin Orthop. 1996;330:98–107.
16. Lohr JF, Uhthoff HK. The pathogenesis of degenerative rotator cuff tears. Orthop Trans. 1987;11:237.
17. Neer CS II: Anterior acromioplasty for classic impingement syndrome in the shoulder: a preliminary report. J Bone Joint Surg. 1972;50A:41–50.
18. Walch G, Levigne C. Treatment of deep surface partial-thickness tears of the supraspinatus in patients under 30 years of age. In: Gazielly DF, Gleyze P, Thomas T, eds. *The Cuff*. Paris: Elsevier; 1997:243–244.
19. Clark JM, Harryman DT II. Tendons, ligaments, and capsule of the rotator cuff. J Bone Joint Surg. 1992;74A:713–725.
20. Nakajima T, Rokuuma N, Hamada K, et al. Histologic and biomechanical characteristics of the supraspinatous tendon: Reference to rotator cuff tearing. J Shoulder Elbow Surg. 1994;3:79–87.
21. Fukuda H, Hamada K, Yamada N, et al. Pathology and pathogenesis of partial-thickness cuff tears. In: Gazielly DF, Gleyze P, Thomas T, eds. *The Cuff*. Paris: Elsevier; 1997:234–237.
22. Yamanaka K, Fukuda H. Ageing process of the supraspinatus tendon with reference to rotator cuff tears. In: Watson MS, ed. *Surgical Disorders of the Shoulder*. Edinburgh: Churchill Livingstone; 1991:247–258.
23. Sonnabend DH, Yu Y, Howlett R, et al. Laminated tears of the human rotator cuff: A histologic and immunochemical study. J Shoulder Elbow Surg. 2001;10:109–115.
24. Andrews JR, Broussard TS, Carson WG. Arthroscopy of the shoulder in the management of partial tears of the rotator cuff: a preliminary report. Arthroscopy. 1985;1:117–122.
25. Cordasco FA, Backer M, Craig EV, et al. The partial-thickness rotator cuff tear: is acromioplasty without repair sufficient? Amer J Sports Med. 2002;30:257–260.
26. Montgomery TJ, Yerger B, Savoie FH. Management of rotator cuff tears: a comparison of arthroscopic debridement and surgical repair. J Shoulder Elbow Surg. 1994;3:70–78.
27. Weber SC. Arthroscopic debridement and acromioplasty versus mini-open repair in the treatment of significant partial-thickness rotator cuff tears. Arthroscopy. 1999;15(2):126–131.
28. Fukuda H, Hamada K, Nakajima T, et al. Partial-thickness tears of the rotator cuff. International Ortho. 1996;20:257–265.
29. Sonnabend D, Watson E. Structural factors affecting the outcome of rotator cuff repair. J Shoulder Elbow Surg. 2002;11:212–218.

30. Gartsman GM, Milne JC. Articular surface partial-thickness rotator cuff tears. J Shoulder Elbow Surg. 1995;4:409–415.
31. Lyons TR, Savoie FH III, Field LD. Arthroscopic repair of partial-thickness tears of the rotator cuff. Arthroscopy. 2001;17(2):219–223.
32. Gschwend N, Ivosevic-Radovanovic D, Patte D. Rotator cuff tear: Relationship between clinical and anatomopathologic findings. Arch Orthop Trauma Surg. 1988;107:7–15.
33. Reilly P, Amis AA, Wallace AL, et al. Supraspinatus tears: propagation and strain alteration. J Shoulder Elbow Surg. 2003;12:134–138.
34. Yamanaka K, Matsumoto T. The joint side tear of the rotator cuff: a followup study by arthrography. Clin Orthop. 1994;304:68–73.
35. Bey MJ, Ramsey ML, Soslowsky LJ. Intratendinous strain fields of the supraspinatus tendon: effect of a surgically created articular-surface rotator cuff tear. J Shoulder Elbow Surg. 2002;11:562–569.
36. Graham SM, Yang BY, McMahon PJ, et al. A threshold rotator cuff tear size may predispose to further tearing: a biomechanical study using an animal model. J Bone Joint Surg, British: unpublished data.
37. Paulos LE, Kody MH. Arthroscopically enhanced "mini-approach" to rotator cuff repair. Amer J Sports Med. 1994;22:19–25.
38. Miller SL, Hazrati Y, Cornwall R, et al. Failed surgical management of partial thickness rotator cuff tears. Orthopedics. 2002;25(11):1255–1257.
39. Tibone J. Surgical treatment of tears of the rotator cuff in athletes. J Bone Joint Surg. 1986;68A:887–891.
40. Roye R, Grana WA, Yates CK. Arthroscopic subacromial decompression: Two- to seven-year follow-up. Arthroscopy. 1995;11:301–306.
41. Tibone J, Jobe FW, Kerlan RK, et al. Shoulder impingement syndrome in athletes treated by an anterior acromioplasty. Clin Orthop. 1985;198:135–140.
42. Gartsman, GM. Arthroscopic acromioplasty for lesions of the rotator cuff. J Bone Joint Surg. 1990;72A(2):75–80.
43. Ogilvie-Harris DJ, Wiley AM. Arthroscopic surgery of the shoulder. J Bone Joint Surg. 1986;68B:201.
44. Nottage WM. Rotator cuff repair with or without acromioplasty. Arthroscopy. 2003;19:229–232.
45. Angelo RL. Controversies in arthroscopic shoulder surgery: arthroscopic versus open Bankart repair, thermal treatment of capsular tissue, acromioplasties—are they necessary? 2003;19: 224–228.
46. Burns TP, Turba JE. Arthroscopic treatment of shoulder impingement in athletes. Amer J Sports Med. 1992;20:13–16.

SUBSCAPULARIS REPAIR: OPEN SURGICAL TECHNIQUE

SUMANT G. KRISHNAN, MD, SCOTT D. PENNINGTON, MD,
WAYNE Z. BURKHEAD, JR, MD

■ HISTORY OF THE TECHNIQUE

The subscapularis muscle is a strong internal rotator of the humerus, especially when the arm is in a position of abduction. It also functions as a dynamic stabilizer of the glenohumeral joint. In concert with the other rotator cuff muscles (especially the infraspinatus), the subscapularis depresses the humeral head, allowing the deltoid to elevate the arm as part of the biomechanical force-couple required for active anterior elevation.[1]

The first report documenting the existence of a subscapularis tendon rupture was by Smith[2,3] in 1834, who documented rotator cuff and associated subscapularis tendon ruptures in seven cadaveric specimens. The first documented repair of a subscapularis rupture came almost a century later. Hauser,[4] in 1954, described a repair technique using bone troughs and transosseous sutures through bone tunnels for the subscapularis tendon. Despite this recognition, subscapularis tendon ruptures as an isolated entity received little attention until the past two decades. Gerber and Krushell[5] described a cohort of patients who sustained an isolated disruption of the subscapularis as a result of a traumatic forced external rotation of the involved arm without a concomitant glenohumeral joint dislocation. The success of the operative treatment described by Gerber et al.[6] for this unique injury has led others to confirm the disability associated with, efficacy of early recognition for, and success of surgical treatment for this condition.

■ CLINICAL PRESENTATION AND EVALUATION

Patients presenting with an isolated tear of the subscapularis tendon typically are younger than patients with the more common degenerative tendinopathy and tearing of the remainder of the rotator cuff.[5,7,8] Most of these patients have suffered a traumatic injury. There are four documented traumatic mechanisms of injury for isolated rupture of the subscapularis tendon[9,10]:

1 Fall directly on the shoulder not associated with a dislocation;
2 Rupture associated with an anterior dislocation of the shoulder;
3 Violent external rotation injury with the arm in an adducted position;
4 Violent hyperextension injury.

Patients usually present with night pain and pain that produces significant functional limitations. They often complain of pain both with the arm at the side and with elevation. Another common complaint is pain and weakness when reaching behind for a wallet in a pants pocket. In the largest reported series, all patients documented pain with the arm below the shoulder, pain with the arm in the overhead position, anterior shoulder pain at night, and weakness of the upper extremity.[6]

Physical Examination

Physical examination of the patient with a subscapularis tendon rupture demonstrates increased external rotation (usually by 10 degrees to 30 degrees) compared to the contralateral side. A positive liftoff or "belly press" test is also present **(Fig. 11-1A,B)**. Recent electromyographic evidence demonstrates that the liftoff appears to preferentially isolate the lower portion of the subscapularis, and the belly press isolates the upper portion of the subscapularis.[11]

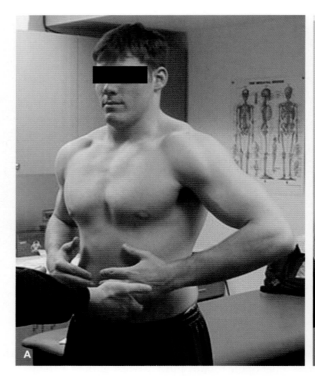
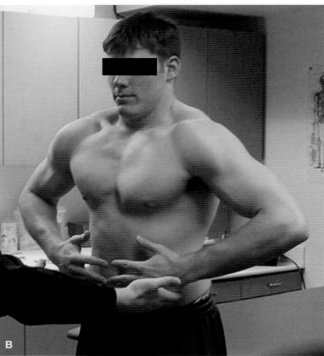

Fig. 11-1. The belly press test. **A:** Right, positive belly press test. Note that the elbow goes posterior to the trunk with the patient unable to maintain internal rotation. **B:** Left, note that the patient is able to maintain internal rotation and the elbow is maintained anterior to the trunk.

Imaging

Plain radiographs are usually normal, though in the chronic case the axillary view may demonstrate static anterior subluxation.[12–14] Magnetic resonance imaging (MRI) or computed tomography (CT) with arthrographic dye are the gold standard tests for radiographic confirmation of the subscapularis tendon tear.[15,16] MRI demonstrates the condition of the tendon, partial or full thickness tearing, and atrophy and fatty degeneration of the muscle.

■ INDICATIONS AND CONTRAINDICATIONS

Surgical repair of the subscapularis is indicated in any full-thickness tear without fatty degeneration of the muscle, unless medically contraindicated. Recent published literature documents the efficacy of early recognition and surgical treatment for this condition due to the pain and functional deficits that may arise from a chronically disrupted tendon.[6,8]

Contraindications to primary repair include complete fatty degeneration of the subscapularis muscle, as in a long-standing chronic situation. In such a case, where primary repair is fraught with a high incidence of rerupture, pectoralis major tendon transfer is the operation of choice.

■ SURGICAL TECHNIQUE

The deltopectoral approach provides maximum exposure to the subscapularis muscle. The tendon is often retracted inferiorly and medially and scarred, requiring extensive mobilization. The axillary nerve can be identified and protected

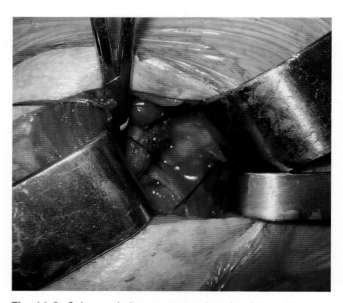

Fig. 11-2. Subscapularis tear retracted to glenoid rim. Note that the conjoined tendon has been released and retracted.

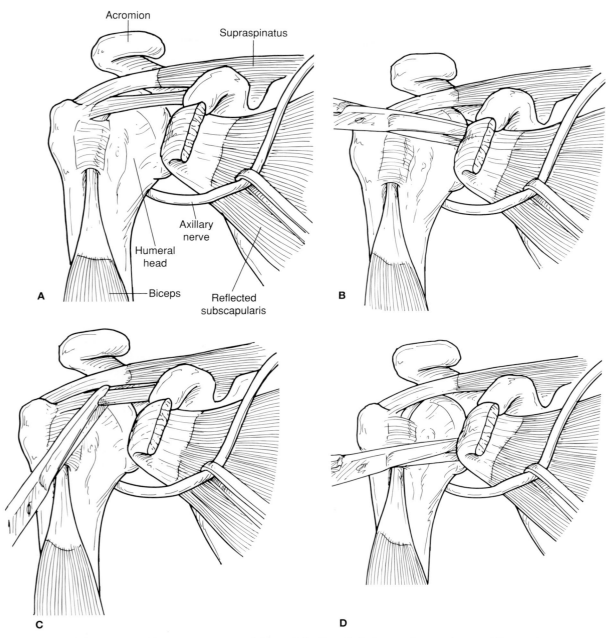

Fig. 11-3. A: Subscapularis prepared for mobilization. **B:** Release of coracohumeral ligament. **C:** Release of anterior capsule. **D:** Release of inferior capsule (protecting axillary nerve).

with this approach. The deltoid splitting approach does not allow safe access to the inferior most reaches of the glenohumeral joint for identification of the axillary nerve or mobilization of the muscle-tendon unit, but is satisfactory for upper subscapularis tears seen in conjunction with anterosuperior cuff lesions.

After identifying the interval between the deltoid and pectoralis major muscles, the clavipectoral fascia is divided at the lateral aspect of the muscular portion of the conjoined tendon. The conjoined tendon is then retracted medially to expose the retracted and torn subscapularis tendon. If the subscapularis is severely scarred and retracted, the conjoined

tendon is divided approximately 4 mm distal to the coracoid process and retracted medially. This permits visualization of the retracted subscapularis tendon, avoiding blind placement of clamps near the neurovascular bundle **(Fig. 11-2)**.

A thin layer of tissue may either be attached to the lesser tuberosity or continue anterior to the tuberosity to the lateral ridge of the bicipital groove. This often is scarred bursa. The edge of the subscapularis tendon is tagged with heavy suture. A 360-degree mobilization of the tendon is performed, especially in chronic cases, starting with the release of any residual inferior muscular attachment **(Fig. 11-3A,B,C,D)**. The humeroscapular interface is released with a

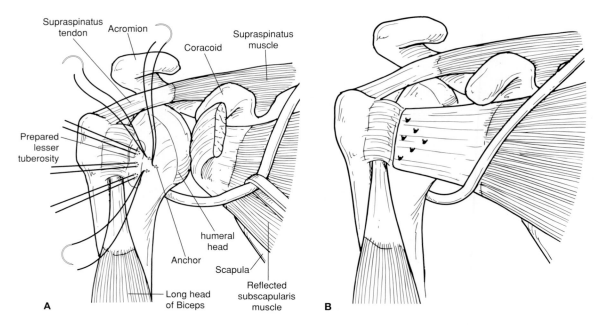

Fig. 11-4. A: Preparation of the bony surface for reattachment of the subscapularis tendon. A burr is used to prepare the lesser tuberosity to a bleeding surface for reattachment of the subscapularis tendon. Suture anchors are placed along the prepared lesser tuberosity in a triangular fashion and sutures are passed through medial portion of subscapularis tendon in a mattress fashion. **B:** Two-row (medial and lateral fixation) repair completed after tying suture anchor mattress sutures by reattachment of lateral portion of tendon with simple sutures.

combination of blunt and sharp dissections. The subscapularis tendon is released superiorly from the coracohumeral ligament attachment and inferiorly from the glenohumeral capsular attachment. An intra-articular release of the anterior glenohumeral capsule completes mobilization of the tendon.

The biceps tendon is frequently found medially subluxed out of its groove with subscapularis ruptures.[17] It is often frayed with evidence of tendon degeneration. When this condition exists, a tenodesis is performed. The technique for the tenodesis involves cauterizing the bicipital groove followed by burring the groove to bleeding bone. The tendon is tenodesed with mattress sutures from one or two Mitek Fastin 5.0 double-loaded suture anchors (DepuyMitek, Johnson & Johnson, Norwood, Mass) in the groove with the tendon at its correct length to restore biceps myotension. When the tendon is normal it can be replaced in the groove and the aperture reconstructed, though this is rarely the case.

To reattach the subscapularis, the lesser tuberosity is exposed and cleaned of soft tissue. A burr is then used to expose bleeding bone at the footprint of the subscapularis where the tendon will make contact with the humerus. Usually, three Mitek Fastin 5.0 double-loaded suture anchors or Mitek G2 suture anchors (DepuyMitek, Johnson & Johnson, Norwood, Mass) are then placed approximately 1 cm apart in the lesser tuberosity and down the anatomic neck of the humerus in a triangular fashion **(Fig. 11-4A,B)**. All sutures from each anchor are placed through the subscapularis tendon and tied in a mattress fashion. The

remaining lateral portion of the tendon can be reinforced with simple transosseous sutures or with sutures through the soft tissue on the lateral aspect of the bicipital groove to "flatten" the lateral portion of the subscapularis tendon against its footprint on the lesser tuberosity **(Fig. 11-5)**. Finally, the shoulder is placed through a gentle range of

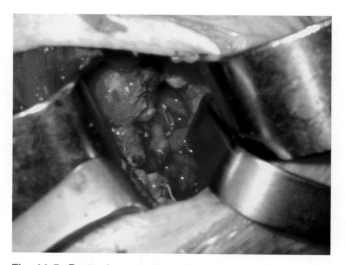

Fig. 11-5. Reattachment of the subscapularis tendon. Mattress sutures from the suture anchors are placed through the subscapularis tendon and tied in place. The lateral portion of the tendon is repaired either through transosseous sutures or to the tissue at the lateral portion of the bicipital groove ("two-row" repair).

motion to determine the safe arcs for postoperative rehabilitation, especially in external rotation. If the conjoined tendon was released for visualization, it is reattached with tendon-to-tendon sutures to the coracoid process. If desired, a suture anchor in the coracoid may also be used, but is usually not necessary.

■ TECHNICAL PERILS AND PITFALLS

Visualization and mobilization of the retracted subscapularis tendon is the most challenging part of this procedure. Tenotomy of the conjoined tendon allows easy access to the entire subscapularis, and surgeons should not hesitate to perform this maneuver if simple retraction of the conjoined tendon does not provide adequate exposure.

During identification and mobilization of the retracted subscapularis, surgeons must pay acute attention to the location of the axillary nerve. The nerve crosses the muscle belly of the subscapularis from proximal-medial to distal-lateral and enters the quadrangular space just inferior to the glenohumeral capsule. When the subscapularis is retracted to the level of the glenoid, the tendon may be closely opposed to the axillary nerve, and great care must be taken during mobilization. Again, if difficulty is encountered during this preparation, release and retraction of the conjoined tendon can provide a much easier approach to the subscapularis with minimal increased morbidity.

The footprint of the subscapularis on the lesser tuberosity is broad based. Consequently, the suture anchors should be used in a mattress fashion and in a triangular fashion to replicate the tendon-to-bone contact. Lateral sutures (through bone or to the soft tissue of the bicipital groove) serve to confirm anatomic restoration of tendon position and to reinforce the repair through a "two-row" medial and lateral fixation technique.

■ REHABILITATION AND RETURN TO SPORTS

Patients are placed into a sling for 4 weeks after surgery if the repair is an isolated subscapularis repair. Otherwise, immobilization is dictated by any other concomitant procedure (such as supraspinatus rotator cuff repair, anterior glenohumeral stabilization, and so forth). Passive range of motion is begun immediately, and external rotation is limited for the first 4 postoperative weeks to 10 degrees less than the passive rotation limit obtained on the operating table (i.e., if 40 degrees of passive rotation are obtained intraoperatively with no tension on the repair, the postoperative passive external rotation is limited to 30 degrees for 4 weeks). Deltoid isometrics are also used to avoid postoperative atrophy of the shoulder girdle musculature.

Following removal of the sling, full active motion is allowed, with resistance exercises begun 10 weeks after the isolated subscapularis repair. Internal rotation strengthening is begun 12 weeks after surgery, and patients are allowed to return to all activities at 6 months after surgery. Full recovery of all strength and return to the previous level of sporting participation usually takes 12 months.

■ CLINICAL OUTCOMES AND RESULTS

Gerber[5,6] reviewed 16 patients with an acute traumatic event and operative confirmation of a subscapularis tendon tear. Three of these patients had undergone previous surgery for their injury. At an average of 43 months postoperatively, 13 of 16 patients were considered to have a good or excellent result. On a visual analog function scale, patients rated their shoulder as 82% of normal. The postoperative Constant score was also 82% of age-matched controls; ranging from 29% to 109%. Operative treatment was deemed cost-effective within the Swiss National Accident Insurance System.

Deutsch et al.[10] reviewed 14 patients at 2 years after surgical treatment of a subscapularis tendon tear. Patients demonstrated decreased pain with sports activities, activities of daily living, anterior shoulder pain at night, and shoulder weakness. Seventy-one percent reported complete relief of preoperative symptoms. All 14 returned to previous employment and 12 of the 14 returned to previous sporting activities.

Brown et al.[9] reported the results of a recent study of surgical treatment of subscapularis tendon ruptures. Ten of 11 patients had good or excellent results at an average of 51 months. Results were best in patients without axillary nerve palsy.

■ CONCLUSION AND FUTURE DIRECTIONS

Patients with a sudden loss of active motion after an external rotation or hyperextension injury should be viewed with a high index of suspicion for a subscapularis tear. Appropriate physical examination maneuvers and confirmatory imaging studies will lead to timely surgical intervention. Meticulous surgical repair combined with a studied rehabilitation program should yield excellent clinical outcomes and should lessen both the length and degree of disability from this shoulder disorder.

Future repairs of the subscapularis and other rotator cuff tendons will likely involve the introduction of factors designed to promote tissue healing to bone—"orthobiologic" products. In addition, the advent of gene therapy has led researchers to begin devising methods to improve the healing rate of tendon to bone. These advances will undoubtedly improve the ability of surgeons to expeditiously return their patients back to preoperative levels of function.

■ REFERENCES

1. Jobe CM. Gross anatomy of the shoulder. In: Rockwood C, Matsen F, eds. *The Shoulder*, 2nd ed. Philadelphia: Saunders, 1998;61–62.
2. Smith SJ. Pathological appearances of seven cases of injury of the shoulder joint, with remarks. London Med Gaz. 1834;14:280.
3. Smith SJ. Pathological appearances of seven cases of injury of the shoulder joint, with remarks. Am J Med Sci. 1835;16:219–224.
4. Hauser EDW. Avulsion of the tendon of the subscapularis muscle. J Bone Joint Surg. 1954;36A:139–141.
5. Gerber C, Krushell RJ. Isolated rupture of the tendon of the subscapularis muscle. J Bone Joint Surg. 1991;73B:389–394.
6. Gerber C, Hersche O, Farron A. Isolated rupture of the subscapularis tendon. J Bone Joint Surg. 1996;78A:1015–1023.
7. McAuliffe TB, Dowd GS. Avulsion of the subscapularis tendon: a case report. J Bone Joint Surg. 1987;69A:1454.
8. Ticker JB, Warner JP. Single-tendon tears of the rotator cuff. Ortho Clin North Am. 1997;28:99–116.
9. Brown T, et al. Surgical treatment of isolated subscapularis tendon ruptures. Paper presented at the American Academy of Orthopaedic Surgeons 67th Annual Meeting; March 2000; Orlando Fla.
10. Deutsch A, Altchek DW, Veltri DM, et al. Traumatic tears of the subscapularis tendon. Am J Sports Med. 1997;25:13–22.
11. Tokish JM, Decker MJ, Ellis HB, et al. The belly-press test for the physical examination of the subscapularis muscle: electromyographic validation and comparison to the lift-off test. J Shoulder Elbow Surg. September–October 2003;12(5):427–430.
12. DePalma AF, Cooke AJ, Prabhaker M. The role of the subscapularis in recurrent anterior dislocations of the shoulder. Clin Orthop. 1967;54:35.
13. Neviaser RJ, Neviaser TJ. Recurrent instability of the shoulder after age 40. J Shoulder Elbow Surg. 1995;4:416–418.
14. Symeonides PP. The significance of the subscapularis muscle in the pathogenesis of recurrent anterior dislocation of the shoulder. J Bone Joint Surg. 1972;54B:476–483.
15. Farin P, Jaroma H. Sonographic detection of tears of the anterior portion of the rotator cuff. J Ultrasound Med. 1996;15:221–225.
16. Patten RM. Tears of the anterior portion of the rotator cuff (the subscapularis tendon): NR imaging findings. Am J Roentgenol. 1994;162:351–354.
17. Walch G, Nove-Jossderand L, Boileau P, et al. Subluxations and dislocations of the tendon of the long head of the biceps. J Shoulder Elbow Surg. 1998;7:100–108.

It is our belief that most subscapularis tears can be arthroscopically repaired. A careful three-sided release can provide sufficient lateral mobility to the subscapularis tendon so that even tears retracted medial to the glenoid can be repaired arthroscopically.

■ REHABILITATION AND RETURN TO SPORTS

After surgery, the arm is placed in a sling with a small pillow. The sling is continuously worn for 6 weeks. Active flexion and extension of the elbow are encouraged. In repairs that involve less than 50% of the subscapularis tendon, passive external rotation is encouraged to up to 30 degrees. In complete subscapularis repairs, passive external rotation is restricted to 0 degrees (straight ahead). After 6 weeks, passive overhead stretching with a rope and pulley is begun, as well as internal rotation stretching. Isotonic strengthening of the rotator cuff, deltoid, and scapular stabilizers is not begun until 12 weeks after surgery. Progressive activities are allowed as strength increases. Unrestricted activities are not allowed until a minimum of 6 months after surgery.

■ OUTCOMES AND FUTURE DIRECTIONS

The senior author (SSB) and Tehrany[26] have reported the results of arthroscopic subscapularis tendon repairs in 25 patients. In this study, eight patients had complete isolated subscapularis tears, six patients had complete subscapularis tears combined with tears of the supraspinatus and infraspinatus tendons, and 11 patients had partial subscapularis tears combined with tears of the supraspinatus and infraspinatus. Preliminary results demonstrated that the UCLA score improved from a preoperative average of 10.7 to a postoperative average of 30.5 after an average follow-up of 10.7 months. UCLA scores were similar in patients with isolated or combined tears and complete and partial tears. Ninety-two percent of patients obtained excellent to good results, while one patient was graded as a fair result and one patient was graded as a poor result. Forward flexion improved markedly, from an average of 96.3 degrees to 146.1 degrees. Ten patients had preoperative radiographic proximal humeral migration. After repair, eight of these ten patients were found to have lasting reversal of their proximal humeral migration.

In our cadaveric study, the subscapularis footprint was found to be widest superiorly, suggesting that the upper subscapularis is likely the strongest and the most important part of the tendon. A recent study by Halder et al.[28] confirmed that the strongest part of the subscapularis insertion was at the superior portion of the footprint.

The surgeon might be tempted to ignore or debride a partial tear involving only the upper subscapularis tendon.

However, we believe that it is important to recognize and repair all complete and partial tears of the subscapularis tendon in order to optimize functional results.

■ SUGGESTED READINGS

Chow CT, ed. *Advanced Arthroscopy*. New York: Springer-Verlag; 2001.
Codman, EA. *The Shoulder*. Boston: Thomas Todd; 1934.
McGinty JB, Burkhart SS, Jackson RW, et al. eds. *Operative Arthroscopy*. Philadelphia: Lippincott Williams & Wilkins; 2003.

■ REFERENCES

1. Inman VT, Saunders JB, Abbott LC. Observations on the function of the shoulder joint. J Bone Joint Surg Am. 1944;26:1–30.
2. Burkhart SS. Current concepts. Reconciling the paradox of rotator cuff repair versus debridement: a unified biomechanical rationale for the treatment of rotator cuff tears. Arthroscopy. 1994;10:4–19.
3. Burkhart SS. Shoulder arthroscopy: new concepts. Clin Sports Med. 1996;15:635–653.
4. Burkhart SS. Arthroscopic debridement and decompression for selected rotator cuff tears. Clinical results, pathomechanics, and patient selection based on biomechanical parameters. Orthop Clin North Am. 1993;24:111–123.
5. Burkhart SS. Arthroscopic treatment of massive rotator cuff tears. Clin Orthop. 2001;390:107–118.
6. Burkhart SS. Fluoroscopic comparison of kinematic patterns in massive rotator cuff tears: a suspension bridge model. Clin Orthop. 1992;284:144–152.
7. Burkhart SS. Arthroscopic treatment of massive rotator cuff tears: clinical results and biomechanical rationale. Clin Orthop. 1991;267:45–56.
8. Biondi J, Bear TF. Isolated rupture of the subscapularis tendon in an arm wrestler. Orthopaedics. 1988;11:647–649.
9. DePalma AF, Cooke AJ, Prabhakar M. The role of the subscapularis in recurrent anterior dislocations of the shoulder. Clin Orthop. 1967;54:35–49.
10. Deutsch A, Altchek DW, Veltri DM, et al. Traumatic tears of the subscapularis tendon: clinical diagnosis, magnetic resonance imaging findings, and operative treatment. Am J Sports Med. 1997;25:13–22.
11. Gerber C, Hersche O, Farron A. Isolated rupture of the subscapularis tendon: results of operative repair. J Bone Joint Surg Am. 1996;78:1015–1023.
12. Gerber C, Krushell RJ. Isolated rupture of the tendon of the subscapularis muscle: clinical features in 16 cases. J Bone Joint Surg Br. 1991;73:389–394.
13. Hauser ED. Avulsion of the tendon of the subscapularis muscle. J Bone Joint Surg Am. 1954;36:139–141.
14. McAuliffe TB, Dowd GS. Avulsion of the subscapularis tendon. J Bone Joint Surg Am. 1987;69:1454–1455.
15. Neviaser RJ, Neviaser TJ, Neviaser JS. Concurrent rupture of the rotator cuff and anterior dislocation of the shoulder in the older patient. J Bone Joint Surg Am. 1988;70:1308–1311.
16. Nove-Josserand L, Levigne C, Noel E, et al. Isolated lesions of subscapularis muscle: apropos of 21 cases. Rev Chir Orthop Reparatrice Appar Mot. 1994;80:595–601.
17. Smith JG. Pathological appearances of seven cases of injury of the shoulder joint, with remarks. London Med Gaz. 1834;14:280–285.
18. Symeonides PP. The significance of the subscapularis muscle in the pathogenesis of recurrent anterior dislocation of the shoulder. J Bone Joint Surg Br. 1972;54:476–483.

19. Ticker JB, Warner JJP. Single-tendon tears of the rotator cuff: evaluation and treatment of subscapularis tears and principles of treatment for supraspinatus tears. Orthop Clin North Am. 1997;28:99–116.

20. Walch G, Nove-Josserand L, Levigne C, et al. Complete ruptures of the supraspinatus tendon associated with hidden lesions of the rotator interval. J Shoulder Elbow Surg. 1994;3:353–360.

21. Warner JJP, Higgins L, Parsons IV IM, et al. Diagnosis and treatment of anterosuperior rotator cuff tears. J Shoulder Elbow Surg. 2001;10:37–46.

22. Sakurai G, Ozaki J, Tomita Y, et al. Incomplete tears of the subscapularis tendon associated with tears of the supraspinatus tendon: cadaveric and clinical studies. J Shoulder Elbow Surg. 1998;7:510–515.

23. Bennett WF. Subscapularis, medial, and lateral head coracohumeral ligament insertion anatomy: arthroscopic appearance and incidence of "hidden" rotator interval lesions. Arthroscopy. 2001;17:173–180.

24. Burkhart SS, Tehrany AM, Klein JR, et al. The subscapularis footprint: an anatomic study. Arthroscopy. Submitted.

24a. Greis PE, Kuhn JE, Schultheis J, et al. Validation of the lift-off test and analysis of subscapularis activity during maximal internal rotation. Am J Sports Med. 1996;24:589–593.

25. Schwamborn T, Imhoff AB. Diagnostik und klassifikation der rotatorenmanschettenlasionen. In: Imhoff AB, Konig U, eds. Schulterinstabilitat-Rotatorenmanschette. Darmstadt: Steinkopf Verlag; 1999:193–195.

25a. Tokish JM, Decker MJ, Ellis HB, et al. The belly-press test for the physical examination of the subscapularis muscle: electromyographic validation and comparison to the lift-off test. J Shoulder Elbow Surg. 2003;12:427–430.

26. Burkhart SS, Tehrany AM. Arthroscopic subscapularis tendon repair: technique and preliminary results. Arthroscopy. 2002;18:454–463.

26a. Barth J, Burkhart SS, De Beer JF. The bear hug sign: a new test for detecting subscapularis tendon tears. Arthroscopy. Accepted for publication; in press.

27. Lo IK, Burkhart SS. The comma sign: an arthroscopic guide to the torn subscapularis tendon. Arthroscopy. 2003;19:334–337.

28. Halder A, Zobitz ME, Schultz F, et al. Structural properties of the subscapularis tendon. J Orthop Res. 2000;18:829–834.

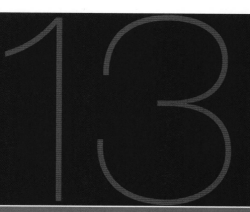

SUBSCAPULARIS RECONSTRUCTION WITH PECTORALIS MAJOR TRANSFER

13

JAY D. KEENER, MD, KEN YAMAGUCHI, MD

■ BACKGROUND

The subscapularis muscle is important for normal shoulder function and stability. It constitutes the sole anterior component of the rotator cuff and is the most powerful of the cuff muscles.[1] The subscapularis is a strong internal rotator of the glenohumeral joint, particularly with the shoulder in an adducted and extended position.[2,3] The dynamic force couple created from the coordinated efforts of the subscapularis and the posterior rotator cuff is critical for normal glenohumeral joint kinematics and stability.[4,5] This force couple has been shown experimentally to be an important contributor to humeral head depression throughout multiple positions of glenohumeral abduction.[6] Loss of subscapularis function commonly results in pain and weakness and occasionally impairment in shoulder function, which may require surgical treatment.[7,8]

Fortunately, subscapularis tendon tears are relatively uncommon. Isolated subscapularis tears are even less frequent. Codman[9] reported involvement of the subscapularis in 3.5% of a series of 200 rotator cuff tears, and Deutsch et al.[8] noted significant involvement of the subscapularis in 4% of a series of 350 rotator cuff tears. Warner et al.[10] noted involvement of the subscapularis tendon in 4.7% of a series of 407 rotator cuff tears. The majority of subscapularis injuries are associated with tears of the superior rotator cuff (anterosuperior cuff tears) as well.[10–12] Isolated subscapularis tears are more commonly associated with trauma in comparison to other types of rotator cuff injuries.[7,13] Traumatic subscapularis tendon tears have been associated with recurrent anterior glenohumeral dislocation in several clinical series.[14–17] Subscapularis deficiency is also a well-documented complication of open anterior instability and prosthetic humeral replacement.

■ HISTORY OF THE TECHNIQUE

Repair of acute subscapularis tears has produced excellent clinical results.[7,18,19] Unfortunately, the diagnosis of isolated subscapularis tears is often delayed or missed.[7] A completely torn subscapularis tendon is prone to retraction and the development of irreversible changes of the muscle. After a delay of several months or longer, repair of the retracted tendon can be very difficult. Inferior clinical results have been reported with delayed repair of subscapularis tears[10,13] and, in many cases, the subscapularis has been found to be irreparable at the time of surgery.[14,20]

Muscle transfers have become useful salvage options for patients with irreparable tears of the subscapularis. Options include transfer of the pectoralis major, pectoralis minor, trapezius, latissimus dorsi, teres major, as well as allograft reconstruction.[11,21–24] The pectoralis major tendon transfer has produced the most reliable clinical results when compared to other reconstructive options. Several characteristics of the pectoralis major make it favorable for reconstruction of the subscapularis. These include muscle bulk (including elderly patients), a robust tendon, location, similarity of function, and tendon excursion. Pectoralis major tendon transfer has been shown to be beneficial in several clinical situations related to subscapularis insufficiency. Successful results have been reported with associated recurrent anterior shoulder instability secondary to subscapularis deficiency,[14] massive posterior rotator cuff tears,[20,23] and for humeral head containment in the setting of anterosuperior migration.[25]

■ EVALUATION

The clinical presentation of patients with subscapularis tears is variable. The majority of subscapularis tears are not isolated but are seen in combination with tears of the superior and posterior cuff. Most patients in this setting are older and present with chronic pain and progressive deterioration of function of the shoulder joint. Acute loss in function in the setting of chronic shoulder symptoms may indicate an acute on chronic rotator cuff injury and should raise the suspicion of subscapularis involvement as well. Isolated injuries of the subscapularis often result from trauma to the shoulder. A forced external rotation moment with or without hyperextension of the adducted shoulder has been reported as a common mechanism of subscapularis injury.[7,8] In these series, the average patient ages were 39 and 50 years, considerably younger than the typical presentation of a massive anterosuperior rotator cuff tear. Anterior shoulder dislocation in the middle-aged patient can result in subscapularis disruption and recurrent instability.[14,17] Subscapularis failure can complicate open instability or prosthetic replacement surgery.

The majority of patients with subscapularis tears will complain of pain that may or may not be localized to the anterior shoulder. Most patients will note increased pain and weakness with both overhead activities and strenuous activities below shoulder level. Isolated tears may produce minimal symptoms and can be easily overlooked. Activities requiring forced internal rotation such as reaching behind the body, placing the hand in a back pocket, or reaching the abdomen are difficult.[18] Sensations of glenohumeral instability are common, especially in more active patients or following prosthetic replacement.

The physical examination of patients with subscapularis tears is significantly influenced by the integrity of the remaining rotator cuff. The majority of patients with isolated tears of the subscapularis can still elevate the arm to the overhead position.[14,18] Tears that also include the posterior cuff often produce significant loss of active elevation due to disruption of the rotator cuff force couple.[10] Isolated subscapularis tears are commonly missed initially and require a high index of suspicion. Subscapularis tears will often result in an increase in external rotation range of motion compared to the opposite shoulder. The abdominal compression and liftoff tests are excellent clinical examination tools that are highly accurate for detecting subscapularis disruption.[2,3,7] However, pain and limited passive range of motion may hinder the accuracy of liftoff test because of the arm position required to perform the maneuver. The strength of the remainder of the rotator cuff should be assessed because of the high prevalence of associated tears of the supraspinatus and infraspinatus muscles. Apprehension in abduction may be seen in those patients with instability. Tears of the subscapularis are often associated with instability of the long head of the biceps tendon.[10,26,27] Biceps provocation tests can clue the clinician to the presence of biceps tendon instability.

Radiographs of the shoulder in patients with isolated subscapularis tears are typically normal. Occasionally subtle anterior translation of the humeral head can be appreciated on the axillary radiograph in patients with subscapularis deficiency. Tears that also include the posterior cuff will often result in superior migration of the humeral head. This is particularly evident on true anteroposterior (AP) radiographs

performed with slight abduction of the shoulder. Tears of the subscapularis can accurately be identified with both ultrasound and magnetic resonance imaging (MRI).[28–31] Associated MRI findings are frequently encountered and fairly specific to subscapularis injuries. These include subluxation or dislocation of the biceps tendon, fluid collections local to the subscapular recess, or subcoracoid bursa and supraspinatus tears.[29,30] MRI evaluation is particularly useful in identifying the degree of tendon retraction and fatty degeneration and atrophy of the subscapularis muscle. Ultrasound examination is more favorable in the postoperative setting because of improved accuracy of rotator cuff imaging over MRI, especially in the setting of implants.[32]

■ SURGICAL INDICATIONS AND CONTRAINDICATIONS

It is appropriate to consider a pectoralis tendon transfer in those patients with pain, instability, and associated impaired function in whom primary subscapularis repair is unlikely to be successful.[11,33] The indication for pectoralis major tendon transfer is primarily related to the likelihood of success of primary subscapularis repair. We prefer to treat all acute subscapularis tears with surgical repair and attempt to repair chronic tears when possible. Most clinical series of primary subscapularis repair demonstrate improved clinical results of repair over reconstruction.[7,8,20,23,34] Primary repair of the subscapularis tendon should be performed when possible. Often a tendon transfer will be performed in conjunction with other reconstructive procedures such as prosthetic replacement of the humeral head (cuff tear arthropathy), repair of massive rotator cuff tears, or in the setting of instability following arthroplasty.

The final decision to perform a tendon transfer instead of, or in addition to, subscapularis repair is best made at the time of surgery. Attempted subscapularis repair in the presence of advanced muscle shortening, atrophy, and fatty infiltration is unlikely to be successful. Preoperative MRI findings that demonstrate retraction of the tendon medial to the edge of the glenoid or fatty infiltration of the subscapularis muscle of grade III or IV have been used as criteria to proceed with pectoralis major tendon transfer.[20] Patients undergoing attempted subscapularis repair should be counseled preoperatively regarding the possibility of pectoralis tendon transfer, based on the severity and chronicity of the injury, preoperative imaging, and intraoperative findings.

Contraindications to performing a pectoralis tendon transfer include the presence of a repairable subscapularis tendon tear or inadequate pectoralis major tissue. The repair is also contraindicated in the medically unstable or in those who are unable to comply with postoperative rehabilitation. Relative contraindications include a massive tear of the anterosuperior and posterior cuff with pseudoparalysis where restoration of functional elevation is unlikely. In addition, the surgeon must be comfortable with the anatomy and surgical dissection of the pectoralis major tissue and the conjoint tendon and the surrounding neurovascular structures.

■ SURGICAL TECHNIQUE

Several variations of the pectoralis major tendon transfer have been described. We prefer a subcoracoid transfer of the sternal head of the pectoralis major muscle. We believe the subcoracoid position best re-creates the mechanical vector of the subscapularis muscle. The sternal head of the pectoralis muscle is usually more robust than the clavicular head and has a fiber orientation that best re-creates the downward pull of the subscapularis muscle.

All surgeries are performed under general anesthesia. Regional anesthetic can be used to supplement postoperative pain control. The patient is positioned beach chair. An extended deltopectoral skin incision is made from the coracoid process extending 12 to 15 cm inferolaterally. Full thickness subcutaneous flaps are elevated with electrocautery. The medial flap is developed to the point of full exposure of the inferior border of the pectoralis muscle superficially. The deltopectoral interval is developed taking the cephalic vein laterally with the deltoid muscle. Dissection proceeds through this interval to the level of the clavipectoral fascia. Fascial adhesions are swept off the lateral aspect of the pectoralis muscle with a dry sponge exposing the insertion of the pectoralis tendon onto the humerus. The clavipectoral fascia is opened inferior to the coracoacromial ligament. This interval is developed inferiorly with blunt dissection lateral to the conjoint tendon. The arm is externally rotated exposing any remaining subscapularis tendon and the anterior humeral circumflex vessels.

A thin layer of tissue often covers the anterior aspect of the humeral head in place of the normal subscapularis tendon. The torn subscapularis tendon usually retracts medially under the conjoint tendon within this layer of fibrous tissue. A fluid-filled bursa may be present anteriorly. The anterior humeral circumflex vessels are identified and ligated with suture. The fibrous tissue/tendon remnant is tagged with a stay suture and released from the humerus at the level of the rotator interval just medial to the lesser tuberosity. The release continues inferiorly as the adducted humerus is progressively externally rotated. Often the inferior fibers of the muscular insertion of the subscapularis will be found attached to the inferior aspect of the lesser tuberosity. This portion of the subscapularis is left intact. The axillary nerve is identified by palpation along the inferior border of the subscapularis muscle. A thin flat retractor or small sponge can be placed between the axillary nerve and subscapularis while the tendon is mobilized. Sharp dissection is used to release the contracted coracohumeral ligament from the superior border of the subscapularis. The muscle is then freed from the anterior glenoid and subscapular fossa. The inferior border of the muscle is mobilized from surrounding adhesions while protecting the axillary nerve and the anterior neurovascular structures. After full release, the integrity of the subscapularis muscle and mobility of the tendon are assessed. If the tissue is judged to be of poor quality or irreparable then the decision is made to proceed with pec-

toralis major tendon transfer. In some cases the inferior portion of the subscapularis tendon can be repaired to the lesser tuberosity with transosseous sutures.

Detailed knowledge of the anatomy of the pectoralis major muscle and tendon is essential when harvesting the muscle. The sternal head of the pectoralis major lies inferior and deep to the clavicular head. The interval between the muscles and the orientation of the tendon can usually be readily identified at the inferior edge. This interval is developed bluntly through the superficial fascia and the fibers are then spread moving laterally toward the tendon. The tendon of the sternal head maintains a constant anatomic relationship to the clavicular head at its humeral attachment. The sternal tendon rotates deep to the clavicular tendon to form the posterior lamina of the pectoralis major insertion. The clavicular tendon remains anterior to the sternal tendon, creating the anterior lamina.[35] The posterior lamina extends more proximally than the anterior lamina. The interval between the two divisions is further developed by sweeping the clavicular head muscle fibers off the sternal tendon with a dry sponge. The deep aspect of the pectoralis major tendon is more tendinous than the superficial surface[35] **(Fig. 13-1)**.

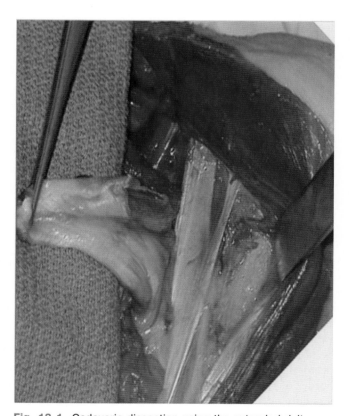

Fig. 13-1. Cadaveric dissection using the extended deltopectoral approach. The pectoralis tendon has been released and the deep surface of the tendon is visualized. The deep tendon surface is wider and more robust in comparison to the superficial surface. (Reprinted with permission from Klepps SJ, Goldfarb C, Flatow E, et al. Anatomic evaluation of the subcoracoid pectoralis major transfer in human cadavers. J Shoulder Elbow Surg. 2001;10(5):453–459.)

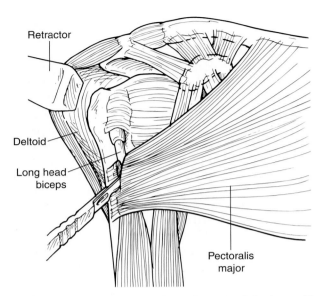

Fig. 13-2. The extended deltopectoral approach is shown. The pectoralis major insertion into the humerus is exposed. The superior portion of the pectoralis major insertion is released, as shown. If the patient has a small pectoralis major muscle, then the entire pectoralis can be released and transferred. (Reprinted with permission from Klepps S, Galatz LM, Yamaguchi K. Subcoracoid pectoralis major transfer: a salvage procedure for irreparable subscapularis deficiency. Tech Shoulder Elbow Surg. 2001;2:85–91.)

The inferior and superior aspects of the sternal tendon are tagged with suture of different colors to allow for correct orientation of the twisted tendon after release. The sternal head tendon is then taken directly off the humerus using a sharp blade **(Fig. 13-2)**. Previous anatomic studies have demonstrated the relationship of the pectoral nerves to the deep surface of the pectoralis major muscle.[35] The muscle can be safely split for a distance of 8.5 cm from the lateral edge of the tendon before risking damage to the medial pectoral nerve. The lateral pectoral nerve is located medial to the pectoralis minor muscle and innervates the upper portion of the pectoralis major. Avoiding dissection medial to the pectoralis minor tendon will protect both pectoral nerves **(Fig. 13-3)**. Resch et al.[23] has shown electromyographically that the pectoralis major muscle can be safely split for a distance of roughly 10 cm without denervation of either the clavicular or sternal heads. Care must be taken when mobilizing the sternal head as the medial pectoral nerve can be as close as 1.2 cm for the inferior border of the pectoralis major.[35] In older patients with a less developed pectoralis major muscle we often mobilize the entire muscle to provide a more robust tendon transfer. The released pectoralis major tendon is then secured with a heavy, braided, nonabsorbable suture. A running, locking stitch is weaved from the tendon edge laterally toward the musculotendinous junction and back down the opposite side.

The medial aspect of the coracoid process is then identified. The insertion of the pectoralis minor tendon is partially released from the coracoid for improved exposure deep to the conjoint tendon. The medial aspect of conjoint tendon is defined and the fascia is opened with blunt dissection. The interval is further developed by sweeping the finger inferiorly. The musculocutaneous nerve can be seen at its entrance on the undersurface of the coracobrachialis. This can often be identified with palpation alone, but we prefer to visualize the nerve prior to tendon transfer. The musculocutaneous nerve enters the deep surface of the conjoint tendon at a variable distance from the coracoid. The average distance from the coracoid tip to the point where the nerve penetrates the coracobrachialis is 6.1 cm (range 3.5 to 10 cm)[35] **(Fig. 13-4)**. In the majority of patients a proximal branch of the musculocutaneous nerve can be identified entering the coracobrachialis muscle. The proximal branch has variable anatomy and must often be released to allow adequate room for the pectoralis major tendon to rest in the subcoracoid position.[35] The released sternal head tendon is then passed deep to the clavicular head and under the conjoint tendon while remaining superficial

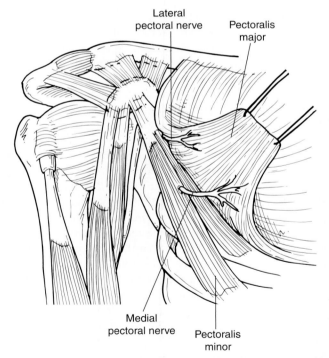

Fig. 13-3. In this case, the entire pectoralis muscle tendon will be used for transfer. The tendon and muscle are mobilized from surrounding soft tissues and off the underlying clavipectoral fascia to the level of the pectoralis minor muscle medially. The medial and lateral pectoral nerves are visualized inserting into the undersurface of the pectoralis major. (Reprinted with permission from Klepps SJ, Galatz LM, Yamaguchi K. Subcoracoid pectoralis major transfer: a salvage procedure for irreparable Subscapularis deficiency. Tech Shoulder Elbow Surg. 2001;2: 85–91.)

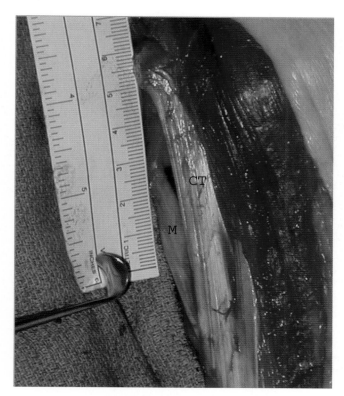

Fig. 13-4. The musculocutaneous nerve is seen deep to the conjoined tendon. The average distance from the coracoid process to the main trunk of the nerve entering the coracobrachialis is 6.1 cm. A proximal branch of the musculocutaneous nerve is often seen entering the coracobrachialis muscle approximately 4.4 cm below the coracoid process. This branch is usually sacrificed to accommodate the transferred pectoralis major tendon. M, musculocutaneous nerve; CT, conjoint tendon. (Reprinted with permission from Klepps SJ, Goldfarb C, Flatow E, et al. Anatomic evaluation of the subcoracoid pectoralis major transfer in human cadavers. J Shoulder Elbow Surg. 2001;10(5):453–459.)

to the musculocutaneous nerve **(Fig. 13-5A,B)**. Excessive tension in the nerve after transfer must be assessed by direct palpation after tendon transfer. Errant placement of the tendon under the musculocutaneous nerve risks neuropraxic injury from tension created by the bulky pectoralis major tendon.

The excursion of the transferred pectoralis major tendon is assessed by tensioning the stay sutures. The edge of the pectoralis tendon can usually be displaced 2 to 3 cm lateral to the bicipital groove with the arm in neutral rotation.[35] The excursion of the transferred tendon usually allows for attachment to the anterolateral aspect of the greater tuberosity. The surface of the greater tuberosity is roughened to a raw surface. The tendon is repaired to the greater tuberosity using transosseous sutures with a wide bone bridge **(Fig. 13-6)**. The repair can be augmented medially with the placement of bone anchors in the lateral aspect of the lesser tuberosity. This also increases the area for tendon-to-bone healing by enlarging the footprint of the repair. The transfer should be tensioned to allow 30 degrees of external

rotation with the arm at the side. The surgical wound is closed over suction drains. A compressive type sterile dressing is placed over the shoulder and upper arm to minimize the risk of hematoma formation.

■ TECHNICAL ALTERNATIVES AND PITFALLS

Great care must be used when mobilizing the subscapularis tendon particularly in the presence of revision surgery. Scarring and adhesions around the subscapularis are a result of both the subscapularis injury as well as prior surgical dissection. We take great care in isolating the axillary nerve prior to complete subscapularis mobilization. The nerve can be tagged with a vessel loop and should be protected with retractors prior to mobilization of the subscapularis and isolation of the conjoint tendon.

Several variations of the pectoralis major transfer have been described. Alternatives include harvesting of the entire or a portion of the pectoralis major muscle. We prefer to transfer the entire muscle in older patients or in those who display little pectoralis major muscle bulk. In those patients with a robust pectoralis major muscle either the sternal or clavicular portion can be utilized. We prefer to transfer the sternal portion because the orientation of this portion of the muscle best re-creates the line of action of the subscapularis muscle. The transferred tendon can be routed either over or beneath the conjoint tendon. We prefer to route the transferred tendon underneath the conjoint tendon to better re-create the downward vector of the subscapularis muscle. Fixation of the transferred tendon can be accomplished with either transosseous sutures or with the use of suture anchors. Both options allow excellent fixation of the tendon to bone. The site of attachment for the transferred tendon is best chosen by the available excursion of the muscle/tendon unit. Either the lesser tuberosity or the anterolateral aspect of the greater tuberosity will re-create the desired mechanical effect of the tendon transfer.

Potential pitfalls of this surgery should first focus on proper patient selection. If possible, the subscapularis muscle should be mobilized and repaired in lieu of performing a muscle transfer. The most predictable functional results are obtained in those patients with an intact or repairable posterior cuff, an intact coracoacromial arch, and a functioning deltoid muscle. When performing a split pectoralis major transfer, it is important to understand the anatomy of the pectoralis muscle tendon insertion to the humerus and to harvest only the desired portion of the tendon. Proper orientation of the twisted sternal portion of the pectoralis major tendon should be maintained when securing the transferred tendon to bone. Care must be taken not to denervate the muscle with medial and deep dissection during mobilization or split of the pectoralis major.

The surgeon must be comfortable with the anatomy and potential complications of dissection medial to the conjoint

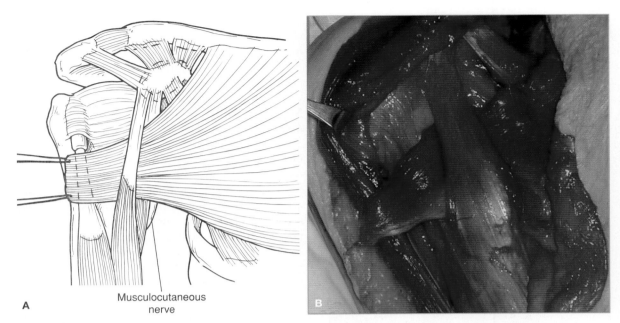

A

Musculocutaneous
nerve

B

Fig. 13-5. **A:** After securing the tendon with a heavy, running stitch, the entire pectoralis major tendon is transferred deep to the conjoint tendon and superficial to the musculocutaneous nerve. (Reprinted with permission from Klepps SJ, Galatz LM, Yamaguchi K. Subcoracoid pectoralis major transfer: a salvage procedure for irreparable subscapularis deficiency. Tech Shoulder Elbow Surg. 2001;2:85–91.) **B:** Cadaveric dissection showing the subcoracoid position of the transferred pectoralis major tendon. Prior to transfer, a running locked Krackow stitch should be placed in the tendon to facilitate transfer and allow repair to the greater tuberosity. (Reprinted with permission from Klepps SJ, Goldfarb C, Flatow E, et al. Anatomic evaluation of the subcoracoid pectoralis major transfer in human cadavers. J Shoulder Elbow Surg. 2001;10(5):453–459.)

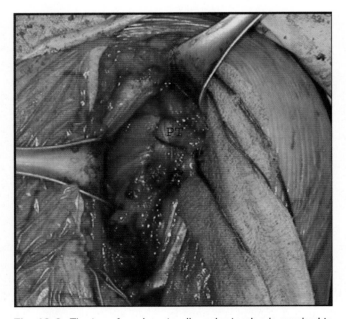

PT

Fig. 13-6. The transferred pectoralis major tendon is repaired to the greater tuberosity over the biceps tendon. Transosseous bone tunnels are used for fixation in the greater tuberosity. PT, pectoralis tendon.

tendon. The musculocutaneous nerve should be identified and remain deep to the transferred tendon to avoid neuropraxic injury. Choosing the proper site of attachment of the transferred tendon is important to avoid overtensioning the repair and limiting external rotation range of motion. Transosseous fixation allows maximal strength of the repaired tendon. Failure of the repair has been reported and is associated with a poor outcome.[24] We prefer to use heavy suture (no. 5 braided nonabsorbable suture) and a running Krackow stitch to maximize the strength of the repair. Hematoma formation is a potential complication of the surgery that can be minimized with the use of suction drains and compressive wraps to the anterior chest and shoulder.

■ REHABILITATION

The rehabilitation following pectoralis tendon transfer is the same as for rotator cuff repair. The shoulder is protected in a sling for 6 weeks. Pendulum and passive range of motion exercises are initiated on the first postoperative day. External rotation range of motion is limited to 10 to 20 degrees or an amount determined by intraoperative assessment of the tension of the transfer for the initial 6 weeks. Early motion helps to prevent scarring of the tendon to the glenoid or the deep surface of the conjoint tendon. Passive elevation to tolerance is allowed with the shoulder in a position of slight internal rotation. The sling can be removed when in a safe environment after 3 weeks.

Active assistive elevation is initiated at 3 weeks if no additional rotator cuff repair was performed but delayed until 6 weeks in the presence of a rotator cuff repair. At 6 weeks, progressive active and passive range of motion is allowed with no limits on external rotation range of motion or combined shoulder motions. Shoulder strengthening exercises are dictated according to concurrent rotator cuff pathology and the return of a functional range of motion. In cases of isolated pectoralis major tendon transfer, rotator cuff strengthening is started with isometrics at 4 weeks, excluding internal rotation. Internal rotation strengthening activities are begun at 8 weeks postsurgery. Progression into higher-level functional activities is initiated as range of motion and strength return.

■ OUTCOMES/FUTURE DIRECTIONS

Transfer of the pectoralis major tendon in the presence of an irreparable subscapularis tear has been successful in many clinical scenarios. However, the clinical results of pectoralis tendon transfer have been less dramatic than direct repair of subscapularis tears.[8,18] Relief of pain and improvement in range of motion, function, and stability of the shoulder have been noted by several authors.[14,20,23] The ultimate restoration in function is likely dependent upon associated pathology of the shoulder such as the presence of a massive tear of the remaining rotator cuff.

Wirth and Rockwood[14] performed a transfer of the clavicular head of the pectoralis major, the pectoralis minor, or both in 13 patients with recurrent anterior stability of the shoulder in the presence of an irreparable subscapularis tear. The surgery also included imbrication and repair of the anterior glenohumeral joint capsule. At 5-year follow-ups 10 of the 13 patients were noted to have a satisfactory result according to a modification of the Neer and Foster grading criteria and the American Shoulder and Elbow Surgeons scale. Patients with satisfactory results had stable shoulders with minimal to no pain and demonstrated an average of 143 degrees of elevation and 43 degrees of external rotation range of motion.[14]

Resch et al.[23] reported the results of 12 patients with chronic subscapularis tears treated with subcoracoid transfer of the upper portion of the pectoralis major muscle. Eight patients had isolated tears of the subscapularis while 4 patients had associated tears of the supraspinatus muscle. At 28-month follow-ups, 9 of the 12 patients had an excellent or good clinical result, 3 had a fair result, and no patient had a poor result. Pain relief following surgery was reliable.

The average functional rating with the use of the Constant and Morley score increased from 26.9% to 67.1% of age and gender adjusted normal values. Subjective assessment of function on a visual analog scale of 0 to 100 improved from 20 preoperatively to 63 at final follow-up.

Jost et al.[20] reported the results of 28 patients (30 shoulders) following transfer of the entire pectoralis major muscle for the treatment of an irreparable subscapularis tear. Twelve shoulders had isolated tears of the subscapularis, while 18 shoulders had an associated tear of the supraspinatus or supraspinatus and infraspinatus. The pectoralis muscle was transferred to the greater tuberosity superficial to the conjoint tendon and associated rotator cuff tears were repaired when possible. At an average follow-up of 32 months, moderate improvements in pain and function were achieved. The mean relative Constant score improved from 47% preoperatively to 70% postoperatively. Significant improvements in pain, flexion range of motion, abduction strength, and function were noted. The presence of an irreparable massive rotator cuff tear was a detriment to the final outcome.[20]

Transfer of the pectoralis major tendon has also been successful for improved containment in patients with anterosuperior migration of the humeral head. Galatz et al.[25] reviewed the results of 14 subcoracoid pectoralis major transfers in a series of complex shoulder cases, all of whom displayed anterosuperior migration of the humeral head due to massive insufficiency of the rotator cuff. While shoulder function remained impaired, most patients had significant relief of pain and improved function with the arm at the waist level. All but one patient demonstrated improved containment of the humeral head under the remaining coracoacromial arch.

Pectoralis major tendon transfers have been successfully performed in many clinical scenarios for the subscapularis deficient shoulder. However, this reconstruction must continue to be considered as a salvage operation. Further studies with larger series of patients are needed to better assess the benefits of the procedure and to identify the optimal surgical candidates. Many variations of the pectoralis major muscle transfer have been described. Further studies are needed to assess which portion of the muscle best re-creates the function of the subscapularis. It remains unproven whether the subcoracoid position of the muscle transfer is superior biomechanically to the supracoracoid position. Optimal fixation of the tendon repair to maximize the chance of tendon-to-bone healing is debated and warrants further investigation.

■ REFERENCES

1. Keating JF, Waterworth P, Shaw-Dunn J, et al. The relative strengths of the rotator cuff muscles: a cadaver study. J Bone Joint Surg Br. 1993;75:137–140.
2. Tokish JM, Decker MJ, Ellis HB, et al. The belly-press test for the physical examination of the subscapularis muscle: electromyographic validation and comparison to the lift-off test. J Shoulder Elbow Surg. 2003;12:427–430.

3. Greis PE, Kuhn JE, Schultheis J, et al. Validation of the lift-off test and analysis of subscapularis activity during maximal internal rotation. Am J Sports Med. 1996;24:589–593.

4. Thompson WO, Debski RE, Boardman ND III, et al. A biomechanical analysis of rotator cuff deficiency in a cadaveric model. Am J Sports Med. 1996;24:286–292.

5. Burkhart SS. Fluoroscopic comparison of kinematic patterns in massive rotator cuff tears: a suspension bridge model. Clin Orthop. 1992;284:144–152.

6. Halder AM, Zhao KD, Odriscoll SW, et al. Dynamic contributions to superior shoulder stability. J Orthop Res. 2001;19:206–212.

7. Gerber C, Hersche O, Farron A. Isolated rupture of the subscapularis tendon. J Bone Joint Surg Am. 1996;78:1015–1023.

8. Deutsch A, Altchek DW, Veltri DM, et al. Traumatic tears of the subscapularis tendon: clinical diagnosis, magnetic resonance imaging findings, and operative treatment. Am J Sports Med. 1997;25:13–22.

9. Codman EA. *The Shoulder: Rupture of the Supraspinatus Tendon and Other Lesions in or About the Subacromial Bursa.* Boston: Thomas Todd; 1934.

10. Warner JJ, Higgins L, Parsons IM, et al. Diagnosis and treatment of anterosuperior rotator cuff tears. J Shoulder Elbow Surg. 2001;10:37–46.

11. Warner JJ. Management of massive irreparable rotator cuff tears: the role of tendon transfer. Instr Course Lect. 2001;50:63–71.

12. Warner JJ, Gerber C. Treatment of massive rotator cuff tears: posterior-superior and anterior-superior. In: Iannotti JP, ed. *The Rotator Cuff: Current Concepts and Complex Problems.* Rosemont, Ill.: American Academy of Orthopaedic Surgeons; 1998:59–94.

13. Mansat P, Frankle MA, Cofield RH. Tears in the subscapularis tendon: descriptive analysis and results of surgical repair. Joint Bone Spine. 2003;70:342–347.

14. Wirth MA, Rockwood CA Jr. Operative treatment of irreparable rupture of the subscapularis. J Bone Joint Surg Am. 1997;79:722–731.

15. Neviaser RJ, Neviaser TJ, Neviaser JS. Concurrent rupture of the rotator cuff and anterior dislocation of the shoulder in the older patient. J Bone Joint Surg Am. 1988;70:1308–1311.

16. Neviaser RJ, Neviaser TJ, Neviaser JS. Anterior dislocation of the shoulder and rotator cuff rupture. Clin Orthop. 1993;291:103–106.

17. Neviaser RJ, Neviaser TJ. Recurrent instability of the shoulder after age 40. J Shoulder Elbow Surg. 1995;4:416–418.

18. Gerber C, Krushell RJ. Isolated rupture of the tendon of the subscapularis muscle: clinical features in 16 cases. J Bone Joint Surg Br. 1991;73:389–394.

19. Hauser ED. Avulsion of the tendon of the subscapularis muscle. J Bone Joint Surg Am. 1954;36A:139–141.

20. Jost B, Puskas GJ, Lustenberger A, et al. Outcome of pectoralis major transfer for the treatment of irreparable subscapularis tears. J Bone Joint Surg Am. 2003;85A:1944–1951.

21. Gerber C, Hersche O. Tendon transfers for the treatment of irreparable rotator cuff defects. Orthop Clin North Am. 1997;28:195–203.

22. Moeckel BH, Altchek DW, Warren RF, et al. Instability of the shoulder after arthroplasty. J Bone Joint Surg Am. 1993;75:492–497.

23. Resch H, Povacz P, Ritter E, et al. Transfer of the pectoralis major muscle for the treatment of irreparable rupture of the subscapularis tendon. J Bone Joint Surg Am. 2000;82:372–382.

24. Gerber A, Clavert P, Millett PJ, et al. Split pectoralis major and teres major tendon transfers for reconstruction of irreparable tears of the subscapularis. Tech Shoulder Elbow Surg. 2004;5:5–12.

25. Galatz LM, Connor PM, Calfee RP, et al. Pectoralis major transfer for anterior-superior subluxation in massive rotator cuff insufficiency. J Shoulder Elbow Surg. 2003;12:1–5.

26. Walch G, Nove-Josserand L, Boileau P, et al. Subluxations and dislocations of the tendon of the long head of the biceps. J Shoulder Elbow Surg. 1998;7:100–108.

27. Bennett WF. Arthroscopic repair of anterosuperior (supraspinatus/subscapularis) rotator cuff tears: a prospective cohort with 2- to 4-year follow-up: classification of biceps subluxation/instability. Arthroscopy. 2003;19:21–33.

28. Teefey SA, Hasan SA, Middleton WD, et al. Ultrasonography of the rotator cuff: a comparison of ultrasonographic and arthroscopic findings in one hundred consecutive cases. J Bone Joint Surg Am. 2000;82:498–504.

29. Li XX, Schweitzer ME, Bifano JA, et al. MR evaluation of subscapularis tears. J Comput Assist Tomogr. 1999;23:713–717.

30. Tung GA, Yoo DC, Levine SM, et al. Subscapularis tendon tear: primary and associated signs on MRI. J Comput Assist Tomogr. 2001;25:417–424.

31. Pfirrmann CW, Zanetti M, Weishaupt D, et al. Subscapularis tendon tears: detection and grading at MR arthrography. Radiology. 1999;213:709–714.

32. Prickett WD, Teefey SA, Galatz LM, et al. Accuracy of ultrasound imaging of the rotator cuff in shoulders that are painful postoperatively. J Bone Joint Surg Am. 2003;85A:1084–1089.

33. Klepps S, Galatz L, Yamaguchi K. Subcoracoid pectoralis major transfer: a salvage procedure for irreparable subscapularis deficiency. Tech Shoulder Elbow Surg. 2001;2:85–91.

34. Burkhart SS, Tehrany AM. Arthroscopic subscapularis tendon repair: technique and preliminary results. Arthroscopy. 2002;18:454–463.

35. Klepps SJ, Goldfarb C, Flatow E, et al. Anatomic evaluation of the subcoracoid pectoralis major transfer in human cadavers. J Shoulder Elbow Surg. 2001;10:453–459.

Part

C

ACROMIOCLAVICULAR JOINT

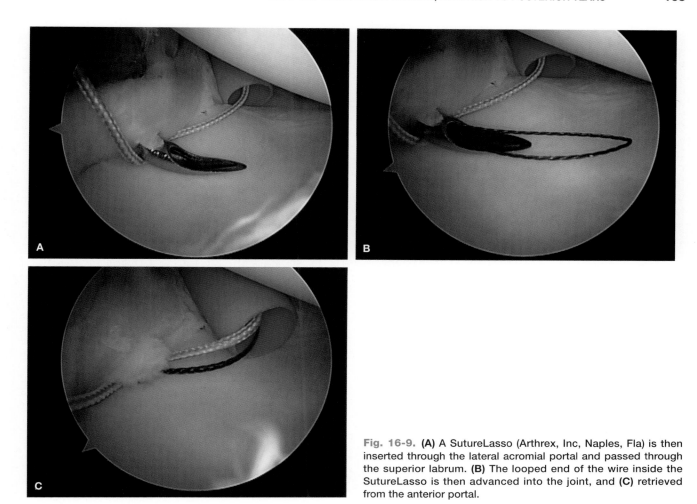

Fig. 16-9. (A) A SutureLasso (Arthrex, Inc, Naples, Fla) is then inserted through the lateral acromial portal and passed through the superior labrum. **(B)** The looped end of the wire inside the SutureLasso is then advanced into the joint, and **(C)** retrieved from the anterior portal.

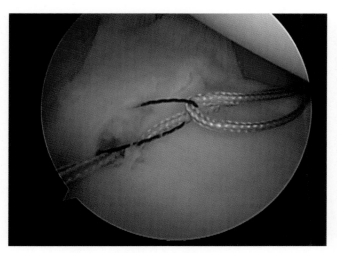

Fig. 16-10. The suture limb is then threaded through the loop of the wire and the wire is pulled out from the lateral acromial portal, thus shuttling one limb of suture through the labrum.

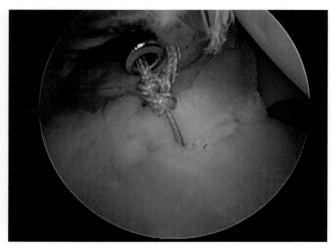

Fig. 16-11. An arthroscopic sliding knot is then used and advanced down to the labrum with a knot pusher.

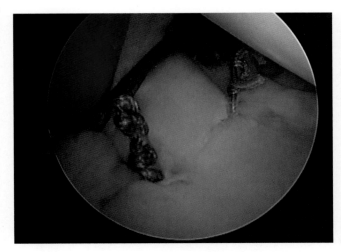

Fig. 16-12. A second anchor is placed anterior to the biceps and knot is tied.

with the SLAP repair. However, this is seldom necessary as the superior labral repair generally restores the proper glenohumeral translation, rotation, and stability.[22–24] This is analogous to the stable knee protecting the meniscal repair.

■ REFERENCES

1. Andrews JR, CarsonWG Jr, Mcleod WD. Glenoid labrum tears related to the long head of the biceps. Am J Sports Med. 1985;13:337–341.
2. Snyder SJ, Karzel RP, Del Pizzo W, et al. SLAP lesion of the shoulder. Arthroscopy. 1990;6:274–279.
3. Yoneda M, Hirooka A, Saito S, et al. Arthroscopic stapling for detached superior glenoid labrum. J Bone Joint Surg Br. 1991;73: 746–750.
4. Field LD, Savoie FH III. Arthroscopic suture repair of superior labral detachment lesions of the shoulder. Am J Sports Med. 1993;21:783–790.
5. Resch H, Golser K, Thoeni H, et al. Arthroscopic repair of superior glenoid labral detachment (the SLAP lesion). J Shoulder Elbow Surg. 1993;2:147–155.
6. Pagnani MJ, Speer KP, Altchek DW, et al. Arthroscopic fixation of superior labral lesions using a biodegradable implant: a preliminary report. Arthroscopy. 1995;11:194–198.
7. Kim SH, Ha KI, Kim SH, et al. Results of arthroscopic treatment of superior labral lesions. J Bone Joint Surg Am. 2002;84A(6): 981–985.
8. Mileski RA, Snyder SJ. Superior labral lesions in the shoulder: pathoanatomy and surgical management. J Am Acad Orthop Surg. 1998;6:121–131.
9. Nam EK, Snyder SJ. Current concepts: clinical sports medicine update. The diagnosis and treatment of superior labral, anterior and posterior (SLAP) lesions. Am J Sports Med. 2003;31:798–810.
10. Snyder SJ, Banas MP, Karzel RP. An analysis of 140 injuries to the superior glenoid labrum. J Shoulder Elbow Surg. 1995;4:243–248.
11. Maffet MW, Gartsman GM, Moseley B. Superior labrum-biceps tendon complex lesions of the shoulder. Am J Sports Med. 1995;23(1):93–98.
12. Burkhart SS, Morgan CD. Technical note: the peel-back mechanism: its role in producing and extending posterior type SLAP lesions and its effect on SLAP repair rehabilitation Arthroscopy. 1998;14:637–640.
13. O'Brien SJ, Pagnani MJ, Fealy S, et al. The active compression test: a new and effective test for diagnosing labral tears and acromioclavicular joint abnormality. Am J Sports Med. 1998;26(5):610–613.
14. Liu SH, Henry MH, Nuccion S, et al. Diagnosis of glenoid labral tears: a comparison between magnetic resonance imaging and clinical examinations. Am J Sports Med. 1996;24(2):149–154.
15. Kim SH, Ha KI, Han KY. Biceps load test: a clinical test for superior labrum anterior and posterior lesions in shoulders with recurrent anterior dislocations. Am J Sports Med. 1999;27(3):300–303.
16. Chandnani VP, Yeager TD, DeBerardino T, et al. Glenoid labral tears: prospective evaluation with MRI imaging, MR arthrography, and CT arthrography. Am J Roentgenology. 161(6):1229–1235.
17. Jee WH, McCauley TR, Katz LD, et al. Superior labral anterior posterior (SLAP) lesions of the glenoid labrum: reliability and accuracy of MR arthrography for diagnosis. Radiology. January 2001;218(1):127–132.
18. Williams MM, Snyder SJ, Buford D Jr. The Buford complex—the "cord-like" middle glenohumeral ligament and absent anterosuperior labrum complex: a normal anatomic capsulolabral variant. Arthroscopy. June 1994;10(3):241–247.
19. McIntyre LF, Caspari RB. The rationale and technique for arthroscopic reconstruction of anterior shoulder instability using multiple sutures. Orthop Clin North Am. January 1993;24(1):55–58.
20. Morgan CD, Bodenstab AB. Arthroscopic Bankart suture repair: technique and early results. Arthroscopy. 1987;3(2):111–122.
21. Speer KP, Warren RF, Pagnani M, et al. An arthroscopic technique for anterior stabilization of the shoulder with a bioabsorbable tack. J Bone Joint Surg Am. December 1996;78(12):1801–1807.
22. Grossman MG, Tibone JE, McGarry MH, et al. A cadaveric model of the throwing shoulder: a possible etiology of superior labrum anterior-to-posterior lesions. J Bone Joint Surg Am. April 2005;87(4):824–831.
23. Panossian VR, Mihata T, Tibone JE, et al. Biomechanical analysis of isolated type II SLAP lesions and repair. J Shoulder Elbow Surg. 2005;14:529–534.
24. Youm T, Tibone JE, ElAttrache NS, et al. Loading the long head of the biceps affects glenohumeral kinematics. Paper presented at: Orthopaedic Research Society Meeting; March 22, 2006; Chicago.

DISORDERS OF THE LONG HEAD OF THE BICEPS

17

■ CHRISTOPHER S. AHMAD, MD

■ HISTORY OF THE TECHNIQUE

Surgical treatment options for long head of biceps tendon disorders have included debridement, tenotomy, and tenodesis. Gilcreest[1] in 1936 described surgical management of a ruptured proximal biceps tendon with suturing the stump of the tendon to the coracoid process. Hichcock and Bechtol[2] described fixation of the tendon in the bicipital groove by creating an osteoperiosteal flap raised from the floor of the groove and securing the tendon deep to this flap with sutures. In 1960, Michele[3] described keystone tenodesis, which placed the proximal biceps into a bony trough created in the bicipital groove followed by covering the trough with a bone block. Froimson[4] in 1974 described keyhole tenodesis, which rolled the tendon into a ball and inserted it into a fashioned "keyhole" in the bicipital groove.

More recently, all arthroscopic biceps tenodesis techniques have been described and especially advocated when concomitant rotator cuff pathology or AC joint pathology are being addressed arthroscopically. Gartsman and Hammerman[5] described an arthroscopic biceps tenodesis technique employing suture anchors. Boileau et al.[6] presented a technique using interference screw fixation with a guide pin drilled through the humerus to tension the biceps within a bony tunnel. Klepps et al.[7] described a technique using interference screw fixation with tensioning of the biceps delivered into a bony tunnel using suture anchors.

An alternative approach to tenodesis that is becoming more popular is simple tenotomy of the biceps tendon. Significant controversy exists regarding both options of tenotomy versus tenodesis for treatment of painful biceps disorders.[4,8–11] Biceps tenodesis has suggested advantages over tenotomy that include maintenance of the length tension relationship, prevention of muscle atrophy, improve-ment of elbow flexion and supination strength, avoidance of cramping pain, and avoidance of cosmetic deformity.[12] Gill et al.,[13] however, reported that simple biceps tenotomy for the treatment of bicipital pathology results in significant reduction in pain and improvement in function. Osbahr et al.[14] evaluated intra-articular biceps tenotomy versus tenodesis. In the majority of patients, cosmetic appearance, the grade of muscle spasms, and the level of anterior shoulder pain were not different for either tenotomy or tenodesis.

Anatomy

The long head of the biceps originates from both the supra-glenoid tubercle and the glenoid labrum with variation in the amount of tendon directly attached to glenoid and the amount attached to labrum.[15,16] The 9-cm long tendon changes its geometry during its course. A recent study showed that the proximal cross-sectional area was 22.7 mm^2 and the distal was 10.8 mm^2.[17] The tendon is flatter and horizontal while on top of the humeral head and then becomes more triangular as it courses inferior into the bicip-ital groove. Once out of the groove, the tendon continues down the anterior aspect of the humerus and becomes mus-culotendinous near the insertion of the deltoid and pec-toralis major tendons. The bicipital portion of the tendon is intra-articular but extra synovial with a synovial sheath that reflects upon itself and encases the tendon. Arm position dictates how much intra-articular tendon is present with the maximum intra-articular tendon in arm adduction and extension, while the minimum is in arm abduction.

Soft tissues stabilize the long head of the biceps within the bicipital groove. At the entrance to the groove, the rota-tor interval and confluence of soft tissue of the supraspinatus and subscapularis bridge the lesser and greater tuberosities. The coracohumeral ligament has bands that insert into the subscapularis, transverse humeral ligament, and the lesser tuberosity, thereby creating a roof overlying the biceps tendon. The superior glenohumeral ligament forms the floor of the rotator interval and creates a pulley that acts as a circular sleeve guiding the long head of biceps into the bicipital groove. The transverse humeral ligament and the falciform ligament from the sternocostal portion of pectoralis major stabilize the tendon within the bicipital groove.

The function of the long head of the biceps remains controversial. Biomechanical studies indicate that the biceps contributes to stability of the glenohumeral joint.[18-20] Itoi et al.[18] reported decreased anterior and posterior displacement as well as decreased external rotation of the humeral head with loading of the biceps tendon. Similarly, Rodosky et al.[20] simulated contractions of the biceps muscle and observed increased torsional stability of the glenohumeral joint. Other studies have suggested that the long head of the biceps functions more with elbow activity and less with shoulder activity.[21,22]

Pathology

Although the function of the long head of the biceps tendon in the shoulder remains controversial, there is less doubt that the biceps tendon can be a significant source of pain.[2,23-30] Biceps disorders have been classified as either biceps instability or biceps tendonitis.[31] Tendonitis is more commonly associated with other shoulder disorders such as rotator cuff disease. Because of the intimate association of the biceps tendon with the rotator cuff, the principal cause of biceps degeneration is attributed to mechanical impingement of the tendon against the coracoacromial arch, similar to rotator cuff impingement.[32-35] The tendon is either atrophic from the degenerative process or hypertrophic in response to the chronic inflammation from the impingement.[22] Synovitis of the biceps tendon most often occurs in the segment within the bicipital groove.[36] Primary bicipital tendonitis is less usual and requires exclusion of rotator cuff pathology for the diagnosis.

Subluxation of the long head of the biceps is most commonly associated with loss of soft tissue restraints from rotator cuff tears.[23,37-40] In the presence of a subscapularis tear, the tendon can sublux medial and deep to the subscapularis. A frank dislocation of the long head of the biceps is nearly always associated with a subscapularis tear.[31]

Rupture of the long head of the biceps tendon typically occurs in the setting of a diseased tendon and a previous history of subacromial impingement. Alternatively, more acute trauma, involving either a powerful supination force or a fall on the outstretched arm, can cause proximal biceps rupture. With partial tearing of the biceps tendon, significant pain and dysfunction is common. In contrast, full thickness traumatic ruptures of the biceps tendon are generally less symptomatic following the acute event.[39,41] Spontaneous or traumatic ruptures of the long head of the biceps generally do not require surgical intervention.

■ INDICATIONS AND CONTRAINDICATIONS

Patients complain of pain localized to the anterolateral aspect of the shoulder, which radiates down the anterior arm into the biceps muscle with extension and internal rotation maneuvers of the arm.[23,25,37-39] Pain at rest and night pain are seen further in the disease progression. The pain may be compounded by concomitant impingement syndrome or rotator cuff tears. Patients with instability of the biceps have painful snapping or clicking in the shoulder typically in overhead positions with internal to external humeral rotation. Because subluxation occurs in the presence of rotator cuff disease, rotator cuff symptoms are usually also present. Frank dislocations of the long head of the biceps usually follow a traumatic event and are most often associated with complete tear of the subscapularis.

The most common examination finding is point tenderness of the biceps tendon within the bicipital groove. Biceps related tenderness can be differentiated from rotator cuff tendonitis by external rotation of the arm. Pain related to the biceps migrates laterally with external rotation of the arm, whereas pain related to rotator cuff tendonitis radiates to the deltoid insertion and does not move with arm rotation. Other specific physical examination tests used to identify pathology of the long head of the biceps tendon include the Speed test,[1,25] the Yergason test,[42] and the biceps instability test.[43] Biceps instability is tested with full abduction and external rotation attempting to elicit a painful click that may be palpable. Because instability of the biceps is often associated with a partial or complete subscapularis rupture, the liftoff[43] and belly-press[44] tests are an essential part of the biceps evaluation. Complete rupture of the long head of the biceps is identified by a cosmetic deformity from the biceps dropping toward the elbow. Shallowness occurs in the anterior portion of the shoulder accompanied by a lump on the anterolateral aspect of the arm.

Radiographic examination should include anteroposterior (AP) views in neutral, internal, and external rotation, an axillary view, and scapular Y-view to assess for associated abnormalities. Ultrasound may dynamically correlate clinical examination with sites of tenderness but is not routine. MRI has the advantages of visualizing the biceps in its groove and surrounding osteophytes as well as assessing associated rotator cuff pathology. Lack of positive findings on MRI does not rule out the presence of significant biceps tendon pathology.

The criterion for biceps tendon management has been outlined by Yamaguchi et al.[22] Reversible changes are considered when degeneration includes less than 25% partial tearing and the tendon has normal position within the bicipital groove. Reversible changes are treated with observation of the biceps and treatment of associated pathology. Irreversible changes include partial thickness tearing or fraying greater than 25%, subluxation of the tendon from the bicipital groove, or reduction in tendon size that is greater than 25%. Additional relative indications for biceps tenotomy or tenodesis are failed subacromial decompression with persistent symptoms attributed to the biceps. Tenodesis is performed for younger patients (less than 55 years) and especially if they are thin. For the older less active patient, tenotomy is performed. Patients must be counseled and accept the possible deformity that can occur if the long head of the biceps retracts into the arm.[6] Biceps tenodesis is generally recommended for younger patients and has been well described using open techniques.[4,11,31]

■ SURGICAL TECHNIQUES

Tenotomy

Standard arthroscopy is performed in either the lateral or beach chair position. Diagnostic arthroscopy is performed to identify all pathology. The anterior portal is created and the biceps is pulled into the joint using a probe for full evaluation. Evaluation of the portion of biceps in the intertubercular groove is required to avoid missing pathology in that part of the tendon. If tenotomy is indicated, a basket instrument or ablation device is used to release the tendon from its attachment on the superior glenoid. A motorized shaver is used to smooth the superior labrum. Concomitant pathology is then addressed such as subacromial decompression and rotator cuff repair.

Arthroscopic Tenodesis

The patient is positioned in the lateral decubitus or beach chair positions and the portals are outlined **(Fig. 17-1)**. A standard posterior portal is created 1 to 2 cm inferior and 1 to 2 cm medial to the posterolateral edge of the acromion. Standard diagnostic arthroscopy is performed and the intra-articular portion of the biceps tendon is visualized. The anterior portal is then created just lateral to the coracoid process, entering

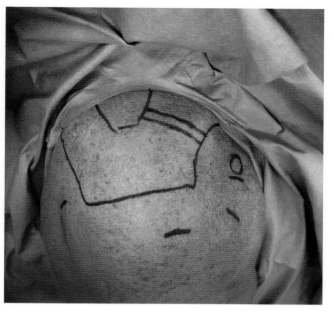

Fig. 17-1. Patient placed in the beach chair position with standard posterior, modified lateral, anterolateral, and anterior portals outlined. (Reprinted with permission from Ahmad CS, ElAttrache NS. Arthroscopic biceps tenodesis. Ortho Clin North Am. 2003; 34:499–506.)

the joint superior to the lateral half of the subscapularis tendon. The biceps tendon is pulled into the joint using a probe to visualize the portion of the biceps that lies within the groove to fully evaluate the tendon. Significant pathology can be missed if the tendon is not drawn into the joint **(Fig. 17-2A,B)**. If significant tearing (greater than 25%), subluxation, or severe tendonitis, demonstrated by hemorrhagic inflammation, is seen, then the decision to perform a tenodesis is made.

Control of the biceps is obtained by percutaneously placing an 18-gauge spinal needle through the proximal biceps

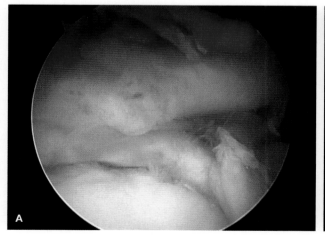 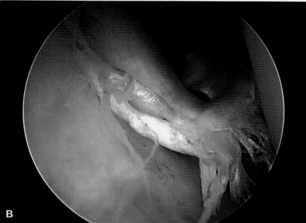

Fig. 17-2. Arthroscopic view of long head of biceps tendon within the glenohumeral joint. **A:** More normal appearance prior to drawing the tendon into the joint. **B:** Significant degeneration of the tendon appreciated following drawing the tendon into the joint. (Reprinted with permission from Ahmad CS, ElAttrache NS. Arthroscopic biceps tenodesis. Ortho Clin North Am. 2003;34:499–506.)

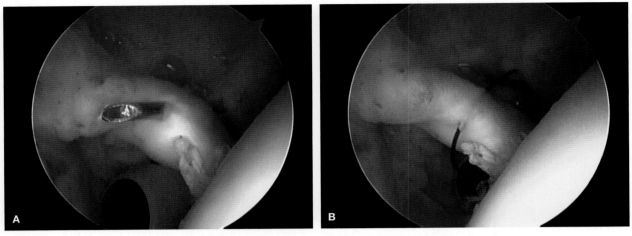

Fig. 17-3. The long head of the biceps is controlled by passing monofilament sutures through a spinal needle introduced percutaneously and retrieved out the anterior portal. **A:** Spinal needle penetrating biceps. **B:** Suture passed and retrieved out anterior portal. (Reprinted with permission from Ahmad CS, ElAttrache NS. Arthroscopic biceps tenodesis. Ortho Clin North Am. 2003;34: 499–506.)

passing no. 0 monofilament sutures **(Fig. 17-3A,B)**. Two sutures are placed and retrieved out the anterior portal. The tenotomy is then performed at the superior labrum using a basket **(Fig. 17-4)**, and the residual stump is debrided to a stable, smooth margin.

Visualization is then changed to the subacromial space. A lateral working portal is established just posterior and 2- to 3-cm lateral to the anterior edge of acromion (Fig. 17-1). Placing this portal more anterior than a typical lateral portal placed at the middle acromion allows better visualization of the bicipital groove. A bursectomy is performed clearing the anterior and lateral gutters of the subacromial space and exposing the greater tuberosity. If necessary, an acromioplasty is performed at this point. The arthroscope is then

placed into the lateral portal. The sutures controlling the tendon are tensioned to pull the tendon out of the defect created in the rotator cuff interval from placement of the anterior cannula. The biceps sheath and falciform ligament of the pectoralis major tendon are identified and transected using an arthroscopic blade or hook electrocautery. Care is taken to avoid damage to the biceps tendon or the traction sutures. The anterior portal cannula is removed and the biceps tendon is delivered out of the skin **(Fig. 17-5)**.

The shoulder and elbow are flexed and the arm positioned in appropriate internal/external rotation to place the biceps directly under the anterior portal to maximize the tendon delivered out of the skin. A portion (10 to 15 mm) may be excised to adjust tendon length for proper tension

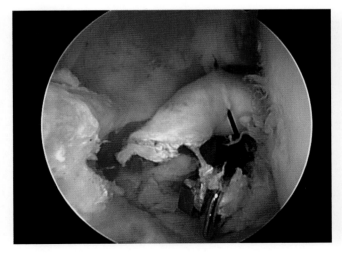

Fig. 17-4. Tenotomy of long head of biceps is performed using basket instruments. (Reprinted with permission from Ahmad CS, ElAttrache NS. Arthroscopic biceps tenodesis. Ortho Clin North Am. 2003;34:499–506.)

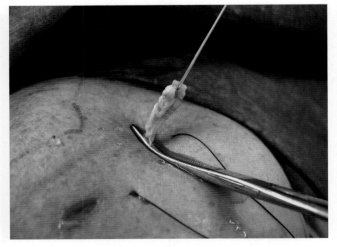

Fig. 17-5. Biceps tendon delivered out the anterior portal and a whipstitch placed. (Reprinted with permission from Ahmad CS, ElAttrache NS. Arthroscopic biceps tenodesis. Ortho Clin North Am. 2003;34:499–506.)

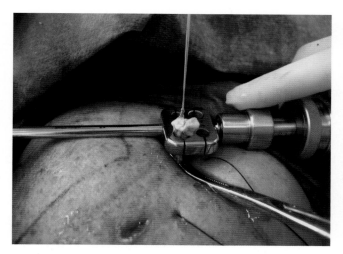

Fig. 17-6. Biceps tendon diameter sized. (Reprinted with permission from Ahmad CS, ElAttrache NS. Arthroscopic biceps tenodesis. Ortho Clin North Am. 2003;34:499–506.)

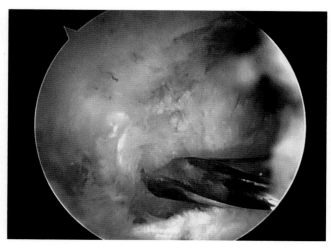

Fig. 17-8. Guide pin placed in bicipital groove. (Reprinted with permission from Ahmad CS, ElAttrache NS. Arthroscopic biceps tenodesis. Ortho Clin North Am. 2003;34:499–506.)

for the tenodesis in the bicipital groove. The length of biceps that is intra-articular has been estimated at 35 mm with the arm adducted to the side.[45] Approximately 20 mm of tendon will be placed in a bone tunnel; therefore, removing an additional 10 to 15 mm restores the appropriate length. The traction sutures are then augmented with a whipstitch of no. 2 nonabsorbable suture for 20 mm (Fig. 17-5). The biceps tendon is then contoured to a uniform shape and the diameter is determined with sizing guides **(Fig. 17-6)**.

An accessory anterolateral portal is created 2 to 3 cm anterior to the anterolateral edge of the acromion (Fig. 17-1). Exact position can be verified with a spinal needle to gain the proper angle on the bicipital groove. The bicipital groove is debrided of soft tissue using a shaver or ablation device **(Fig. 17-7)**. With the arm slightly externally rotated for the

proper angle, a 2.4-mm guide pin is placed in the center of the bicipital groove perpendicular to the surface of the bone **(Fig. 17-8)**. The bone tunnel is then created using a cannulated reamer, the same diameter as the tendon, to a depth of 25 to 30 mm **(Fig. 17-9)**.

The anterior portal cannula is exchanged for an 8.25-mm clear cannula, which accommodates the interference screw and driver. An interference screw is chosen 1 mm smaller than the hole drilled and placed on the Bio-Tenodesis driver (Arthrex, Inc, Naples, Fla). The biceps tendon is controlled by passing the whipstitch suture through the cannulation of the driver **(Fig. 17-10)**. With the tendon drawn tight against the driver, the driver and tendon are inserted into the bone tunnel. The screw is then advanced over the tip of the driver with constant tension on the graft into the bone tunnel. The

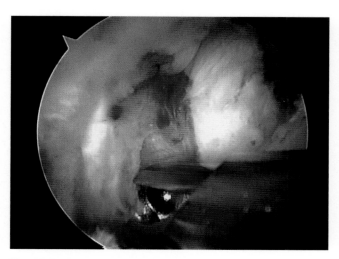

Fig. 17-7. Bicipital groove debrided. (Reprinted with permission from Ahmad CS, ElAttrache NS. Arthroscopic biceps tenodesis. Ortho Clin North Am. 2003;34:499–506.)

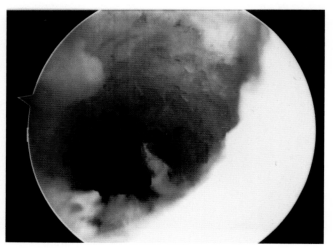

Fig. 17-9. Bone tunnel created in bicipital groove. (Reprinted with permission from Ahmad CS, ElAttrache NS. Arthroscopic biceps tenodesis. Ortho Clin North Am. 2003;34:499–506.)

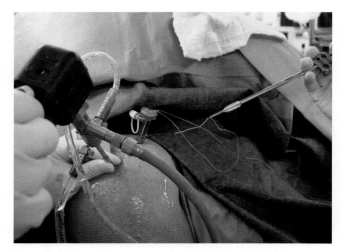

Fig. 17-10. Interference screw on Bio-Tenodesis screwdriver with sutures being passed through the cannulation of the driver with a wire passer. (Reprinted with permission from Ahmad CS, ElAttrache NS. Arthroscopic biceps tenodesis. Ortho Clin North Am. 2003;34:499–506.)

suture controlling the graft is then tied over the screw with standard knot tying techniques. This creates secondary fixation from the sutures **(Fig. 17-11)**.

■ TECHNICAL ALTERNATIVES AND PITFALLS

Arthroscopic biceps tenodesis is technically demanding. As an alternative, open tenodesis may be preferred. If a mini-open rotator cuff repair is being performed, tenodesis is accomplished through the mini-open deltoid splitting approach. The biceps may be released from the glenoid dur-

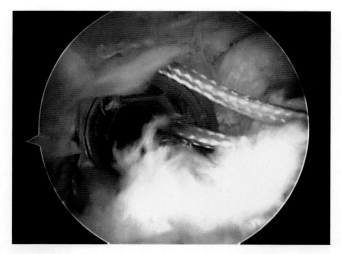

Fig. 17-11. Interference screw placement with fixation is achieved by both the interference screw and the sutures. (Reprinted with permission from Ahmad CS, ElAttrache NS. Arthroscopic biceps tenodesis. Ortho Clin North Am. 2003;34:499–506.)

ing the arthroscopic portion of the case. The arm is externally rotated and abducted to position the bicipital groove underneath the deltoid split. The transverse humeral ligament is divided in line with the groove, and the biceps tendon is identified and delivered out through the deltoid split.

When a mini-open rotator cuff repair is not being performed, a subpectoral inferior axillary approach may be employed. The incision is placed in the axilla, centered on the inferior border of the pectoralis major tendon. The biceps and coracobrachialis are identified and the overlying fascia is incised longitudinally. A Hohmann retractor is placed under the pectoralis major to retract the muscle proximal and lateral. The long head of the biceps is delivered. With either the mini-open or the subpectoralis approach, the next step is determining the length of the biceps for appropriate tension. At the location of the intended tenodesis, 25 mm is added to the biceps and the remaining tendon is excised. Fixation is now obtained similar to the arthroscopic technique, but now with direct visualization.

■ REHABILITATION AND RETURN TO SPORTS

For patients undergoing combined rotator cuff repair and biceps tenodesis, postoperative rehabilitation is focused on protecting the rotator cuff repair. Full passive shoulder and elbow motion is performed during the first 6 weeks, with avoidance of shoulder extension and internal rotation. Active shoulder motion begins at 6 weeks and is continued for 3 months when resistive exercises begin. For patients undergoing isolated tenodesis, full passive and active assisted shoulder motion exercises are begun immediately. Active biceps flexion, however, is avoided for 6 weeks. At 6 weeks, full, unlimited, active elbow motion and resistive exercises are allowed. Aggressive strengthening for elbow flexion and supination is initiated at 12 weeks.

■ OUTCOMES AND FUTURE DIRECTIONS

Several methods of open biceps tenodesis have been previously reported with excellent outcome.[2,4,8,9,11,26,31] The open techniques require a separate deltopectoral incision, which potentially increases postoperative pain and is cosmetically less appealing. The goals of arthroscopic techniques are to achieve equal fixation strength with less morbidity. Arthroscopic rotator cuff repairs are being performed more frequently, which also favors a concomitant arthroscopic biceps tenodesis.

Three different arthroscopic biceps tenodesis techniques have been previously reported.[5-7] Gartsman and Hammerman[5] described a technique that uses bone anchors for fixation. Boileau et al.[6] described a technique that requires passage of a guide pin from anterior to posterior through the humerus, which facilitates tensioning the graft into a tunnel with fixation achieved by using an interference screw. This technique has potential risk to the neurovascular structures. Klepps et al.[7] described a technique that uses a bone anchor to deliver and temporarily hold the biceps into the bone tunnel while the interference screw is placed.

The current technique presented reduces the technical challenge while providing optimum biologic environment for healing. Biomechanical testing in cadavers of interference screw fixation, using the tenodesis driver, has demonstrated fixation strength from 220 to 280 N with displacements of 4 to 6 mm under cyclic loading, which compares to the open bone tunnel technique of approximately 240 N with 8-mm displacement.[12] Romeo[12] compared open subpectoral and arthroscopic tenodesis techniques with 17 patients in each group with 7 months follow-up. There was no difference found in American Shoulder and Elbow Surgeon Simple Shoulder Test or Visual Analog Scale testing. There was a 6% reoperation rate of persistent shoulder pain in both groups. Longer follow-up is required to fully compare the different techniques.

The proximal biceps tendon is a significant source of shoulder pain, and that may be treated with either biceps tenotomy or tenodesis. Biceps tenodesis has suggested advantages over tenotomy that include maintenance of the length tension relationship, prevention of muscle atrophy, maintenance of elbow flexion and supination strength, avoidance of cramping pain, and avoidance of cosmetic deformity. The recent advancement of arthroscopic tenodesis techniques has provided sufficient fixation strength while easing technical demands and minimizing neurovascular injury risk. With our newer techniques and better understanding of proximal biceps tendon pathology, the indications for tenodesis are evolving and longer-term follow-up is required to fully evaluate the outcome of these procedures.

■ REFERENCES

1. Gilcreest EL. Dislocation and elongation of the long head of the biceps brachii: an analysis of six cases. Ann Surg. 1936;104:118–136.
2. Hichcock HH, Bechtol CO. Painful shoulder: observations on role of tendon of long head of biceps brachii in its causation. J Bone Joint Surg Am. 1948;30:263–273.
3. Michele AA. Bicipital tenosynovitis. Clin Orthop. 1960;18:261–267.
4. Froimson AI. Keyhole tenodesis of biceps origin at the shoulder. Clin Orthop. 1975 Oct;(112):245–249.
5. Gartsman GM, Hammerman SM. Arthroscopic biceps tenodesis: operative technique. Arthroscopy. 2000;16(5):550–552.
6. Boileau P, Krishnan SG, Coste JS, et al. Arthroscopic biceps tenodesis: a new technique using bioabsorbable interference screw fixation. Arthroscopy. 2002;18(9):1002–1012.
7. Klepps S, Hazrati Y, Flatow E. Arthroscopic biceps tenodesis. Arthroscopy. 2002;18(9):1040–1045.
8. Becker DA, Cofield RH. Tenodesis of the long head of the biceps brachii for chronic bicipital tendinitis: long-term results. J Bone Joint Surg Am. 1989;71(3):376–381.
9. Berlemann U, Bayley I. Tenodesis of the long head of biceps brachii in the painful shoulder: improving results in the long term. J Shoulder Elbow Surg. 1995;4(6):429–435.
10. Curtis AS, Snyder SJ. Evaluation and treatment of biceps tendon pathology. Orthop Clin North Am. 1993;24(1):33–43.
11. Dines D, Warren RF, Inglis AE. Surgical treatment of lesions of the long head of the biceps. Clin Orthop. 1982 Apr;(164):165–171.
12. Romeo AA. Biceps tenodesis. Presented at: Annual Meeting of the American Society for Sports Medicine; 2002; Orlando, Fla.
13. Gill TJ, McIrvin E, Mair SD, et al. Results of biceps tenotomy for treatment of pathology of the long head of the biceps brachii. J Shoulder Elbow Surg. 2001;10(3):247–249.
14. Osbahr DC, Diamond AB, Speer KP. The cosmetic appearance of the biceps muscle after long-head tenotomy versus tenodesis. Arthroscopy. 2002;18(5):483–487.
15. Cooper DE, Arnoczky SP, O'Brien SJ, et al. Anatomy, histology, and vascularity of the glenoid labrum: an anatomical study. J Bone Joint Surg Am. 1992;74(1):46–52.
16. Vangsness CT Jr, Jorgenson SS, Watson T, et al. The origin of the long head of the biceps from the scapula and glenoid labrum: an anatomical study of 100 shoulders. J Bone Joint Surg Br. 1994;76(6):951–954.
17. McGough RL, Debski RE, Taskiran E, et al. Mechanical properties of the long head of the biceps tendon. Knee Surg Sports Traumatol Arthrosc. 1996;3(4):226–229.
18. Itoi E, Kuechle DK, Newman SR, et al. Stabilising function of the biceps in stable and unstable shoulders. J Bone Joint Surg Br. 1993;75(4):546–550.
19. Pagnani MJ, Deng XH, Warren RF, et al. Role of the long head of the biceps brachii in glenohumeral stability: a biomechanical study in cadavera. J Shoulder Elbow Surg. 1996;5(4):255–262.
20. Rodosky MW, Harner CD, Fu FH. The role of the long head of the biceps muscle and superior glenoid labrum in anterior stability of the shoulder. Am J Sports Med. 1994;22(1):121–130.
21. Levy AS, Kelly BT, Lintner SA, et al. Function of the long head of the biceps at the shoulder: electromyographic analysis. J Shoulder Elbow Surg. 2001;10(3):250–255.
22. Yamaguchi K, Riew KD, Galatz LM, et al. Biceps activity during shoulder motion: an electromyographic analysis. Clin Orthop. 1997 Mar;(336):122–129.
23. Burkhead WZ, Arcand MA, Zeman C, et al. The biceps tendon. In: Rockwood CAJ, Matsen FA, eds. *The Shoulder*. Philadelphia: WB Saunders; 1998:1009–1063.
24. Meyer AW. Spontaneous dislocation and destruction of long head of biceps brachii. Arch Surg. 1928;17:493–506.
25. Neviaser RJ. Lesions of the biceps and tendinitis of the shoulder. Orthop Clin North Am. 1980;11(2):343–348.
26. O'Donoghue DH. Subluxing biceps tendon in the athlete. Clin Orthop. 1982(164):26–29.
27. Pfahler M, Branner S, Refior HJ. The role of the bicipital groove in tendopathy of the long biceps tendon. J Shoulder Elbow Surg. 1999;8(5):419–424.
28. Post M, Benca P. Primary tendinitis of the long head of the biceps. Clin Orthop. 1989 Sep;(246):117–125.
29. Walch G, Nove-Josserand L, Boileau P, et al. Subluxations and dislocations of the tendon of the long head of the biceps. J Shoulder Elbow Surg. 1998;7(2):100–108.
30. Warren RF. Lesions of the long head of the biceps tendon. Instr Course Lect. 1985;34:204–209.
31. Sethi N, Wright R, Yamaguchi K. Disorders of the long head of the biceps tendon. J Shoulder Elbow Surg. 1999;8(6):644–654.
32. Burns WC II, Whipple TL. Anatomic relationships in the shoulder impingement syndrome. Clin Orthop. 1993 Sep;(294):96–102.
33. Neer CS II. Anterior acromioplasty for the chronic impingement syndrome in the shoulder: a preliminary report. J Bone Joint Surg Am. 1972;54(1):41–50.
34. Neer CS II. *Shoulder Reconstruction*. Philadelphia: WB Saunders; 1990.
35. Neviaser TJ. The role of the biceps tendon in the impingement syndrome. Orthop Clin North Am. 1987;18(3):383–386.

36. Neviaser TJ, Neviaser RJ, Neviaser JS. The four-in-one arthroplasty for the painful arc syndrome. Clin Orthop. 1982(163):107–112.

37. Burkhead WZ. The biceps tendon. In: Rockwood CA, Matsen FAI, eds. *The Shoulder*. Philadelphia: WB Saunders; 1990:791–836.

38. Burkhead WZ. The biceps tendon. In: Rockwood CAJ, Matsen FAI, eds. *The Shoulder*. 2d ed. Philadelphia: WB Saunders; 2000:1009–1063.

39. Habermeyer P, Walch G. The biceps tendon and rotator cuff disease. In: Burkhead WZ, ed. *Rotator Cuff Disorders*. Baltimore: Williams and Wilkins; 1996:142–159.

40. Slatis P, Aalto K. Medial dislocation of the tendon of the long head of the biceps brachii. Acta Orthop Scand. 1979;50(1):73–77.

41. Warren RF. Lesions of the long head of the biceps tendon. Instr Course Lect. 1985;30:204–209.

42. Yergason RM. Supination sign. J Bone Joint Surg. 1931;13:160.

43. Gerber C, Krushell RJ. Isolated rupture of the tendon of the subscapularis muscle. Clinical features in 16 cases. J Bone Joint Surg Br. 1991;73(3):389–394.

45. Mazzocca AD, Romeo AA. Arthroscopic biceps tenodesis in the beach chair position. Oper Tech Sports Med. 2003;11(1):6–14.

44. Gerber C, Hersche O, Farron A. Isolated rupture of the subscapularis tendon. J Bone Joint Surg Am. 1996;78:1015–1023.

COMPLEX AND SALVAGE STABILIZATION

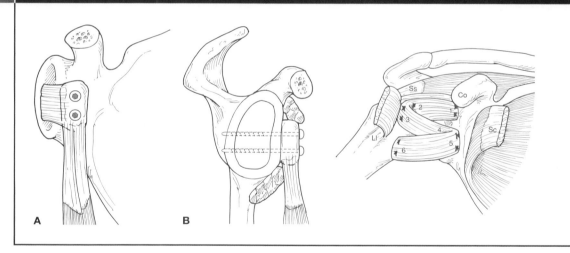

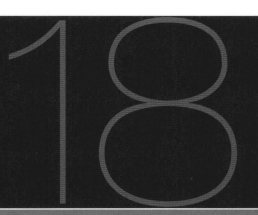

MODIFIED BRISTOW, LATARJET, AND ALLOGRAFT CAPSULAR RECONSTRUCTION

G. RUSSELL HUFFMAN, MD, MPH, JAMES E. TIBONE, MD

The goal of any surgical technique treating glenohumeral instability is to afford a stable shoulder while preserving glenohumeral range of motion. The surgical approach to the patient's instability is directed by the anatomy of the instability and by the functional demands placed upon the shoulder. For cases of traumatic anterior shoulder instability, either open or arthroscopic Bankart repairs remain the surgical procedure of choice. Failure rates for arthroscopic procedures approach the success obtained with open Bankart repairs with failure rates averaging 3% to 5%.[1,2] The success of an "anatomic" instability repair, however, diminishes with the chronicity of glenohumeral instability and with the development of deficient anatomic restraints to instability.

There are several instances in which anterior capsulolabral reconstructions fail to address the anatomy of instability. The Bankart reconstruction fails to provide sufficient long-term shoulder stability in cases of: (a) severe glenoid bone loss; (b) engaging Hill-Sachs lesions; and (c) glenohumeral capsule attenuation from prior thermal treatment, failed instability surgery, connective tissue disorders, and chronic recurrent instability. This chapter discusses options to treat complex shoulder instability in cases of glenoid and humeral bone loss and in cases of capsular insufficiency.

■ PATIENT EVALUATION

All patients should undergo a thorough history specifically addressing the onset and events surrounding their initial dislocation episode, the chronicity and number of instability events, positions that cause apprehension, current level of activity, and any prior stabilization procedures. It is extremely helpful to obtain copies of operative reports and intraoperative arthroscopy photos to better understand the status of the shoulder.

The physical examination focuses on ascertaining the direction of instability: anterior, inferior, posterior, or multidirectional. Additionally, associated pathology including superior labrum, anterior to posterior (SLAP) lesions, rotator cuff tears, scapulothoracic dysfunction, and neurological findings should be evaluated particularly after prior surgical treatment. The load and shift test is the preferred method for quantifying the degree of anterior instability as well as determining the competence and presence of the anterior band of the inferior glenohumeral ligament. In the anesthetized patient, obtaining a locked dislocation after the load and shift indicates a large bony lesion that may preclude Bankart repair. When treating patients with capsular attenuation, a careful assessment of restraints to anterior, posterior, and inferior translation is important. The posterior load and shift test and an assessment for inferior instability with observation of a sulcus sign in adduction and neutral rotation as well as in adduction and external rotation will indicate competency of the coracohumeral ligament, superior glenohumeral ligament, and rotator interval. If the sulcus sign is positive only in neutral rotation, then the interval is competent. If the sulcus remains positive after external rotation, the interval is loose and provides insufficient restraint to inferior instability. Generalized ligamentous laxity should also be assessed in each patient and comparison with the contralateral shoulder is essential in making the correct diagnosis.

Glenoid bone loss has been reported with an incidence as high as 80% and humeral impaction fractures in 70% of cases of chronic, recurrent anterior glenohumeral instability.[3] Many of the bony glenoid lesions involve less than 20% of the glenoid width and may be treated with more standard approaches to instability surgery than discussed in this chapter.[4] In most instances, glenoid and humeral bone loss are evident with standard radiographs. A true glenohumeral anteroposterior (AP) projection and an internal rotation AP will reveal significant Hill-Sachs lesions. An apical oblique view is also useful in visualizing Hill-Sachs lesions.[5] Although the axillary lateral radiograph is an important part of the initial trauma evaluation of a patient with shoulder instability, this view fails to adequately identify or to quantify sufficiently the degree of glenoid bone loss.[6] The West-Point lateral[7] or the glenoid profile lateral as described by Bernegeau et al.[6] more accurately defines anterior inferior glenoid bone loss in all cases of traumatic instability. With the appropriate use of AP and the glenoid profile view, identification of bony defects is possible without the use of additional imaging modalities. However, when quantifying glenoid bone loss, computed tomography (CT) is the most precise imaging modality. In cases of revision instability surgery in which the amount of glenoid loss is uncertain, a CT scan may be useful. Additionally, in cases of combined glenoid and humeral bone loss, use of preoperative CT may allow the surgeon to appropriately plan for both anterior stabilization procedures as well as for addressing humeral bone loss. Magnetic resonance imaging (MRI) is not necessary in the routine assessment of instability patients. However, an MRI allows assessment of capsular integrity after thermal capsulorrhaphy and is useful in the preoperative assessment of the rotator cuff in patients over 40 with a history of traumatic instability.

All patients should undergo examination under anesthesia, including anterior and posterior load and shift, as well as assessment of inferior instability. The routine use of arthroscopic examination allows precise measurement of glenoid bone loss[8] and an additional assessment of the appropriateness of arthroscopic stabilization techniques. The failure rate of arthroscopic stabilization when glenoid bone loss exceeds one fifth the glenoid width is 60%.[8] Additionally, dynamic assessment of engaging Hill-Sachs lesions may be confirmed arthroscopically. In cases of capsular attrition from failed thermal capsulorrhaphy or failed instability procedures in patients with generalized ligamentous laxity, proceeding directly to open surgical treatment is appropriate.

■ MODIFIED BRISTOW TECHNIQUE

History of the Technique

In 1958 Helfet[9] first described a technique of suturing the tip of the coracoid to the glenohumeral capsule and to the periosteum of the anterior glenoid in cases of recurrent anterior glenohumeral instability. Mead and Sweeney[10] modified the procedure in 1964 to include rigid fixation of the bone block to the anterior glenoid rim with a screw. The transferred short head of the biceps and coracobrachialis provide a dynamic restraint to inferior and anterior instability, particularly in positions of glenohumeral abduction and external rotation. Additional restraint is provided by passing the bone block and conjoined tendon between the inferior one third and superior two thirds of the subscapularis, which prevents

the subscapularis from ascending above the inferior aspect of the humeral head during abduction and shoulder external rotation. There is debate over the effectiveness of the bony process in providing an osseous restraint to dislocation.

Indications and Contraindications

Indications for the modified Bristow procedure include treatment of anterior instability in patients with bony glenoid defects exceeding 20% of the inferior glenoid diameter, patients with failed prior stabilization procedures and bony glenoid or humeral head deficits, and patients participating in contact sports with failed prior stabilization procedures. The procedure allows for preservation of external rotation. Coracoid transfer procedures should not be viewed as the initial stabilization procedure in patients with traumatic anterior instability in the absence of substantial glenoid defects or engaging humeral defects. In these instances, either an arthroscopic or open Bankart procedure should be utilized depending upon the technical abilities of the surgeon and the activity level of the patient. Contraindications to performing the Bristow include subscapularis tears and glenoid defects exceeding one third of the anterior glenoid.

Surgical Technique

General anesthesia is used for this procedure. Supplemental regional blocks allow for lowered narcotic use and for the procedure to be performed in an outpatient setting when qualified anesthesia personnel are available. In cases in which the amount of anterior glenoid bone loss is questionable or additional diagnoses are suspected, the patient is placed in the lateral decubitus position and undergoes arthroscopic evaluation. The amount of bone loss is determined by identifying the bare spot in the center of the glenoid. A probe with markings is then used to measure the distance from the posterior aspect of the glenoid to the bare spot. This distance should be the same as the distance from the bare spot to the anterior aspect of the glenoid. The amount of anterior glenoid bone loss can then be measured **(Fig. 18-1)**. In addi-

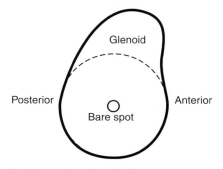

Fig. 18-1. Technique of arthroscopic assessment of anteroinferior glenoid bone loss measured at the bare spot. (Adapted from Burkhart SS, Debeer JF, Tehrany AM, et al. Quantifying glenoid bone loss arthroscopically in shoulder instability. Arthroscopy. 2002;18:488–491.)

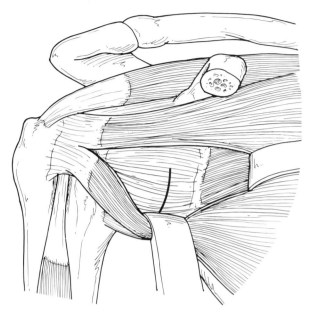

Fig. 18-8. The anterior capsule is exposed through a subscapularis split (alternatively the subscapularis can be retracted through an L-shaped incision). The capsule is incised vertically with a retractor placed inferiorly to protect the axillary nerve and a medial retractor exposing the medial glenoid neck.

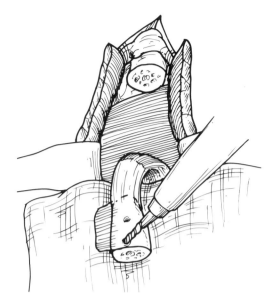

Fig. 18-9. The coracoid process is predrilled with a 2.5-mm drill inferiorly and superiorly prior to placement along the glenoid rim. A towel is placed behind the coracoid during drilling. The lateral attachment of the coracoacromial ligament is left attached to the coracoid process for repair to the anterior glenohumeral capsule.

The optimal position is for the block to be placed below the glenoid equator and flush with the glenoid rim. Excessive medial displacement greater than 0.5 cm should not be tolerated. Similarly, lateral overhang of the process is poorly tolerated and should be contoured to match the concavity of the remaining glenoid surface with a high-speed burr. The superior hole is then drilled in a bicortical fashion through the superior coracoid hole and through the posterior glenoid cortex. Care should be taken when drilling the superior hole to ensure that the drill exits the posterior glenoid well below the spinoglenoid notch to avoid iatrogenic injury to the suprascapular nerve. After measuring and tapping the hole, a 30- to 40-mm partially threaded screw is inserted. This should not be overtightened as the coracoid process can be fractured. A washer may be used but is often unnecessary. The inferior screw is subsequently placed in a similar fashion **(Fig. 18-10A,B,C)**.

The lateral capsular flap is then repaired to the lateral edge of the coracoacromial ligament with an interrupted layer of nonabsorbable suture. It is important to perform this step with the arm in maximum external rotation. Next, the subscapularis is reapproximated with several no. 0 braided absorbable sutures if a subscapularis split has been performed. The repair should be performed to allow adequate excursion of the subscapularis around the transferred coracoid and conjoined tendon to permit full external motion. If an L-shaped subscapularis exposure was performed, then no. 2 braided nonabsorbable sutures are used to reapproximate the subscapularis tendon to the lateral

tendinous insertion that was preserved during exposure. Closure of the deltopectoral interval is typically not necessary. The deep dermal layer and cutaneous layers are closed with buried absorbable sutures. Steri-strips and a sterile bandage are applied to the wound. A drain is not routinely used.

Postoperative Care

Patients are kept in a sling for 2 weeks following surgery. Immediate shoulder motion is permitted within the lesser arc of shoulder motion (hand visible at all times) with supervised physical therapy. Resisted shoulder motion and greater arc motion is permitted after 6 weeks or after radiographic evidence of osseous union. At 6 weeks, active shoulder motion against light resistance is permitted. At 3 months, weight lifting is permitted within the lesser arc of shoulder motion, and passive external rotation stretching under the supervision of a physical therapist is initiated. At 6 months full activities including contact sports are permitted.

Pitfalls and Complications

Successful utilization of the Latarjet technique of stabilization for traumatic anterior shoulder instability relies upon proper patient selection as well as adherence to pertinent technical aspects of the procedure. Important technical points to which the surgeon should adhere include: stable screw fixation of bone block laid flat in a subequatorial position with the coracoid flush to the anterior glenoid rim;

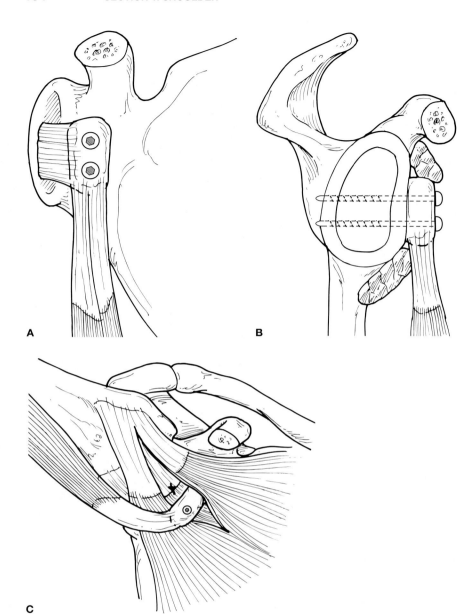

Fig. 18-10. A: Placement of the bone block along the inferior half of the glenoid, secured with two partially threaded screws. The coracoacromial ligament is retained for repair to the lateral portion of the glenohumeral capsule. **B:** Side view of screw placement. **C:** A sling effect is created by placing the bone block between the inferior one third and superior two thirds of the subscapularis.

preservation of the inferior third of the subscapularis; and suturing of the lateral capsular flap to the coracoacromial ligament with the shoulder in full external rotation. Complications with the Latarjet include fracture of the coracoid block. Use of a 4.5-mm fully threaded cortical screw requires overdrilling of the coracoid process with a 4.5-mm drill to compress the coracoid process. However, overdrilling with such a large drill may lead to unwanted fracture at the drill hole. Preferably, a 3.2-mm drill should be used with a partially threaded screw to allow compression of the transferred coracoid process. If the glenoid neck and inferior coracoid process are not prepared for with complete soft tissue removal and gentle decortication, nonunion may occur. Lateral overhang of the coracoid process has been associated with glenohumeral osteoarthritis.[14] Finally, loss

of external rotation may occur if the coracoacromial ligament is not sutured to the glenohumeral capsule with the arm in maximum external rotation or the subscapularis is not preserved allowing early active external rotation during the postoperative period.

ALLOGRAFT CAPSULAR RECONSTRUCTION

History of the Technique

Patients with attenuated or absent glenohumeral capsule pose one of the greatest challenges in the surgical management of glenohumeral instability. Patients with attenuated capsule fall into two broad categories: patients failing prior multiple stabilization procedures, including arthroscopic thermal capsulorrhaphy; and patients with connective tissue disorders including Ehlers Danlos syndrome. Glenohumeral capsular augmentation and reconstruction have been described with autogenous hamstring or long head of the biceps tendons, autogenous iliotibial band, and reconstructions using Achilles, tibialis anterior, and hamstring allograft.[15,16] Our preference for capsular reconstruction is with tibialis anterior allograft.

Evaluation

Careful patient evaluation preoperatively helps the surgeon plan in advance to obtain necessary allograft or for patient counseling and preparation of potential autogenous graft sites. Evaluation begins with ascertaining a history of instability including: the initial instability episode, whether it was traumatic or atraumatic, voluntary or involuntary; the activity level of the patient; family history of connective tissue disorders; the number and nature of instability occurrences; and the specifics of prior surgical treatment. Physical examination should focus on the direction of apprehension and glenohumeral instability, the competence of the coracohumeral ligament and rotator interval, an assessment of generalized ligamentous laxity, and assessment of deltoid and rotator cuff function. In cases of prior failed thermal treatment, an MRI with intra-articular contrast may help the treating surgeon quantify the amount of remaining capsule.

Indications

Indications for allograft capsular reconstruction include cases of failed treatment for multidirectional instability, failures after anterior instability reconstruction with insufficient capsule for standard capsulolabral reconstruction, and cases of attenuated capsule after thermal capsular capsulorrhaphy. Over the past several years, iatrogenic capsular insufficiency and attenuation have become more common from thermal damage incurred during arthroscopic thermal capsulorrhaphy. Although it is important to perform an inferior capsular shift in these patients,[17] the capsular tissue quality may be insufficient to provide adequate joint stability. McFarland et al.[18] showed that after thermal capsular treatment, the morphologic collagen structure of the capsule is altered up to 16 months later.

Absolute contraindications to allograft capsular reconstruction include active glenohumeral joint infections, patients with recurrent voluntary subluxations, and cases of instability coupled with brachial plexus injury. Although capsular augmentation may be appropriate for selected patients with connective tissue disorders and pathologic ligamentous laxity, patients with sufficient capsular tissue should undergo a standard inferior capsular shift and labral repair when possible, even if additional allograft capsular augmentation is required.

Surgical Technique

The patient is positioned supine with a single folded towel placed under medial border of the ipsilateral scapula. The patient is brought to the lateral edge of the table and the operative extremity is placed on a hand board. The surgeon stands in the axilla and the assistant toward the head. A regional block may be administered for additional analgesia depending upon the comfort and skill of the anesthesiologist. Prior to surgical preparation, a careful examination under anesthesia is performed, assessing for anterior and posterior instability using the load and shift test. Inferior instability is assessed using the sulcus sign with inferior traction applied in adduction with neutral rotation and subsequently with external rotation to assess the competency of the coracohumeral ligament. This examination is repeated at the end of the reconstruction to assess the adequacy of conferred glenohumeral stability. Stability of the patient's contralateral shoulder is also assessed under anesthesia preoperatively.

A straight incision is made extending inferiorly from the coracoid process roughly 5 cm in length in line with the axillary fold. The incision is carried through the subcutaneous fat. Athletic males may have little subcutaneous fat, and when possible the dissection should maintain the fascial integrity of the underlying deltoid and pectoralis major muscles. Subcutaneous flaps are made with Metzenbaum scissors over the deltoid and pectoralis fascia. Self-retaining retractors or hand-held retractors are used to retract the skin and subcutaneous tissues. The cephalic vein is identified and retracted laterally with the deltoid. Hand-held retractors are placed to retract the deltoid laterally and the pectoralis major medially. The clavipectoral fascia is incised lateral to the conjoint tendon. The dissection should be blunt at this level and maintained lateral to the conjoint tendon as the musculocutaneous nerve often penetrates the muscle bellies of the coracobrachialis and short head of the biceps from 5 to 7 cm distal to the coracoid process. Either a self-retaining Hawkins-Bell retractor (DePuy Inc, Warsaw, Ind) or hand-held retractors are placed laterally under the deltoid and medially under the conjoint tendon. We prefer hand-held retractors as less continuous pressure is placed on the musculocutaneous nerve. It is important to identify and protect the axillary nerve at this point in the procedure. The arm is adducted and only moderately externally rotated enough to bring the lesser tuberosity into the operative field without placing tension on the axillary nerve.

The subscapularis tendon is then identified and released using a needle-tipped electrocautery. A 1-cm cuff of subscapularis is left laterally for repair later, and an L-shaped incision is made in the subscapularis with the needle-tipped cautery beginning in the rotator interval. The inferior third of the subscapularis and its insertion on the humerus is preserved. Care is taken to separate the capsule from the subscapularis and preserve any remnants of capsule. Dissection of the interval between the subscapularis and underlying capsule is most easily performed medially using a needle-tipped electrocautery device and blunt dissection. This step is critical and is typically possible even in cases in which the capsule is extremely thin and attenuated. Several interrupted sutures are placed to tag the tendon of the subscapularis once the superior two third of the muscle and tendon are released. The dissection of the subscapularis off of the anterior capsule proceeds medially over the glenoid neck and inferiorly into the axillary recess. A single-pronged retractor may be placed within the subscapularis, inferior to the inferior capsule and inferior glenoid neck to afford exposure to the inferior capsule and protect the axillary nerve. A three-pronged retractor is placed outside the capsule along the medial aspect of the anterior glenoid neck. The rotator interval is plicated prior to making a capsular incision with 1 or 2 no. 2 FiberWire sutures (Arthrex, Inc, Naples, Fla). A glenoid-based T-shaped capsular incision is then performed with a scalpel to expose the glenoid rim, labrum, and medial glenoid neck.

An inferior capsular shift is subsequently performed. We perform a glenoid-based shift, although a humeral-based shift may work as well. In shoulders in which the capsule is missing or incomplete, the split should be at the equator of the glenoid. In cases in which the labrum is not detached, the capsule is separated from the labrum and the shifted capsule is sutured to the labrum with no. 2 braided nonabsorbable suture. Next, three anchors are placed along the anterior glenoid rim. If the labrum is medially displaced or insufficient to hold suture, the inferior capsule is advanced superiorly to the inferior anchor first and to the middle and superior anchors subsequently. The superior leaf of the capsule is sewn over the inferior leaf with an interrupted layer of no. 2 FiberWire or equivalent braided, nonabsorbable suture.

When the capsule is attenuated or absent and in cases where a prior shift has failed, an anterior tibialis allograft is thawed. It is cut into two equal limbs each measuring roughly 10 cm. Two additional anchors are placed medial to the glenoid rim on the glenoid neck at the 2 and 4 o'clock positions. The first graft is placed inferiorly and looped back around the sutures from the inferior anchor **(Fig. 18-11)** that are tied around the midportion of this graft. Alternatively, the needles may be left on the anchors and placed through the midportion of each graft. However, we have found that placing the suture through the allograft does not enhance fixation and is more difficult to perform medially on the glenoid neck than simply tying the sutures around the allograft. The inferior graft will reconstruct the inferior and middle glenohumeral ligament complexes. The second allograft section is placed superiorly and looped around the sutures of the middle glenoid anchor. The sutures are then tied and cut.

Three additional anchors are then placed laterally in the humeral head, one inferiorly, one in the midportion, and a third superiorly. To facilitate this, the lateral capsule is opened with a T-shaped incision. The lateral capsule, if sufficient, is reapproximated and imbricated into the allograft capsular reconstruction upon closure. With the arm in neu-

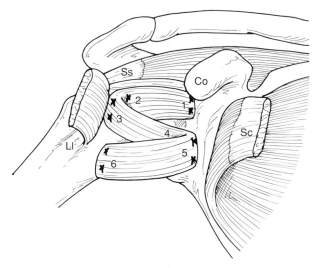

Fig. 18-11. Placement of allograft around anchor sutures in two anchors placed medially in the anterior glenoid neck.

tral rotation to a few degrees of external rotation, the inferior limb is tensioned and sutured laterally to the inferior anchor. Initially, the shoulder is overtightened to allow for subsequent creep of the allograft. In this patient population, increased laxity should be expected after operative reconstruction. For this reason, the reconstruction is performed in less than maximum external rotation. Subsequently, the superior limb of the inferior graft and the inferior limb of the superior graft are sutured laterally to the middle humeral anchor. The superior limb of the superior graft is then tensioned and tied to the superior humeral anchor laterally. The inferior limb is subsequently advanced superiorly and sutured to the middle limb with interrupted nonabsorbable suture. Similarly the middle limbs are sutured together and then to the superior limb **(Fig. 18-12)**. If possible, the superior

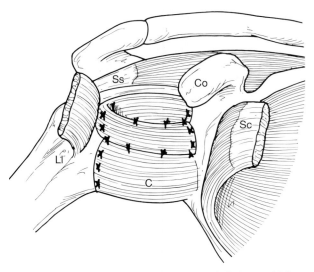

Fig. 18-12. Final suturing of inferior allograft limb to middle and middle to superior.

and inferior limbs should be imbricated to the underlying capsule. Shoulder stability is then gently retested with a load and shift test. Inferior instability is examined with gentle inferior traction in neutral and external rotation to compare with the preoperative sulcus sign. All anchor sutures are cut at this stage and any excess tendon is trimmed laterally.

The subscapularis is repaired with interrupted no. 2 non-absorbable sutures. One or two absorbable sutures reapproximate the split portion of the subscapularis inferiorly. The skin is closed with absorbable sutures placed subcuticularly. Steri-strips and a sterile dressing are applied. A drain is not typically required.

Rehabilitation

Allograft glenohumeral capsule reconstruction is a salvage procedure for the majority of patients undergoing this treatment. For this reason, limited goals and prolonged immobilization are essential to ensure a successful outcome. Patients are placed in a sling in the operating room and remain in the sling for 6 weeks postoperatively. Elbow and wrist motion are initiated immediately. No physical therapy is initiated during this time. After 3 months, gentle stretching exercises under the supervision of a therapist are initiated when indicated. Full activity is permitted at 6 months.

Pitfalls and Complications

Alternatives to allograft capsular reconstruction include performing an inferior capsular shift when adequate capsule remains. Massoud et al.[17] have shown that even after thermal capsular necrosis, inferior capsular shift may be successful without further capsular reconstruction. However, in cases of prior failed stabilization, intrinsic connective tissue disorders, and after failed thermal capsulorrhaphy, autograft or allograft augmentation of the capsular shift is advised. Alternatives to tibialis anterior allograft reconstruction include other allograft sources including hamstring and Achilles, autograft hamstrings, iliotibial band, or long head of the biceps tendon. The anterior tibialis allograft is reliable for this procedure as it has superior tensile strength compared to hamstring tendons, is readily available as a graft source, and it has adequate length to use a single graft with no associated donor morbidity.

Complications to this procedure arise with undertensioning of the reconstruction. Patients undergoing this procedure have a history of multidirectional instability, connective tissue disease, or failed prior stabilization and tend to stretch after the reconstruction. The allograft reconstruction should be viewed as an adjunct to a properly tensioned inferior capsular shift to ensure biologic healing and sustainable results after reconstruction. Failure to properly diagnose the pattern of instability preoperatively and with an examination under anesthesia may also lead to inferior results.

■ REFERENCES

1. Kim S-H, Ha K, Cho Y, et al. Arthroscopic anterior stabilization of the shoulder: two to six-year follow-up. J Bone Joint Surg. 2003;85A:1511–1518.
2. Bankart ASB. The pathology and treatment of recurrent dislocation of the shoulder joint. Br J Surg. 1949;26:23–29.
3. Edwards TB, Boulahia A, Walch G. Radiographic analysis of chronic anterior shoulder instability. Arthroscopy. 2003;19:735–739.
4. Sugaya H, Moriishi J, Dohi M, et al. Glenoid rim morphology in recurrent anterior glenohumeral instability. J Bone Joint Surg. 2003;85A:878–884.
5. Sloth C, Just SL. The apical oblique radiograph in examination of acute shoulder trauma. Eur J Radiol. August 1989;9(3):147–151.
6. Bernageau J, Patte D, Bebeyre J, et al. Interet du profil glenoidien dans les luxations recidivates de l'epaule. Rev Chir Orthop. 1976;62(suppl II):142–147.
7. Itoi E, Lee S-K, Amrami KK, et al. Quantitative assessment of classic anteroinferior bony Bankart lesions by radiography and computed tomography. Am J Sports Med. 2003;31:112–118.
8. Burkhart SS, Debeer JF, Tehrany AM, et al. Quantifying glenoid bone loss arthroscopically in shoulder instability. Arthroscopy. 2002;18:488–491.
9. Helfet AJ. Coracoid transplantation for recurring dislocation of the shoulder. J Bone Joint Surg. 1958;40B:198–202.
10. Mead NC, Sweeney HJ. Bristow procedure. Spectator Letter, The Spectator Society, July 9, 1964.
11. Hovelius L, Korner L, Lundberg B, et al. The coracoid transfer for recurrent dislocation of the shoulder: technical aspects of the Bristow-Latarjet procedure. J Bone Joint Surg. 1983;65A:926.
12. Latarjet M. A propos du traitement des luxations recidivantes de l'epaule. Lyon Chir. 1954;49:994–1003.
13. Edwards BT, Walch G. The Latarjet procedure for recurrent anterior shoulder instability: rationale and technique. Op Tech Sports Med. 2002;10:25–32.
14. Allain J, Goutallier D, Glorion C. Long-term results of the Latarjet procedure for the treatment of anterior instability of the shoulder. J Bone Joint Surg. 1998;80A:841–852.
15. Iannotti JP, Antoniou J, Williams GR, et al. Iliotibial band reconstruction for treatment of glenohumeral instability associated with irreparable capsular deficiency. J Shoulder Elbow Surg. 2002;11:618–623.
16. Warner JP, Venegas AA, Lehtinen JT, et al. Management of capsular deficiency of the shoulder: a report of three cases. J Bone Joint Surg. 2002;84A:1668–1671.
17. Massoud SN, Levy O, Copeland SA. Inferior capsular shift for multidirectional instability following failed laser-assisted capsular shrinkage. J Shoulder Elbow Surg. 2002;11(4):305–308.
18. McFarland EG, Kim TK, Banchasuek P, et al. Histologic evaluation of the shoulder capsule in normal shoulders, unstable shoulders, and after failed thermal capsulorrhaphy. Am J Sports Med. 2002;30:636–642.

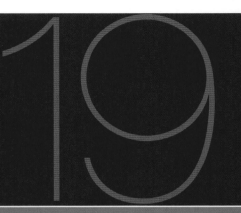

HUMERAL HEAD BONY DEFICIENCY (LARGE HILL-SACHS)

ANTHONY MINIACI, MD, FRCSC, PAUL A. MARTINEAU, MD, FRCSC

■ HISTORY OF THE TECHNIQUE

Bony defects of the posterior-superior aspect of the humeral head occur commonly in association with anterior glenohumeral dislocation. One of the first descriptions of these lesions was by Flower[1] in 1861, with many subsequent investigators reporting on these bony defects of the humeral head.[2–5] In 1940, Hill and Sachs,[6] two radiologists, reported that these defects were actually compression fractures produced when the posterolateral humeral head impinged against the anterior rim of the glenoid.

Since then, Hill-Sachs lesions have been found to occur with an incidence between 32% and 51% at the time of initial anterior glenohumeral dislocation.[6–9] In shoulders sustaining a Hill-Sachs lesion at the initial dislocation, there exists a statistically significant association with recurrent dislocation.[10]

Although Hill-Sachs lesions are common after anterior glenohumeral dislocations, there are relatively few papers describing specific treatments for these humeral head defects. In general, specific surgical procedures to address Hill-Sachs lesions have not been recommended in the initial surgical management of recurrent anterior dislocations because the majority of these lesions are small to moderate in size and do not routinely cause significant symptoms of instability. In fact, Bankart[11] himself did not ascribe any significance to Hill-Sachs lesions observing "nothing can be done about them if they are found."

Nevertheless, a certain subset of patients exists with more significant bony defects and ongoing symptoms of "instability" and/or painful clicking, catching, or popping, sometimes occurring even after surgical procedures are directed at treating their anterior instability. Rowe et al.[12] found a 76% incidence of Hill-Sachs lesions in patients evaluated for recurrent anterior dislocation of the shoulder after surgical repair,

and stated "a Hill-Sachs lesion of the humeral head may play a role in the development of recurrent dislocation after surgical repair."

The concept of "articular arc length mismatch" has been recently put forth to explain the ongoing sensation of catching or popping arising with the shoulder in the abducted and externally rotated position in patients with large Hill-Sachs lesions.[13] Furthermore, many of the patients with these symptoms have undergone previous anterior stabilization procedures. This phenomenon occurs mainly in a position of abduction and external rotation of the shoulder. In this position, a large "engaging" Hill-Sachs lesion encounters the anterior glenoid rim, resulting in the rim "dropping into" the Hill-Sachs lesion. This phenomenon can and does occur in the presence of intact or repaired glenohumeral ligaments. The sudden loss of a segment of articular arc on the humeral side of the joint presents an abrupt "flat spot" to the glenoid, causing an uneasy sensation in the patient that feels much like subluxation.

It is also important to differentiate between "engaging" and "nonengaging" Hill-Sachs lesions.[14] In an engaging Hill-Sachs lesion, the long axis of the defect is parallel to the anterior glenoid with the shoulder in a functional position of abduction and external rotation. This leads to the Hill-Sachs lesion engaging or catching the corner of the glenoid. Conversely, a nonengaging Hill-Sachs lesion is one that either fails to engage the glenoid in a functional arm position or engages the glenoid only in a nonfunctional arm position. In the first type of nonengaging lesion, the long axis of the Hill-Sachs lesion is tangential to the anterior glenoid with the shoulder in a functional position of abduction and external rotation. The Hill-Sachs defect passes diagonally across the anterior glenoid with external rotation; therefore, there is continual contact of the articulating surfaces and no engagement of the Hill-Sachs lesion by the anterior glenoid. In the second type of nonengaging lesion, the Hill-Sachs defect "engages" only in a position that is considered "nonfunctional" (i.e., shoulder in some degree of extension, or in abduction of less than 70 degrees). Since symptoms are greatest if the engagement occurs with the shoulder in a functional position, involving a combination of flexion, abduction, and external rotation, this second group of Hill-Sachs lesions, while technically engaging, has been defined as functionally nonengaging.

Hence, when a patient has symptomatic anterior instability associated with an engaging Hill-Sachs lesion with an articular-arc deficit, treatment must be directed at both repairing the Bankart lesion, if present, and preventing the Hill-Sachs lesion from engaging the anterior glenoid.

We believe that the treatment of symptomatic anterior glenohumeral instability, involving an engaging Hill-Sachs lesion with an articular-arc deficit, can best be accomplished with a technique of anatomic allograft reconstruction of the humeral head using a side and size-matched humeral head osteoarticular allograft. This technique involves an anatomic reconstruction, which eliminates the structural pathology, while maintaining the range of motion of the glenohumeral joint.

■ INDICATIONS AND CONTRAINDICATIONS

The indications for anatomic allograft reconstruction of the humeral head are ongoing symptomatic anterior glenohumeral instability or painful clicking, catching, or popping in a patient with a large engaging Hill-Sachs lesion. We have most commonly used this technique as a secondary procedure in patients who have failed previous soft-tissue stabilization procedures. However, if a large engaging Hill-Sachs lesion is identified prior to undergoing initial surgical treatment, this technique could be performed as part of the primary anterior stabilization procedure. In patients at high risk of redislocation (e.g., epilepsy with recurrent anterior instability and large Hill-Sachs defects) this procedure can be performed at the primary operation.

Contraindications to this procedure include routine medical co-morbidities precluding an elective surgical procedure with general anesthetic, existing infection, or presence of a nonengaging Hill-Sachs lesion.

■ PREOPERATIVE PLANNING

All patients are initially evaluated with complete history and physical examination. Specifics of the history include questioning for the mode of onset and timing of initial symptoms and for the details of present symptoms including pain, frequency, instability, and level of function. In addition, all previous surgical procedures performed on the

shoulder should be noted. Most patients will give a history of recurrent dislocations or multiple surgical attempts to correct the instability. The patients have usually sustained glenohumeral dislocations as a result of significant trauma. Another group of patients that can be encountered is patients with grand mal seizures and recurrent anterior dislocations. These patients usually have fairly large Hill-Sachs defects and significant apprehension about the use of their arms. As a result of the violence of the dislocations, the amount of bone pathology present, and the inability to predict the onset of epileptic events, it is worth considering treating this group of patients with an allograft reconstruction of the humeral head defect at the index procedure as soft tissue repairs alone may not be enough to prevent recurrent injury.

Physical examination should focus on inspection for previous scars, a thorough determination of active and passive range of motion, evaluation of the integrity and strength of the rotator cuff, and a detailed examination for glenohumeral laxity in the anterior, posterior, and inferior directions. Examination for apprehension should be performed in multiple positions as the group of patients with large Hill-Sachs lesions usually exhibits apprehension that often occurs with the arm in significantly less than 90 degrees abduction/90 degrees external rotation.

Preoperative imaging includes a comprehensive plain film evaluation with anteroposterior (AP), true AP, axillary, and Stryker Notch views of the involved shoulder (Fig. 19-1). All patients require a preoperative axial imaging study (computed

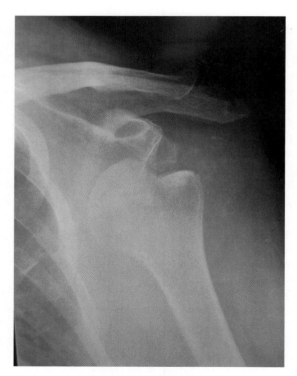

Fig. 19-1. AP x-ray of shoulder demonstrating a large Hill-Sachs lesion.

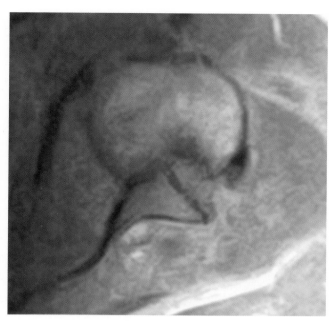

Fig. 19-2. Axial MRI image demonstrating large engaging Hill-Sachs lesion.

tomography [CT] or magnetic resonance imaging [MRI]) to more fully define the bony architecture of the glenoid and humeral head and specifically the details of the Hill-Sachs lesion **(Fig. 19-2)**. One must be careful in the interpretation of these studies since the plane of the Hill-Sachs defect is oblique to the plane of the axial image. Therefore, the size of these defects is often underestimated in standard axial imaging. Three-dimensional reconstruction can be a useful tool to aid in more clearly defining the size and location of the defect and to provide an estimation of the amount of the articular surface involved.

Allograft sizing can be accomplished using plain radiographs with magnification markers or using CT or MRI scan data. However, appropriate sizing of the proximal humeral allograft requires a specific protocol to be arranged between the surgeon and the supplying tissue bank.

A fresh-frozen side and size-matched osteoarticular humeral head allograft is obtained from a reputable, certified tissue bank. The graft serves mainly a structural function, and cartilage viability is probably not essential for success. The availability of fresh frozen tissue can be problematic, and therefore in the past we have performed the procedure using irradiated grafts. However, in two cases using irradiated grafts we have observed partial collapse of the grafts, which required reoperation and screw removal. Therefore, our present protocol favors the use of fresh frozen tissue. If different size grafts or femoral head grafts are used, they may not match the curvature of the native humeral head exactly and often need to be trimmed to obtain fit. Nevertheless, if there are no humeral allografts available, then the use of nonmatched humeral grafts or femoral heads is certainly possible and reasonable.

■ SURGICAL TECHNIQUE

After the administration of a general anesthetic, the patient is positioned in the modified beach chair position with the involved upper extremity draped free. An extended deltopectoral approach is used, taking the cephalic vein laterally with the deltoid muscle. Deltoid detachment is not routinely required. The lateral border of the conjoined tendon is identified and gently retracted medially to expose the underlying subscapularis tendon. A coracoid osteotomy is not usually performed. Tag sutures are placed in the lateral aspect of the subscapularis tendon, and the entire tendon is transected vertically 0.5 cm medial to its insertion onto the lesser tuberosity. Care is taken to avoid injury to the axillary nerve. The interval between the subscapularis and the anterior capsule is then carefully developed using sharp dissection, continuing medially to the neck of the glenoid. The inferior capsule is then further isolated using careful blunt dissection. Alternatively, the capsule and subscapularis can be left together as one complex; however, we find it simpler and easier to expose the humeral head and repair the capsulolabral structures separately. A laterally based capsulotomy is made with the vertical limb in line with the subscapularis incision and continuing superiorly. The anterior-inferior capsule is then released off the surgical neck of the humerus with intra-articular dissection using a periosteal elevator. A humeral head retractor is placed into the glenohumeral joint, allowing inspection of the glenoid and anterior/inferior capsulolabral structures for any pathology. If a Bankart lesion is found, it is repaired using either bony drill holes or suture anchors, but the sutures are left untied until completion of the allograft reconstruction.

The humeral head retractor is withdrawn and the humerus is brought into maximal external rotation to expose the Hill-Sachs lesion. Unroofing the synovial expansion of the supraspinatus, which overlies the tendon of the long head of the biceps, will allow the humerus to be more fully externally rotated, allowing better visualization and access to the Hill-Sachs lesion. A flat narrow retractor is then placed in a position over the reflected undersurface of the subscapularis tendon and behind the neck of the humerus on the posterior rotator cuff in order to lever out the humeral head and present the Hill-Sachs lesion for reconstruction **(Fig. 19-3)**.

With the Hill-Sachs lesion adequately exposed, a microsagittal saw is used to smooth and reshape the defect into a chevron-type configuration, so that the piece of matching allograft humeral head to be inserted will resemble a "deep-dish slice of pie" shape **(Fig. 19-4)**. The base and side of the defect can then be further smoothed using a hand rasp to achieve precise, flat surfaces. The base (x), height (y), length (z), and rough outside partial circumference (c) of the defect are then measured to the nearest millimeter **(Fig. 19-5)**. Knowing which quadrant of the humeral head is involved, a corresponding piece is cut from the matched humeral head allograft that is 2 to 3 mm larger in all dimensions than the measured defect. The allograft segment is then provisionally placed into the Hill-Sachs defect and resized in all three

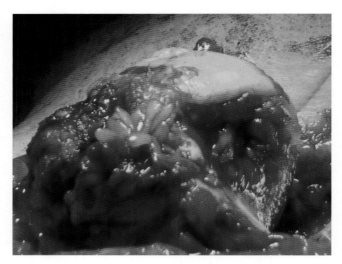

Fig. 19-3. Intraoperative exposure of large Hill-Sachs lesion to be reconstructed.

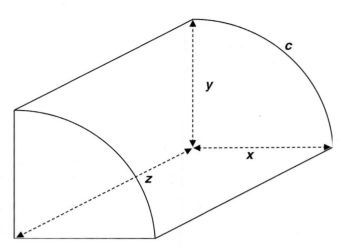

Fig. 19-5. Schematic representation of required measurements of the defect and graft. Base (x), height (y), length (z), and rough outside partial circumference (c) of the defect are then measured to the nearest millimeter.

planes. Excess length is then carefully trimmed with the microsagittal saw. It is very important to also reshape the graft in the other two planes. Fine-tuning of graft size is then continued in one plane at a time until a perfect size match is achieved in all planes including base (x), height (y), length (z), and outside partial circumference (c).

The allograft segment is placed into the defect and aligned so as to achieve a congruent articular surface. It is next provisionally secured in place with two or three smooth 0.045-inch Kirschner wires **(Fig. 19-6)**. The wires are then sequentially replaced with 3.5-mm fully threaded cortical screws placed in a lag fashion. The screw heads are countersunk so that they are below the level of the articular surface **(Fig. 19-7A,B)**.

The joint is irrigated and taken through a range of motion to ensure that the reconstructed humeral head provides a

smooth congruent articulating surface. The capsulotomy is closed with absorbable suture, tying any previously placed sutures used to repair the capsulolabral pathology if present. The subscapularis tendon is then reapproximated to its stump anatomically, without shortening, using nonabsorbable suture. The conjoined tendon, deltoid, and pectoralis major muscles are allowed to return to their normal anatomic positions and the deltopectoral interval is not closed. A routine subcutaneous and skin closure is then performed, a sterile dressing is applied, and the arm is placed into a shoulder immobilizer.

■ TECHNICAL ALTERNATIVES AND PITFALLS

Several techniques have been described in the literature to address symptomatic engaging Hill-Sachs lesions. These

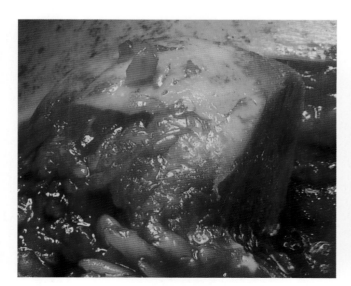

Fig. 19-4. Reshaping of Hill-Sachs lesion to prepare to receive allograft.

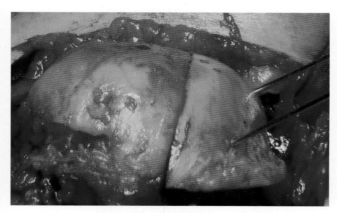

Fig. 19-6. Anatomic allograft reconstruction of Hill-Sachs defect with humeral allograft provisionally held in place with two Kirschner wires.

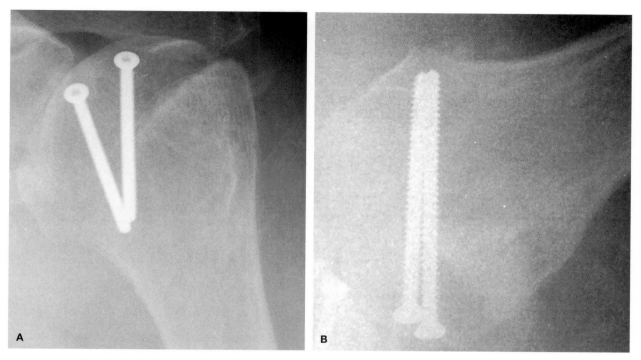

Fig. 19-7. A: AP x-ray of shoulder demonstrating anatomic allograft reconstruction of Hill-Sachs defect fixed with two countersunk cortical screws. **B:** Axillary view of shoulder demonstrating anatomic allograft reconstruction of Hill-Sachs defect fixed with two countersunk cortical screws.

include: (a) open anterior procedures, such as open capsular shift,[15] designed to limit external rotation such that the humeral head defect is kept from engaging[13]; (b) rotational proximal humeral osteotomy[16]; (c) transfer of the infraspinatus into the defect to render the lesion essentially extra-articular[17] or (d) filling in of the Hill-Sachs defect so that it can no longer engage, using either a corticocancellous iliac graft[18] or a femoral head osteoarticular allograft.[19] If the defect is severe, prosthetic replacement, using either hemiarthroplasty or total shoulder arthroplasty is recommended,[20] especially in the setting of chronic dislocations.

In the case of posterior glenohumeral dislocation, Gerber et al.[21,22] have reported on the successful reconstruction of the humeral head by elevation of the depressed cartilage and subchondral buttressing with cancellous bone graft, as well as femoral head osteoarticular allograft reconstruction of the humeral head defect.

Complications that occurred in our series of humeral osteoarticular allograft reconstruction of the Hill-Sachs lesions included radiographic follow-up evidence of partial graft collapse in two of 18 patients, early evidence of osteoarthritis in three patients (marginal osteophytes), and one mild subluxation (posterior). Hardware complications developed in two patients who complained of pain with extreme external rotation. The screws were removed at approximately 2 years postoperatively in both patients, thereby relieving their symptoms.

■ REHABILITATION/RETURN TO SPORTS RECOMMENDATIONS

After surgery, patients are given a sling for comfort and allowed full passive range of motion immediately as tolerated. Due to the subscapularis detachment, we protect against active and resisted internal rotation for a period of 6 weeks. Following the initial 6-week period, patients are allowed terminal stretching and strengthening exercises. The shoulders are imaged with repeat radiographs at 6 weeks and 6 months, and with CT scans at 6 months to assess for consolidation and incorporation of the graft.

■ OUTCOMES AND FUTURE DIRECTIONS

Between 1995 and 2001, we performed and reviewed this procedure in 18 patients who had failed previous attempts at surgical stabilization. Fifteen patients had a history of traumatic anterior glenohumeral instability related to sports, and three patients had instability related to seizures or other trauma. All had posterolateral humeral head defects (Hill-Sachs lesions) that comprised greater than 25% of the humeral head. One patient had both anterior and posterior humeral head defects from bidirectional shoulder instability sustained as a result of a seizure disorder. No patients had true multidirectional instability. Since then we have performed humeral osteoarticular allografting as a primary procedure for patients with seizure disorders with anterior instability and for patients judged to be at high risk of failure of isolated capsulolabral repair due to the extensive size of their Hill-Sachs defect.

Patients in the formal review were assessed preoperatively and postoperatively with a detailed history, physical examination, and radiographic evaluation, including plain films and axial imaging (CT and/or MRI) as well as with validated clinical evaluation measures (Constant-Murley shoulder scale, Western Ontario Shoulder Instability Index (WOSII), and SF-36).

Findings at the time of surgery included nine patients with recurrent Bankart lesions, nine with capsular redundancy only, no patients with subscapularis tears, one patient with posterior glenoid erosion, and three with anterior glenoid deficiency (<20%), which was not reconstructed.

Mean length follow-up was 50 months (range 24 to 96 months). There were no episodes of recurrent instability. Sixteen of 18 (89%) patients returned to work. The average Constant-Murley score postoperatively was 78.5. The WOSII, which is a validated quality-of-life scale specific to shoulder instability utilizing a visual analog scale response format, decreased and patients were significantly improved.

Overall, this represents the first reported series of anatomic allograft reconstruction of Hill-Sachs defects for recurrent traumatic anterior instability following failed repairs. This technique has been shown to be effective for a difficult problem with few available treatment options. The patients demonstrated improvement in stability, loss of apprehension, and high subjective approval, allowing return to near normal function with no further episodes of instability. Although infrequently a cause for clinical concern, Hill-Sachs defects can be the source of significant disability and recurrent instability in a subset of patients. One should consider anatomic allograft reconstruction of these defects as a viable treatment alternative.

■ SUGGESTED READINGS

Burkhart SS, Danaceau SM. Articular arc length mismatch as a cause of failed Bankart repair. Arthroscopy. 2000;16:740–744.

Gerber C, Lambert SM. Allograft reconstruction of segmental defects of the humeral head for the treatment of chronic locked posterior dislocation of the shoulder. J Bone Joint Surg Am. 1996;78:376–382.

Rowe CR, Zarins B, Ciullo JV. Recurrent anterior dislocation of the shoulder after surgical repair: apparent causes of failure and treatment. J Bone Joint Surg Am. 1984;66:159–168.

■ REFERENCES

1. Flower WH. On the pathological changes produced in the shoulder-joint by traumatic dislocations, as derived from an examination of all specimens illustrating this injury in the museums of London. Trans Pathol Soc London. 1861;12:179.
2. Broca A, Hartman H. Contribution a l'etude des luxations de l'epaule. Bull Soc Anat Paris. 1890;4:312.
3. Caird FM. The shoulder joint in relation to certain dislocations and fractures. Edinburgh Med J. 1887;32:708.
4. Hermodsson I. Roentgenologischen studien uber die traumatischen und habituellen schulterverrenkugen nach vorn und nach unten. Acta Radiol. 1934;Suppl. 20:1.
5. Perthes G. Ueber ergebnisse der operationen bei habitueller schulterluxation, mit besonderer berucksichtigung unseres verfahrens. Dtsch Z Chir. 1925;194:1.
6. Hill HA, Sachs MD. The groove defect of the humeral head: a frequently unrecognized complication of dislocations of the shoulder joint. Radiology. 1940;35:690–700.
7. Calandra JJ, Baker CL, Uribe J. The incidence of Hill-Sachs lesions in initial anterior shoulder dislocations. Arthroscopy. 1989;5:254–257.
8. Hovelius L. Anterior dislocation of the shoulder in teen-agers and young adults: five-year prognosis. J Bone Joint Surg Am. 1987;69:393–399.
9. Simonet WT, Cofield RH. Prognosis in anterior shoulder dislocation. Am J Sports Med. 1984;12:19–24.
10. Hovelius L, Augustini BG, Fredin H, et al. Primary anterior dislocation of the shoulder in young patients: a ten-year prospective study. J Bone Joint Surg Am. 1996;78:1677–1684.
11. Bankart BA. Discussion on recurrent dislocation of the shoulder. J Bone Joint Surg Br. 1948;30:47.
12. Rowe CR, Zarins B, Ciullo JV. Recurrent anterior dislocation of the shoulder after surgical repair: apparent causes of failure and treatment. J Bone Joint Surg Am. 1984;66:159–168.
13. Burkhart SS, Danaceau SM. Articular arc length mismatch as a cause of failed Bankart repair. Arthroscopy. 2000;16:740–744.
14. Burkhart SS, De Beer JF. Traumatic glenohumeral bone defects and their relationship to failure of arthroscopic Bankart repairs: significance of the inverted-pear glenoid and the humeral engaging Hill-Sachs lesion. Arthroscopy. 2000;16:677–694.
15. Neer CS, Foster CR. Inferior capsular shift for involuntary inferior and multidirectional instability of the shoulder: a preliminary report. 1980. J Bone Joint Surg Am. 2001;83A:1586.
16. Weber BG, Simpson LA, Hardegger F. Rotational humeral osteotomy for recurrent anterior dislocation of the shoulder associated with a large Hill-Sachs lesion. J Bone Joint Surg Am. 1984;66:1443–1450.
17. Connolly JF. Humeral head defects associated with shoulder dislocations—their diagnostic and surgical significance. AAOS Instr Course Lect. 1972;21:42–54.
18. Branes J. Tratamiento de las luxaciones recidivantes de la articulation escapulo humeral. Paper presented at: IV Congress of Simposia Latino Americana Orthopedica y Traumatologica. Santiago, Chile. 1969.
19. Yagishita K, Thomas BJ. Use of allograft for large Hill-Sachs lesion associated with anterior glenohumeral dislocation: a case report. Injury. 2002;33:791–794.
20. Pritchett JW, Clark JM. Prosthetic replacement for chronic unreduced dislocations of the shoulder. Clin Orthop Relat Res. 1987;216:89–93.
21. Gerber C. L'instabilite posterieur de l'epaule.Cahiers d'enseignement de la SOFCOT. Paris, Expansion Scientifique Francaise, 1991;223–245.
22. Gerber C, Lambert SM. Allograft reconstruction of segmental defects of the humeral head for the treatment of chronic locked posterior dislocation of the shoulder. J Bone Joint Surg Am. 1996;78:376–382.

MISCELLANEOUS

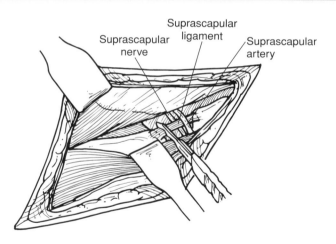

Suprascapular
nerve

Suprascapular
ligament

Suprascapular
artery

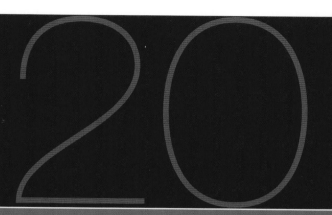

PECTORALIS MAJOR MUSCLE REPAIR

JULIO PETILON, MD, JON K. SEKIYA, MD

■ HISTORY OF THE TECHNIQUE

Rupture of the pectoralis major muscle is rare, with only approximately 150 reported cases in the literature since its first description by Patissier in 1822.[1,2] However, over half of these cases have been identified in the past 30 years. Initially associated with work-related accidents, this condition is now more common among weight lifters and athletes participating in strenuous activities. With society's increased interest in fitness and sport it is likely that this injury may become more prevalent.

Operative treatment of a ruptured pectoralis major muscle ensures the best outcome in terms of patient satisfaction, strength, cosmesis, and return to athletic activity.[1-13] A meta-analysis performed by Bak et al.[1] revealed 88% of patients treated surgically had excellent or good results versus 27% treated nonoperatively. Another study of 22 patients using objective isokinetic testing demonstrated that the peak torque in those treated surgically returned to 99% of that of the uninjured side compared to only 56% in the patients managed nonoperatively.[14] Since the majority of ruptures occur at the myotendinous junction, emphasis of repair is placed on anatomic reapproximation of the ruptured tendon to its insertion site on the humerus. Several techniques for surgical repair have been described. Nevertheless, because of its rarity most results are based on only a few subjects. Furthermore, lack of standardized objective values makes it difficult to compare several of these techniques.

Schepsis et al.[3] described a trough and drill hole technique using a modified Kessler grasping stitch for successfully repairing six acute injuries (less than 2 weeks after injury) and seven chronic injuries. Their results demonstrated an average overall 96% subjective rating in the acute group, 93% in the chronic group, and 51% in the nonoperative group. Objective isokinetic testing after treatment revealed 102% adduction strength in the acute group (when compared to the uninjured side), 94% in the chronic group, and 71% in the nonoperative group. Furthermore, there were no statistically significant subjective or objective differences between the acute or chronically injured patients.

This technique has also been described successfully in the treatment of a 13-year delayed repair and a rupture associated with an anterior shoulder dislocation.[15,16] Miller et al.[17] reported successful repair of an acute complete tendinous rupture using bone anchors. The 19-year-old patient was able to return to collegiate football. Other authors have performed successful repairs by attaching the tendon to the humerus with periosteal sutures.[5,7,9]

Another popular technique described in the literature is the reattachment of the ruptured tendon to the humerus with the use of heavy sutures and drill holes. Kretzler and Richardson[8] achieved good success using two rows of drill holes at the site of insertion in 15 patients. Strength was fully restored in 13 of the patients, with the remaining patients reporting significant improvements. Two patients who were repaired approximately 5.5 years after the injury who did not return to full strength showed significant improvement via Cybex evaluation. One demonstrated an increase in horizontal adduction strength from 50% to 80%, and the other from 60% to 84%. Deformity and range of motion were also corrected. Similar results have been reported by other authors.[18,19] Muscle belly tears occur less frequently and can usually be treated conservatively. However, direct surgical repair has also been described with good results.[7]

■ INDICATIONS AND CONTRAINDICATIONS

Pectoralis major muscle tears can often be diagnosed clinically. The physician must have a good understanding of the typical history and findings on physical examination. Up to 50% of patients may be initially misdiagnosed or there may be a delay in accurate diagnosis.[14] Patients often present with a history related to a specific incident where they report a tearing sensation at the site of injury with or without a "pop." Furthermore, they describe a limited range of motion, swelling, ecchymosis, and weakness. Patients may self-treat this injury as a strain with rest and ice until swelling and bruising resolve and then seek medical evaluation secondary to persistent weakness and asymmetry.

Classical physical findings consist of ecchymosis and swelling over the arm and axilla, a palpable defect and weakness in adduction, and internal rotation of the affected arm **(Fig. 20-1)**. Comparison should always be made to the uninjured side. The classical webbed appearance of a thinned out anterior axilla can be accentuated by abducting the arm 90 degrees. A visual deformity may be enhanced by contraction of the muscle or resisted adduction of the arm as the injured muscle retracts medially and occasionally pulls overlying soft tissue in cases where adhesions have formed. When all of these characteristics are present, one must assume a rupture has occurred. However, classical findings may be masked when there is moderate to severe swelling. Furthermore, the investing fascia of the pectoralis major muscle, which prevents further retraction of the ruptured tendon, may be present as a palpable cord and mistaken for an intact tendon (Carr et al., unpublished data, 2004). Imaging modalities may assist with diagnosis and help provide additional clinical information. Conventional radiographs should always be ordered to rule

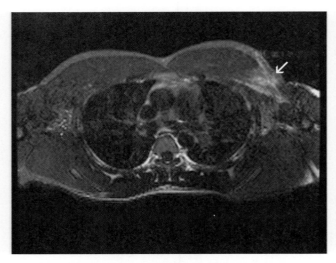

Fig. 20-2. Axial T2-weighted MRI scan of bilateral upper extremities. Rupture of the left pectoralis major muscle *(arrow)* is easily identified and distinguished from the intact muscle on the opposite side.

out any avulsions, fractures, or dislocations. The characteristic finding of a ruptured pectoralis major muscle would be soft tissue swelling and the absence of the pectoralis major shadow. Further evaluation would consist of magnetic resonance imaging (MRI), the modality of choice for a detailed assessment of this injury. We recommend axial cuts to include the contralateral pectoralis major muscle for comparison to the injured side **(Fig. 20-2)**. MRI has been described to accurately determine the grade and site of injury with great sensitivity.[20–22]

The literature supports surgical repair of complete distal pectoralis major muscle ruptures. A complete rupture is defined as the total disruption of either the clavicular or more commonly the sternal head, or the combination of the two, at the tendon insertion site or myotendinous junction. This provides the best results, especially in patients that are active and desire continuation of athletic activities. In older sedentary individuals, nonoperative management may be a reasonable option since it will not likely limit the performance of normal activities of daily living. This will, however, leave the patient with a cosmetic defect and a noticeable strength deficit. Therefore, the level of activity and cosmetic desires should be discussed during surgical evaluation. Comorbid conditions must also be evaluated and considered along with the risks and benefits of surgery for each individual patient.

Some authors argue that diagnosis and repair should occur within 2 months of the injury.[1,7,9,11] They believe that delayed correction is more difficult and results in significant cosmetic and strength deficits. Nevertheless, many other authors have described repairs in patients from 3 months to 13 years out from the injury that provided comparable results with patients treated acutely.[3,6,10,13–15,23,24] It is our opinion that although delayed repair may require additional

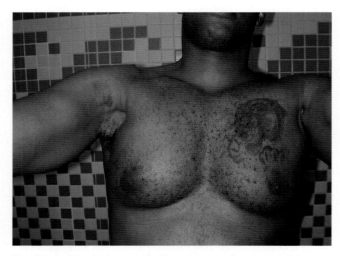

Fig. 20-1. Physical exam finding of a complete acute right pectoralis major muscle rupture. Note the ecchymosis, deformity, and loss of contour of the right anterior chest wall and axilla when compared with the left side.

steps and a larger incision during surgery secondary to adhesions and retraction of the tendon, surgical repair still results in a dramatic improvement in strength.

■ SURGICAL TECHNIQUE

The patient is placed in a modified beach chair position with the head of the table elevated approximately 30 degrees to 45 degrees, which will reduce venous pressure and bleeding. A sandbag or bump should be placed under the medial scapula of the affected side to improve surgical exposure. The affected arm and shoulder are prepped and draped free to allow full range of motion during the procedure. A general anesthetic with muscle relaxation is used to facilitate mobilization of the injured muscle and tendon. This is especially helpful in chronic cases where adhesions and retraction of the torn muscle often require additional mobilization. A variation of the standard deltopectoral incision is made. The proximal extent is made slightly more medial at the level of the coracoid process, which may allow access to the retracted tendon and ends slightly more lateral distally for better access to the pectoralis major insertion site. The incision is often extended proximally and distally in chronic ruptures to facilitate the soft tissue dissection and mobilization of the tendon. The pectoralis major muscle is made up of two broad sheets, the clavicular and sternal heads, which converge and rotate 90 degrees onto each other prior to inserting, just lateral to the bicipital groove. The most inferior muscle fibers end superiorly and posteriorly to the clavicular head. Consequently, this orientation places the sternal head at a mechanical disadvantage and provides a possible explanation for why it is most commonly injured.[6] As a result, the anterior lamina of the tendon, composed of the clavicular head, is often found intact. Furthermore, the anterior fascia of the pectoralis major tendon, which is continuous with the brachial fascia, is frequently undamaged and can be mistaken as an intact tendon. Occasionally, this must be incised to allow better exposure and access to the ruptured sternal portion of the tendon, which is posterior and usually retracted medial to the clavicular insertion. With chronic ruptures, scar tissue formation may also give a false impression of an intact tendon.

After the incision is made, the groove between the deltoid and pectoralis major muscles is developed down to the deltopectoral interval. Note that the internervous plane lies between these two muscles, with the axillary nerve supplying the deltoid and the medial and lateral pectoral nerves innervating the pectoralis major muscle. The cephalic vein is identified and retracted laterally. Adhesions in chronic cases are often present to the overlying subdermal layers and chest wall, spanning the injury pattern, and must be released during initial dissection. Blunt dissection is continued inferior and medial to the clavicular head, which is often intact. Once the ruptured tendon is identified, it is freshened with a

scalpel. It is then mobilized and stay sutures are placed to assist with traction and tension. Mobilization deep to the muscle must be done with care not to injure the medial and lateral pectoral nerves that enter the muscle on its deep surface medially.

Next, the insertion site must be exposed, which lies lateral to the bicipital groove and can be palpated through the inferior portion of the incision. If only the sternal head is torn, the insertion site will be located posterior to the tendon insertion of the anterior laminae. If both heads are ruptured, residual fibers lateral to the long head of the biceps may help mark the insertion site. Care must be taken not to injure or breech the biceps tendon.

Reapproximation of the torn tendon to its anatomical insertion site is achieved by either the use of suture anchors or the bone trough technique. The suture anchor technique is favored in patients with acute tears and good bone quality where the repair can be accomplished under little tension. In these cases, a burr is utilized to create a 3- to 5-cm (to match patient tendon width) by 1-cm area of bleeding bone at the insertion site. Decortication must be avoided or poor suture anchor pullout strength will result. We have had good results with anchors composed of no. 2 or no. 5 braided, nonabsorbable suture. Three to five anchors are evenly placed along the insertion site. One limb of the suture is brought through the tendon and muscle fascia to create a Krackow or modified Kessler grasping stitch. The other end is sutured through the tendon with a single throw and advanced through the sliding anchor, slowly pulling the sutured tendon to its insertion site. With the arm in adduction and neutral rotation, the suture is tied. The remaining sutures are placed and tensioned in a similar fashion **(Fig. 20-3)**. Tension of the repair should be tested and allow approximately 30 degrees of abduction and neutral rotation without undue

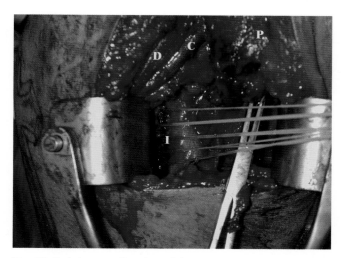

Fig. 20-3. Intraoperative view of the suture anchor technique for a pectoralis major muscle repair. Note the five evenly spaced anchors with suture along the insertion site *(I)* and the ruptured pectoralis major muscle *(P)* held by forceps. D, deltoid; C, cephalic vein.

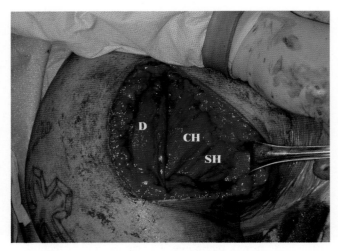

Fig. 20-4. Intraoperative view of a repaired sternal head *(SH)* rupture under an intact clavicular head *(CH)* of the pectoralis major muscle. D, deltoid.

tension. Any remaining tendon at the insertion site is over-sewn to the repaired rupture **(Fig. 20-4)**.

In cases of chronic ruptures, poor bone quality, or where the repair must be achieved under tension, we prefer utilizing the bone trough technique. As above, a burr is used to produce a 3-cm bony trough at the tendon insertion site, while undercutting the superior portion. Three to five equally spaced drill holes are made approximately 1 cm lateral to the trough using a 2-mm drill bit. Using a strong no. 2 braided, nonabsorbable suture, the tendon is grasped in a similar fashion as above and passed through the trough and drill holes. The sutures are then tied over the bone bridge between two approximating drill holes, with the arm held in adduction and neutral position. Again, any remaining distal tendon is sutured over the repair site.

Intramuscular tears are rare, and most of these injuries can be managed conservatively with good results. This usually consists of rest, initial immobilization, and physical therapy advancing to resisted strengthening by 6 weeks. However, failure of nonoperative care may require surgical repair. In these situations, the muscle is repaired using a modified Kessler technique with no. 2 braided, nonabsorbable sutures in three layers. We begin in the posterior fascia of the medially torn muscle, followed by the middle layer, and lastly place sutures through the anterior fascia and muscle to provide three layers of interlocking sutures that can evenly distribute the demanding load of the muscle. These sutures are then tied to the distal portion of the tendon or muscle. Prior to closure, the wound site is copiously irrigated. A standard closure is performed, and the arm is placed in a sling.

The patient is usually admitted overnight for observation and intravenous antibiotics. Neurovascular status and patient comfort are frequently assessed. The following morning the patient is discharged in a sling, with adequate analgesics, and instructed on a standardized postoperative rehabilitative protocol.

■ TECHNICAL ALTERNATIVES AND PITFALLS

The bone trough technique, which is likely the most popular among orthopedists, can certainly be used for all patients with acute or chronic ruptures. In contrast, however, we believe the suture anchor technique should be limited to patients with good bone quality and repairs that do not require extreme tension. Both extreme tension and poor cortical strength may lead to the failure of this technique.

Adequate tension during the repair is critical. Proper positioning of the arm as described above and good grasping suture techniques have provided us with the best results. Some surgeons, however, prefer to suture the repair with the arm in internal rotation, which is acceptable, as long as the proper tension is applied. Overtightening may result in decreased range of motion or failure of the repair during postoperative rehabilitation. In contrast, poor tension may result in persistent weakness.

The use of two rows of drill holes at the insertion site has achieved good results in the literature. However, we prefer to provide a direct bed where the tendon may be repaired. Although direct suturing of the torn tendon to the remaining tuft of muscle at the insertion site has also been reported, we are concerned that it does not provide a strong enough anchor for most repairs. Additionally, there may not be an adequate amount of remaining tendon at the insertion site.

■ REHABILITATION

The patient is instructed to wear the sling for 4 to 6 weeks at all times, including sleep, except when doing prescribed rehabilitative exercises. Those patients requiring an extensive mobilization of the muscle and/or those who are repaired under tension are usually protected in a sling for the full 6 weeks. A home program is established once the patient is discharged. The patient is immediately started on passive pendulum exercises and passive forward elevation up to 130 degrees with the arm adducted. Active and passive range of motion of the neck, elbow, wrist, and hand are to be performed several times a day. An icing program is also implemented. However, during this period, any active abduction, forward elevation, and external rotation are to be avoided.

By 6 weeks, the sling should be discontinued and gentle passive range of motion can begin in all planes of shoulder motion to pain tolerance. A periscapular strengthening program and isometric strengthening exercises can also be added at this time. Nevertheless, the patient is restricted from performing any active internal rotation, shoulder adduction, or horizontal adduction to allow the repair to fully heal. At three months after surgery, the patient should be near full range of motion and ready to commence a strengthening regimen. Progressive, resisted strengthening exercises are begun and include horizontal adduction, shoulder adduction, internal rotation, and forward elevation with the use of arm bands and pulleys. Periscapular strengthening is continued and rotator cuff strengthening exercises may begin. The patient is advised not to perform any dips, push-ups, bench press, flies, or military press. At 6 months, the patient may be slowly advanced to using light weights with high repetitions for dumbbell bench press and push-ups are begun. Between 9 to 12 months postoperatively, the patient is returned to full activities and may include all types of weight exercises to continue strengthening. Nevertheless, heavy weight, low repetition exercises involving the pectoralis major muscle are discouraged indefinitely (particularly with flat barbell bench press).

OUTCOMES AND FUTURE DIRECTIONS

The results of surgical repair of pectoralis major muscle injuries can return a patient to full strength and function as well as reduce any cosmetic deformity. The subjective result according to Schepsis et al.[3] for patients operatively treated for acute ruptures demonstrated a 94% return of their strength compared to preinjury levels, 95% of pain relief, 84% of cosmetic satisfaction, and 96% overall satisfaction. In comparison, the chronic ruptures revealed an average 90% return of strength, 89% pain relief, 84% cosmetic satisfaction, and 93% overall satisfaction. The differences between these two groups were not found to be statistically significant. In contrast, the nonoperative group reported an average 67.5% return of strength, 65% pain relief, 56% cosmetic satisfaction, and 51% overall satisfaction. All three groups regained full range of motion. Objective isokinetic testing was performed at three angular velocities (60, 180, 240 deg/sec) and compared to the uninjured side. Patients in the acute and chronic groups treated operatively had peak torques between 74% and 110%, work per repetition between 82% and 108%, and fatigue indexes between 102% and 121% compared to the nonoperative group, which demonstrated values between 63% and 75%, 58% and 82%, and 52% and 78% in the respective categories. Bak et al.[1] performed a meta-analysis that further confirmed the superior results of surgery when compared to conservative treatment (88% versus 27% with excellent or good results). When corrected for repairs delayed more than 16 weeks, outcome results were noted to be 90% excellent or good. They stated that there was a significant difference in results when comparing acute (0 to 8 weeks) repairs to chronic ruptures (9 to 52 weeks). Outcomes for the acute group were reported as 58% excellent and 31% good compared to 17% excellent and 67% good in the chronic group. As a result, they concluded that a delay in surgery increased the risk of complications during the repair secondary to scar formation and retraction of the muscle. Therefore, it is suggested to perform surgical repair as acutely as possible. Nevertheless, repair of a chronic rupture still provides a significant improvement in strength, function, and cosmesis.

It is possible that current research in tendon healing may implement treatment and improve outcomes. The concentration of research focuses on the use of growth factors, which appear to affect angiogenesis, and the recruitment of essential factors necessary for the process of tendon healing. Although the role and effect of these factors are still under considerable study, several primary reports have described significant positive results in tendon strength and accelerated healing time.[25,26] In addition, the use of gene transfer has been recommended as an ideal method for the delivery of these factors.[26] These biological interventions, if successful, have the potential to significantly improve our results of surgical repair with pectoralis major muscle injuries.

REFERENCES

The views expressed in this chapter are those of the authors and do not reflect the official policy or position of the Department of the Navy, Department of Defense, or the United States Government.

1. Bak K, Cameron EA, Henderson IJ. Rupture of the pectoralis major: a meta-analysis of 112 cases. Knee Surg Sports Trauma Arthrosc. 2000;21:113–119.
2. Quinlan JF, Molloy M, Hurson BJ. Pectoralis major tendon ruptures: when to operate. Br J Sports Med. 2002:36:226–228.
3. Schepsis AA, Grafe MW, Jones HP, et al. Rupture of the pectoralis major muscle: outcome after repair of acute and chronic injuries. Am J Sports Med. 2000;28:9–15.
4. Park JY, Espiniella JL. Rupture of pectoralis major muscle: a case report and review of literature. J Bone Joint Surg. 1970;52:577–581.
5. Zeman SC, Rosenfeld RT, Lipscomb PR. Tears of the pectoralis major muscle. Am J Sports Med. 1979;7:343–347.
6. Wolfe SW, Wickiewicz TL, Cavanaugh JT. Rupture of the pectoralis major muscle: an anatomic and clinical analysis. Am J Sports Med. 1992;20:587–593.
7. McEntire JE, Hess WE, Coleman SS. Rupture of the pectoralis major muscle: a report of eleven injuries and review of fifty-six. J Bone Joint Surg Am. 1972;54:1040–1046.
8. Kretzler HH Jr, Richardson AB. Rupture of the pectoralis major muscle. Am J Sports Med. 1989;17:453–458.
9. Berson BL. Surgical repair of pectoralis major rupture in an athlete: case report of an unusual injury in a wrestler. Am J Sports Med. 1979;7:348–351.
10. Liu J, Wu JJ, Chang CY, et al. Avulsion of the pectoralis major tendon. Am J Sports Med. 1992;20:366–368.
11. Rijnberg WJ, Van Linge B. Rupture of the pectoralis major muscle in body-builders. Arch Othop Trauma Surg. 1993;112:104–105.
12. Pavlik A, Csepai D, Berkes I. Surgical treatment of pectoralis major rupture in athletes. Knee Surg Sports Trauma Arthrosc. 1998;6:129–133.
13. Roi GS, Respizzi S, Dworzak F. Partial rupture of the pectoralis major muscle in athletes. Int J Sports Med. 1990;11:85–87.
14. Hanna CM, Glenny AB, Stanley SN, et al. Pectoralis major tears: comparison of surgical and conservative treatment. Br J Sports Med. 2001;35:202–206.
15. Anbari A, Kelly JD IV, Moyer RA. Delayed repair of a ruptured pectoralis major muscle: a case report. Am J Sports Med. 2000;28: 254–256.
16. Arciero RA, Cruser DL. Pectoralis major rupture with simultaneous anterior dislocation of the shoulder. J Shoulder Elbow Surg. 1997;6:318–320.
17. Miller MD, Johnson DL, Fu FH, et al. Rupture of the pectoralis major muscle in a collegiate football player: use of magnetic

resonance imaging in early diagnosis. Am J Sports Med. 1993;21:475–477.

18. Orava S, Sorasto A, Aalto K, et al. Total rupture of pectoralis major muscle in athletes. Int J Sports Med. 1984;5:272–274.

19. Dunkelman NR, Collier F, Rook JL, et al. Pectoralis major muscle rupture in windsurfing. Arch Phys Med Rehab. 1994;74:819–821.

20. Connell DA, Potter HG, Sherman MF, et al. Injuries of the pectoralis major muscle: evaluation with MR imaging. Radiology. 1999;210:785–791.

21. Carrino JA, Chandnanni VP, Mitchell DB, et al. Pectoralis major muscle and tendon tears: Diagnosis and grading using magnetic resonance imaging. Skeletal Radiol. 2000;29:305–313.

22. Ohashi K, El-Khoury GY, Albright JP, et al. MRI of complete rupture of the pectoralis major muscle. Skeletal Radiol. 1996;25:625–628.

23. Scott BW, Wallace WA, Barton MA. Diagnosis and assessment of pectoralis major rupture by dynamometry. J Bone Joint Surg Br. 1993;74:111–113.

24. Lindenbaum BL. Delayed repair of a ruptured pectoralis major muscle. Clin Orthop. 1975;109:120–121.

25. Molloy T, Wang Y, Murrel G. The roles of growth factors in tendon and ligament healing. Sports Med. 2003;33:381–394.

26. Zhang F, Lineweaver WC. Growth factors and gene transfer with DNA strand technique in tendon healing. J Long Term Eff Med Implants. 2002;12:105–112.

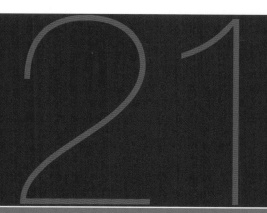

SUPRASCAPULAR NERVE DECOMPRESSION

ORR LIMPISVASTI, MD, RONALD E. GLOUSMAN, MD

■ HISTORY OF THE TECHNIQUE

Thomas first described suprascapular nerve palsy in the French literature in 1936.[1] Since that description, there have been many reports in the English literature describing the pathoanatomy, clinical findings, and treatment of suprascapular neuropathy.[2–5] The suprascapular nerve is primarily a motor nerve that originates from the fifth, sixth, and occasionally fourth cervical nerve root. Although there are rarely cutaneous sensory fibers, branches of the nerve receive afferent sensory input from the glenohumeral joint, acromioclavicular joint, and the coracohumeral ligament. Suprascapular neuropathy can result from nerve traction, extrinsic compression, direct trauma, or a primary neuropathy. The suprascapular nerve is particularly prone to injury as it crosses through the suprascapular notch to supply the supraspinatus muscle and then again at the spinoglenoid notch as it travels into the infraspinatus fossa.

Traction injury at the suprascapular notch and spinoglenoid notch is a common etiology of neuropathy in overhead athletes. Repetitive stretching of the nerve can occur as it courses through a confined space, leading to direct nerve injury or injury to the vascular supply of the nerve. This mechanism can be exacerbated by extreme positions of abduction and retraction found in overhead sports (volleyball, baseball, tennis). Extrinsic compression of the suprascapular nerve can also occur at the spinoglenoid notch secondary to ganglion cysts. These ganglion cysts are often associated with glenohumeral pathology such as labral tears.

The natural history of suprascapular neuropathy is not well documented, but in the athletic population, there can be a significant number of asymptomatic athletes with clinically evident suprascapular neuropathy.[6–8] One study in volleyball players suggests that athletes can remain asymptomatic despite findings of atrophy and weakness on clinical

examination.[8] Symptomatic suprascapular neuropathy without evidence of a compressive lesion should be initially treated with nonoperative treatment. Martin et al.[2] reported that 80% of their patients treated nonoperatively improved without the need for nerve decompression. Nonoperative treatment in their study included strengthening of the deltoid, rotator cuff, and periscapular muscles for a minimum of 6 months while avoiding exacerbating activities. Other conservative measures include anti-inflammatory medications and the selective use of corticosteroid injections. Patients who have symptoms refractory to conservative management may be candidates for suprascapular nerve decompression.

Many different techniques have been described to decompress the nerve at the suprascapular notch. An anterior approach starting medial to the coracoid has been described to reach the suprascapular notch.[9] The increased risk of iatrogenic neurovascular injury with this dissection has led most authors to advocate either a superior or posterior approach to access the suprascapular nerve. The superior approach is a trapezius-splitting approach advocated by Vastamaki and Goransson.[10] The trapezius is split in line with its fibers directly above the suprascapular notch, and the supraspinatus muscle is retracted posteriorly to visualize the notch. The topographical landmarks for the superior approach have been defined in a recent cadaveric study.[11] The posterior approach, advocated by Post and Grinblat,[3] is the one most commonly used in our practice to visualize the suprascapular notch. This approach involves elevation of the trapezius from the scapular spine. For open decompression of the suprascapular nerve at the spinoglenoid notch, a posterior approach through the deltoid is generally recommended.[4] This approach can either utilize a split of the deltoid in line with its fibers or a release of the posterior deltoid from the spine. Subsequent inferior retraction of the infraspinatus muscle exposes the spinoglenoid notch. Although the surgical approaches described may vary, the actual decompression of the nerve generally includes the release of the transverse scapular ligament, spinoglenoid ligament, or both ligaments. Some authors have also advocated osseous decompression of a stenotic notch.

■ INDICATIONS AND CONTRAINDICATIONS

The first step toward determining the appropriate treatment for suprascapular nerve entrapment is confirming diagnosis. The subjective complaints of the patient can vary significantly, especially in overhead athletes. Many asymptomatic overhead athletes have well-documented suprascapular neuropathy on clinical examination. Symptomatic patients frequently describe a poorly localized discomfort or ache over the posterior and lateral aspects of the shoulder. Whether this pain is from injury to the sensory branches of the posterior glenohumeral joint or secondary to rotator cuff deficiency is unknown. Pathology at the suprascapular notch is generally more symptomatic with regard to weakness and pain than pathology at the spinoglenoid notch. By the time the suprascapular nerve has reached the spinoglenoid notch, it has already given off its motor branches to the supraspinatus and received afferent fibers from the posterior joint capsule.

Objective findings vary with the progression of the disease and the location of nerve entrapment. The location of suprascapular nerve injury as it travels through the suprascapular notch and the spinoglenoid notch determines the location of muscle atrophy **(Fig. 21-1)**. Nerve pathology at the spinoglenoid notch will present with atrophy isolated to the infraspinatus muscle. Although wasting of the infraspinatus may be less symptomatic, it is generally more visible than atrophy of the supraspinatus due to the overlying trapezius

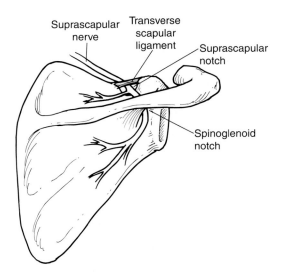

Fig. 21-1. The suprascapular nerve passes beneath the transverse scapular ligament in the suprascapular notch and around the base of the scapular spine through spinoglenoid notch.

muscle. Weakness of the supraspinatus and infraspinatus can often be clinically detected even though weakness may not be a primary subjective complaint of the athlete. Pain in the posterior shoulder can sometimes be reproduced with cross-body adduction and internal rotation; however, this should be differentiated from pathology at the acromioclavicular joint. There can also be point tenderness to palpation over the suprascapular notch or posterior joint line.

Concomitant and precipitating pathology in the overhead athlete can include glenohumeral instability, scapular dyskinesis, and labral pathology. Posterior and superior labral pathology has been associated with spinoglenoid notch cysts and suprascapular nerve compression. Careful examination of glenohumeral stability as well as scapulothoracic mechanics is warranted when evaluating a shoulder with suprascapular neuropathy.

The differential diagnosis of suprascapular nerve palsy includes primary mononeuropathy, cervical radiculopathy, brachial plexitis (Parsonage-Turner syndrome), quadrilateral space syndrome, thoracic outlet syndrome, rotator cuff disease and neoplasm, or other compressive mass. Clinically, we have found that proximal neuropathies such as cervical radiculitis and brachial plexopathy are generally more common etiologies confounding diagnosis of suprascapular nerve entrapment.

Diagnostic studies are important to confirm the diagnosis of suprascapular neuropathy. Plain radiography can be useful for determining the morphology of the suprascapular notch. A 15-degree caudal-oblique anteroposterior (AP) view of the scapula can give a good assessment of the notch morphology. Magnetic resonance imaging (MRI) can be especially helpful in ruling out concomitant pathology or unusual causes of suprascapular neuropathy. Ganglion cysts and other compressive lesions such as tumors can be readily identified with MRI. Atrophy of the rotator cuff muscle and intra-articular pathology such as labral tears are also well visualized with an MRI. We commonly utilize MR arthrography in overhead athletes when there is clinical suspicion of labral and rotator cuff pathology due to its increased accuracy.

Nerve conduction studies and electromyography provide essential information on the location and severity of suprascapular nerve palsy. Electrodiagnostic studies can identify whether the motor dysfunction is isolated to the infraspinatus or also involves the supraspinatus, facilitating the location of the lesion. Positive findings include denervation potential fibrillations, spontaneous activity, and prolonged motor latencies. Normal mean latency from Erb's point to the supraspinatus is 2.7 ms and 3.3 ms to the infraspinatus.[12,13] Although false-negative findings can be present, our practice is to avoid surgical decompression in the face of normal electrodiagnostic studies without an obvious compressive lesion.

Nonoperative treatment is the initial treatment of choice for suprascapular nerve compression in the absence of a compressive lesion. We generally recommend a minimum of 6 to 12 months of rest, physical therapy, and judicious use of anti-inflammatory medications. Avoiding exacerbating activities and strengthening of the rotator cuff and scapular stabilizers often gives good relief and return to function.

Our indication for open surgical decompression in the absence of a compressive lesion is a high level of diagnostic certainty (clinical presentation and diagnostic studies) as well as a failure of nonoperative treatment for at least 6 months. Concomitant pathology such as a labral tear or compressive lesion (ganglion cyst) can lead to earlier surgical intervention. If the suprascapular neuropathy is thought to be symptomatic secondary to a ganglion cyst or labral tear, we generally prefer arthroscopic cyst decompression and labral repair as indicated before performing an open surgery with greater morbidity.

Absolute contraindications to open suprascapular nerve decompression include asymptomatic overhead athletes with clinical findings of atrophy. The natural history of this population is that they will tend to remain asymptomatic.[8] We also avoid prophylactic surgical decompression of the nerve when a cyst is present on MRI because image-guided aspiration techniques and arthroscopic techniques are less invasive. Relative contraindications include pain in the absence of atrophy and weakness or the lack of positive electrodiagnostic studies.

Preoperative planning includes confirming the diagnosis and localizing the lesion. We prefer to limit the decompression to either the suprascapular notch or the spinoglenoid notch. Arthroscopy is performed before open decompression to complete diagnostic examination of the glenohumeral joint and treat any contributing intra-articular pathology.

■ SURGICAL TECHNIQUE

Arthroscopy followed by open suprascapular nerve decompression is performed as an outpatient surgery. Although we commonly use both general and regional anesthesia during many of our shoulder surgeries, we do not use regional anesthesia during this procedure because it can compromise an accurate neurologic examination during the postoperative period. After general anesthesia is induced, careful physical examination of the shoulder is performed to assess range of motion and glenohumeral stability. The patient is positioned in the lateral decubitus position for both arthroscopy of the shoulder as well as the open decompression. We utilize a bean bag holder and posts to secure the patient. The entire upper extremity including the scapula are prepped and draped with the arm in longitudinal traction at approximately 45 degrees of abduction and 30 degrees of flexion.

Diagnostic arthroscopy is performed through the standard posterior portal incision. An anterior-superior portal is established using an outside-in technique, and an anterior cannula is placed to facilitate instrumentation. After complete diagnostic arthroscopy, careful examination of the integrity of the superior and posterior labrum is performed. If a cyst is present on an MRI, cyst decompression can be performed at this time using a small arthroscopic periosteal elevator. The elevator is

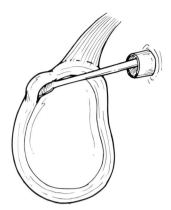

Fig. 21-2. Intraarticular decompression of the cyst is carefully performed through the glenolabral junction.

advanced along the glenolabral junction or through the labral tear if present **(Fig. 21-2)**. Extreme care must be taken during this maneuver due to the proximity of the suprascapular nerve. The average distances of the suprascapular nerve to the superior rim of the glenoid and the posterior rim of the glenoid are 2.9 cm and 1.8 cm respectively.[14] Elevation of the labrum beyond 1 cm is generally not necessary, and a viscous, yellow cyst fluid typically extravasates from the opening with minimal separation. The presence of the cystic fluid is a helpful indicator of cyst decompression. The labrum is repaired in standard fashion using bioabsorbable suture anchors with simple or mattress suture configuration. Other pathology within the glenohumeral joint or subacromial space can be addressed before completion of arthroscopy.

Surgical decompression of the suprascapular nerve at the suprascapular notch is performed in the same position following arthroscopy. The arm is taken off of traction and allowed to rest at the patient's side. A posterior approach is used to access the suprascapular notch, as it does not damage the muscle of the trapezius. The scapular spine can be palpated as a landmark even in well-muscled individuals. A 10-cm transverse incision is made parallel and slightly superior to the scapular spine **(Fig. 21-3)**. Electrocautery is used to achieve hemostasis. The trapezial insertion and periosteum are sharply elevated from the scapular spine. The interval between the undersurface of the trapezius and the supraspinatus is identified. The trapezius is gently retracted cephalad with a wide retractor, while blunt dissection is carefully performed along the surface of the supraspinatus muscle toward the suprascapular notch **(Fig. 21-4)**. During blunt dissection, care must be taken not to injure the suprascapular vessels as they course over the ligament. Gentle inferior retraction of the supraspinatus muscle exposes the suprascapular ligament and notch. Once the suprascapular vessels, nerve, and ligament have all been identified and well visualized, the ligament is carefully released medial to the nerve and artery **(Fig. 21-5)**. If there is a cyst in close proximity to the nerve, it can be decompressed or resected at this time. In a small portion of

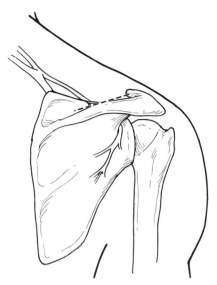

Fig. 21-3. A ten-centimeter transverse incision is made parallel and slightly superior to the scapular spine.

patients, the suprascapular ligament can be partially or completely ossified. In that case, a small Kerrison rongeur can be used to resect the ossified ligament. We do not routinely perform osseous decompression of the suprascapular notch. The trapezius is then reattached to the scapular spine using no. 2 nonabsorbable suture through small drill holes as necessary. The wound is closed in layers and a sling is used for immobilization. The duration of use of the sling is for 1 to 2 weeks postoperatively for comfort unless there is a concomitant intra-articular repair performed.

If the clinical examination and diagnostic studies point to the spinoglenoid notch as the primary site of nerve injury, we do not perform release of the suprascapular ligament. A posterior deltoid approach is used to access the spinoglenoid notch. Patient positioning is the same as for suprascapular ligament release. The skin incision is made along the Langer

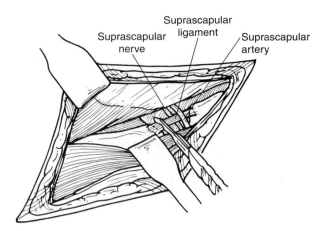

Fig. 21-5. The suprascapular nerve, vessels, and ligament are identified. The ligament is then carefully released medial to the nerve and artery.

lines approximately 3 cm medial to the posterolateral corner of the acromion. The deltoid can be split in line with its fibers starting at the scapular spine and extending distally 5 cm **(Fig. 21-6)**. Further distal extension of the deltoid split can risk injury to the axillary nerve. Alternatively, the deltoid origin can be sharply elevated from the scapular spine, leaving a cuff of tissue to later effect closure through drill holes in the spine. This approach allows increased exposure and includes a longitudinal deltoid split at the raphe between the middle and posterior deltoid heads **(Fig. 21-7)**. The choice of utilizing a deltoid detachment versus an isolated deltoid split in our practice is based on surgeon preference and the need for increased exposure to the spinoglenoid notch. The infraspinatus can then be identified and retracted inferiorly to expose the spinoglenoid notch. Careful dissection exposes the suprascapular nerve as it courses around the base of the scapular spine. Entrapment of the nerve by a ganglion cyst

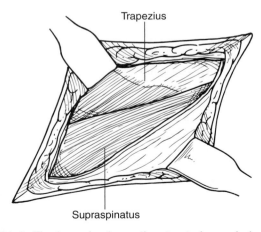

Fig. 21-4. The trapezius is gently retracted superiorly with a wide retractor, while blunt dissection is carefully performed along the surface of the supraspinatus muscle toward the suprascapular notch.

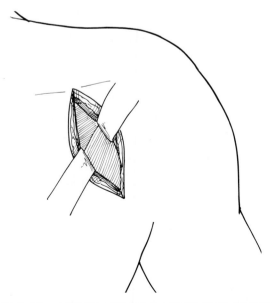

Fig. 21-6. The deltoid is split in line with its fibers beginning at the scapular spine and extending distally up to 5 cm.

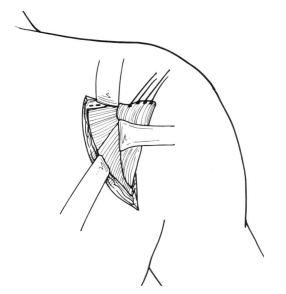

Fig. 21-7. The deltoid origin can also be sharply elevated from the scapular spine to increase the exposure.

or the spinoglenoid ligament can be addressed at this point. If a cyst is present, it can be removed and the ligament excised sharply **(Fig. 21-8)**. Care should be taken to protect the neurovascular structures during nerve decompression. We do not recommend osseous decompression of the spinoglenoid notch except in the case of an obvious bone spur that is impinging on the nerve. If the deltoid was taken down off of the scapular spine, it is reattached with nonabsorbable sutures though small drill holes. The deltoid fascia is reapproximated and the skin and subcutaneous tissue closed in layers. A sling is used postoperative for comfort only.

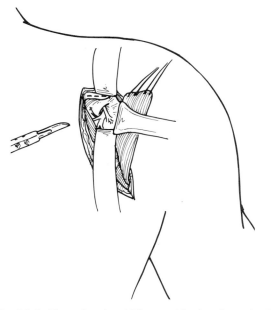

Fig. 21-8. The spinoglenoid ligament is sharply excised.

■ TECHNICAL ALTERNATIVES AND PITFALLS

The decompression of the suprascapular nerve at the suprascapular notch can also be performed through a superior approach that utilizes a trapezius split. The topographical landmarks for this approach have been defined in a cadaveric study; the suprascapular ligament is typically located 1.3 cm posterior to the posterior border of the clavicle, 2.9 cm medial to the acromioclavicular joint, and approximately 4 cm deep to the skin.[11] A skin incision along the Langer line over this point is made, followed by a split in the trapezius muscle in line with its fibers. The supraspinatus muscle can then be retracted posteriorly to expose the suprascapular notch. Nerve decompression and ligament release can be performed in the same fashion as when utilizing the posterior approach.

If a ganglion cyst is compressing the suprascapular nerve, an alternative approach to arthroscopic or open decompression is to utilize an image-guided aspiration technique. Computed tomography, sonography, and interactive MRI-guided aspiration techniques have been reported as useful in the treatment of symptomatic glenoid labral cysts.[15,16] The disadvantage is the inability to address the labral pathology that may be causing the cyst.

■ REHABILITATION/RETURN TO SPORTS RECOMMENDATIONS

The postoperative rehabilitation is based upon the pathology found and treatment rendered. The sling is generally worn for comfort for 1 to 2 weeks, after which point, range of motion exercises are initiated. If a concomitant labral repair is performed for a tear or intra-articular cyst decompression, then the rehabilitation includes a limitation in range of motion depending upon the size and location of the tear. Strengthening exercises for the rotator cuff and scapular stabilizers are started after 3 to 4 weeks. Overhead athletes can begin a progressive throwing program once rotator cuff strength is symmetrical and scapular stabilization and rhythm have normalized. Although most patients can return to daily work activities by 3 months following surgery, overhead athletes may require 4 to 6 months to achieve enough strength and control in their shoulders to return to play.

■ OUTCOMES AND FUTURE DIRECTIONS

Our results for operative suprascapular nerve decompression are similar to those reported in the literature.[2,3] Clinical results for pain relief are typically better than restoration of significant atrophy and weakness. Patients treated earlier in the disease process also tend to fare better after both surgical and nonoperative treatment. The careful selection of patients is critical for a successful outcome. Patients without electrodiagnostic changes before surgery often have a less reliable clinical improvement. Improvement in image-guided cyst aspiration techniques may help prevent significant suprascapular nerve palsies secondary to compressive ganglion cysts. An increased clinical awareness of this entity in the athletic population will hopefully decrease the need for suprascapular nerve decompression in the future.

■ REFERENCES

1. Thomas A. La paralysie du muscle sous-epineux. Presse Med. 1936;64:1283–1284.
2. Martin SD, Warren RF, Martin TL, et al. Suprascapular neuropathy: results of non-operative treatment. J Bone Joint Surg. 1997; 79A:1159–1165.
3. Post M, Grinblat E. Suprascapular nerve entrapment: diagnosis and results of treatment. J Shoulder Elbow Surg. 1993;2:190–197.
4. Romeo AA, Rotenberg DD, Bach BR. Suprascapular neuropathy. J Am Acad Orthop Surg. 1999;7:358–367.
5. Safran MR. Nerve injury about the shoulder in athletes, Part 1. Am J Sports Med. 2004;32:803–819.
6. Cummins CA, Messer TM, Schafer MF. Infraspinatus muscle atrophy in professional baseball players. Am J Sports Med. 2004; 32:116–120.
7. Ferretti A, Cerullo G, Russo G. Suprascapular neuropathy in volleyball players. J Bone Joint Surg. 1987;69:260–263.
8. Ferretti A, De Carli A, Fontana M. Injury of the suprascapular nerve at the spinoglenoid notch: the natural history of infraspinatus atrophy in volleyball players. Am J Sports Med. 1998;26: 759–763.
9. Murray JWG. A surgical approach for entrapment neuropathy of the suprascapular nerve. Orthop Rev. 1974;3:33–35.
10. Vastamaki M, Goransson H. Suprascapular nerve entrapment. Clin Orthop. 1993;297:135–144.
11. Weinfield AB, Cheng J, Nath RK, et al. Topographic mapping of the suprascapular ligament: a cadaver study to facilitate suprascapular nerve decompression. Plast Reconstr Surg. 2002;110: 774–779.
12. Khalili AA. Neuromuscular electrodiagnostic studies in entrapment neuropathy of the suprascapular nerve. Orthop Rev. 1974;3: 27–28.
13. Kraft GH. Axillary, musculocutaneous and suprascapular nerve latency studies. Arch Phys Med Rehabil. 1972;53:383–387.
14. Shishido H, Kikuchi S. Injury of the suprascapular nerve in shoulder surgery: an anatomic study. J Shoulder Elbow Surg. 2001;10: 372–376.
15. Hashimoto BE, Hayes AS, Ager JD. Sonographic diagnosis and treatment of ganglion cysts causing suprascapular nerve entrapment. J Ultrasound Med. 1994;13:671–674.
16. Winalski CS, Robbins MI, Silverman SG. Interactive magnetic resonance image-guided aspiration therapy of a glenoid labral cyst. J Bone Joint Surg. 2001;83A:1237–1242.

2

ELBOW

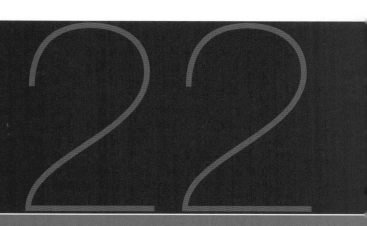

■ DIAGNOSTIC ARTHROSCOPY AND LOOSE BODY REMOVAL

■ GLEN A. MCCLUNG, MD, LARRY D. FIELD, MD, FELIX H. SAVOIE III, MD

■ HISTORY OF THE TECHNIQUE

In 1932 Michael Burman[1] concluded that the elbow joint was "unsuitable for examination" arthroscopically. Since that time advances in arthroscopy and equipment have made elbow arthroscopy safe and effective in the management of a variety of elbow disorders. Elbow arthroscopy is a technically demanding procedure that requires a thorough knowledge of the neurovascular anatomy of the elbow. The original indications for elbow arthroscopy only included the diagnosis and removal of loose bodies. As techniques have advanced, the indications for elbow arthroscopy have expanded to include the treatment of synovitis, osteochondritis dissecans, capsular contractures, arthritis, fractures, lateral epicondylitis, and instability.[2–5]

Elbow arthroscopy was originally performed with the patient in the supine position and the hand suspended to traction. Because of poor access to the posterior aspect of the elbow, Poehling et al.[6] popularized the prone position for elbow arthroscopy. The lateral decubitus position has been advocated by O'Driscoll and Morrey.[3] The arm is positioned with the involved side up, the elbow flexed at 90 degrees, and the arm supported by a padded bolster. This position allows better access to both anterior and posterior compartments.

■ INDICATIONS AND CONTRAINDICATIONS

The indications for elbow arthroscopy include the removal of loose bodies,[2,7–12] removal of osteophytes secondary to osteoarthritis,[13,14] radial head resection,[15] release of capsular contractures and adhesions,[16,17] and the resection of symptomatic plica.[18,19] Other indications include the treatment of osteochondritis dissecans,[2,20–22] fractures,[2,23,24] lateral epicondylitis,[25,26] instability,[27] septic arthritis,[5] synovectomy,[5,23] and evaluation of patients with chronic elbow pain.[2]

Multiple studies have demonstrated the effectiveness of elbow arthroscopy for the diagnosis and treatment of loose bodies. Success rates have been reported in the 90% range.[7,8,10,11] Elbow arthroscopy for loose bodies is indicated in symptomatic patients who fail to respond to conservative treatment. The operating surgeon should attempt to determine the etiology of the loose body. Loose bodies are often a result of osteochondritis dissecans. Other causes include trauma, arthritis, or synovial osteochondromatosis. It is essential that the operating surgeon determine the source of loose bodies, since the outcome of the patient will be determined by the disease, not just the removal of loose fragments.[22]

Prior to taking a patient to the operating room for the removal of loose bodies, a careful history and physical examination must be performed. A history of prior surgeries should be obtained, particularly those involving release or transposition of the ulnar nerve. Physical examination should include range of motion, stability, and neurovascular exam. The ulnar nerve should be evaluated during elbow flexion to ascertain subluxation or dislocation of the nerve. Loose bodies are commonly located in the coronoid fossa, the olecranon fossa, and the posterior lateral gutter, and access to these sites must be obtainable by the surgeon. A complete and thorough evaluation of the joint is necessary because loose bodies can migrate to any area of the elbow.

■ PORTALS

A thorough knowledge of the neurovascular anatomy of the elbow and its three-dimensional relationship to the surface

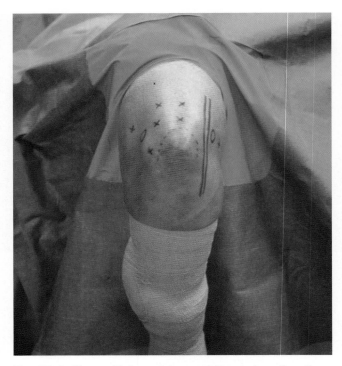

Fig. 22-1. The multiple portals are delineated on the elbow. Surface landmarks including the ulnar nerve marked by the long, parallel lines, the medial and lateral epicondyles marked by the circles, and the various portals marked by the x's are shown in this patient's left elbow in the prone position.

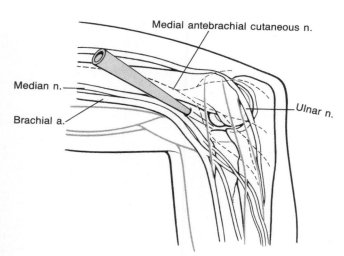

Fig. 22-2. The proximal anterior-medial portal located approximately 2 cm's superior and 2 cm's anterior to the medial epicondyle is marked along with relevant neurovascular structures.

anatomy is required to perform elbow arthroscopy. There are eight access portals that are utilized in elbow arthroscopy. These are determined by neurovascular and musculotendinous anatomy about the elbow. Arthroscopic treatment of the elbow may require the use of several of these portals since the elbow is a highly constrained joint. As the complexity of arthroscopic procedures of the elbow have increased, the number of portals utilized have also increased with an emphasis on the proximal anterior portals.

Surface landmarks are marked on the skin prior to creating portals **(Fig. 22-1)**. Important landmarks to outline are the radial head, olecranon, lateral epicondyle, medial epicondyle, and ulnar nerve. Prior to making portals, the joint must be distended with 20 to 30 ml of sterile saline. This can be done by placing an 18-guage spinal needle either in the olecranon fossa or the soft spot bounded by the lateral epicondyle, olecranon, and radial head. Neurovascular structures are displaced away from the joint with distention of the joint, which gives an additional margin of safety.[28,29]

Poehling et al.[6] first described the proximal anteromedial portal in 1989. This portal is located 2 cm proximal to the medial epicondyle and just anterior to the medial intermuscular septum **(Fig. 22-2)**. The medial intermuscular septum is identified by palpation, and the portal is made anterior to the septum so that the ulnar nerve is not injured. The blunt trocar is introduced into the portal, anterior to the septum, and aimed toward the radial head while maintaining contact with the anterior surface of the humerus. This allows the brachialis

muscle to remain anterior and protect the median nerve and brachial artery. The trocar enters the elbow through the tendinous origin of the flexor-pronator group and medial capsule.[30]

The proximal anteromedial portal has been recommended as the initial portal utilized with the patient in the prone or lateral decubitus position.[6,28] This portal is thought to offer safer access and better visualization of the joint. In addition, fluid extravasation may be less with this portal compared to the anterolateral portal.[28] Visualization of the entire anterior aspect of the joint including the anterior capsule, trochlea, capitellum, coronoid process, radial head, and medial and lateral gutters can be obtained with this portal.

The primary structure at risk with this portal is the posterior branch of the medial antebrachial cutaneous nerve.[31] This nerve is located approximately 2.3 mm from the trocar. With the elbow in flexion, the median nerve is relatively safe, protected by the brachialis muscle, being located on average a distance of 12.4 to 22 mm from the trocar.[28,31] The path of the trocar aims distally and is in a parallel orientation to the median nerve, making injury to the nerve less likely. The ulnar nerve is located on average a distance of 12 to 23.7 mm from the portal.[28,31] The ulnar nerve is not at risk as long as the portal is made anterior to the intermuscular septum. Contraindications to the use of this portal are a history of subluxation or transposition of the ulnar nerve from its groove.[28,31,32] Care must be taken to ensure that the ulnar nerve is not subluxed prior to anteromedial portal placement. This portal may be used in these circumstances only if the nerve is identified prior to trocar entry.

The anteromedial portal, first described by Andrews and Carson,[23] is positioned 2 cm distal and 2 cm anterior to the medial epicondyle **(Fig. 22-3)**. With the elbow flexed to 90 degrees, the blunt trocar is aimed at the center of the joint, passing through the flexor-pronator origin and the brachialis muscle before entering the joint capsule anterior to the medial collateral ligament. This portal may also be established by using an inside-out technique with the arthroscope

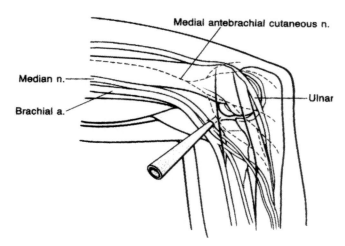

Fig. 22-3. The standard anterior-medial portal is delineated being approximately 2 cm's distal and 2 cm's anterior to the medial epicondyle. Pertinent neurovascular structures are delineated in this illustration well.

in the lateral portal.[28] The entire anterior compartment of the elbow can be visualized from this portal, especially the lateral structures. The medial antebrachial cutaneous nerve is at greatest risk of being injured, located on average 1 mm from the portal.[31] The median nerve is in closer proximity to this portal, being located on average a distance of 7 to 14 mm.[29,31] Lindenfeld[28] reports an average distance of 22 mm from the portal to the median nerve if this portal is established 1 cm anterior to the medial epicondyle.

The proximal anterolateral portal, described by Stothers et al.,[31] Field et al.,[33] and Savoie and Field[34] is positioned 2 cm proximal and 1 to 2 cm anterior to the lateral epicondyle (Fig. 22-4). This portal may be used as the initial portal in elbow arthroscopy. The blunt trocar is aimed toward the center of the joint, while maintaining contact with the anterior humerus, and pierces the brachioradialis muscle, brachialis muscle, and lateral joint capsule before entering

the anterior compartment. This portal allows visualization of the anterior compartment, specifically the lateral and anterior aspects of the radial head and capitellum, lateral gutter, anterior ulnohumeral joint, and anterior elbow capsule.

The structures at risk on the lateral side are the posterior branch of the lateral antebrachial cutaneous nerve and the radial nerve. The trocar in the proximal anterolateral portal lies on average 6.1 mm from the posterior branch of the antebrachial cutaneous nerve.[31] This portal was developed because of the proximity of the radial nerve to the standard anterolateral portal. With the elbow in 90 degrees of flexion and distended with fluid, the radial nerve is located an average distance of 9.9 to 14.2 mm from the proximal anterolateral portal in contrast to 4.9 to 9.1 mm from the standard anterolateral portal.[31,33]

The standard anterolateral portal, first described by Andrews and Carson[23] in 1985, is located 3 cm distal and 1 cm anterior to the lateral epicondyle (Fig. 22-4). The blunt trocar is aimed toward the center of the joint and passed through the extensor carpi radialis brevis muscle and lateral joint capsule before entering the joint. This portal can also be established with an inside-out technique using the arthroscope in the anteromedial or proximal anteromedial portal. The arthroscope is advanced to the capsule lateral to the radial head. The arthroscope is then removed from the cannula and replaced with a blunt rod that tents the overlying skin. The skin is incised over the rod, and a cannula is positioned over the rod and placed into the joint. It is imperative when using this technique that the blunt rod enters the capsule lateral to the radial head rather than anterior to it in order to avoid injury to the radial nerve.[28,31,32]

The anterolateral portal offers visualization of the anterior medial aspect of the joint, including the coronoid process, trochlea, coronoid fossa, and medial aspect of the radial head. Visualization of the lateral joint is better with the proximal anterolateral portal.[33] This portal is also useful as a working portal with arthroscope in the proximal anteromedial portal especially for procedures on the radial head.

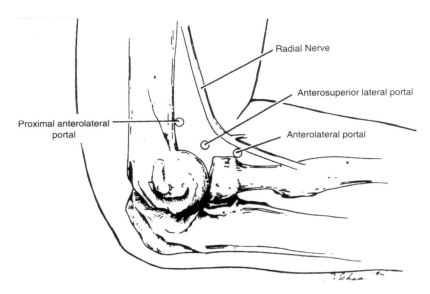

Fig. 22-4. Three primary lateral portals being the proximal anterolateral portal, the anterior superior lateral portal and the distal anterolateral portal are delineated in this figure along with their proximity to the radial nerve.

Lynch et al.[29] have shown the anterolateral portal to be located 2 mm from the posterior antebrachial cutaneous nerve. The radial nerve lies 4.9 to 9.1 mm from this portal with the elbow in 90 degrees of flexion and the joint distended with fluid.[31,33] Because of its proximity and increase risk to the radial nerve, most authors recommend a more proximal entry for this portal.

The midlateral portal is located in the center of the triangular area bordered by the olecranon, lateral epicondyle, and the radial head. This portal is also known as the direct lateral portal or soft spot portal. The blunt trocar passes through the anconeus muscle and the posterior capsule and into the joint. This is the same path that an 18-gauge needle takes for initial distension of the joint. The midlateral portal offers visualization of the radial-ulnar joint as well as the inferior aspect of the radial head and capitellum.

Instrumentation of the lateral gutter and posterior radiocapitellar joint may be utilized with this portal. There is minimal risk to neurovascular structures with this portal. The posterior antebrachial cutaneous nerve, approximately 7 mm away,[35] is the only structure at risk. Because of leakage of fluid into the soft tissues, it is advisable to delay this portal until the end of the operation.[4,31,32]

The straight posterior or transtriceps portal is located 3 cm proximal to the tip of the olecranon in the midline posteriorly[4,36] **(Fig. 22-5)**. This portal allows visualization of the entire posterior compartment as well as the medial and lateral gutters.[30] The blunt trocar is advanced toward the olecranon fossa through the triceps tendon and posterior joint capsule. With the arthroscope in the posterolateral portal, the straight posterior portal can be used for distal humeral fenestration with a drill or burr in ulnohumeral arthroplasty to access the anterior compartment of the elbow.[32] This portal may also be used for instrumentation in removal of loose bodies and excision of olecranon spurs.[30]

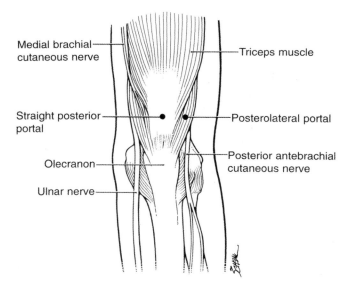

Fig. 22-5. The two standard posterior portals most commonly utilized in the elbow are delineated in this figure.

The posterolateral portal is located 3 cm proximal to the olecranon tip and just lateral to the triceps tendon (Fig. 22-5). The blunt trocar is advanced toward the olecranon fossa, passing lateral to the triceps tendon to enter the joint through the posterolateral capsule. This is performed with the elbow held in 45 degrees of flexion in order to relax the triceps and posterior capsule.[31] Triceps tendon injury can be avoided by remaining close to the posterior humeral cortex with the blunt trocar. This portal is approximately 20 mm from the medial antebrachial cutaneous nerve and 25 mm from the posterior antebrachial cutaneous nerve.[29] The posterolateral portal allows excellent visualization of the posterior compartment of the elbow as well as medial and lateral gutters. In examining the medial gutter from this portal, the operating surgeon must be aware of the location of the ulnar nerve, which lies just superficial to the medial capsule.[6,32]

Access to the posterolateral aspect of the elbow can be obtained anywhere between the soft spot portal to the standard posterolateral portal, 3 cm proximal to the olecranon tip. The posterolateral II portal is usually placed just lateral to the olecranon process and can be moved proximally or distally as needed. Visualization through this portal usually consists of distally the posterior radiocapitellar joint and proximally across the olecranon into the olecranon fossa. It may be used for excision of lateral olecranon spurs, resection of posterolateral plica, and debridement of the radial aspect of the ulnohumeral joint. The triceps tendon and ulnohumeral cartilage are at risk with placement of this portal.[34]

■ SURGICAL TECHNIQUE

Elbow arthroscopy can be performed under general or regional anesthesia. General anesthesia allows for complete muscle relaxation and flexibility of the patient.[6] In an awake patient with regional anesthesia, the prone or lateral decubitus position may be poorly tolerated.[30] Neurologic function can also be monitored postoperatively with general anesthesia alone.

Regional anesthesia with a scalene, axillary, or Bier intravenous regional block may also be used if the patient cannot undergo general anesthesia. The axillary block does not always achieve complete anesthesia about the elbow. Regional anesthesia may limit operative time secondary to longevity of the anesthetic agent or the intolerance of the patient to the tourniquet in a Bier block.

In the supine position, first reported by Andrews and Carson,[23] the patient lies supine with the shoulder over the edge of the operating table. The shoulder is abducted to 90 degrees and is in neutral rotation with 90 degrees of elbow flexion. The elbow is suspended by a traction device that is attached to either the hand or forearm **(Fig. 22-6)**.

There are several advantages of the supine position in elbow arthroscopy.[37] The supine position allows the anesthesiologist easier access to the patient's airway, and there is more flexibility to the choice of anesthesia. The conceptualization of the intra-articular anatomy is facilitated with the

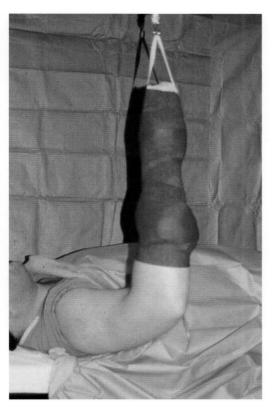

Fig. 22-6. Arthroscopy may be performed in the supine position as noted with the elbow suspended to overhead traction as noted in this right elbow.

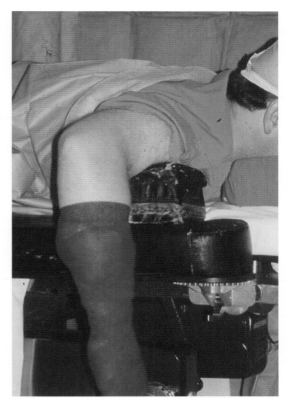

Fig. 22-7. Elbow arthroscopy may be performed in the prone position with a bolster under the upper arm as noted in this figure.

elbow in the supine position, with the elbow joint in a more familiar anatomic orientation. Conversion of an arthroscopic procedure to an open procedure is readily facilitated in the supine position when required.

Disadvantages of the supine position include the requirement for a traction device with the assistance of a second person to stabilize the arm during arthroscopy. Manipulation of the elbow is more difficult with the overhead traction device. Finally, this position provides poor access to the posterior compartment of the elbow joint.

In response to the disadvantages of the supine position, Poehling et al.[6] described the prone position for elbow arthroscopy. The patient is placed prone on the operating table over chest rolls to ensure adequate ventilation. The shoulder is abducted to 90 degrees and the arm is supported by an arm positioner or an arm board **(Fig. 22-7)**. The arm board is placed parallel to the operating table, centered at the shoulder. A sandbag, foam support, or rolled blankets are placed under the upper arm to elevate the shoulder and allow the elbow to rest in 90 degrees of flexion.

Advantages of the prone position are improved access and visualization of the posterior compartment of the elbow. Because the forearm hangs freely from the arm board, the elbow is easily manipulated from near full flexion to full extension. In the prone position the anterior aspect of the elbow is facing inferiorly toward the floor, which allows neurovascular structures to fall anteriorly away from

the joint. This provides an additional margin of safety when establishing portals. No special equipment or additional personnel are needed because the elbow position on the arm board is stable. The prone position, like the supine position, allows for easy conversion to an open procedure.[38]

Disadvantages of the prone position are mostly from an airway and patient positioning consideration. Chest rolls, protective padded face masks, and pillows are needed to pad all prominences susceptible to pressure sores during the procedure. Regional anesthesia is usually not well tolerated by the patient. If general anesthesia becomes necessary secondary to failure of the block or patient anxiety, repositioning of the patient is required. Open approaches to the medial and lateral sides are readily accessible; however, an anterior approach would require repositioning.

The lateral decubitus position, first described by O'Driscoll and Morrey,[3] combines the advantages of the supine and prone position while avoiding some of the pitfalls of each position. The patient is placed in the lateral decubitus position with the arm positioned in an arm holder or over a bolster. The shoulder is flexed to 90 degrees and internally rotated, and the elbow flexed 90 degrees over a padded bolster **(Fig. 22-8)**.

The surgical procedure is performed with the elbow in the prone position and thus provides the same advantages of the prone position. The lateral decubitus does allow for easier patient positioning, and patients can tolerate the lateral decubitus position better if regional anesthesia is needed.

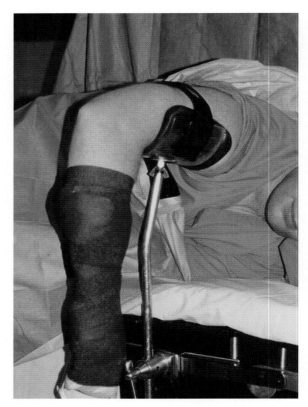

Fig. 22-8. Prone positioning of the elbow may also be accomplished by placing the patient in the lateral decubitus position and using the elbow support device.

This position allows better access to the airway and is easier to convert from regional to general anesthesia if required. Disadvantages include the use of a padded bolster and the possibility of needing to reposition if an open procedure is required.

The proximal anteromedial is the initial portal established unless history of ulnar nerve transposition or subluxation prohibits its use. This portal is located 2 cm proximal to the medial epicondyle and anterior to the intermuscular septum. A no. 11 knife blade is used to incise skin only while a hemostat dissects to the joint capsule. With the elbow in 90 degrees of flexion, a small blunt trocar and cannula for the 4.5-mm arthroscope is aimed toward the radial head while maintaining contact with the anterior aspect of the humerus. Once inside the joint, an egress of fluid confirms intra-articular placement. A 4.5-mm, 30-degree arthroscope is introduced into the cannula with the inflow connected to the bridge on the scope.

With the arthroscope in the proximal anteromedial portal the entire anterior compartment of the elbow can be evaluated. From lateral to medial this includes examination of the lateral gutter, capitellum, radial head, anterior capsule, trochlea, coronoid process, and if properly placed, medial gutter. The arthroscopic evaluation initially includes inspection of the radiocapitellar joint through a range of motion in pronation and supination. This is performed to ensure that the radial head is congruent with the capitellum and that no subluxation exists and to evaluate the articular cartilage of

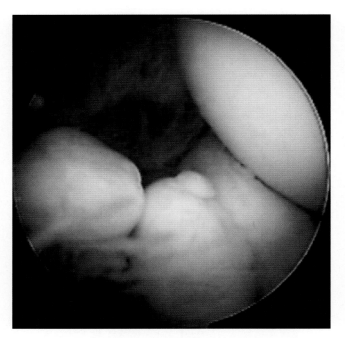

Fig. 22-9. In this view from the proximal anterior medial portal multiple loose bodies are noted anterior to the radiocapitellar joint.

the radial head. The arthroscope is then advanced anterior to the radiocapitellar joint and the lens is rotated to visualize the capsule and undersurface of the extensor muscles. The ulnohumeral articulation is evaluated next by retracting and rotating the arthroscope so that the coronoid process is in view. By rotating the lens superiorly the attachment of the capsule to the humerus is visible.

Loose bodies are commonly found in the anterior compartment in the coronoid fossa **(Fig. 22-9)**. Once the loose body is identified, a lateral portal is established using a spinal needle. For removing loose bodies the proximal anterolateral portal is preferred. The spinal needle is placed 2 cm proximal and 1 to 2 cm anterior to the lateral epicondyle, aiming toward the center of the joint. Once intra-articular placement is confirmed arthroscopically, the spinal needle is removed and a no. 11 blade knife is used to incise skin only in order to avoid damage to cutaneous nerves. A blunt trocar and cannula are then advanced into the joint, while maintaining contact with the anterior humerus to avoid injury to the radial nerve. A grasper with teeth is introduced into the proximal anterolateral portal and used to remove the loose bodies **(Fig. 22-10)**. It may be necessary to "pin or stab" the loose body with an 18-gauge spinal needle, inserted through midanterolateral or anteromedial portal site, in order to provide resistance for grasping. The loose body should be rotated as it is being brought through the soft tissue so that it does not get lost. For larger loose bodies the portal may have to be enlarged in order to accommodate the size of the fragment. Otherwise, the loose body may need to be removed piece by piece.

Once the loose bodies in the anterior compartment are removed, the posterior compartment is addressed. The cannula in the proximal anteromedial portal is left in place and

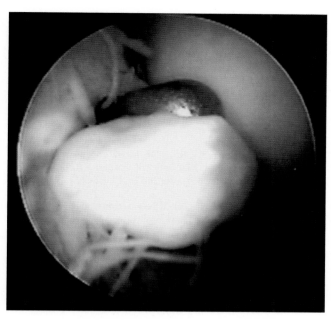

Fig. 22-10. These loose bodies may be removed from an antero-lateral portal using a grasping device.

the inflow is attached so that the loose bodies are pushed to the posterior compartment. In the posterior compartment, loose bodies are usually located in the olecranon fossa **(Fig. 22-11)**. The straight posterior portal is established using a no. 11 blade knife 3 cm proximal from the olecranon process and in the midline posteriorly. The blunt trocar and cannula are directed toward the olecranon fossa. Once loose bodies are identified, the posterolateral portal is established by placing a spinal needle 3 cm proximal to olecranon process and lateral to

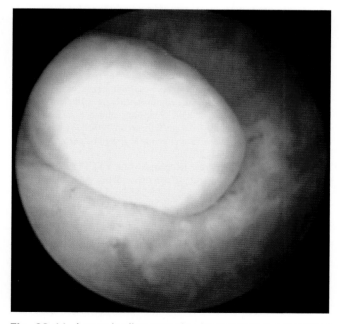

Fig. 22-11. Loose bodies may also be noted in the posterior aspect of the elbow. This loose body is located in the center of the olecranon fossa.

the triceps. Once the spinal needle is determined to be in the appropriate position arthroscopically, a no. 11 blade knife is used to incise only skin and a blunt trocar and cannula are introduced into the posterior compartment. Usually a motorized shaver is necessary to débride soft tissue in order to obtain full access to the olecranon fossa. The loose bodies can be removed from either the straight posterior or posterolateral portal. The tip of the olecranon should be carefully evaluated because this is often a source for loose bodies. The arthroscope is next directed toward the medial gutter. Using the opposite hand the surgeon applies pressure in an alternating fashion to the soft tissues posterior to the medial epicondyle in a distal to proximal direction. This maneuver should "milk" any loose bodies from the medial gutter. "Hidden" loose bodies are often found in the posterolateral gutter.

The scope is then directed down the lateral gutter where the midlateral or soft spot portal is established by first using a spinal needle to confirm placement intra-articularly. Usually a soft tissue plica or synovium may need to be débrided for adequate visualization. This portal is useful in location and removal of loose bodies as well as the location of osteochondritis dissecans. Once all loose bodies have been removed, Steri-strips are placed over the portals and a compressive dressing is placed on the extremity. Neurovascular checks are performed in the recovery room.

■ TECHNICAL ALTERNATIVES AND PITFALLS

Loose body removal from the elbow is the most successful and ideal indication for elbow arthroscopy. The success often depends on the cause of the loose body. Most pitfalls in elbow arthroscopy relate to damage to neurovascular structures with a prevalence ranging from 0% to 14% in the literature.[29,36,39-43] Most nerve injuries are transient and can be caused from extravasation of fluid or local anesthetic,[23] compression from the arthroscopic sheaths, direct injury from the trocar, or overaggressive joint distension. Injury to the radial, median, anterior interosseous nerve, medial antebrachial cutaneous, and ulnar nerve have all been reported.[23,29,41-46] In a review of 473 consecutive elbow arthroscopies, Kelly et al.[40] found 10 patients (2.5%) with transient nerve palsies.

Many nerve injuries are associated with the use of the anterolateral and anteromedial portals because of their close proximity to neural structures. The radial nerve, posterior interosseous nerve, and superficial branch of the radial nerve have been injured during placement of the anterolateral portal.[29,41,46] Injuries of the median and anterior interosseous nerve during placement of the anteromedial portal have been reported.[23,29,43] Neuroma formation can result from superficial cutaneous being injured.[29]

In order to avoid nerve injuries, knowledge of neurovascular anatomy and careful portal placement are critical. The prone position allows neurovascular structures to fall anteriorly away from the joint. Fluid distension of the joint and flexing the elbow to 90 degrees has been documented to increase the distance between neurovascular structures and portals.[28,29] When making a portal, the knife blade should cut only through skin. The skin should drag across the blade instead of making a stab incision. This prevents injuries to the superficial cutaneous nerves.

Other complications in elbow arthroscopy are iatrogenic articular cartilage injury, infection, persistent drainage of portals, synovial fistula formation, and problems associated with the tourniquet. Complications such as arthrofibrosis, reflex sympathetic dystrophy, and thromboembolism are less frequently seen.[45]

■ REHABILITATION

Postoperatively, the patient is usually placed in a compressive dressing and may use the extremity as tolerated. On postoperative day one the patient is started on a home exercise program of active and active assisted range of motion. This program includes flexion, extension, supination, and pronation. The patient is seen in the office 1 week after surgery and his or her progress is monitored so that full range of motion is attained.

■ OUTCOMES AND FUTURE DIRECTIONS

Probably one of the most successful operations in elbow arthroscopy is removal of symptomatic loose bodies. Several authors have reported on the beneficial effects of removal of loose bodies. As mentioned previously, the physician should attempt to determine the cause of the loose bodies. In many cases, simply removing loose fragments will not improve the outcome of the patient. This point is illustrated by O'Driscoll and Morrey's[2] review of 71 elbow arthroscopies in which 24 elbows had loose bodies. Fourteen patients with a primary diagnosis of loose bodies and another four patients with loose bodies secondary to osteochondritis dissecans improved after arthroscopic removal of their loose bodies. Patients with loose bodies secondary to posttraumatic arthritis, primary degenerative disease, synovial chondromatosis, or idiopathic flexion contracture did not improve with simple removal of loose bodies.

The indications of elbow arthroscopy continue to expand as surgical techniques improve. Elbow arthroscopy decreases the morbidity of an open procedure while allowing the operating surgeon a complete evaluation of the joint. With careful attention to detail and meticulous surgical technique, elbow arthroscopy can be performed safely with minimal risk of complications.

■ REFERENCES

1. Burman M. Arthroscopy of the elbow joint: a cadaver study. J Bone Joint Surg. 1932;14:349.
2. O'Driscoll SW, Morrey BF. Arthroscopy of the elbow: diagnostic and therapeutic benefits and hazards. J Bone Joint Surg Am. 1992;74:84–94.
3. O'Driscoll SW, Morrey BF. Arthroscopy of the elbow. In: Morrey BF, ed. *The Elbow and Its Disorders* 2nd ed. Philadelphia: Saunders; 1993:120–130.
4. Poehling GG, Ekman EF, Ruch DS. Elbow arthroscopy: introduction and overview. In: McGinty JB, Caspari RB, Jackson RW, et al., eds. *Operative Arthroscopy*, 2nd ed. Philadelphia: Lippincott-Raven; 1996:821–828.
5. Wiesler ER, Poehling, GG. Elbow arthroscopy: introduction, indications, complications, and results. In: McGinty JB, Burkhart SS, Jackson RW, et al., eds. *Operative Arthroscopy*, 3rd ed. Philadelphia: Lippencott-Raven; 2003:661–664.
6. Poehling GG, Whipple TL, Sisco L, et al. Elbow arthroscopy: a new technique. Arthroscopy. 1989;5:222–224.
7. Boe S. Arthroscopy of the elbow: diagnosis and extraction of loose bodies. Acta Orthop Scand. 1986;57:52–53.
8. McGinty J. Arthroscopic removal of loose bodies. Orthop Clin North Am. 1982;13:313–328.
9. Morrey BF. Arthroscopy of the elbow. In: Anderson LD, ed. *Instructional Course Lectures*, Vol. 35. Roesmont, Ill.: American Academy of Orthopaedic Surgeons; 1986:102–107.
10. O'Driscoll SW. Elbow arthroscopy for loose bodies. Orthopaedics. 1992;15:855–859.
11. O'Driscoll SW. Elbow arthroscopy: loose bodies. In: Morrey BF, ed. *The Elbow and Its Disorders*, 3rd ed. Philadelphia: Saunders; 2000:510–514.
12. Savoie FH. Arthroscopic management of loose bodies of the elbow. Oper Tech Sports Med. 2001;9(4):241–244.
13. O'Driscoll SW. Arthroscopic treatment for osteoarthritis of the elbow. Orthop Clin North Am. 1995;26:691–706.
14. Ogilvie-Harris DJ, Gordon R, MacKay M. Arthroscopic treatment for posterior impingement in degenerative arthritis of the elbow. Arthroscopy. 1995;11:437–443.
15. Menth-Chiari WA, Ruch DS, Poehling GG. Arthroscopic excision of the radial head: clinical outcome in 12 patients with posttraumatic arthritis after fracture of the radial head or rheumatoid arthritis. Arthroscopy. 2001;17(9):918–923.
16. Byrd JW. Elbow arthroscopy for arthrofibrosis after type I radial head fractures. Arthroscopy. 1994;10:162–165.
17. Jones GS, Savoie FH. Arthroscopic capsular release of flexion contractures (arthrofibrosis) of the elbow. Arthroscopy. 1993;9:277–283.
18. Antuna SA, O'Driscoll SW. Snapping plicae associated with radiocapitellar chondromalacia. Arthroscopy. 2001;17(5):491–495.
19. Clarke R. Symptomatic lateral synovial fringe of the elbow joint. Arthroscopy. 1988;4:112–116.
20. Baumgarten TE, Andrew JR, Satterwhite YE. The arthroscopic evaluation and treatment of osteochondritis desiccants of the capitellum. Am J Sports Med. 1998;26:520–523.
21. Ruch DS, Cory JW, Poehling GG. The arthroscopic management of osteochondritis dissecans of the adolescent elbow. Arthroscopy. 1998;14(8):797–803.
22. Savoie FH, Field LD. Basics of elbow arthroscopy. Tech Orthop. 2000;15(2):138–146.
23. Andrews JR, Carson WG. Arthroscopy of the elbow. Arthroscopy. 1985;1:97–107.
24. Moskal JH, Savioe FH, Field LD. Elbow arthroscopy in trauma and reconstruction. Orthop Clin North Am. 1999;30:163–177.
25. Baker CL Jr, Murphy KP, Gottlob CA, et al. Arthroscopic classification and treatment of lateral epicondylitis: two-year clinical results. J Shoulder Elbow Surg. 2000;9(6):475–482.

26. Smith AM, Castle JA, Ruch DS. Arthroscopic resection of the common extensor origin: anatomic considerations. J Shoulder Elbow Surg. 2003;12(4):375–379.

27. Smith JP III, Savoie FH, Field LD. Posterolateral rotatory instability of the elbow. Clin Sports Med. 2001;20(1):47–58.

28. Lindenfield TN. Medial approach in elbow arthroscopy. Am J Sports Med. 1990;18:413–417.

29. Lynch GJ, Meyers JF, Whipple TL, et al. Neurovascular anatomy and elbow arthroscopy: inherent risks. Arthroscopy. 1986;2:191–197.

30. Lyons TR, Field LD, Savoie FH. Basics of elbow arthroscopy. In: Price CT, ed. *Instructional Course Lectures*, Vol. 49. Rosemont, Ill.: American Academy of Orthopaedic Surgeons; 2000:239–246.

31. Stothers K, Day B, Reagan WR. Arthroscopy of the elbow: anatomy, portal sites, and a description of the proximal lateral portal. Arthroscopy. 1995;11:449–457.

32. Plancher KD, Peterson RK, Breezenoff L. Diagnostic arthroscopy of the elbow: set-up, portals, and technique. Oper Tech Sports Med. 1998;6:2–10.

33. Field LD, Altchek DW, Warren RF, et al. Arthroscopic anatomy of the lateral elbow: a comparison of three portals. Arthroscopy. 1994;10:602–607.

34. Savoie FH, Field LD. Anatomy. In: Savoie FH, Field LD, eds. *Arthroscopy of the Elbow*. New York: Churchill Livingstone; 1996:3–24.

35. Aldolfsson L. Arthroscopy of the elbow joint: a cadaveric study of portal placement. J Shoulder Elbow Surg. 1994;3:53–61.

36. Poehling GG, Ekman EF. Arthroscopy of the elbow. In: Jackson DW, ed. *Instructional Course Lectures*, Vol. 44. Rosemont, Ill.: American Academy of Orthopaedic Surgeons; 1995:217–228.

37. McKenzie PJ. Supine position. In: Savoie FH, Field LD, eds. *Arthroscopy of the Elbow*. New York: Churchill Livingstone; 1996:35–39.

38. Rubin CJ. Prone or lateral decubitus position. In: Savoie FH, Field LD, eds. *Arthroscopy of the Elbow*. New York: Churchill Livingstone; 1996:41–47.

39. Andrews JR, Baumgarten TE. Arthroscopic anatomy of the elbow. Orthop Clin North Am. 1995;26:671–677.

40. Kelly EW, Morrey BF, O'Driscoll SW. Complications in elbow arthroscopy. J Bone Joint Surg Am. 2001;83:25–34.

41. Papilion JD, Neff RS, Shall LM. Compression neuropathy of the radial nerve as a complication of elbow arthroscopy: a case report and review of the literature. Arthroscopy. 1988;4:284–286.

42. Rodeo SA, Forester RA, Weiland AJ. Neurologic complications due to arthroscopy. J Bone Joint Surg Am. 1993;75:917–926.

43. Ruch DS, Poehling GG. Anterior interosseous nerve injury following elbow arthroscopy. Arthroscopy. 1997;13:756–758.

44. Casscells SW. Neurovascular anatomy and elbow arthroscopy: inherent risks [Editor's comment]. Arthroscopy. 1986;2:190.

45. Small NC. Complications in arthroscopy: the knee and other joints. Arthroscopy. 1986;2:253–258.

46. Thomas MA, Fast A, Shapiro DL. Radial nerve damage as a complication of elbow arthroscopy. Clin Orthop. 1987;215:130–131.

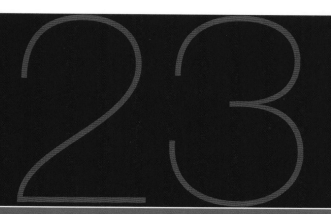

MANAGEMENT OF THE ARTHRITIC AND STIFF ELBOW AND OSTEOCHONDRITIS DESSICANS OF THE CAPITELLUM

RAFFY MIRZAYAN, MD, DANIEL C. ACEVEDO, BS, CHRISTOPHER S. AHMAD, MD, NEAL S. ELATTRACHE, MD

■ HISTORY OF THE TECHNIQUE

Primary osteoarthritis (OA) of the elbow is uncommon and accounts for less than 10% of joints involved in primary osteoarthritis.[1] Historically, osteoarthritis of the elbow has been reported mostly in elderly men involved in an occupation requiring manual labor. These patients can often tolerate significant motion loss with pain only at end range. In an active patient with work or athletic activities requiring extremes of flexion and extension, end-arc motion loss and pain are not tolerated as well. The previously reported motion arc of 30 to 130 necessary for activities of daily living is frequently not sufficient for these patients.[2] This disease of the "active elbow" is the result of repetitive forceful axial loading in hyperextension and hyperflexion, which results in olecranon and coronoid impingement and capsular injury. It is commonly seen in boxers and football linemen, as well as laborers who use jackhammers.

Contractures are a result of degenerative arthritis, post-traumatic arthritis, and chronic overuse injuries of the elbow.[3] Elbow contractures are initially treated nonoperatively with physical therapy. After failure of nonoperative treatment, surgical management is pursued. Traditionally, surgical management involved open surgery in the anterior cubital fossa to perform anterior capsulectomies, distal biceps brachii tendon lengthening, and brachialis muscle transfers.[4] Jones and Savoie[4] then described a lateral incision technique in 1990 that allowed more complete evaluation and resection of osteophytes of both anterior and posterior parts of the joint. Mansat and Morrey[5] described a limited lateral approach known as the column procedure. This procedure elevated muscles of the lateral supracondylar ridge to access the joint for capsulectomy and debridement of the joint. These surgical methods produced some improvement

in the range of motion of the elbow. The limitation of these approaches is that it is difficult to reach the posteromedial aspect of the elbow. This is usually the location of osteophytes and posteromedial capsular/ligamentous contractures that can limit flexion. If elbow flexion is severely limited, these procedures will not sufficiently release the elbow to allow increased flexion. It also places the ulnar nerve at risk, as it is not directly visualized and cannot be protected.

Contractures from posterior osteophytic changes were seen to have persistent blockage to extension despite debridement of the posterior aspects of the joint. Kashiwagi[6] originally described a procedure that fenestrated the olecranon fossa to create communication between the olecranon and coronoid fossae to alleviate the posterior bony block contributing to elbow contracture. Morrey[7] later modified this technique into a procedure described as open ulno-humeral arthroplasty. Others elevated the triceps tendon in order to remove loose bodies and osteophytes from the anterior capsule through the humeral fenestration.[8] These techniques were used for successful treatment of elbow contractures and have been recently modified for arthroscopic use.

Hotchkiss[9] has described a medial approach to address open release of the stiff elbow. The advantage of this approach is that the ulnar nerve is easily identified and can be released or transposed if necessary. In addition, if flexion is severely limited, the posterior bands of the ulnar collateral ligament can be released to increase flexion. The exposure is performed in the "over-the-top" fashion, where the flexor pronator mass is elevated off the anterior aspect of the medial epicondyle. The anterior band of the ulnar collateral ligament is not transected. The anterior capsule is sharply excised and the posterior compartment can also be addressed.

In the 1990s, arthroscopic surgery became an option for capsular release in elbow contractures, removal of loose bodies, as well as radial head resections.[4,10,11] Arthroscopy offers many advantages for the treatment of elbow contractures including: minimal trauma to surrounding soft tissues, immediate postoperative range of motion exercises, and minimal postoperative scarring.[8] This surgical technique requires an experienced surgeon and great attention to detail. The use of arthroscopy to treat elbow contractures is becoming more popular as surgeons are gaining more experience in elbow arthroscopy. O'Driscoll and Morrey[12] first described arthroscopy for the removal of loose bodies causing mechanical impairment. More recent studies have described arthroscopic techniques for early osteophyte formation and contractures.[4,13] Arthroscopic radial head resection has also been described with satisfactory results.[14]

■ INDICATIONS AND CONTRAINDICATIONS

Indications for arthroscopic management of the arthritic elbow include pain, which has failed nonoperative measures including injections, physical therapy, and anti-inflammatory medications. Mechanical symptoms, including locking which is due to loose bodies or uneven surfaces from chondral wear, can be managed arthroscopically. Limitation in range of motion can also be improved arthroscopically. In general, 100-degree arcs of flexion (30 degrees to 130 degrees) and rotation (50 degrees each of pronation and supination) allow most activities of daily living.[2] These parameters are not tolerated as well with a younger and athletic population in order to perform their sporting activities. Thus, they should be used as guidelines, but each patient's needs for range of motion requirements should be assessed individually. When patients have a flexion contracture of greater than 30 degrees, arthroscopic debridement, osteophyte excision with or without capsular release will restore most of the range of motion.

The senior author's (NSE) personal treatment algorithm for open versus arthroscopic management depends on the amount of flexion present in the elbow and whether the ulnar nerve is involved. If the elbow cannot be flexed greater than 110 degrees preoperatively or there is ulnar nerve involvement, then an open medial, over-the-top approach, as described by Hotchkiss,[9] is performed in order to address the ulnar nerve, resect olecranon osteophytes, release the posterior medial capsule, as well as debride coronoid osteophytes and release the capsule anteriorly. Otherwise, arthroscopic management is successful in addressing loose body removal, osteophyte excision, capsular release, and radial head resection. The best results are obtained if an adequate amount of midarc joint space is still seen on preoperative radiographs.

Contraindications to performing this procedure arthroscopically include: late infectious arthritis, severe arthritis with significant, diffuse joint space loss, and ankylosis of the joint. In addition, submuscular transposition of the ulnar nerve is a contraindication for anteromedial portal placement.

■ SURGICAL TECHNIQUE

Anesthesia

A general anesthetic is used for this procedure. Muscle paralysis is not required. It is helpful to see muscle twitches if the instrumentation gets too close to a nerve. A preoperative nerve block for pain control is not performed. Since the proximity of neural structures make them susceptible to injury, a nerve block would not allow a surgeon to know if a postoperative deficit is due to nerve injury from the surgery or from the nerve block. If a nerve block is desired for postoperative pain management, it is best performed in the postoperative area, after the patient has been awakened and a thorough neurovascular examination has been performed and documented. A subclavicular block is the block of choice for the elbow, as an intrascalene block does not properly affect the ulnar nerve distribution. If desired, an indwelling catheter is left in place after induction of a nerve block in order to provide continuous pain control. The patient can then be admitted and monitored and started on a continuous passive motion machine with adequate pain

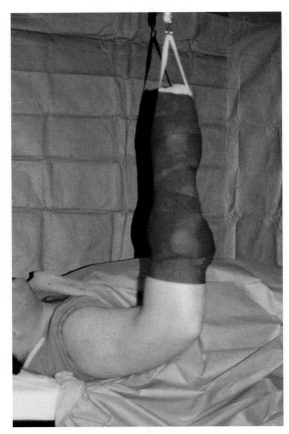

Fig. 23-1. Supine position with arm in traction.

control. Alternatively, the procedure can be done as an out-patient and the catheter is not left in.

Patient Positioning

Patient positioning depends on surgeon preference and previous experience with a particular position. Supine, lateral decubitus, and prone positions have all been described and used with good success. The supine position **(Fig. 23-1)** is useful if the majority of the operation is performed in the anterior compartment. This position allows for easier orientation of anatomic landmarks in the anterior compartment. Supine position is especially useful if an open procedure is anticipated following arthroscopy.

Surface Landmarks and Portal Placement

It is extremely important to draw out anatomic landmarks prior to elbow arthroscopy **(Fig. 23-2A,B,C)**. The course of the ulnar nerve should be palpated and outlined. It is important to examine the patient preoperatively and assess for ulnar nerve subluxation to prevent injury to the nerve. The medial and lateral margins of the triceps tendon, lateral and medial

epicondyles, lateral and medial columns (and the medial intermuscular septum), and the radial head are outlined. The anteromedial portal is created 2 cm proximal and 1 cm anterior to the medial epicondyle. This portal should be placed anterior to the medial intermuscular septum to prevent injury to the ulnar nerve. The direct posterior portal is made through the triceps tendon 2 cm proximal to the tip of the olecranon. The posterolateral portal is created at the same level as the direct posterior portal just at the lateral margin of the triceps tendon. The anterolateral portal is created 2 cm proximal and 1 cm anterior to the radiocapitellar joint. A soft spot portal is also placed in the middle of a triangle drawn from the lateral epicondyle, radial head, and olecranon. This allows improved access to the radial head if a resection is planned.

Arthroscopy

After the landmarks are drawn, the limb is Esmarched and the tourniquet is inflated. The joint is first insufflated with 30 to 40 cc of normal saline **(Fig. 23-3)**. This allows the distention of the capsule and pushes vital neurovascular structures away from the joint line. The arthroscope sheath with a blunt obturator is introduced through the anterolateral

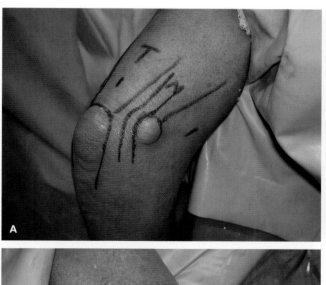
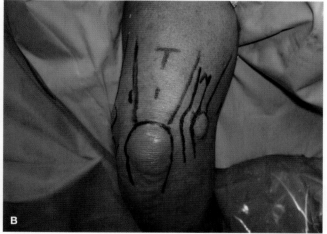
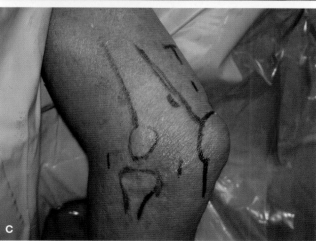

Fig. 23-2. Anatomic landmarks: **(A)** medial view, **(B)** posterior view, **(C)** lateral view.

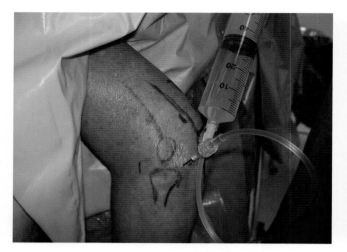

Fig. 23-3. Joint is insufflated with normal saline.

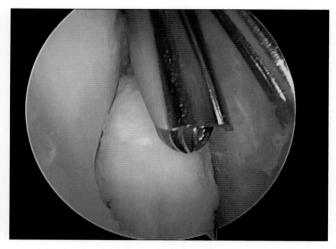

Fig. 23-5. The coronoid osteophyte is burred down.

portal. It is preferable to start with this portal since in cases where a submuscular ulnar nerve transposition has been performed, the anteromedial portal cannot be used as the first portal. The outflow on the arthroscope sheath is left open and when a gush of fluid is expressed out of it, intra-articular placement is confirmed. The anteromedial portal is then created by an inside-out or outside-in technique. The anterior compartment is usually difficult to visualize due to thickened scar tissue and synovitis. A shaver is introduced through the lateral cannula and scar tissue and synovitis is debrided. Care should be taken to avoid excessive suction on the shaver. It is often better to remove the wall suction from the shaver and allow drainage by gravity. This will prevent premature excision of the capsule, which can lead to extravasation of fluid into the muscle and poor visualization. It is extremely helpful to place retractors into the anterior compartment to help retract the capsule while work is being completed on other structures (Fig. 23-4).

A bur is then used to remove the osteophyte off of the coronoid process (Fig. 23-5). There is a cartilage cap on the osteophyte as well as the coronoid process facing the articular surface, which protects the bur from damaging the articular surfaces of the humerus. The coronoid should be excised to the level of capsular insertion. The cartilage cap is then excised with a shaver or a sharp instrument such as an elevator, Freer, or even the shaver. A capsulotomy is begun from medial to lateral, and capsular release is performed with a shaver. The capsule is shaved off the humeral origin. It is crucial to have very little suction, if any, in order to prevent inadvertently grasping neural structures. The radial nerve can be found at the lateral border of the brachialis muscle.

Localized lateral, radiocapitellar tenderness preoperatively and Outerbridge grade IV chondral changes at the time of arthroscopy are indications for a radial head resection (Fig. 23-6). The bur is placed through the lateral portal and excision of the head is started anteriorly and carried posteriorly (Fig. 23-7). The assistant can pronate and supinate

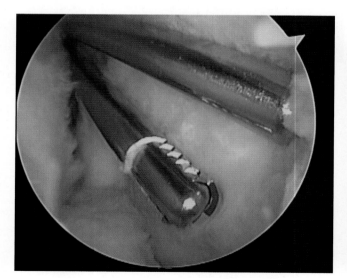

Fig. 23-4. A switching stick is used as a retractor. The capsule is retracted away from the shaver.

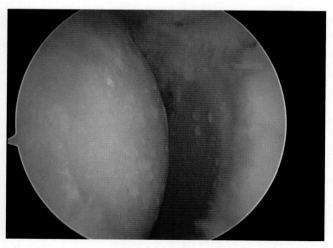

Fig. 23-6. Grade IV chondromalacia of the radiocapitellar joint capitellum to the left and radial head on the right.

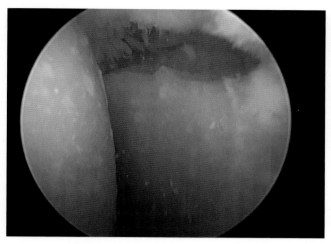

Fig. 23-7. Radial head resection is started from the anterolateral portal and carried out from anterior to posterior.

the forearm and deliver the radial head to the bur. The cartilage cap will protect the lesser sigmoid notch against injury from the bur. When the bur no longer reaches parts of the radial head and forearm rotation no longer aids in the resection, accessory portals are used between the lateral portal already present and the soft spot portal. A spinal needle can aid the proper portal placement. The radial head is resected back to the radial neck. The lesser sigmoid notch can serve as a guide to the proper amount of resection **(Fig. 23-8)**. There should be no bone contacting the lesser sigmoid notch.

The posterior compartment is addressed last. The arthroscope is placed through the posterolateral portal and a shaver through the direct posterior portal. Upon initial entrance into the joint, there is excessive scar tissue, which prevents adequate visualization. The shaver and the arthroscope should be directed toward the olecranon fossa, and the scar tissue should be excised with the shaver until adequate visualization is obtained. Oftentimes multiple loose bodies

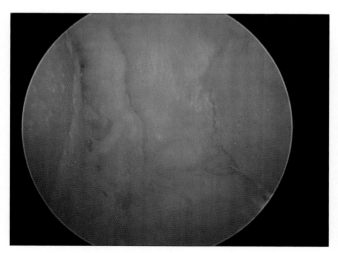

Fig. 23-8. Image after radial head resection. The lesser sigmoid notch guides the amount of radial head resection and to prevent excessive resection of the radial neck.

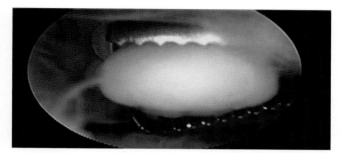

Fig. 23-9. Toothed grasper removing a loose body.

are seen in the posterior compartment and olecranon fossa. A toothed grasper is used to remove loose bodies, which allows even better visualization **(Fig. 23-9)**. Osteophytes can then be seen at the tip of the olecranon, in the olecranon fossa, as well as below the fossa where the tip of the olecranon has been impinging **(Fig. 23-10)**. The assistant flexes and extends the elbow slowly to allow the surgeon to see the osteophytes of the tip of the olecranon and to assess sites of impingement against the humerus. The medial and lateral gutters are inspected to ensure that there are no loose bodies present **(Fig. 23-11)**. An Outerbridge-Kashiwagi (OK) procedure is not routinely performed.

■ TECHNICAL ALTERNATIVES AND PITFALLS

Traditionally, diagnostic arthroscopy is first performed in the anterior compartment, followed by the posterior compartment. Occasionally, when treating elbows with stiffness and arthrosis, the anterior capsule is less pliable and does not push away from the anterior cortex. Therefore, the procedure is started in the posterior compartment first. In addition, an arthroscopic OK procedure may be performed **(Fig. 23-12)**. This allows the surgeon visualization of the

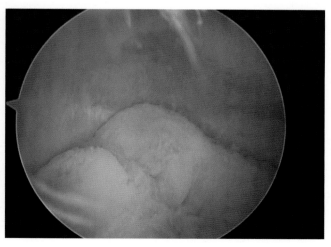

Fig. 23-10. Olecranon tip spur.

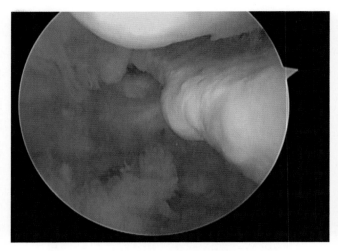

Fig. 23-11. Medial gutter without loose bodies.

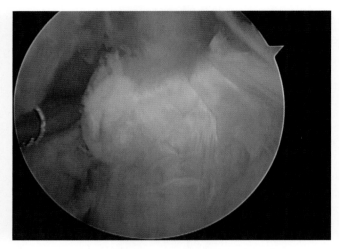

Fig. 23-13. Thickened anterior humeral spur at the coronoid fossa.

anterior compartment as a switching stick is introduced from the anteromedial portal. The arthroscope can then be withdrawn and placed over the switching stick safely into the anterior compartment. The OK procedure is not a necessary part of the procedure for a successful outcome. It merely allows for better visualization and safer instrument placement. Another advantage of performing the OK procedure is that it allows for an instrument to be placed from the posterior compartment and push the anterior capsule away from the humerus acting as a retractor in order to improve visualization. An end-cutting bur is used to perform the OK procedure. Alternatively, the protective sheath around the end of the bur can be trimmed off. Normally, the layer of bone separating the olecranon and coronoid fossae is very thin (approximately 1 to 2 mm). In patients with arthrosis and stiffness, the layer of bone is thickened. In addition, if there are osteophytes anteriorly by the coronoid fossa, it may seem thicker when the bone is being burred **(Fig. 23-13)**. Care must be taken to avoid violating the medial and lateral

columns to prevent stress risers, which can lead to distal humerus fractures. Capsular release is the last step performed in order to prevent fluid extravasation. In addition to a shaver, an arthroscopic basket can also be used to perform a capsulotomy. The basket can be used by first separating the capsule from the muscle fibers and then removing small fragments of the capsule in a piecemeal fashion.

The alternative to doing arthroscopic management of the arthritic elbow is to perform the procedure in an open fashion. The column procedure as described by Mansat and Morrey[5] is the most widely accepted method of performing this procedure for regaining motion. If the ulnar nerve is involved or flexion is limited to less than 115 degrees, the medial over-the-top approach as described by Hotchkiss[9] can be used.

■ REHABILITATION

Rehabilitation should be initiated as soon as possible after the procedure. Patients may be admitted for overnight observation and pain control and started on a continuous passive motion machine (CPM), which can be continued at home after the patient is discharged. A splint is not applied after surgery, and only a soft dressing is placed to allow early range of motion. The patients are referred to physiotherapy where initially the goal is to reduce swelling and help manage pain. Active and active-assist range of motion for both flexion-extension and pronation-supination are emphasized.

■ OUTCOMES AND RESULTS

Elbow contractures have been treated with open surgical techniques with favorable results. The outcomes of recent arthroscopic surgical techniques have been seen to be comparable.

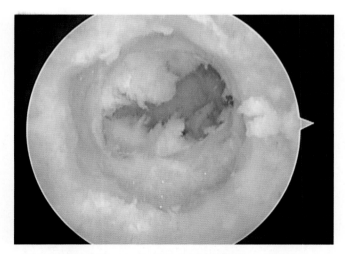

Fig. 23-12. Arthroscopic Outerbridge-Kashiwagi procedure.

This surgical technique also offers the advantages of minimal surgical incisions, faster recovery and rehabilitation, and fewer complications.[8]

Open surgical techniques, such as the column procedure described by Mansat and Morrey[5] were used for extrinsic contractures of the elbow. This series showed that 89% of the patients had increased range of motion, and 82% were considered to have had a satisfactory result. However, this series showed that 26% had a delayed loss of motion some time after the procedure. Morrey[7] also described ulnohumeral arthroplasty for the treatment of elbow stiffness caused by osteoarthritis. His initial data showed that this procedure improved flexion, extension, and pain in osteoarthritis. He reported an 86% patient satisfaction. Long-term analysis of the patients revealed an increase in the arc of elbow flexion from 79 degrees to 101 degrees and 76% were relieved of pain. This series also demonstrated that 28% of the patients had ulnar nerve symptoms after the procedure.[15]

In a series described by Aldridge et al.[16] with patients who had open anterior release of the elbow, the main difference was seen to be in improvement of extension of the elbow. This series illustrated that better results were afforded with continuous passive motion used immediately after the procedure for up to four weeks. Most of the complications were neuropathies. These open procedures have afforded improvements in elbow contracture but are more invasive than arthroscopic measures.

Arthroscopy has achieved desirable results in the treatment of contractures of the elbow. The first case of arthroscopic release was described by Nowicki and Shall.[3] The arthroscopic release of the anterior capsule showed no complications or residual symptoms. The patient in this case report was able to return to semiprofessional volleyball one month after the arthroscopic procedure. Jones and Savoie[4] then went on to report the results of the use of arthroscopic surgery for posttraumatic and arthritic contractures. The flexion contractures were reduced from a mean of 38 degrees to 3 degrees. The study showed an increase in average flexion from 106 degrees to 138 degrees. Increases in supination from 45 degrees to 84 degrees, and in pronation from 80 degrees to 88 degrees were seen as well. This study showed one complication—posterior interosseous nerve palsy. In 1995, Kim et al.[17] used arthroscopic surgery to remove loose bodies, excise osteophytes, excise the radial head, and perform abrasion arthroplasty. Satisfactory results were achieved in 92% of patients with improvements in the range of motion by an average of 24 degrees from elbows with previous limitation of motion. A median nerve palsy was seen in two of the patients involved in this study, but the symptoms resolved one month postoperatively.

A retrospective study by Timmerman and Andrews[18] showed that in 19 cases of posttraumatic arthrofibrosis treated with arthroscopy, 84% had a good to excellent result. The average extension increased from 29 degrees to 11 degrees and average flexion increased from 123 degrees to 134 degrees. In this series of patients, 14 were involved in sports and 11 returned to previous levels of sporting activity after the procedure. The only failure in this study was due to a case of severe arthritis. In 1998 Phillips and Strasburger[19] described a series involving the arthroscopic treatment of 15 posttraumatic and ten degenerative arthritis induced contractures of the elbow. The average increase in the arc of motion was 41 degrees. All patients in this series showed increases in motion and decreases in pain throughout follow-up. There were no neurovascular complications in this study. Ball et al.[20] described a more recent study of treatment of the posttraumatic elbow. Arthroscopic surgery improved flexion from an average of 117.5 degrees to 133 degrees and extension from an average of 35.4 degrees to 9.3 degrees. All of the patients studied were satisfied with their results. Pain was decreased in some, but six out of 14 continued to have pain despite the procedure. Most of the patients had a primary loss of extension of the elbow; therefore, this study cannot be extrapolated for patients with primary loss of flexion.

Arthroscopic surgery has also been used to treat osteoarthritis. Degenerative arthritis of the elbow with predominantly posterior involvement was treated with arthroscopic surgery in a series reported by Ogilvie-Harris et al.[21] Fourteen out of 21 of these patients were classified postoperatively as excellent and seven as good, based on the 100-point elbow scoring system by Morrey.[7] Fourteen of these patients returned to full activity after the surgery. Savoie et al.[13] used arthroscopic ulnohumeral arthroplasty to treat restricted arthritic elbows. Their patients showed a 49-degree improvement of average flexion, 32-degree improvement of average extension, and an 81-degree improvement of the average arc of motion. This improvement in the range of motion was seen to be better than similar open surgical techniques described by Morrey[7] and Kashigawi.[6] Every patient in this study believed that the surgery was beneficial. All had decreased amounts of pain, and 33% had complete relief of pain. Using the Andrews and Carson scoring system, the patients in this study overall had good to excellent results in improvement of elbow motion and pain control.[13] The complication rate was 13%. This was comparable to the rate of complications seen in open ulnohumeral arthroplasty.

Contractures in the elbow have been seen to result from radiocapitellar degeneration and loose bodies in or around the elbow joint.[8] Radial head fractures can cause degeneration of the radiocapitellar joint, which can lead to pain and loss of motion.[10] Posttraumatic arthritis secondary to radial head fractures can be an indication for excision of the radial head. Arthroscopy allows for direct visualization of the radiocapitellar joint. Field and Savoie[10] reviewed the results of arthroscopic radial head excisions and found a study where 34 out of 37 were successful. They also reviewed the results of 24 patients in which some had radial head excisions in addition to fenestration of the posterior fossa of the elbow. Twenty-three of 24 had success with an increase in average flexion from 90 degrees to 139 degrees and average extension from 40 degrees to 8 degrees.

The removal of loose bodies has also been performed arthroscopically with success. Removal of loose bodies was seen to improve pain in 85%, elbow locking in 92%, and swelling of the elbow in 71% in a series reported by Ogilvie-Harris and Schemitsch.[11] The procedure showed an 89% improvement overall; however, it was unsuccessful in improving crepitus and the procedure was seen to result in no improvement of the range of motion for a third of the patients. Loose body removal from the posterior fossa showed the greatest benefit. Only two cases of neuropraxia were seen in this trial with no other major complications.

The use of arthroscopic surgery for the treatment of contractures in the elbow as well as radial head resection is promising. The literature shows favorable outcomes in range of motion and pain with rarely reported complications. The use of arthroscopic surgery requires the surgeon to have experience to achieve desirable results. This surgical technique has the advantage of minimal incisions, faster recovery, and better visualization of intra-articular structures.

■ TREATMENT OF CAPITELLAR OSTEOCHONDRITIS DISSECANS

Panner's disease is an osteochondrosis of the capitellum which affects individuals younger than 10 years of age.[22] Radiographic features include fissuring, irregularity, and fragmentation of the capitellum, followed by reossification and resolution of symptoms. Panner's disease is usually self-limited and must be differentiated from osteochondritis dissecans (OCD).

In skeletally immature athletes, repetitive stresses to the elbow that create radiocapitellar joint compression forces result in cartilage and bony damage manifesting as capitellar OCD.[23-26] Patients with capitellar OCD typically have a history of repetitive activity such as throwing or gymnastics. Symptoms include lateral elbow pain often associated with stiffness. Locking and catching suggests the presence of intra-articular loose bodies. Physical exam most commonly demonstrates loss of motion with 15 degrees to 20 degrees flexion contracture. Crepitus and tenderness may be elicited over the radiocapitellar joint. Plain radiographs often demonstrate fragmented subchondral bone with lucencies and irregular ossification of the capitellum. Loose bodies may also be seen in the elbow joint on plain radiographs. Magnetic resonance imaging (MRI) may further delineate the avascular segment and loose bodies **(Fig. 23-14)**.

Initial treatment consists of activity modification, avoidance of throwing or other related sports, nonsteroidal anti-inflammatory drugs, and bracing for acute symptoms. This

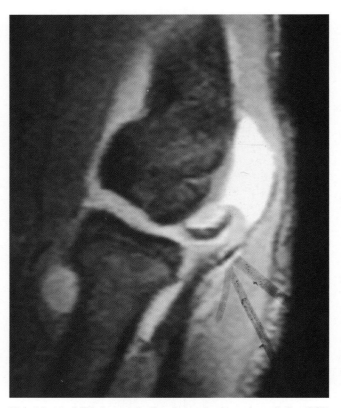

Fig. 23-14. MRI demonstrating loose body and capitellar OCD lesion. (From Ahmad C, ElAttrache N. Mosaicplasty for capitellar osteochondritis dissecans. In: Yamagachi K, King G, McKee M, O'Driscoll S, eds. *Advanced Reconstruction Elbow*. Rosemont, Illinois: American Academy of Orthopaedic Surgeons. In press.)

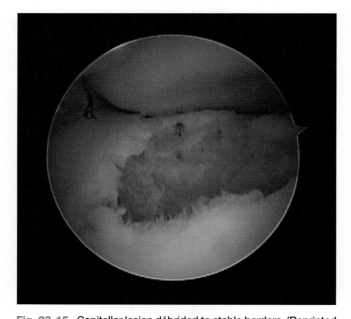

Fig. 23-15. Capitellar lesion débrided to stable borders. (Reprinted with permission from Ahmad C, ElAttrache N. Mosaicplasty for capitellar osteochondritis dissecans. In: Yamagachi K, King G, McKee M, O'Driscoll S, eds. *Advanced Reconstruction Elbow*. Rosemont, Illinois: American Academy of Orthopaedic Surgeons. In press.)

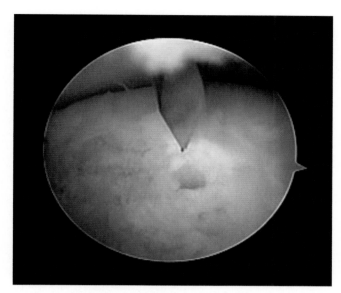

Fig. 23-16. Drilling with smooth pin. (Reprinted with permission from Ahmad C and ElAttrache N. Mosaicplasty for capitellar osteochondritis dissecans. In: Yamagachi K, King G, McKee M, O'Driscoll S, eds. *Advanced Reconstruction Elbow*. Rosemont, Illinois: American Academy of Orthopaedic Surgeons. In press.)

is followed by physical therapy to regain strength and motion. Younger skeletally immature patients have a better prognosis for nonoperative treatment than older patients. Surgery is indicated for patients who fail nonoperative treatment.

Capitellar OCD lesions have been classified based on status and stability of the overlying cartilage.[27,28] Lesions with stable and attached cartilage are treated with drilling. Higher

grade lesions are treated with removal of loose bodies, contouring of affected cartilage back to a stable rim **(Fig. 23-15)**, and then drilling to introduce marrow elements and create a fibrocartilage healing response **(Fig. 23-16)**. **Figure 23-17A,B** demonstrates bleeding from drill sites.

Mosaicplasty is indicated for large capitellar lesions that allow the radial head to engage the lesion as observed during arthroscopy. These lesions typically involve the lateral aspect of the capitellum, resulting in loss of the lateral buttress to the radial head. Advanced stages of OCD that involve degenerative changes of the radial head and deformity of the capitellum are relative contraindications to mosaicplasty.

A midlateral working portal is used to establish healthy stable cartilage borders. The elbow is then flexed to 90 to 100 degrees and a spinal needle is introduced through the onconeus for an exact perpendicular approach to the lesion. The recipient site is then drilled, creating the desired diameter tunnel for the osteochondral graft **(Fig. 23-18)**. The donor osteochondral graft is then harvested from the intercondylar notch of the knee arthroscopically. The plug is then introduced into the recipient site and impacted flush with the surrounding cartilage **(Fig. 23-19)**. The process of osteochondral grafting is repeated until the lesion is adequately replaced **(Figs. 23-20 and 23-21)**. If the entire lesion is not fully resurfaced, the remainder is treated with drilling.

Physical therapy is then instituted to regain range of motion while avoiding strengthening that may compromise the healing response. Gentle resistance exercises are initiated at 3 months with greater resistance at 4 months. For throwing athletes, a throwing program is started at 5 months. Full effort throwing is achieved at 6 months.

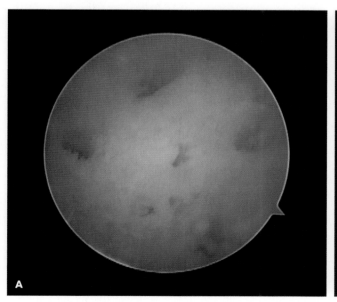
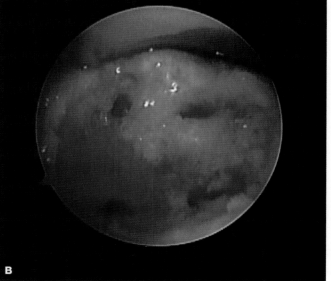

Fig. 23-17. A: Completed drilling. **B:** Bleeding confirmed from the drill sites. (Reprinted with permission from Ahmad C and ElAttrache N. Mosaicplasty for capitellar osteochondritis dissecans. In: Yamagachi K, King G, McKee M, O'Driscoll S, eds. *Advanced Reconstruction Elbow*. Rosemont, Illinois: American Academy of Orthopaedic Surgeons. In press.)

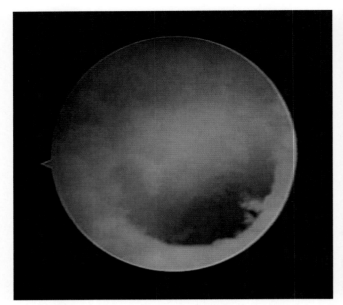

Fig. 23-18. Recipient site for osteochondral autograft drilled. (Reprinted with permission from Ahmad C and ElAttrache N. Mosaicplasty for capitellar osteochondritis dissecans. In: Yamagachi K, King G, McKee M, O'Driscoll S, eds. *Advanced Reconstruction Elbow*. Rosemont, Illinois: American Academy of Orthopaedic Surgeons. In press.)

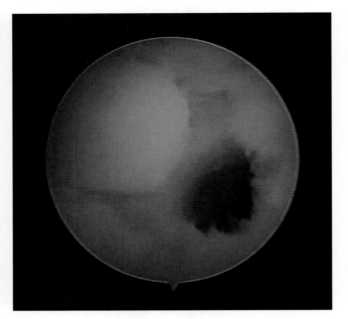

Fig. 23-20. Second recipient site drilled for osteochondral autograft. (Reprinted with permission from Ahmad C and ElAttrache N. Mosaicplasty for capitellar osteochondritis dissecans. In: Yamagachi K, King G, McKee M, O'Driscoll S, eds. *Advanced Reconstruction Elbow*. Rosemont, Illinois: American Academy of Orthopaedic Surgeons. In press.)

Several short-term studies have observed favorable return to competitive athletics with debridement and marrow stimulation when indicated.[27,29–34] No reports are available for all arthroscopic mosaicplasty treatment for capitellar OCD. The senior author has performed seven cases of arthroscopic mosaicplasty for elbow OCD with good to excellent patient satisfaction and return to activity in six patients. There were no complications. The unsatisfied patient had arthritic

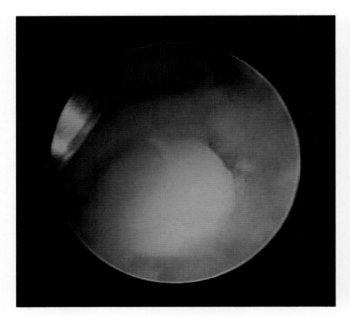

Fig. 23-19. First osteochondral autograft placed and impacted flush with adjacent surface. (Reprinted with permission from Ahmad C and ElAttrache N. Mosaicplasty for capitellar osteochondritis dissecans. In: Yamagachi K, King G, McKee M, O'Driscoll S, eds. *Advanced Reconstruction Elbow*. Rosemont, Illinois: American Academy of Orthopaedic Surgeons. In press.)

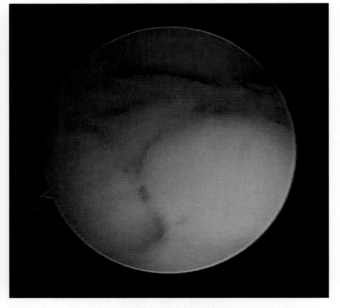

Fig. 23-21. Completed mosaicplasty. (Reprinted with permission from Ahmad C and ElAttrache N. Mosaicplasty for capitellar osteochondritis dissecans. In: Yamagachi K, King G, McKee M, O'Driscoll S, eds. *Advanced Reconstruction Elbow*. Rosemont, Illinois: American Academy of Orthopaedic Surgeons. In press.)

changes involving the radial head and significant deformity of the capitellum that contributed to the poor result.

■ REFERENCES

1. Doherty M, Preston B. Primary osteoarthritis of the elbow. Ann Rheum Dis. 1989 48(9):743–747.
2. Morrey BF, Askew LJ, Chao EY. A biomechanical study of normal functional elbow motion. J Bone Joint Surg Am. 1981;63:872–877.
3. Nowicki KD, Shall LM. Arthroscopic release of a posttraumatic flexion contracture in the elbow: a case report and review of the literature. Arthroscopy. 1992; 8(4):544–547.
4. Husband JB, Hastings H. The lateral approach for operative elbow release of post-traumatic contracture of the elbow. J Bone Joint Surg. 1990;72A:1353–1358.
5. Mansat P, Morrey BF. The column procedure: a limited lateral approach for extrinsic contracture of the elbow. J Bone Joint Surg. 1998; 80A(11):1603–1615.
6. Kashiwagi D. Intraarticular changes of the osteoarthritic elbow, especially about the fossa olecrani. J Jpn Orthop Assoc. 1978;52:1367–1382.
7. Morrey BF. Primary degenerative arthritis of the elbow: treatment by ulnohumeral arthroplasty. J Bone Joint Surg. 1992;74B:409–413.
8. Savoie FH, Field LD, Hartzhog CW. Arthroscopic treatment of ankylosis of the elbow. In: Baker CL, Plancher KD, eds. Operative Treatment of Elbow Injuries. New York: Springer; 2002:177–184.
9. Hotchkiss RN. In: Green DP, Pederson WP, eds. Green's Operative Hand Surgery, 4th ed. New York: Churchill-Livingstone; 1999:667–682.
10. Field LD, Savoie FH. Arthroscopic radial head resection. In: Baker CL, Plancher KD, eds. Operative Treatment of Elbow Injuries. New York: Springer; 2002:185–194.
11. Ogilvie-Harris DJ, Schemitsch E. Arthroscopy of the elbow for removal of loose bodies. Arthroscopy. 1993;9(1):5–8.
12. O'Driscoll SW, Morrey BF. Arthroscopy of the elbow: diagnostic and therapeutic benefits and hazards. J Bone Joint Surg. 1992;74(1):84–94.
13. Savoie FH, Nunley PD, Field LD. Arthroscopic management of the arthritic elbow: indications, techniques, and results. J Shoulder Elbow Surg. 1999;8:214–219.
14. Menth-Chiari WA, Poehling GG, Ruch DS. Arthroscopic resection of the radial head: technical note. Arthroscopy. 1999;15:226–230.
15. Antuna SA, Morrey BF, Adams RA, et al. Ulnohumeral arthroplasty for primary degenerative arthritis of the elbow. J Bone Joint Surg. 2002;84A(12):2168–2173.
16. Aldridge JM, Atkins TA, Gunneson EE, et al. Anterior release of the elbow for extension loss. J Bone Joint Surg. 2004;86A(9):1955–1960.
17. Kim S, Kim H, Lee J. Arthroscopy for limitation of motion of the elbow. Arthroscopy. 1995;11(6):680–683.
18. Timmerman LA, Andrews JR. Arthroscopic treatment of post-traumatic elbow pain and stiffness. Am J Sports Med. 1994;22(2):230–235.
19. Phillips BB, Strasburger S. Arthroscopic treatment of arthrofibrosis of the elbow joint. Arthroscopy. 1998;14(1):38–44.
20. Ball CM, Meunier M, Galatz LM, et al. Arthroscopic treatment of post-traumatic elbow contracture. J Shoulder Elbow Surg. 2002;11:624–629.
21. Ogilvie-Harris DJ, Gordon R, Mackay M. Arthroscopic treatment for posterior impingement in degenerative arthritis of the elbow. Arthroscopy. 1995;11(4):437–443.
22. Panner H. An affection of the capitulum humeri resembling Calvé-Perthes' disease of the hip. Acta Radiol. 1927;8:617–618.
23. Douglas G, Rang M. The role of trauma in the pathogenesis of the osteochondroses. Clin Orthop Relat Res. 1981;158:28–32.
24. Jackson DW, Silvino N, Reiman P. Osteochondritis in the female gymnast's elbow. Arthroscopy. 1989;5(2):129–136.
25. Ruch DS, Poehling GG. Arthroscopic treatment of Panner's disease. Clin Sports Med. 1991;10(3):629–636.
26. Singer KM, Roy SP. Osteochondrosis of the humeral capitellum. Am J Sports Med. 1984;12(5):351–360.
27. Baumgarten TE, Andrews JR, Satterwhite YE. The arthroscopic classification and treatment of osteochondritis dissecans of the capitellum. Am J Sports Med. 1998;26(4):520–523.
28. Difelice G, Meunier M, Paletta GJ. Elbow injury in the adolescent athlete. In: Altchek D, Andrews J, eds. The Athlete's Elbow. Philadelphia: Lippincott Williams & Wilkins; 2001:231–248.
29. Bojanic I, Ivkovic A, Boric I. Arthroscopy and microfracture technique in the treatment of osteochondritis dissecans of the humeral capitellum: report of three adolescent gymnasts. Knee Surg Sports Traumatol Arthrosc. 2005. [E pub ahead of print].
30. Brownlow HC, O'Connor-Read LM, et al. Arthroscopic treatment of osteochondritis dissecans of the capitellum. Knee Surg Sports Traumatol Arthrosc. 2006;14(2):198–202.
31. Byrd JW, Jones KS. Arthroscopic surgery for isolated capitellar osteochondritis dissecans in adolescent baseball players: minimum three-year follow-up. Am J Sports Med. 2002;30(4):474–478.
32. Krijnen MR, Lim L, Willems WJ. Arthroscopic treatment of osteochondritis dissecans of the capitellum: report of 5 female athletes. Arthroscopy. 2003;19(2):210–214.
33. McManama GB Jr, Micheli LJ, Berry MV, et al. The surgical treatment of osteochondritis of the capitellum. Am J Sports Med. 1985;13(1):11–21.
34. Ruch DS, Cory JW, Poehling GG. The arthroscopic management of osteochondritis dissecans of the adolescent elbow. Arthroscopy. 1998;14(8):797–803.

24

VALGUS EXTENSION OVERLOAD

■ JAMES R. ANDREWS, MD, RENEÉ S. RILEY, MD

■ HISTORY OF THE TECHNIQUE

Bennett,[1] in 1941, described elbow pathology he had noted in baseball pitchers, reporting loose bodies and osteophytes of the coronoid and olecranon tip. He anecdotally reported that removal relieved symptoms and allowed return to play. The spectrum of symptoms and pathology associated with valgus extension overload of the elbow was described by Waris[2] in 1946 in his article on 17 elite javelin throwers. He described the debilitating posteromedial elbow pain sometimes associated with loss of extension, which required between 4 weeks and 1 year of rest before return to play. He reported radiographic changes in the olecranon in 12 of 17 cases. He concluded that these changes were due to the repetitive trauma of throwing.

Slocum,[3] in 1968, classified elbow injuries into three categories: medial tension overload, lateral compression overload, and extension overload. He concluded that the combination of these in the baseball pitcher led to the excessive wear in the joint.

King et al.,[4] in 1969, reported on a series of 50 professional baseball pitchers and noted a 50% incidence of elbow flexion contracture. They coined the term "medial elbow stress syndrome" and noted attenuated medial structures leading to the compression of the lateral compartment and loose body formation. They also noted loose bodies posteriorly, but hypothesized that this was not due to the force of hyperextension jamming the olecranon into its fossa, because of the high incidence of flexion contracture in pitchers. Rather, they thought that the valgus stress was the culprit, leading to impingement of the medial aspect of the olecranon against the wall of the olecranon fossa.

Indelicato et al.,[5] in 1979, reported that 20 out of 25 professional baseball pitchers were able to return to competitive throwing following open excision of osteophytes and removal of loose bodies through a medial approach. Wilson et al.,[6] in 1983, coined the term "valgus extension overload" and reported on five pitchers who underwent excision of posteromedial osteophytes through a posterolateral approach, and all returned to their previous level of competition.

With the advent of elbow arthroscopy, open treatment of valgus extension overload is primarily of historic interest, except in cases where arthroscopy is contraindicated or when another open procedure is being performed (e.g., ulnar collateral ligament reconstruction). Andrews and Timmerman,[7] in 1995, reported on 72 professional baseball players who underwent elbow surgery. Sixty-eight percent of those treated with arthroscopic excision of posteromedial olecranon osteophytes returned to the same or higher level of competition.

Reddy et al.,[8] in 2000, reported that posterior olecranon impingement was the most common diagnosis in 187 elbow arthroscopies performed at the Kerlan-Jobe Clinic from 1991–1997. They noted that 92% of the patients contacted rated their results as good or excellent at an average of 42 months follow-up, and 85% of professional athletes returned to their previous level of competition. There was no mention, however, of the reoperation rate in this patient population.

■ INDICATIONS AND CONTRAINDICATIONS

Valgus extension overload describes a constellation of pathologies in the elbow of the throwing athlete as a result of the repetitive forces exerted during the throwing motion. Medial compartment distraction is accompanied by lateral compartment compression and posterior compartment impingement. The most common presentation is pain secondary to impingement of the posteromedial olecranon tip and the medial aspect if the trochlea, sometimes associated with loss of extension due to osteophyte formation. Valgus extension overload can also be present with changes in the lateral compartment due to compressive forces. Loose bodies can cause painful catching and locking. The throwing athlete will often complain of pain with ball release as well as diminished velocity or loss of ball control, usually with early release and high pitches.[9]

On physical examination, flexion contracture is a common finding, but it is not necessarily pathologic in the throwing athlete. The valgus extension overload test is performed by repeatedly forcing the elbow from slight flexion rapidly into extension while applying a valgus stress. This should reproduce pain in the posteromedial aspect of the elbow from impingement of the posteromedial olecranon tip on the medial wall of the olecranon fossa. From a pathophysiologic standpoint, this is associated with valgus overload with or without instability, and forced hyperextension. Radiographs may show the olecranon osteophyte or loose bodies. A posterior osteophyte may be seen on a routine lateral view. The best view for showing the posteromedial osteophyte is an oblique axial view with the elbow flexed to 110 degrees **(Fig. 24-1)**, although it is not always visualized on radiographs.

Indications for surgery include the clinical history and physical exam findings described above with or without radiographic evidence of osteophyte formation. The athlete should have failed a course of nonoperative management and be unable to throw effectively due to posteromedial elbow

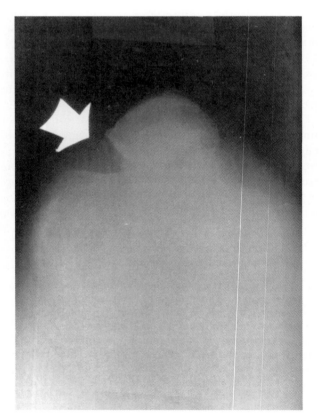

Fig. 24-1. Axial view of the elbow showing articulation of olecranon with trochlea and posteromedial olecranon osteophyte on profile.

pain or locking from loose bodies. Conservative treatment in the face of a posteromedial olecranon osteophyte has not had a high success rate in our experience; but in general, we do recommend a 6-week period of rest and strengthening exercises, including a rotator cuff protocol, followed by an interval throwing program. This is beneficial for overall general conditioning and improves results postoperatively if surgery is required.[6] Often, the surgical procedure can be delayed until the end of the season, depending on whether the athlete is able to tolerate the symptoms and to play effectively.

Contraindications to surgical treatment with arthroscopy include any condition that does not allow distention of the joint or access to the joint otherwise, such as bony or fibrous ankylosis. Also, conditions that place the neurovascular structures at increased risk for injury are relative contraindications. These include previous ulnar nerve transposition, which precludes the use of an anteromedial portal, and severe deformities, which distort anatomy, such as rheumatoid arthritis. Any condition that increases the risk for infection, such as cellulitis of the overlying skin, is a contraindication.

■ SURGICAL TECHNIQUES

Anesthesia

General anesthesia is commonly used for elbow arthroscopy for several reasons. It provides complete muscle relaxation and is most comfortable for the patient. It also allows for a reliable neurovascular exam immediately following the procedure, which is important because most of these operations are performed on an outpatient basis and prolonged observation is not feasible. Some surgeons advocate the use of intravenous regional anesthesia, but we do not recommend its use for the above reason and because the use of a double tourniquet can compromise exposure.

Patient positioning is very important during elbow arthroscopy to ensure adequate visualization of the joint. We use the supine position **(Fig. 24-2)** because of the ease of general anesthesia and conversion to an open procedure, if necessary. It is our opinion that the structures are in a more anatomic orientation in this position as well. Other alternatives include the prone and lateral decubitus positions.

Surface Anatomy

The identification of palpable surface structures about the elbow is crucial prior to arthroscopy. A marking pen should be used to outline the medial and lateral epicondyles, which should be easily palpated. The radial head can be identified by supinating and pronating the forearm. The olecranon tip is subcutaneous and should be marked as well **(Fig. 24-3A,B)**. The ulnar nerve can be felt just posterior to the medial epicondyle. It is crucial to make sure that the nerve does not sublux anteriorly and to review the surgical history to confirm that the nerve has not been transferred during a previous procedure.

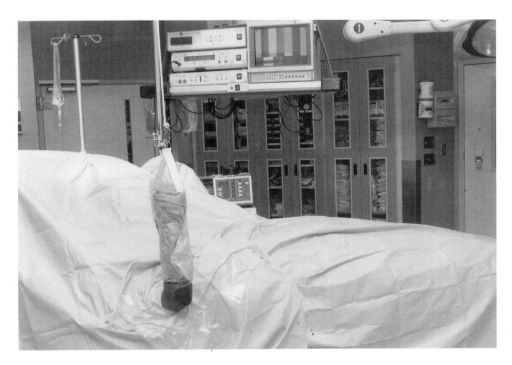

Fig. 24-2. Supine positioning, with arm prepared and draped, suspended from a pulley system.

Anterolateral Portal

The anterolateral portal is established after the joint is distended by injecting saline into the lateral soft spot. The anterolateral portal is located in a different "soft spot" approximately 2 cm proximal and 1 cm anterior to the lateral humeral epicondyle. A spinal needle is placed first to ensure egress of fluid before making the skin incision. The incision is superficial, and a hemostat is used to spread the soft tissues. Care must be taken to avoid the cutaneous nerves in the region, including the lateral antebrachial and the posterior antebrachial cutaneous nerves. To establish the anterolateral portal, the blunt trocar and sheath for a 4.0-mm 30-degree arthroscope are inserted into the portal site. An assistant should apply pressure to the syringe, injecting saline into the lateral soft spot. This will distend the joint and move the neurovascular structures away from the capsule. The trocar should be directed toward the center of the elbow, and the capsule is trapped against the distal humerus and then punctured to enter the joint. This is necessary to avoid damage to the anterior neurovascular structures. The radial nerve is also at risk, and the arthroscope may pass from 4 mm to 7 mm posterior to it. This distance is closer to 7 mm when the joint is distended.

Anteromedial Portal

Often, with isolated posterior pathology, an anteromedial portal is not necessary. Especially in throwers, this portal is not

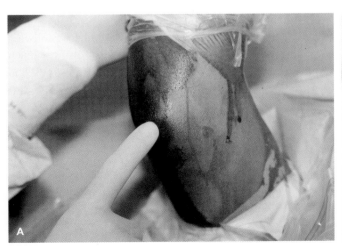 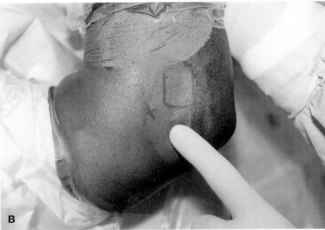

Fig. 24-3. A: Medial side of the elbow, with structures marked, including olecranon tip, medial epicondyle, and ulnar nerve. B: Lateral side of the elbow with structures marked, including the radial head and lateral epicondyle.

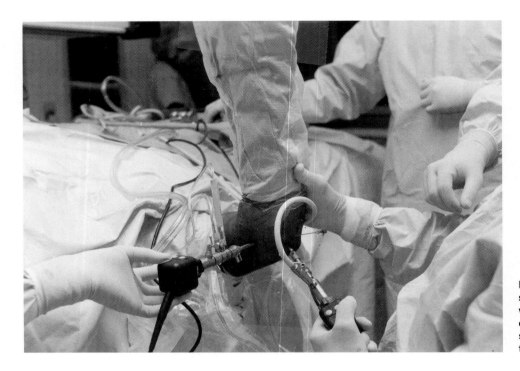

Fig. 24-4. The 2.7-mm arthroscope in the direct lateral portal, with light source attached (blue cord), and the 4.0-mm arthroscope supplying inflow through the anterolateral portal.

established unless it is absolutely needed, to avoid neurovascular risk and the surgical trauma to the medial soft tissues. If it is necessary, the anteromedial portal is established under direct needle visualization approximately 2 cm proximal and 2 cm anterior to the medial epicondyle. The portal passes between 6 and 14 mm from the median nerve and, on average, 17 mm posteromedial to the brachial artery.[10] The medial antebrachial cutaneous nerve can lie as close as 1 mm from the portal.

Direct Lateral Portal

The direct lateral portal is established in the spot where the initial spinal needle was placed to distend the joint, in the soft spot bordered by the radial head, lateral epicondyle, and olecranon. A skin incision is made, and the 2.7 mm arthroscope is introduced because the lateral compartment is such a small space. We find it helpful to have the 4-mm arthroscope remain in the anterolateral portal with the inflow coming through the larger scope, which allows for better distention of the joint **(Fig. 24-4)**. There is little danger to neurovascular structures with this portal, which passes through the anconeus muscle.

Accessory Lateral Portal

The accessory lateral portal is established for instrumentation if debridement is needed in the lateral compartment. It is located approximately 1.5 cm distal to the direct lateral portal and is established with needle localization. Risk to critical structures is minimal.

Posterolateral Portal

The posterolateral portal is located approximately 3 cm proximal to the tip of the olecranon along the lateral border of the triceps. To establish the portal, the 2.7-mm arthroscope in the direct lateral portal is used to visualize the pos-

terolateral capsule adjacent to the olecranon tip, and a spinal needle is used to localize the site. Once it is visualized, the skin incision is made, and the soft tissues are spread using a hemostat. A 4.0-mm blunt trocar is introduced. The elbow can be extended about 30 degrees to 40 degrees of flexion to facilitate entry into the joint. The posterior antebrachial and lateral brachial cutaneous nerves are at risk.

Straight Posterior Portal

The straight posterior portal is located approximately 2 cm from the olecranon tip and midline to the posterolateral portal. It is a triceps-splitting portal. It is established with needle localization with the elbow flexed 20 degrees to 30 degrees. The posterolateral and posterior portals should be as close to a 90-degree angle to each other as possible. This portal is used to resect the posterior olecranon osteophyte in valgus extension overload and is also useful for removing loose bodies. The ulnar nerve is at risk with this portal, and careful attention should be paid to frequent reorientation of the anatomy when working in this area of the elbow.

Procedure

The patient is positioned supine, with a tourniquet placed as high on the arm as possible. The arm is suspended from a traction device with a hook and loop fastener gauntlet and elastic wrap. The elbow should be flexed 90 degrees and the shoulder abducted 90 degrees. This usually requires about 5 lbs of traction. The surgeon sits on a rolling stool on the radial side of the arm, while an assistant sits on the ulnar side. The surface landmarks are outlined using a sterile marking pen.

The tourniquet is inflated to 250 mm Hg. Exsanguination is not necessary because the arm has been suspended during preparation and draping. A pressure sensitive arthroscope is used to prevent overdistention. A spinal needle is introduced into the lateral soft spot between the lateral epicondyle, radial head, and olecranon. Saline is injected through a syringe connected to intravenous tubing. Another spinal needle is introduced into the site for the anterolateral portal, and fluid egress is noted. The portal is then established while an assistant holds pressure on the syringe of saline, and the 4.0-mm arthroscope is introduced. From this portal, the distal humerus, trochlea, and coronoid process can be inspected. An anteromedial portal is established under direct visualization using a spinal needle for localization. The anterior compartment is inspected for any loose bodies, osteophyte formation, or chondral damage to the radial head, capitellum, or coronoid process. A valgus stress test with the elbow at 70 degrees of flexion is helpful to evaluate for ulnar collateral ligament insufficiency. An opening of greater than 1 to 2 mm between the coronoid process and the trochlea is suggestive of VCL laxity, but this arthroscopic exam must be correlated with history and physical exam. The arthroscope is introduced into the anteromedial portal to best visualize the capitellum and radial head. Care should be taken to leave the cannulae in the joint when changing portals to prevent multiple passes of trocars, which increases risk to neurovascular structures and extravasation of fluid into the soft tissues. If loose bodies are present, they should be removed through the anterolateral portal with the arthroscope in the anteromedial portal. Loose body removal should be the last procedure performed through this portal because it sometimes leads to fluid extravasation.

With the 4.0-mm arthroscope in the anterolateral portal, a direct lateral portal should be established for the 2.7-mm arthroscope. The fluid is introduced through the 4.0-mm scope, while the smaller scope is used to actually view the tight lateral compartment. The radial head, capitellum, trochlear notch, and trochlear ridge can be seen through this portal. If any debridement is needed, an accessory lateral portal is established about 1 cm distal to the direct lateral portal. Instrumentation is introduced through this portal for debridement or removal of loose bodies.

The elbow is then extended to 30 degrees of flexion, and the posterolateral portal is established under direct visualization with the 2.7-mm arthroscope. The 4.0-mm arthroscope is introduced through the posterolateral portal. An accessory straight posterior portal is then established with needle localization. These two portals should be as far apart as possible without risking damage to the ulnar nerve. The optimal placement to facilitate triangulation while working in the posterior compartment allows instruments placed in the portals to meet at a 90-degree angle at the olecranon tip **(Fig. 24-5)**.

The posterior compartment is inspected for loose bodies, olecranon osteophyte, and the "kissing lesion" on the posteromedial trochlea. A shaver is introduced through the straight posterior portal to debride soft tissue from the olecranon tip and fossa so that the entire olecranon tip is visualized.

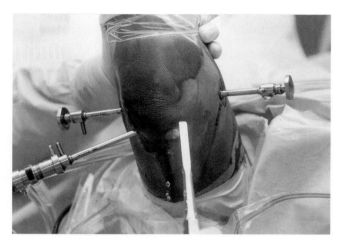

Fig. 24-5. Excision of posteromedial olecranon osteophyte. The 4.0-mm arthroscope is in the posterolateral portal, and the osteotome is in the straight posterior portal. Note that the scope and the osteotome are at approximately right angles to each other.

A small osteotome is used to excise the osteophyte **(Fig. 24-6A),** taking care to remove fragments with a grasper as soon as they become loose **(Fig. 24-6B).** The remainder of the olecranon tip is smoothed using a 5.5-mm bur. How much of the olecranon tip should be removed is not clear. Therefore, we remove only enough bone to allow full extension of the elbow without impingement, which is usually 3 to 5 mm. Chondromalacia of the posteromedial trochlea is debrided of any unstable cartilage flaps, and abrasion chondroplasty is performed in some cases, depending on the severity of the lesion.

A lateral radiograph of the elbow is taken intraoperatively to ensure that no loose bony fragments remain in the joint or soft tissues and to assess the adequacy of the olecranon excision **(Fig. 24-7)**. A drain is placed through a cannula in the anterolateral portal, and portal sites are closed using nylon sutures. A bulky dressing is applied, and the tourniquet is released.

Postoperative Care

The extremity is elevated and iced, and immediate motion is begun. Particular attention is paid to maintaining extension that was achieved in the operating room. The drain is removed in the recovery area in patients who are released the same day, or on postoperative day 1 in patients who stay in the hospital overnight.

■ TECHNICAL ALTERNATIVES AND PITFALLS

Open excision of an olecranon osteophyte is an alternative to elbow arthroscopy for the treatment of valgus extension overload. This is usually done through a medial incision, and usually in conjunction with another open procedure. The

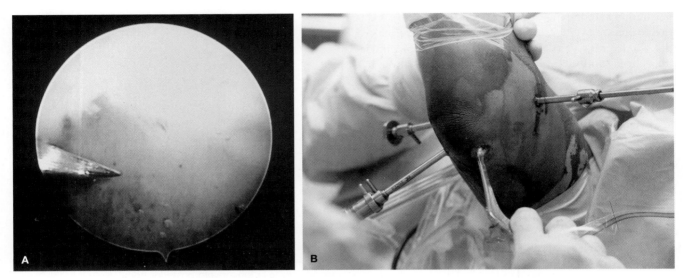

Fig. 24-6. **A:** Arthroscopic view of osteotomy of olecranon tip. **B:** Removal of osteotomized ole-cranon tip with a grasper through the straight posterior portal.

procedure can also be done through a posterolateral anconeus approach, or through a triceps splitting approach. We commonly perform open olecranon excision through a posteromedial arthrotomy in patients who are undergoing ulnar collateral ligament reconstruction. It is performed with an osteotome and bur, much the same as it is through the arthroscope. Visualization is best through the arthroscope or using an open posteromedial approach. In the absence of a concomitant open procedure, elbow arthroscopy is the standard for treatment of valgus extension overload.

Variations in techniques of elbow arthroscopy relate mostly to patient positioning. The prone position was introduced by Poehling et al.[11] in 1989 **(Fig. 24-8)**. They reported better stability of the arm in this position and better access to the posterior compartment when compared to the supine position. There is no need for a suspension system. Also, the anterior neurovascular structures are in a dependent position and fall away from the anterior capsule, which would theoretically decrease the risk of injury. This has not been proven clinically, however.

Another position described by O'Driscoll and Morrey[12] is the lateral decubitus position, in which the patient is placed with the operative side up and the arm supported on a padded bolster **(Fig. 24-9)**. This position is an attempt to combine the benefits of the prone and supine positions. The arm is more stable and the posterior compartment more easily visualized, as in the prone position, but general anesthesia is better administered, although not as easily as in the supine position.

There are advantages and disadvantages to the supine position relative to the other two. First, general anesthesia is easier to administer in this position, and there is no need for chest and pelvic rolls. There is not as much concern over pressure points as there is with the other methods. In our

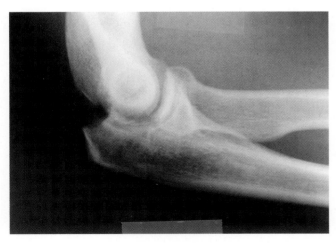

Fig. 24-7. Intraoperative lateral radiograph showing adequate olecranon tip excision and no loose bodies.

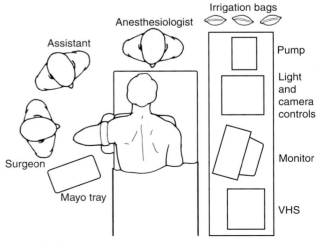

Fig. 24-8. Diagram of operating room setup for prone positioning.

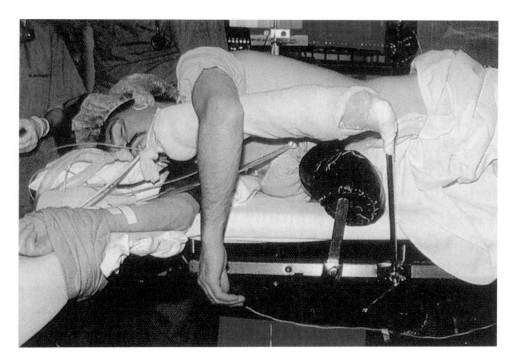

Fig. 24-9. Setup for the lateral decubitus position.

experience, the structures in the elbow are in a more anatomic orientation in this position, but this is probably dependent on the surgeon and what he or she becomes accustomed to. If conversion to an open procedure is necessary, the supine position allows for this without breaking to reposition.

There are some disadvantages of the supine position. A suspension device is required, and stability of the elbow during certain portions of the procedure must be provided by an assistant holding the arm. The posterior compartment can be more difficult to visualize in this position, but with the addition of a few pounds of traction, it is accessible. Basically, the surgeon should use the position with which he or she is most comfortable and with which he or she has the most experience.

In a patient who is diagnosed with isolated valgus extension overload, a meticulous history, physical exam, and diagnostic work-up should be performed to rule out an injury to the ulnar collateral ligament (UCL), as these two pathologies often coexist. Andrews and Timmerman[7] reported on 72 professional baseball players who had undergone elbow surgery. Of those who had arthroscopic posteromedial olecranon excision, 41% required reoperation. Five of the 13 reoperations were ulnar collateral ligament reconstructions. We speculated on whether the osteophyte excision led to increased strain on the UCL or whether mild medial laxity caused the osteophyte formation, and the UCL injury was overlooked at first. We now believe that the UCL injury likely precedes osteophyte formation in most cases.

This hypothesis is supported by the findings of Ahmad et al.[13] who performed a cadaveric study in which seven elbows were tested with two valgus loads at 30 degrees and 90 degrees of flexion. The tests were carried out first with the ulnar collateral ligament intact, then with a partial tear, and lastly, with a complete tear. Pressure-sensitive film was placed in the posteromedial compartment of the elbow during testing, and the contact area between the olecranon and posteromedial trochlea was noted to be decreased by 18.5% in the elbows with partial tears and by 39.7% in those with complete tears, when compared with the intact elbows. The pressure was increased by 11.9% with a partial tear and 72.4% with a complete tear.

We have looked at UCL strain in relation to olecranon excision in a cadaver model.[14] Five cadaver elbows were tested with a valgus stress at six different flexion angles at baseline and after resection of the medial olecranon in 2 mm increments, up to 8 mm. The last, "worst case scenario" test was done with 8 mm of medial and 5 mm of posterior olecranon excision. There were no significant differences in strain between the different levels of osteotomy. Despite these findings, we still resect only enough olecranon to allow full extension of the elbow without impingement. We also have a high index of suspicion for UCL injury in any overhead athlete with posteromedial elbow pain, and perform a careful physical exam and diagnostic workup to evaluate the UCL before scheduling an operation for isolated valgus extension overload.

■ REHABILITATION/RETURN TO SPORTS

Motion is begun immediately following surgery. The goals are to reestablish painless range of motion, retard muscle atrophy, and decrease inflammation. However, overzealous active range of motion within the first 5 days following surgery can lead to drainage from the posterior portal and even fistula formation. This is why it is essential to suture the portal sites and go

TABLE 24-1	Postoperative Rehabilitation Following Posterior Compartment Elbow Arthroplasty

I. Phase I: Immediate motion phase
   Goals: Improve/regain full ROM
        Decrease pain/inflammation
        Retard muscular atrophy
   A. Day 1–4
      ■ ROM to tolerance (extension/flexion and supination/pronation) (Often full elbow extension is not capable due to pain.)
      ■ *Gentle* overpressure into extension
      ■ Wrist flex/ext stretches
      ■ Gripping exercises (putty)
      ■ Isometrics elbow ext/flex
      ■ Compression dressing, ice 4–5 times daily
   B. Day 5–10
      ■ ROM exercises to tolerance (at least 20–90°)
      ■ Overpressure into extension
      ■ Joint mobilization to reestablish ROM
      ■ Wrist flex/ext stretches
      ■ Continue isometrics
      ■ Continue use of ice, compression to control swelling
   C. Day 11–14
      ■ ROM exercises to tolerance (at least 10–100°)
      ■ Overpressure into extension (3–4 times daily)
      ■ Continue joint mobilization techniques
      ■ Initiate light dumbbell program (PREs): biceps, triceps, wrist flex/ext, sup/pronators
      ■ Continue use of ice postexercise

II. Phase II: Intermediate phase
   Goals: Improve strength/power/endurance
        Increase ROM
        Initiate functional activities
   A. Week 2–4
      ■ Full ROM exercises (4–5 times daily)
      ■ Overpressure into elbow extension
      ■ Continue PRE program for elbow and wrist musculature
      ■ Initiate shoulder program (esp ER, RTC)
      ■ Continue joint mobilization
      ■ Continue ice postexercise
   B. Week 4–7
      ■ Continue all exercises listed above
      ■ Initiate light upper body program
      ■ Continue use of ice postactivity

III. Phase III: Advanced strengthening program
   Goals: Improve strength/power/endurance
        Gradual return to functional activities
   Criteria to enter Phase III
      ■ Full nonpainful ROM
      ■ Strength >75% of contralateral side
      ■ No pain or tenderness
   A. Week 8–12
      ■ Continue PRE program for elbow and wrist
      ■ Continue shoulder program
      ■ Continue stretching for elbow/shoulder
      ■ Initiate interval program and gradually return to sport activities

ROM, range of motion; PRE, passive resistance exercise.

slowly with early range of motion. Elbow extension is regained slowly due to pain. By postoperative day 14, range of motion should be 10 degrees to 110 degrees, and in most cases, full range is obtained by 3 weeks. A strengthening program is initiated, with isometrics during the first 2 weeks and isotonic exercises starting during weeks 3 or 4. Most throwing athletes can begin an interval throwing program by 10 weeks. Starting a throwing program too early can initiate calcification in the posterior aspect of the elbow and a recurrence of symptoms. The specific rehabilitation protocol following arthroscopy for valgus extension overload is outlined in **Table 24-1**.[15]

■ OUTCOMES AND FUTURE DIRECTIONS

In our experience, arthroscopic treatment of valgus extension overload in professional throwing athletes has yielded mediocre results with a high reoperation rate when players return to competition. A large part of the problem in our early experience was because concomitant pathologies were overlooked. We believe that our heightened index of suspicion for concomitant injury to the ulnar collateral ligament is yielding improved results and decreasing our reoperation rate.

■ SUGGESTED READINGS

Cain EL, Andrews JR. Elbow arthroscopy in the throwing athlete. In: McGinty JB, Burkart SS, Jackson RW, et al., eds. *Operative Arthroscopy*. Philadelphia: Lippincott Williams & Wilkins; 2003:697–707.
Cain EL, Dugas JR, Wolf RS, et al. Elbow injuries in throwing athletes: a current concepts review. Am J Sports Med. 2003;31: 621–635.
Soffer SR. Diagnostic arthroscopy of the elbow. In: Andrews JR, Timmerman LA, eds. *Diagnostic and Operative Arthroscopy*. Philadelphia: WB Saunders; 1997: 169–181.

■ REFERENCES

1. Bennett GE. Shoulder and elbow lesions of the professional baseball pitcher. JAMA. 1941;117:510–514.
2. Waris W. Elbow injuries of javelin throwers. Acta Chir Scand. 1946;93:563–575.
3. Slocum, DB. Classification of elbow injuries from baseball pitching. Tex Med. 1968;64:48–53.
4. King JW, Brelsford HJ, Tullos HS. Analysis of the pitching arm of the professional baseball pitcher. Clin Orthop. 1969;67:116–123.
5. Indelicato PA, Jobe FW, Kerlan RK, et al. Correctable elbow lesions in professional baseball players: a review of 25 cases. Am J Sports Med. 1979;7:72–75.
6. Wilson FD, Andrews JR, Blackburn TA, et al. Valgus extension overload in the pitching elbow. Am J Sports Med. 1983;11:83–88.
7. Andrews JR, Timmerman LA. Outcome of elbow surgery in professional baseball players. Am J Sports Med. 1995;23: 407–413.

8. Reddy AS, Kvitne RS, Yocum LA, et al. Arthroscopy of the elbow: a long-term clinical review. Arthroscopy. 2000;16: 588–594.

9. Andrews JR, Whiteside JA, Buettner CM. Clinical evaluation of the elbow in throwers. Oper Tech Sports Med. 1996;4:77–83.

10. Andrews JR, Carson WG. Arthroscopy of the elbow. Arthroscopy. 1985;1:97–107.

11. Poehling GG, Whipple TL, Sisco L, et al. Elbow arthroscopy: a new technique. Arthroscopy. 1989;5:222–224.

12. O'Driscoll SW, Morrey BF. Arthroscopy of the elbow. J Bone Joint Surg. 1992;74A:84–94.

13. Ahmad CS, Park MC, ElAttrache NS. Elbow medial collateral ligament insufficiency alters posteromedial olecranon contact. Paper presented at: American Orthopaedic Society for Sports Medicine 29th Annual Meeting; 2003; San Diego. Am J Sports Med. 2004;32:1607–1612.

14. Andrews JR, Heggland EJ, Fleisig GS, et al. Relationship of ulnar collateral ligament strain to amount of medial olecranon osteotomy. Am J Sports Med. 2001;29:716–721.

15. Wilk KE, Azar FM, Andrews JR. Conservative and operative rehabilitation of the elbow in sports. Sports Med Arthrosc Rev. 1995;3:237–258.

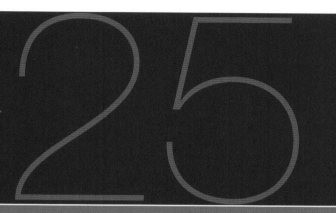

REPAIR OF DISTAL BICEPS TENDON RUPTURES

AUGUSTUS D. MAZZOCCA, MD, JAMES BICOS, MD, ANTHONY A. ROMEO, MD, ROBERT A. ARCIERO, MD

■ HISTORY OF THE TECHNIQUE

Ruptures of the distal biceps tendon have received increased attention recently. This trend is probably the result of increased demands placed on the upper extremities as well as increased activity in the middle-aged population. Treatment options have expanded in an effort to use modern fixation methods to return patients to work or athletic activities quicker.

Historically, a single extensile anterior exposure was used to reinsert the avulsed tendon. Boyd and Anderson[1] subsequently described a two-incision technique designed to minimize anterior exposure and limit the risk to neurovascular structures in proximity to the tuberosity. Their two-incision technique introduced heterotopic ossification and proximal radioulnar synostosis as new complications. In 1985, Morrey et al.[2] modified Boyd's original approach by splitting the supinator and avoiding subperiosteal dissection. These modifications led to a decrease in the rate of heterotopic bone formation and synostosis.

Modifications in the method of fixation have also been proposed. Single incision techniques have been revived with the advent of suture anchors. These procedures utilize a Henry exposure and secure the tendon to the cortical surface of the tuberosity and not into a tunnel or trough. Benefits of the single incision technique include decreased morbidity as well as technical ease in use of the suture anchors. Biomechanical studies have shown that the suture anchor techniques are not as stiff or strong when compared to fixation over a bone bridge.[3] However, in cyclic loading, the suture anchors have performed adequately to allow early passive range of motion (ROM).[4]

In an attempt to combine both a single incision and the use of a tunnel to place the tendon into, Bain et al.[5] have described a technique using the EndoButton (Smith and Nephew, Hamburg, Germany). Studies evaluating its stiffness and strength are ongoing, but the EndoButton has performed well in other applications. However, potential complications in passing a Beath pin through the radius, approximating the length of the suture loop, and "flipping" of the device on the posterior cortex can make it a challenging technical procedure. Furthermore, cyclic loading early on might lead to pistoning of the tendon in the tunnel and impaired healing.

Bioabsorbable interference screw fixation has become popular, especially around the knee. Multiple studies testing the biomechanical properties of bioabsorbable interference screws have been performed. They have routinely shown that the constructs fail by graft slippage past the screws but at a level equal to or greater than other fixation methods.[6-8] In cyclical loading models, the screws have performed favorably as well. On a histological level, direct tendon healing to bone has been observed with interference screw fixation.[6,7] A mature fibrocartilage intratunnel, direct ligamentous insertion can be found at 9 to 12 weeks.[9] When indirect methods of tendon fixation are used, healing progresses via a zone of vascular, highly cellular fibrous tissue that matures through orientation of collagen fibers over a period of 12 to 26 weeks.[10,11]

With the development of new equipment, a bioabsorbable screw can be delivered into a prepared socket without the need for passage of a needle or suture through the socket. The combination of intratunnel fixation, a bioabsorbable device, and a single anterior approach provides an attractive alternative to other techniques. These technical advances provide the surgeon with yet another useful option for fixation of the avulsed distal biceps tendon.

Stringent anatomical dissection and biomechanical evaluation of the techniques mentioned have pointed to a combination approach for fixation of the distal biceps tendon in a high-demand upper-extremity patient (paraplegic, laborer, and athlete). This chapter will describe the two-incision technique, as well as a technique that uses a single incision, interference screw, and EndoButton, allowing immediate active postoperative motion for early return to activity and a decrease in postoperative stiffness or heterotopic ossification.

■ PREOPERATIVE EVALUATION

Patients with complete distal biceps tendon ruptures usually report feeling a sudden, sharp, painful tearing sensation in the antecubital region of the elbow when an unexpected extension force was applied to the flexed/supinated arm. Occasionally, pain is also present in the posterolateral aspect of the elbow. The acute pain subsides in a few hours and is replaced by a dull ache; with chronic ruptures, weakness and fatigue occur with repetitive flexion and supination activities. Physical examination reveals tenderness in the antecubital fossa, and a defect usually can be palpated there. Active flexion of the elbow causes the biceps muscle belly to retract proximally, accentuating the defect in the antecubital fossa. If the biceps tendon can be palpated in the antecubital fossa, a partial rupture of the distal biceps tendon should be considered. Ecchymosis and swelling usually are evident in the antecubital fossa and along the medial aspect of the arm and proximal forearm.

Plain radiographs generally do not show any bony changes, although irregularity and enlargement of the radial tuberosity and avulsion of a portion of the radial tuberosity have been reported with complete ruptures of the distal biceps tendon. Magnetic resonance imaging (MRI) can be helpful to distinguish complete from partial ruptures and to differentiate partial rupture from tendinosis, tenosynovitis, hematoma, and brachialis contusion.

■ INDICATIONS AND CONTRAINDICATIONS

Operative and nonoperative treatment courses are always presented to the patient. Nonoperative treatment involves pain control and introduction of early range of motion when able. Once full range of motion is established, strengthening begins concentrating on supination. The University of Connecticut uses an isokinetic dynamometer to establish strength deficits at the initiation of rehabilitation and at the end. Patients are counseled that they

will lose approximately 25% to 35% of their supination strength. They are also instructed to perform all activities that are important to them. If they are unable to perform any of these functions, operative treatment is once again strongly recommended.

The indications for operative fixation of an acute distal biceps tendon rupture are in patients who cannot tolerate a loss of supination strength. These patients are counseled on the risks and benefits of operative treatment, which include but are not limited to infection, nerve damage, wound breakdown, stiffness, heterotopic ossification, and continued pain. The pre-, intra-, and postoperative course is explained in detail to the patient. The timing of the procedure is also a factor. We do not urgently operate on these cases. With this procedure a safe single incision without the necessity of tendon graft or augmentation can be executed between 1 and 4 weeks. If the patient is outside of this time period, consent and the operative plan should include the potential for tendon graft or augmentation.

■ SURGICAL TECHNIQUE

Anesthesia

The surgical technique to restore the distal biceps does not present any unique problems for the anesthesiologist. We prefer laryngeal mask airway (LMA) as it provides excellent coverage without having the incidence of nausea and vomiting associated with general endotracheal anesthesia. Due to our concern for the neurovascular structures, we prefer to place a nerve block for postoperative pain control after the procedure and after the first postoperative neurovascular examination. This is generally an outpatient procedure, and the patient is sent home to recover after initial stabilization.

Approaches

Two main approaches to the operative procedure exist: The two-incision (modified Boyd-Anderson) and one incision volar approach. Most fixation techniques can be used for each of the approaches described without difficulty.

Modified Boyd-Anderson Approach (Azar Technique)

The Boyd-Anderson surgical approach has been described multiple times in the literature.[1,2] A transverse 3- to 4-cm incision is made over the anterior aspect of the elbow along the flexion crease. The deep fascia is incised, with care taken to identify and protect the lateral antebrachial cutaneous nerve, which lies lateral to the distal biceps tendon. Usually, it is retracted 5 to 7.5 cm proximal to the elbow. A heavy no. 5 or no. 2 nonabsorbable suture is passed through the tendon so that its

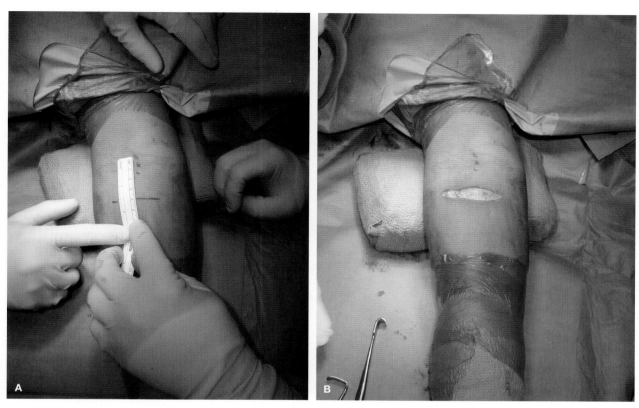

Fig. 25-1. A: Placement of longitudinal or horizontal incision starting 3 cm distal to the skin crease at the antecubital fossa. **B:** Example of horizontal incision.

ends emerge on the avulsed surface. Then a curved Kelly clamp is used to locate the tunnel between the radius and ulna through which the tendon originally passed, taking care not to violate the ulnar periosteum. The elbow is flexed and a second incision is made on the posterolateral aspect of the elbow for the Boyd approach. The interval is developed between the lateral border of the ulna and the anconeus and extensor carpi ulnaris. The anconeus is stripped from the bone subperiosteally. The dissection is deepened to the interosseous membrane, and the supinator muscle overlying the radial head is sharply incised, exposing the radial head. Pronation of the forearm protects the deep branch of the radial nerve as it enters the forearm in the substance of the supinator muscle and brings the radial tuberosity into view. A 0.25-inch osteotome or small bur is used to create a trough in the radial tuberosity and two to three holes are drilled in the margin. With a curved Kelly clamp, the ends of the sutures in the tendon are passed between the radius and ulnar and are brought out through the second incision. Traction on the sutures will advance the tendon into the posterolateral incision. The ends of the sutures are brought out through the holes in the tuberosity and, with the elbow flexed, are securely tied over the bony bridge between the holes. Reinforcing sutures can be placed through the tendon into the adjacent soft tissues if necessary. The two incisions are closed in routine fash-

ion and the elbow is immobilized in a posterior plaster splint with the elbow flexed to 100 degrees and the forearm supinated 45 degrees.

Volar Single Incision Approach

With the volar single incision approach the patient is positioned supine on the operating room table with all anatomical protuberances padded. The arm is placed on a padded arm board with a tourniquet placed as close to the axilla as possible to allow room for an extensile approach if needed. If this is impossible secondary to patient habitus, then a sterile tourniquet is used.

The incision can be horizontally placed 3 to 4 cm distal to the skin crease at the antecubital fossa (better cosmesis) **(Fig. 25-1A)**. The incision can also be placed in a longitudinal fashion (Fig. 25-1B). This approach is a modification of an anterior longitudinal Henry approach with extension along the antecubital fossa if needed. The subcuticular tissue is dissected with Metzenbaum scissors to avoid injury to the lateral antebrachial cutaneous. The plane of the dissection should be in the direction of the incision, which also parallels the superficial sensory nerve **(Fig. 25-2A)**.

The muscular interval between the pronator teres and brachioradialis is bluntly developed to the level of the lacertus fibrosis and surrounding hematoma or scar. Directly in the plane of the dissection lies a series of veins (Leash of

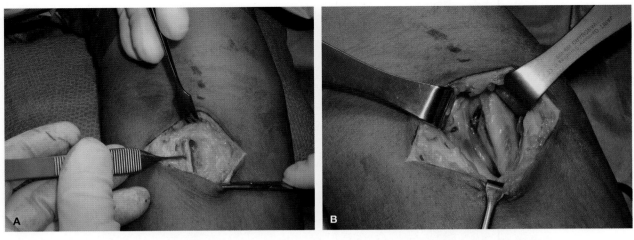

Fig. 25-2. A: The lateral antebrachial cutaneous nerve found in the muscular interval between the brachioradialis and pronator teres. **B:** Special attention is given to the deep venous plexus deeper (Leash of Henry).

Henry) (Fig. 25-2B) and the recurrent branch of the radial artery, which must be addressed by suture ligature, coagulation, or retraction. The frayed edge of the tendon should be found at this level or proximally.

Preparation of the Distal Biceps Tendon

Anatomical evaluation has revealed that the distal biceps tendon attaches on the ulnar side of the tuberosity in a 2 mm by 14 mm ribbonlike configuration after rotating 90 degrees from the musculotendinous junction **(Fig. 25-3)**. Depending on the chronicity of the tear, the biceps tendon is usually retracted from the tuberosity with a bulbous end. The tendon is then measured and trimmed to an 8-mm thickness. If the tendon end is frayed with degenerated collagen, up to 1 cm can be resected from the end with no ill effects.

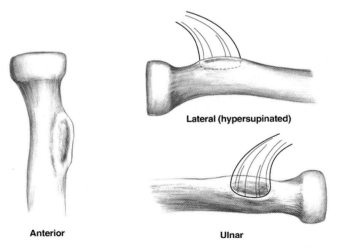

Lateral (hypersupinated)

Anterior   **Ulnar**

Fig. 25-3. Example of the ribbonlike native structure of the distal biceps tendon inserting on the ulnar side of the tuberosity.

Two no. 2 FiberWire (Arthrex, Inc., Naples, Fla) sutures are then placed in the distal tendon (Krackow or whipstitch fashion) **(Fig. 25-4A)**. The first suture is started 12 mm proximal to the end of the tendon, travels distally, then returns proximally after securing the EndoButton, 2 to 3 mm from the distal stump of the tendon (Fig. 25-4B). The tails of this suture are cut. The second suture then starts distally, captures the EndoButton, travels proximally 12 mm, then returns distally (Fig. 25-4C). One end of this suture should be left long and the other short. The long "tail" will be placed through the cannulated portion of the interference screw and will be tied to the short "tail" after insertion (Fig. 25-4D,E). The FiberWire suture has a Kevlar core, allowing it to have the strength of a no. 5 nonabsorbable braided suture but the size of a no. 2. This strength and durability is critical when using the Arthrex Biotenodesis driver (Arthrex, Inc, Naples, Fla), as the metal end can damage and prematurely cut standard braided suture. The remaining outside two holes in the EndoButton are then loaded with two different colors no. 2 FiberWire sutures (Fig. 25-4F). These will be used to pass the EndoButton through the distal cortex.

Bicipital Tuberosity Preparation

The arm is placed in maximal supination and extension to adequately visualize the tuberosity. It is important to visualize the entire tuberosity. The tunnel can be occasionally placed too proximal when using the two-incision approach and looking for the ridge. Care should be taken with the deep tissues not to retract too vigorously on the radial side of the proximal radius as the posterior interosseous nerve can be damaged. The tuberosity is generally covered with a fibrous layer of immature scar. This should be removed for visualization. A Beath pin with an eyelet is placed into the center of the tuberosity and drilled through both cortices.

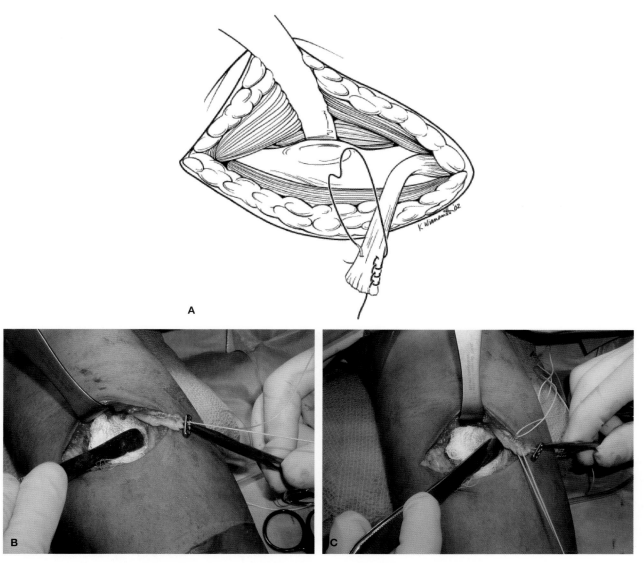

Fig. 25-4. A: Placement of nonabsorbable FiberWire in a Krackow/whipstitch configuration in the distal biceps tendon. **B:** Attachment of EndoButton (Smith and Nephew) to distal biceps tendon. **C:** Second no. 2 FiberWire placed distally at first.

First, an 8-mm cannulated reamer (Arthrex, Inc, Naples, Fla) is used to prepare an 8-mm tunnel through the proximal cortex only (12 to 15 mm) **(Fig. 25-5A)**. A 4.5 cannulated reamer is then used to drill though the distal cortex. Care must be used not to continue reaming after penetrating the cortex, as damage to the dorsal soft tissues may occur. Copious irrigation is used to remove all bone reamings and fragments. The two sutures placed onto the lateral holes of the EndoButton (traction sutures) are then placed into the eyelet of the Beath pin (Fig. 25-5B). The arm is flexed and the Beath pin is pushed through the soft tissue, penetrating the dorsal skin. This pin is placed as ulnarly as possible to avoid damage to the neurovascular structures. One of the sutures is pulled until the EndoButton passes

the distal cortex, the second suture is the toggled, and the EndoButton is deployed **(Fig. 25-6A)**. A portable radiographic image is obtained (mini C-arm) to confirm that the EndoButton is deployed and that there is no intervening soft tissue in the way (Fig. 25-6C,D).

Tenodesis

The tenodesis driver consists of a cannulated handle and post. Sutures from the end of the prepared tendon can be passed through the driver after the chosen screw has been placed onto the driver. The post is used to insert the tendon into the bottom of the socket and hold the tendon in place while the interference screw is advanced over it via a

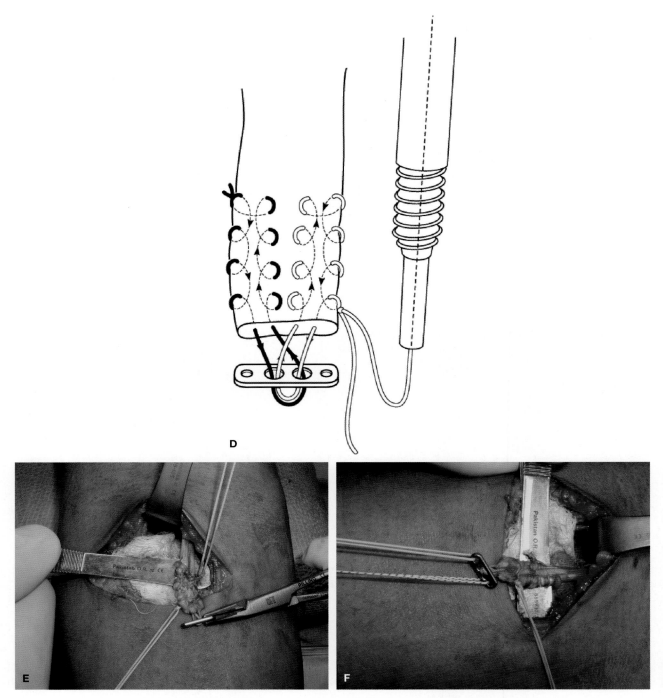

D

E

F

Fig. 25-4. (*Continued*) **D,E:** Orientation of suture, EndoButton, and interference screw. **F:** Final suture and EndoButton configuration with passing sutures placed in the outside holes of the EndoButton.

threaded mechanism (Fig. 25-6B). To perform the tenodesis, one limb of the FiberWire suture is then placed through the tenodesis driver with the 8-mm by 12-mm screw attached (Fig. 25-6D). The driver is then inserted into the 8-mm hole, making sure that the tendon is on the ulnar side of the tuberosity **(Fig. 25-7A)**. While the tendon is stabilized with an Addison forceps, the screw is advanced via the tenodesis driver as described above (Fig. 25-7B). After the screw is inserted and the tenodesis driver is removed, the suture passing through the cannulated screw is tied to the outside of the interference screw. This allows an interference fit of the tendon to bone in addition to a suture anchor effect **(Fig. 25-8)**. Three modes of fixation now exist (interference fit, EndoButton, and suture anchorlike fixation) that allow this method to have superior strength and cyclic load characteristics.

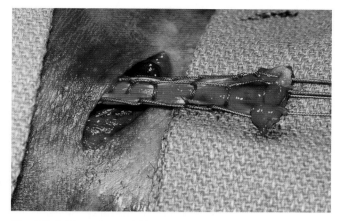

Fig. 26-4. The retracted biceps tendon is milked into the field. Two Bunnell sutures or a Krackow lock stitch are placed in the end of the tendon. (With permission, Mayo Foundation.)

pronated. The ulna is never exposed **(Fig. 26-6)**.[34] A high-speed bur is used to evacuate a 1.5-cm wide and 1-cm deep defect in the radial tuberosity **(Fig. 26-7)**. Three holes 7 to 8 mm apart and at least 5 mm from the edge of the excavation are then placed. The tendon is delivered through the second incision and the sutures are placed through the holes in the tuberosity. The tendon is carefully introduced into the excavation formed in the tuberosity and, with the forearm in the neutral position, the sutures are pulled tight and secured. The wounds are closed in layers with a suction drain inserted in the depths of the wound both anteriorly and posteriorly. The elbow is placed in 90 degrees of flexion with forearm rotation between neutral and supination. A compressive dressing is applied.

Late Reconstruction

The individual needs of the patient and the goals of any late surgical procedure must be carefully balanced. If the patient's

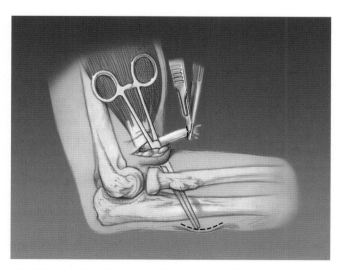

Fig. 26-5. A blunt instrument is introduced in the tract of the biceps tendon, and the skin is indented on the volar aspect of the proximal forearm. An incision is made over this instrument. (With permission, Mayo Foundation.)

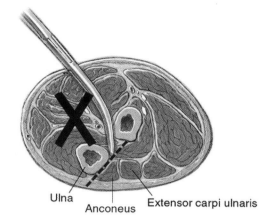

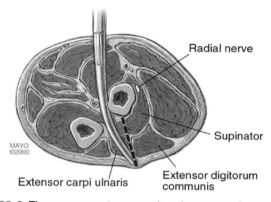

Fig. 26-6. The common extensor and supinator muscles are then split to expose the radial tuberosity. The ulna is not exposed. Full pronation of the forearm brings the tuberosity into the field. (With permission, Mayo Foundation.)

occupation and residual strength do not require improvement of supination endurance, simple reinsertion into the brachialis muscle is performed. While rarely indicated, this surgical procedure is easy, improves flexion strength, and is essentially free of complications. Postoperative rehabilitation is similar to that previously described except that no limitation is placed on pronation and supination in the early postoperative course.

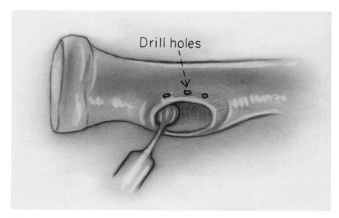

Fig. 26-7. The radial tuberosity is excavated using a high-speed bur. Osseous bridges of 5 to 7 mm from the edge and 7 mm between the holes is ideal. (With permission, Mayo Foundation.)

If, after careful discussion with the patient, improved supination strength is found to be required, several reconstructions have been reported. A fascia lata graft has been described by Hovelius and Josefsson.[22] Others have used a free autogenous semitendinous tendon. If the tendon is retracted and shortened, which is typical, some form of breech augmentation is required. Although we experienced very favorable results, we have abandoned the Ligament Augmentation Device (LAD) in favor of an autologous Achilles tendon graft **(Fig. 26-8)**. This is a very satisfying tissue ideally suited for this reconstruction. The fleck of calcaneus bone is trimmed and embedded into excavated radial tuberosity or it is excised. Then with the elbow flexed to 45 to 60 degrees the Achilles fascia is draped over the biceps muscle and the tendon stump is sewn into the muscle. This offers a very gratifying reconstruction allowing a more aggressive rehabilitation program.

Partial (Incomplete) Distal Biceps Rupture

Partial rupture of the distal biceps tendon is increasingly being recognized. Nielsen[35] documented a case in which the lacertus fibrosus was thought to have initially ruptured with a secondary elongation of the biceps tendon. Chevallier[21] reported an event of first a biceps tendon rupture with secondary stretch of the lacertus fibrosus. My experience suggests that first, a partial rupture of the biceps tendon occurs and the second episode of pain completes the rupture. Later, a secondary stretch or disruption of the lacertus fibrosis may occur.

Diagnosis of partial or impending rupture of the biceps tendon is not easy. The history of forced eccentric contracture is typical, and overuse may have preceded this event. Pain subsides but does not completely abate. Weakness and fatigue are prominent, and crepitus with forearm rotation is common. Distinction from bicipital tubercle bursitis may be difficult, especially because the two conditions can coexist. One of the two patients with cubital bursitis reported by

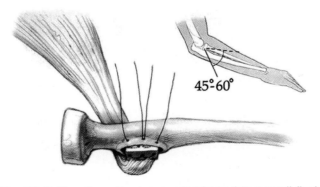

Fig. 26-8. The allograft calcaneus is trimmed to a small fleck measuring 1.3 by 0.8 cm and containing the Achilles tendon allograft attachment. The calcaneus bone is embedded into the excavated tuberosity. Sutures are placed through the tendon and bone and secured to the tuberosity. With the elbow flexed 40 to 60 degrees the flare of the tendon fascia is secured to the biceps with a Bunnell stitch in the tendon remnant if it exists. (With permission, Mayo Foundation.)

Karanjia and Stiles[23] was a woman. She was noted at surgery to have distal biceps tendon degeneration in association with the bursitis. It is possible that the cubital bursitis was a reaction to the partial rupture.

The treatment of the partial tendon rupture may best be understood by considering the pathology of a degenerative tendon. Reimplantation of the remaining portion of the tendon to the radial tuberosity does not reliably relieve pain.[36] Complete removal of the remaining fibers, converting the problem to a complete tear, trimming of the distal tendon, and then reattachment as if this were an acute event is the treatment of choice. Since the tendon is only partially detached, we perform this procedure through the dorsal incision of the two-incision technique. The anterior exposure is not usually necessary.

Technical Alternatives

Because of concern over the development of ectopic bone associated with the two-incision technique and with the advent of suture anchors, the anterior exposure using these anchors is gaining in popularity. If the procedure is done promptly, the tract of the biceps tendon is still present and is easily identified. If performed late (more than 2 weeks after injury), this tract may be obliterated, making the exposure more difficult.[37]

We have no personal experience with these devices for this problem. The specific technique varies according to three variables: exposure, type of anchor used, and method of reattachment. The exposure is usually through a limited anterior approach. Usually two or three suture anchors are used most often directly into the unprepared tuberosity.

■ POSTOPERATIVE MANAGEMENT AND REHABILITATION

After surgery the patient is placed in a posterior splint for approximately 5 days with the elbow flexed to 80 degrees and the forearm in neutral rotation. Following this, for distal biceps tendon repairs, gentle assisted active motion is encouraged, allowing the elbow to resume a full arc of motion over the next 10 days. At about 2 weeks gentle active motion is allowed without weights, and functional activities are avoided with the operated extremity. At 3 to 4 weeks activities of daily living are allowed as tolerated. At 6 to 8 weeks muscle strengthening exercises are begun with 1 lb weight and progressing to 10 lb at 8 to 12 weeks. After 12 weeks activity as tolerated is allowed, and full activity without restriction is permitted 6 months after surgery.

For allograft reconstruction the time frame is doubled. Thus, strengthening exercises are begun after approximately 3 months, and full activity without restriction is allowed 1 year after surgery.

Results

Excellent results are expected with surgical management of the acute rupture. Nontreated distal biceps rupture results in a loss of about 20% flexion and 40% supination strength.[17] Morrey et al.[17] conducted isometric strength assessment tests on seven patients at least 15 months after the two-incision technique. The strength restoration approached normal in flexion and supination. The objective measurements of restoration of normal strength has been reaffirmed using Cybex testing for not only strength but also endurance.[4] Nontreated distal biceps rupture results in a loss of about 20% flexion and 40% supination strength.[17]

Complications

Until recently, there were no individual reports specifically dealing with the complications of surgical treatment for distal biceps tendon rupture in the English literature. Transient radial nerve palsy with reattachment to the tuberosity has been[16,38] and continues to be occasionally noted.[10,32] As mentioned, the use of suture anchors has become of interest to prevent injury to the nerve.

The possibility of ectopic bone formation after the two-incision approach is well known. We have not had a complete osseous bridge at Mayo after 73 surgical procedures performed in the acute or subacute period. The possibility of this complication continues to exist, even after anterior approaches with suture anchors **(Fig. 26-9)**. If the two-incision technique is used, it must be emphasized that the tuberosity is exposed by a muscle splitting approach and the ulna is never visualized (Fig. 26-6).

The Mayo experience with 73 procedures was recently reported by Kelly et al.[39] Of these 73 cases, 70% were treated as described above and four had a minimal amount of ectopic bone or calcification localized in the tendon in one but did not limit motion. One patient had rerupture, one a transient radial nerve palsy, and three lost forearm rotation of 20, 30, and 20 degrees respectively. Of the nine treated with an anterior exposure and secured to the tuberosity, two had transient paresthesias of the radial nerve and one developed

a small amount of ectopic bone with no consequences on motion.

If an osseous bridge does develop, successful resection can be undertaken about 8 to 9 months after the initial surgery.[40] Some cases of extensive involvement of the interosseous space as well as site of attachment pose rather significant challenges of treatment (Fig. 26-9). In some instances the biceps repair can be intimately associated with the ectopic bone. Removing the osseous bar resulted in detachment of the biceps tendon, which then required reattachment into the tuberosity. A good result may be anticipated, but the rehabilitation must begin anew. If a bridge is excised, irradiation with 700 centigray (cGy) may be administered, but in my practice there is little tendency for recurrence of the ectopic bone.

■ REFERENCES

1. Johnson AB. Avulsion of biceps tendon from the radius. NY Med J. 1897;66:261–262.
2. Acquaviva M. Rupture du tendon inférieur du biceps brachial droit à son insertion sur la tubérosité bicipitale: Tenosuture succès opératoire. Marseilles Med. 1898;35:570–576.
3. Giugiaro A, Proscia N. Le rotture del tendine distale e del tendine del capo breve del bicipite brachiale. Minerva Ort. 1957;8(3):57–65.
4. Agins HJ, Chess JL, Hoekstra DV, et al. Rupture of the distal insertion of the biceps brachii tendon. Clin Orthop. 1988;234:34-38.
5. Baker BE, Bierwagen D. Rupture of the distal tendon of the biceps brachii. J Bone Joint Surg. 1985;67A:414–417.
6. Bourne MH, Morrey BF. Partial rupture of the distal biceps tendon. Clin Orthop. 1981;291:143–148.
7. Hang DW, Bach BR Jr, Bojchuk J. Repair of chronic distal biceps brachii tendon rupture using free autogenous semitendinosus tendon. Clin Orthop. 1996;(323):188–191.
8. Leighton MM, Bush-Joseph CA, Bach BR Jr. Distal biceps brachii repair: results of dominant and nondominant extremities. Clin Orthop. 1995;(317):114–121.
9. Le Huec JC, Moinard M, Liquois F, et al. Distal rupture of the tendon of biceps brachii: evaluation by MRI and the results of repair. J Bone Joint Surg. 1996;78B(5):767–770.
10. Louis DS, Hankin FM, Eckenrode JF, et al. Distal biceps brachii tendon avulsion: a simplified method of operative repair. Am J Sports Med. 1986;14:234–236.
11. Straugh RJ, Michelson H, Rosenwasser MP. Repair of rupture of the distal tendon of the biceps brachii: review of the literature and report of three cases treated with a single anterior incision and suture anchors. Am J Orthop. 1997;26(2):151–156.
12. McReynolds IS. Avulsion of the insertion of the biceps brachii tendon and its surgical treatment. J Bone Joint Surg. 1963;45A:1780–1781.
13. Bauman GI. Rupture of the biceps tendon. J Bone Joint Surg. 1934;16:966–967.
14. Postacchini F, Puddu G. Subcutaneous rupture of the distal biceps brachii tendon. J Sports Med. 1975;15(2):81–90.
15. Baker BE. Operative vs. nonoperative treatments of disruption of the distal tendon of biceps. Orthop Rev. 1982;11:71–74.
16. Dobbie RP. Avulsion of the lower biceps brachii tendon: analysis of fifty-one previously reported cases. Am J Surg. 1941;51:662–683.
17. Morrey BF, Askew LJ, An KH, et al. Rupture of the distal biceps tendon: biomechanical assessment of different treatment options. J Bone Joint Surg. 1985;67A:418–421.

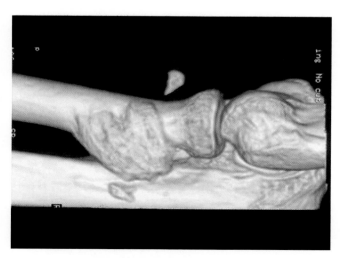

Fig. 26-9. Moderately extensive ectopic bone after the two-incision technique. (With permission, Mayo Foundation.)

18. Bennett BS. Triceps tendon rupture. J Bone Joint Surg. 1962;44A(4):741–744.

19. Davis WM, Yassine Z. An etiologic factor in the tear of the distal tendon of the biceps brachii. J Bone Joint Surg. 1956;38A(6):1365–1368.

20. Debeyre J. Desinsertion du tendon inferieur du biceps brachial. Mem Acad Chir. 1947;74:339–340.

21. Chevallier CH. Sur un gas de desinsertion du tendon bicipital inferieur. Mem Acad Chir. 1953;79:137–139.

22. Hovelius L, Josefsson G. Rupture of the distal biceps tendon. Acta Orthop Scand. 1977;48:280–282.

23. Karanjia ND, Stiles PJ. Cubital bursitis. J Bone Joint Surg. 1988;70B:832-833.

24. Cirincione RJ, Baker BE. Tendon ruptures with secondary hyperparathyroidism: a case report. J Bone Joint Surg. 1975;57A:852–853.

25. Preston FS, Adicoff A. Hyperparathyroidism with avulsion at three major tendons. N Engl J Med. 1961;266(19):968–971.

26. Murphy KJ, McPhee I. Tears of major tendons in chronic acidosis with elastosis. J Bone Joint Surg. 1965;47A(6):1253–1258.

27. Wener JA, Schein AJ. Simultaneous bilateral rupture of the patello tendon and quadriceps expansions in systemic lupus erythematosus: a case report. J Bone Joint Surg. 1974;56A(4):823–824.

28. Seiler JG III, Parker LM, Chamberland PD, et al. The distal biceps tendon: two potential mechanisms involved in its rupture: arterial supply and mechanical impingement. J Shoulder Elbow Surg. 1995;4(3):149–156.

29. Jaslow IA, May VR. Avulsion of the distal tendon of the biceps brachii muscle. Guthrie Clin Bull. 1946;15:124.

30. Lee HG. Traumatic avulsion of tendon of insertion of biceps brachii. Am J Surg. 1951;82:290–292.

31. Platt H. Observations of some tendon ruptures. Br Med J. 1931;1:611.

32. Norman WH. Repair of avulsion of insertion of biceps brachii tendon. Clin Orthop. 1985 Mar;(193):189–194.

33. Boyd HB, Anderson MD. A method for reinsertion of the distal biceps brachii tendon. J Bone Joint Surg. 1961;43A(7):1041–1043.

34. Failla JM, Amadio PC, Morrey BF, et al. Proximal radioulnar synostosis after repair of distal biceps brachii rupture by the two incision technique: report of four cases. Clin Orthop. 1990;253:133–136.

35. Nielsen K. Partial rupture of the distal biceps brachii tendon: a case report. Acta Orthop Scand. 1987;58(3):287–288.

36. Conwell HE, Alldredge RH. Ruptures and tears of muscles and tendons. Am J. Surg. 1937;35(1):22–33.

37. Hook FR, Mazet R Jr. Avulsion of the biceps tendon from its radial insertion. US Nav Med Bull. 1942;40(2):409–411.

38. Meherin J, Kilgore BS Jr. The treatment of rupture of the distal biceps brachii tendon. Am J Surg. 1960;99:636–638.

39. Kelly EW, Morrey BF, O'Driscoll SW. Complications of repair of the distal biceps tendon with the modified two-incision technique. J Bone Joint Surg Am. 2000 Nov;82(11):1575–1581.

40. Failla JM, Amadio PC, Morrey BF. Posttraumatic proximal radioulnar synostosis: results of surgical treatment. J Bone Joint Surg. 1989;71A:1208–1213.

RUPTURE OF THE TRICEPS TENDON

BERNARD F. MORREY, MD

■ HISTORY OF THE TECHNIQUE

Rupture of the triceps tendon is rare.[1-3] Anzel et al.[4] reported that 85% of the 1,015 tendon injuries treated at the Mayo Clinic involved the upper extremity. Of this group of 856, only eight instances of triceps tendon injury were reported, and four of these were due to laceration. Since the first report of Partridge[5] in 1868, as of 2000, fewer than 50 instances have been recorded in the English literature.[6-9] Unlike ruptures of the distal biceps tendon, this may occur both in men and women with a female to male ratio of 2:3. The mean age of occurrence is about 33 years, but rupture has been observed in a broader spectrum of ages including children (aged seven) to adolescents in whom the olecranon physis has just closed,[10] to individuals in their eighties.[11]

Rupture of the triceps tendon may occur either spontaneously, after trauma, or after surgical release and reattachment. Two types of traumatic episodes may be implicated. The most common event is a deceleration force imparted to the arm during extension as the triceps muscle is contracting. This usually occurs during a fall, but avulsion has been reported due to simple, uncoordinated triceps muscle contraction against a flexing elbow.[12,13] The association of triceps tendon avulsion[14] or tear[7] associated with body builders is consistent with the observation of muscle unit damage associated with eccentric contractures in the unconditioned muscle.[15,16] The possibility of anabolic steroid usage must also be considered in this type patient. A direct blow to the posterior aspect of the triceps at its insertion in varying positions also has been reported in several instances[17-19] but is probably an uncommon mechanism of injury.

■ PREDISPOSING CONDITIONS

Triceps rupture is uncommon in body builders and is much less common than distal biceps rupture. Clayton[11] has suggested that olecranon bursitis may predispose to triceps tendon rupture. Disruption of the triceps also may occur spontaneously with minimal trauma in individuals who are compromised by a systemic disease process,[20] such as with renal osteodystrophy and secondary hyperparathyroidism.[21,22] Although the pathophysiology of this association has not been completely explained, an increased amount of elastic fibers in the tendons of patients with renal osteodystrophy undergoing dialysis has been reported.[23] Calcification due to the chronic hypercalcemia of secondary hyperparathyroidism may be yet another explanation for the associated tendon ruptures in this group of patients.[20] Ruptures also have been reported in association with steroid treatment for lupus erythematosus[19] and chronic acidosis,[23] in individuals with osteogenesis imperfecta tarda,[24] and with Marfan syndrome.[25] Diabetes has been recently implicated in a patient with triceps rupture at the musculotendinous junction.[26] Triceps deficiency occurring after total elbow replacement is obviously a problem of exposure, and repair and is discussed elsewhere.

■ INDICATIONS AND CONTRAINDICATIONS

The history is commonly that of a fall on the outstretched hand. Pain at the site of tendinous attachment is a consistent finding. A palpable defect is present in some instances, depending on the extent of triceps retraction. Injury to the muscular tendinous junction results in pain proximal to the olecranon.[6,8] Some loss of extension power is universally observed. Some active elbow extension may be present, but extension against gravity is not possible with a complete rupture.

Three sites of failure have been demonstrated experimentally as well as clinically: the muscle belly, the musculotendinous junction, and the osseous tendon insertion.[27] For this particular injury, the failure has occurred almost universally at the site of attachment to the olecranon, although failure at the musculotendinous junction has occasionally been reported.[26,28,29]

Associated injuries also have been reported. Several instances of concurrent fracture of the radial head have been noted,[20,30] and a recent report of six such injuries suggests that the association may be more common than is appreciated.[31] I have not diagnosed this combination in my practice. A single report of fracture of the wrist[32] along with fracture of the radial head supports the case for the mechanism of injury being a fall on the outstretched hand.

The diagnosis of a partial rupture may be difficult. Pain is not dysfunctional, thus, a number of patients present several weeks after the acute event.[33] Further, some weak residual extension power may be provided by the anconeus/triceps expansion. This effect can be negated by observing the inability to extend the arm overhead against gravity. The roentgenogram is of considerable benefit for diagnosis of this injury in some because flecks of avulsed bone are apparent on the lateral film.[34,35]

Partial tendon rupture can be treated nonoperatively according to some.[17,20,36] Special care must be taken, however, to be ensured that the injury is, in fact, a partial rupture, since a missed complete disruption can cause marked functional impairment. This results in reconstructive procedures that are less reliable than treatment of the acute injury.

Immediate surgery is the treatment of choice for complete rupture. At the time of exploration, the tendinous portion of the triceps is usually involved and retracted within the muscle.[20,32] However, complete disruption of the entire extension mechanism is uncommon as continuity laterally with the anconeus is usually maintained.

■ SURGICAL TECHNIQUE

Immediate repair with a posterior incision just lateral to the midline is the treatment of choice. No. 5 nonabsorbable suture is placed in Bunnell fashion in the torn tendon and then through crisscrossed holes in the proximal ulna **(Fig. 27-1)**. If the avulsion has occurred with a sufficiently large fleck of bone, however, reattachment with a screw and washer is an acceptable alternative.[10] Some have described concurrent reconstructive options, but this is not necessary in the acute, less than 2-week injury. If the lesion has been overlooked or treatment delayed by several weeks or months, one of the reconstructive procedures described below is carried out. I favor the anconeus slide for minimal tissue deficiency, and the allograft Achilles tendon for more extensive soft tissue deficiencies.

Several reconstructive procedures for delayed reconstruction have been reported for individual cases. Bennett[37] and Farrar and Lippert[34] describe a forearm fascial flap to reconstruct the triceps mechanism. The classic

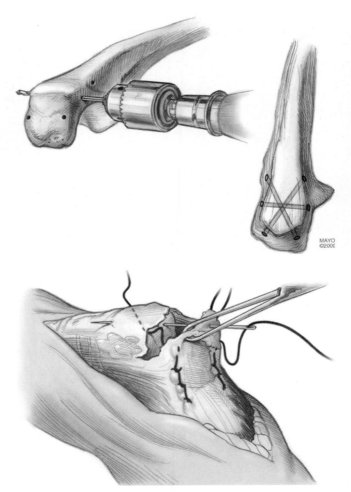

Fig. 27-1. For acute triceps tendon avulsion, no. 5 nonabsorbable suture is passed through the avulsed tendon in a crisscrossed pattern and into the olecranon through bone holes. (With permission from the Mayo Foundation.)

triceps fascial turndown procedure is not reliable in my opinion[11] for those with soft tissue deficiency at the point of attachment. To take full advantage of the lateral expansion, an anconeus slide has proven effective alone or in conjunction with repair. Finally, the allograft Achilles tendon has recently proven to be particularly attractive in those with marked deficiency. The fascial expansion can be used to securely envelope the triceps muscle, and the calcaneus can be trimmed and secured directly over the olecranon **(Fig. 27-2)**.

■ REHABILITATION

In all reconstructive options the construct is secured with the elbow flexed about 40 to 60 degrees. After surgery the arm is protected at 90 degrees for 3 weeks. Gentle active motion is begun. We have found that recovery, even for acute repair, is slow, possibly taking 6 months to gain 80 percent of normal strength.

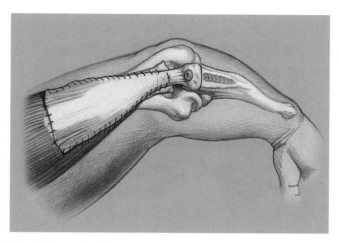

Fig. 27-2. An Achilles tendon allograft with calcaneal bone provides an ideal reconstructive unit. The calcaneus attachment is fashioned and screwed to the olecranon. With the elbow at 20 to 30 degrees flexion, the triceps is brought distally and the Achilles fascia is brought proximally and secured. The proximal aspect of the graft is secured with multiple no. 1 interrupted and running sutures.

■ RESULTS AND MAYO EXPERIENCE

The results of immediate or delayed repair have ultimately been universally good. In most instances, marked improvement in strength and full motion has been restored.

We have recently reviewed our experience at the Mayo Clinic with 15 triceps injuries treated in the period 1977–1997. Eleven (73%) occurred as a result of a fall. Only two had avulsed with a fleck of bone and five had avulsions that spared the lateral aspects of the attachment. All but two did well with various methods of repair. It was observed, however, that recovery requires at least 6 months.[30]

■ COMPLICATIONS AND RESIDUAL DEFICITS

Few complications have been reported other than delayed recovery, variable loss of extension strength, and olecranon bursitis.[38]

■ REFERENCES

1. Brickner WM, Milch H. Ruptures of muscles and tendons. Int Clin. 1928;2:94.
2. Haldeman KO, Soto-Hall R. Injuries to muscles and tendons. JAMA. 1935;104(26):2319–2324.
3. Platt H. Observations of some tendon ruptures. Br Med J. 1931;1:611–615.
4. Anzel SH, Covey KW, Weiner AD, Lipscomb R. Disruption of muscles and tendons: An analysis of 1,014 cases. Surgery 1959;45(3):406–414.
5. Partridge R. A case report of a case of ruptured triceps cubiti. Med Times Gaz. 1868;1:175.
6. Aso K, Torisu T. Muscle belly tear of the triceps. Am J Sports Med. 1984;12:485–487.
7. Herrick RT, Herrick S. Ruptured triceps in a powerlifter presenting as cubital tunnel syndrome: a case report. Am Sports Med. 1987;15(5):514–516.
8. O'Driscoll SW. Intramuscular triceps rupture. Can J Surg. 1992;35(2):203–206.
9. Searfoss R, Tripi J, Bowers W. Triceps brachii rupture: case report. J Trauma. 1976;16(3):244–246.
10. Viegas SF. Avulsion of the triceps tendon. Orthop Rev. 1990;19(6):533–536.
11. Clayton ML, Thirupathi RG. Rupture of the triceps tendon with olecranon bursitis: a case report with a new method of repair. Clin Orthop. 1984;184:183–185.
12. Bauman GI. Triceps tendon rupture. J Bone Joint Surg. 1934;16:966–967.
13. Maydl K. Ueber subcutane Muskel und Sehnenzerreissungen, sowie RissFracturen mit berucksichtigung der Analogen, durch directe gewalt Enstandenen und offenen Verletzungen. Deut Zschr Chir. 1883;17:306–361, 1883;18:35–139.
14. Sherman OH, Snyder SJ, Fox JM. Triceps tendon avulsion in a professional body builder: a case report. Am J Sports Med. 1984;12(4):328–329.
15. Louis DS, Peck D. Triceps avulsion fracture in a weightlifter. Orthopedics. 1992;15(2):207–211.
16. O'Reilly K, Worhal M, Meredith C, et al. Immediate and delayed ultrastructural changes in skeletal muscle following eccentric exercise. Med Sci Sports Exerc. 1986;18(suppl):S42.
17. Anderson KJ, LeCoco JF. Rupture of the triceps tendon. J Bone Joint Surg. 1957;39A(2):444–446.
18. Penhallow DP. Report of a case of ruptured triceps due to direct violence. NY Med J. 1910;91:76–77.
19. Wener JA, Schein AJ. Simultaneous bilateral rupture of the patello tendon and quadriceps expansions in systemic lupus erythematosus: a case report. J Bone Joint Surg. 1974;56A(4):823–824.
20. Preston FS, Adicoff A. Hyperparathyroidism with avulsion at three major tendons. N Engl J Med. 1961;266(19):968–971.
21. Cirincione RJ, Baker BE. Tendon ruptures with secondary hyperparathyroidism: a case report. J Bone Joint Surg. 1975;57A(6):852–853.
22. Fery A, Sommelet J, Schmitt D, et al. Avulsion bilaterale simultanee des tendons quadricipital et rotulien et rupture du tendon tricipital chez un hemodialyse hyperparathyroidien. Rev Chir Orthop. 1978;64(2):175–181.
23. Murphy KJ, McPhee I. Tears of major tendons in chronic acidosis with elastosis. J Bone Joint Surg. 1965;47A:1253–1258.
24. Match RM, Corrylos EV. Bilateral avulsion fracture of the triceps tendon insertion from skiing with osteogenesis imperfecta tarda. Am J Sports Med. 1983;11(2):99–102.
25. Schutt RC, Powell RL, Winter WG. Spontaneous ruptures of large tendons. Paper presented at: American Academy of Orthopedic Surgeons Annual Meeting; January 25, 1982; New Orleans.
26. Wagner JR, Cooney WP. Rupture of the triceps muscle at the musculotendinous junction: a case report. J Hand Surg. 1997;22A(2):341–343.
27. McMaster PE. Tendon and muscle ruptures: clinical and experimental studies on causes and locations of subcutaneous ruptures. J Bone Joint Surg. 1933;15:705–722.
28. Gilcreest EL. Rupture of muscles and tendons. JAMA. 1925;84(24):1819–1822.
29. Montgomery AH. Two cases of muscle injury. Surg Clin (Chicago). 1920;4(4):871–877.
30. Van Riet RP, Morrey BF, Ho E, et al. Surgical treatment of distal triceps rupture. J Bone Joint Surg. 2003;85A(10):1961–1967.
31. Levy M, Fishel RE, Stern GM. Triceps tendon avulsion with or without fracture of the radial head: a rare injury? J Trauma. 1978;18(9):677–679.
32. Lee MLH. Rupture of triceps tendon. Br Med J. 1960;2:197.

33. Inhofe PD, Moneim MS. Late presentation of triceps rupture: a case report and review of the literature. Am J Ortho. 1996;25(11):790–792.

34. Farrar EL III, Lippert FG III. Avulsion of the triceps tendon. Clin Orthop. 1981;161:242–246.

35. Tarsney FF. Rupture and avulsion of the triceps. Clin Orthop. 1972;83:177–183.

36. Debeyre J. Desinsertion du tendon inferieur du biceps brachial. Mem Acad Chir. 1948;74:339–340.

37. Bennett BS. Triceps tendon rupture. J Bone Joint Surg. 1962;44A (4):741–744.

38. Pantazopoulos T, Exarchou E, Stavrou Z, et al. Avulsion of the triceps tendon. J Trauma. 1975;15(9):827–829.

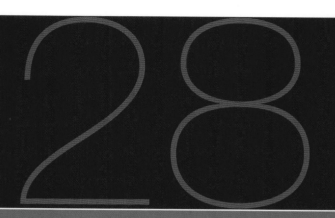

MEDIAL AND LATERAL EPICONDYLITIS: OPEN TREATMENT

USHA S. MANI, MD, ADRIENNE J. TOWSEN, MD, MICHAEL G. CICCOTTI, MD

■ HISTORY OF THE TECHNIQUE

Epicondylitis is one of the most common conditions to affect the elbow in adults. The term epicondylitis does not accurately reflect the disease process, which histologically involves tendon degeneration and an incomplete reparative process rather than inflammatory changes. The term tendinosis is more appropriate when describing this disorder.[1]

The majority of literature available on epicondylitis strongly supports nonsurgical treatment. Greater than 90% of patients with either medial or lateral disease will improve with conservative measures such as anti-inflammatory medications, activity modification, counterforce bracing, local corticosteroid injections, and physical therapy modalities. The small percentage of patients who do not respond to a focused nonsurgical treatment program become candidates for surgical treatment.[1-3]

Historically, a multitude of procedures have been proposed over the past 75 years for the treatment of refractory epicondylitis. Lateral epicondylitis has received the majority of that focus. In 1927, Hohmann described release of the common extensor origin at the lateral epicondyle.[4] Since then, there have been modifications of this original description, as well as alternative procedures put forth in the literature. Release of the extensor origin with or without release of the annular ligament, percutaneous release of the common extensor origin, lengthening of the distal extensor carpi radialis brevis tendon, arthroscopic debridement of the tendon, and, most recently, the use of radiofrequency probes through a limited exposure are all documented ways of surgically handling this problem.[5,6] There has been less literature devoted to medial epicondylitis; however, it is generally agreed that the same surgical principles used on the lateral side apply to the medial side.

Currently, the most widely used open procedure both laterally and medially involves the general principles of exposing

the tendon, excising the pathologic portion, repairing the resultant defect, and reattaching any elevated tendon origin back to the epicondyle. In this chapter we will describe the technique in detail from indications to intraoperative pearls and pitfalls to postoperative rehabilitation and finally outcomes and future directions.

■ INDICATIONS AND CONTRAINDICATIONS

As previously mentioned, the majority of patients with epicondylitis about the elbow do not require surgical management. When evaluating a patient for either medial or lateral elbow pain, it is imperative to rule out other problems that may produce symptoms similar to epicondylitis. The differential diagnosis of lateral epicondylitis most commonly includes posterior interosseous nerve entrapment, radiocapitellar joint disease, including arthrosis and osteochondritis dessicans, and radiculopathy due to cervical spine disease. Primary ulnar neuropathy and ulnar collateral ligament pathology are other etiologies for medial elbow symptoms that can mimic medial epicondylitis. Once diagnosed with medial or lateral epicondylitis, a supervised course of nonoperative treatment should be carried out for a minimum of 3 to 6 months.[1,7]

Nonoperative treatment begins with activity modification. It is often necessary to completely refrain from the offending activity for a short period of time. It is also beneficial to examine technique and equipment use, especially with racket sports. Possible alterations in one or both of these areas may prevent recurrent episodes of epicondylitis. Although the disease process is more of a tendinosis and not a tendonitis, a 2- to 4-week course of anti-inflammatory medication is effective in many patients for the concomitant synovitis. If there has been night pain or no response to anti-inflammatories,

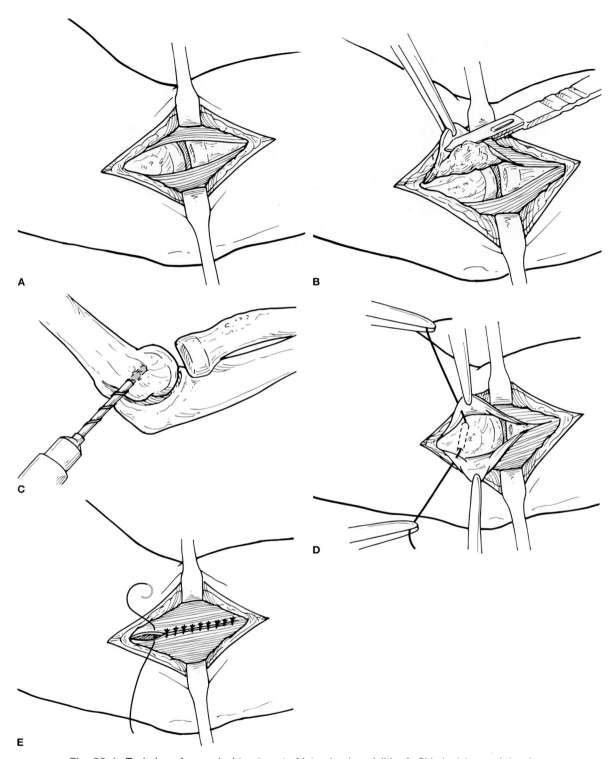

Fig. 28-1. Technique for surgical treatment of lateral epicondylitis. **A:** Skin incision and development of extensor interval. **B:** Excision of pathologic tissue. **C:** Drilling of lateral epicondylar bone tunnel. **D:** Reattachment of extensor origin to lateral epicondyle. **E:** Side-to-side repair of extensor origin. (Modified from Ciccotti MG, Lombardo SJ. Lateral and medial epicondylitis. In Jobe FW, ed. *Operative Techniques in Upper Extremity Injuries in Sports*. St. Louis, MO: CV Mosby; 1996: 431–446.)

then a cortisone injection may also be provided. The use of ice and counterforce braces may also be helpful as part of the treatment regimen. Patients are initiated on a course of physical therapy for flexibility and strengthening. Modalities such as ultrasound, iontophoresis, or electrical stimulation can provide added benefit.[2,8]

If a patient has had all other possible etiologies ruled out and exhibits persistent symptoms that interfere with activities of daily living or optimal athletic performance, in spite of such a focused nonsurgical program for 3 to 4 months, then surgery should be considered. Those patients who have structural injury such as clinically or radiographically identified tearing or detachment of the extensor or flexor-pronator origins may require surgery sooner.

■ SURGICAL TECHNIQUES

Our preferred open surgical treatment for lateral and medial epicondylitis involves the same general principles of removing degenerative tendon, providing an environment for healing tissue, and restoring the tendon origin anatomically.

Lateral Epicondylitis

The choice of anesthetic varies from patient to patient; however, if the patient's medical history allows, general anesthesia is utilized. The use of regional anesthesia may not allow a thorough postoperative neurologic check. The patient is positioned supine with the arm on an arm board or hand table. A tourniquet is applied to the upper arm as high as possible. The arm is draped freely in a standard sterile fashion.

A 5- to 7-cm curvilinear incision is made, just anterior to the lateral epicondyle (Fig. 28-1A,B,C,D). There should be equal exposure proximal and distal to the level of the epicondyle. Anterior and posterior subcutaneous flaps are then sharply developed. Care should be taken to avoid branches of the lateral antebrachial cutaneous nerve.

The common extensor origin is then completely delineated. The interval between the extensor carpi radialis longus and the extensor digitorum communis is developed to expose the extensor carpi radialis brevis tendon. The origin of this tendon is split longitudinally so that the area of pathology can be identified. The diseased portion of the tendon is sharply debrided. A rongeur is used to roughen the surface of the lateral epicondyle, thereby creating a bleeding bed. Care should be taken not to excise too much bone. At this time a firm reattachment of the extensor carpi radialis brevis tendon is performed. A 5/64-inch drill bit is used to create a V-shaped tunnel, drilled perpendicular to the long axis of the extended arm. A heavy suture is passed through the posterior margin of the extensor tendon, through the bony tunnel from posterior to anterior, and finally through the anterior margin of the tendon. The remainder of the tendon is reapproximated with absorbable stitches. The subcutaneous tissue is then closed in a standard fashion, and a running subcuticular

stitch is used in the skin. A soft dressing is placed on the elbow, followed by a posterior splint with the elbow at 90 degrees and the forearm and wrist in neutral.[3,9,10]

Medial Epicondylitis

The anesthesia and positioning is the same for medial epicondylitis as previously described for lateral epicondylitis. The concern with regional anesthesia is greater on the medial side considering the close proximity of the ulnar nerve to the operative field.

A 5- to 7-cm oblique incision is made centered just anterior to the medial epicondyle (Fig. 28-2A,B,C). Anterior and posterior flaps are created bluntly, being careful to avoid the medial antebrachial cutaneous nerve. The common flexor origin is identified. The ulnar nerve may not need to be seen; however, care should be taken to identify its position just posterior to the epicondyle, and it must be protected. Concurrent ulnar nerve or ulnar collateral ligament pathology should be addressed and managed appropriately if symptoms are present. The pronator teres flexor carpi radialis interval is incised. This can be developed either longitudinally or transversely depending on the location of pathologic tissue. Usually the abnormal tissue is fairly focal, lending itself to a longitudinal split. The degenerated tissue is sharply excised. The ulnar collateral ligament lies just deep to the flexor-pronator mass. Care must be taken not to violate this ligament. It should also be inspected for any abnormalities.

A rongeur is used to prepare the medial epicondyle by removing any remaining fibrous tissue and creating a bleeding surface. Multiple small drill holes can be made in the epicondyle to aid in this process. A V-shaped bone tunnel is created as described above for lateral epicondylitis, perpendicular to the longitudinal axis of the humerus. The tendon is reattached in the same fashion as on the lateral side with a stitch through the posterior portion of the tendon, through the tunnel from posterior to anterior, and then through the anterior portion of the tendon. The remainder of the interval is closed with absorbable stitches. The subcutaneous tissue is closed with absorbable suture, and a subcuticular closure completes the case. A standard dressing is placed over the wound followed by a well-padded posterior plaster splint with the elbow at 90 degrees and the forearm and wrist neutral.[10-12]

■ REHABILITATION AND RETURN TO SPORTS

The postoperative rehabilitation for both lateral and medial epicondylitis follows the same general protocol. The plaster splint is removed at 7 to 10 days after surgery. Progressive elbow range of motion is initiated at that point. Gentle passive and active range of motion of the elbow, wrist, and hand is the primary focus of a supervised therapy program during

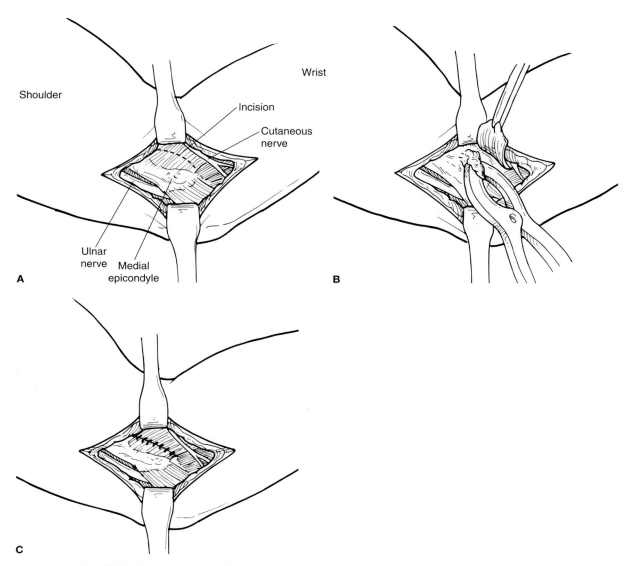

Fig. 28-2. Technique for surgical treatment of medial epicondylitis. **A:** Skin incision and intended incision of common flexor-pronator origin. **B:** Distal reflection of common flexor-pronator origin with debridement of pathologic tissue. **C:** Reattachment of common flexor-pronator origin to medial epicondyle. (Modified from Jobe FW, Ciccotti MG. Lateral and medial epicondylitis of the elbow. J Am Acad Orthop Surg. 1994;2:1–8.)

weeks 2 through 4. During the first 4 weeks, lifting and resisted wrist and finger extension (lateral) or resisted wrist flexion and forearm pronation (medial) are avoided. At 4 weeks, light, resisted isometric exercises begin. Then at 6 weeks from surgery, the patient may start progressive resistance strengthening, including isotonic exercises. Shoulder range of motion and strengthening exercises are included at this time. An overall body conditioning is also carried out. Any equipment or technique enhancement is considered as well. A sport or work simulation can be performed at 10 to 12 weeks to ensure that the patient is prepared to return. Full return to lifting activities or sports is not recommended until 4 to 6 months postoperatively.[1–3]

■ TECHNICAL ALTERNATIVES AND PITFALLS

Alternative operative treatments for epicondylitis include arthroscopic debridement, percutaneous release of the epicondyle, and the use of a radiofrequency probe through a limited open exposure.

Some advocate the arthroscopic approach when concurrent intra-articular pathology is suspected. The technique involves release of the extensor carpi radialis brevis tendon with debridement of the lateral epicondyle and lateral condylar ridge. Proposed advantages include preservation of the common extensor origin, the ability to evaluate for other intra-articular pathology, and a shorter rehabilitation. Opponents of this technique feel that it may not allow thorough debridement of the epicondyle, and the lateral ulnar collateral ligament may be at risk. There is also concern for postoperative functional deficits because of the inability to reattach the released portion of extensor carpi radialis brevis tendon. The arthroscopic approach is not advocated on the medial side.[2,3]

Percutaneous release of the medial or lateral epicondyle is another option discussed in the literature. Baumgard and Schwartz[14] reported excellent results in 91.4% of patients treated with this technique (35 lateral, 6 medial). However, most feel the technique is contraindicated on the medial side due to concerns about the medial antebrachial cutaneous nerve and the ulnar nerve.[15]

A newer technique that has gained some popularity recently involves the use of a radiofrequency probe to create healing tissue in the region of pathology. A limited open exposure is used either medially or laterally. The probe is used on the tendon in several locations at different depths, forming a three-dimensional grid. Concern about thoroughness of debridement has been expressed. No published results are available at this time.[6,12]

■ SURGICAL OUTCOME

The results of operative management for lateral epicondylitis are favorable. Nirschl and Pettrone[9] found that 85% of patients were able to return to full activity without pain and an overall improvement in 97% of the patients. A small percentage of patients (10%–12%) had significant improvement, but still noted pain during aggressive activities. About 2% to 3% of patients had persistent symptoms despite operative treatment. A review of 1,200 patients with lateral epicondylitis over a 10-year period at the Kerlan Jobe Clinic showed that although 95% of the patients were treated successfully with nonoperative treatment, of the 39 patients requiring surgical intervention, 94% reported significant improvement in symptoms. Objective outcome studies revealed that 15% had grip dynamometer deficits and 100% had some isokinetic deficits. At the Rothman Institute, a review of 24 patients treated surgically for recalcitrant lateral epicondylitis also revealed similar results, with 96% of patients having an overall good to excellent result. All athletes returned to their preinjury level of sports competition.[2,3]

Although most patients with medial epicondylitis may be successfully managed with conservative treatment, surgical intervention does provide reliable pain control and return to preinjury level of activity. A review of 35 patients with refractory medial epicondylitis by Vangsness and Jobe[12] revealed that 86% of patients treated surgically noted good or excellent results with no limitation in the use of their elbows. Fourteen patients, who required an ulnar nerve submuscular

transposition, had no persistent symptoms. Nineteen of 20 athletes returned to their previous level of performance. No significant side-to-side differences with regard to grip strength and isokinetic testing were demonstrated postoperatively. Gabel and Morrey[8,11] found 87% good to excellent results in a review of 26 patients treated operatively for medial epicondylitis. Patients with severe coexistent ulnar nerve symptoms had a less favorable outcome than compared to a 96% good to excellent result in patients with absent or minor ulnar nerve symptoms. Baumgard and Schwartz[14] demonstrated that in a small series of six patients 83% had excellent results with percutaneous release of the common flexor origin for medial epicondylitis.

Overall, surgical treatment for epicondylitis results in high patient satisfaction. Pain relief and return to normal activity level are the expected outcomes. Some patients may have mild residual strength deficits, but these do not typically interfere with functional activities.

■ CONCLUSION

Epicondylitis of the elbow is a relatively common disorder caused by both occupational and sports-related activities. Epicondylitis may be associated with other elbow pathology and must be carefully evaluated in order to provide successful treatment. Although the majority of patients respond well to conservative management, surgical intervention for recalcitrant epicondylitis provides reliable pain control and return to previous level of activity. When operative treatment is performed, it is important to adhere to the general principles of removing degenerative tendon, anatomically restoring the tendon, and addressing concomitant pathology.

■ REFERENCES

1. Ciccotti MG. Epicondylitis in the athlete. AAOS Instr Course Lect. 1999;48;375–381.
2. Ciccotti MG, Charlton WPH. Epicondylitis in the athlete. Clin Sports Med. 2001;20(1):77–93.
3. Ciccotti MG, Lombardo SJ. Lateral and medial epicondylitis of the elbow. In: Jobe FW, Pink MM, Glousman RE, et al., eds. *Operative Techniques in Upper Extremity Sports Injuries.* St Louis: Mosby Year Book; 1996:431–446.
4. Hohmann G. Uber den tennisellboggen. Verhand longer der deutschen orthopaedischen gesselschaft. Kong. 1926;21:349–353.
5. Coonrad RW, Hooper WR. Tennis elbow: its course, natural history, conservative and surgical management. J Bone Joint Surg. 1973;55A(6):1177–1182.
6. Nirschl RP. Muscle and tendon trauma: tennis elbow tendinosis. In: Morrey BF, ed. *The Elbow and Its Disorders*, 3rd ed. Philadelphia: WB Saunders; 2000:523–535.
7. Kraushaar BS, Nirschl RP. Current concepts review: tendinosis of the elbow (tennis elbow). J Bone Joint Surg. 1999;81A(2):259–277.
8. Gabel GT, Morrey BF. Medial epicondylitis. In: Morrey BF, ed. *The Elbow and Its Disorders*, 3rd ed. Philadelphia: WB Saunders; 2000:537–542.

9. Nirschl RP, Pettrone FA. Tennis elbow: the surgical treatment of lateral epicondylitis. J Bone Joint Surg. 1979;61A(6):832–839.

10. Spencer GE, Herndon CH. Surgical treatment of epicondylitis. J Bone Joint Surg. 1953;35A(2):421–424.

11. Gabel GT, Morrey BF. Operative treatment of medial epicondylitis. J Bone Joint Surg. 1995;77A(7):1065–1069.

12. Vangsness CT, Jobe FW. Surgical treatment of medial epicondylitis. J Bone Joint Surg Br. 1991;73B:409–411.

13. Ciccotti MG, Ramani MN. Medial epicondylitis. Sports Med Arthrosc Rev. 2003;11(1):57–62.

14. Baumgard SH, Schwartz DR. Percutaneous release of the epicondylar muscles for humeral epicondylitis. Am J Sports Med. 1982;10(4):233–236.

15. Wittenberg RH, Schaal S, Muhr G. Surgical treatment of persistent elbow epicondylitis. Clin Ortho Rel Res. 1992 May;(278):73–79.

ULNAR COLLATERAL LIGAMENT RECONSTRUCTION

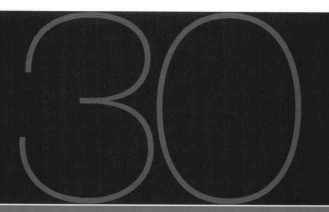

■ CHRISTOPHER S. AHMAD, MD, RAFFY MIRZAYAN, MD, NEAL S. ELATTRACHE, MD

■ HISTORY OF THE TECHNIQUE

Injury to the elbow ulnar collateral ligament (UCL) from valgus forces was first described in a javelin thrower in 1946 by Waris.[1] The injury then became well recognized in overhead throwing athletes with baseball pitchers at highest risk. Jobe et al.[2] developed the original UCL reconstruction and described the technique with initial results in 1986. The technique utilized a tendinous transection and reflection of the flexor-pronator mass, submuscular transposition of the ulnar nerve, and creation of humeral tunnels that penetrated the posterior cortex **(Fig. 30-1)**. This technique offered excellent exposure at the expense of morbidity to the flexor-pronator mass and ulnar nerve. Since that initial report, modifications in the surgical technique have been made to ease technical demands and decrease soft tissue morbidity. A muscle splitting approach has been developed to avoid detachment of the flexor-pronator mass with or without subcutaneous transposition of the ulnar nerve.[3] Modifications in bone tunnel creation have also been made, which direct the tunnels anterior on the humeral epicondyle to avoid risk of ulnar nerve injury while the graft remains passed in a figure-eight fashion.[3] Further changes in bone tunnel configuration have also been developed to reduce the number of tunnels and facilitate easier graft tensioning.[4,5] Results with these modified techniques have proven effective in returning high-level athletes back to throwing.

■ INDICATIONS AND CONTRAINDICATIONS

Patients with a diagnosis of UCL insufficiency that fail nonoperative treatment are candidates for reconstruction.

Accurate diagnosis is based on a history of medial elbow pain during the late cocking/early acceleration phase of throwing. Chronic injuries present gradually, often with painful symptoms occurring only when throwing greater than 50% to 75% of maximal effort, accompanied with inaccurate ball placement. Acute injuries may present suddenly with a pop, sharp pain, and inability to continue throwing. Physical examination features that support the diagnosis include point tenderness elicited directly over the UCL or toward its insertion site at the sublime tubercle. Valgus instability is tested with the patient's elbow flexed between 20 degrees and 30 degrees to unlock the olecranon from its fossa as valgus stress is applied. The milking maneuver is performed by either the patient or the examiner by pulling on the patient's thumb to create valgus stress with the patient's forearm supinated and elbow flexed beyond 90 degrees. The moving valgus stress test is a modification of the milking maneuver where valgus stress is applied while the elbow is moved through an arc of flexion and extension. For both tests, the subjective feeling of apprehension, instability, or localized pain to the UCL indicates UCL injury.

Imaging studies confirm the diagnosis. Valgus stress radiographs may be used to document excessive medial joint line opening, and an opening greater than 3 mm has been considered diagnostic of valgus instability.[2,3,6] Conventional magnetic resonance imaging (MRI) delineates the UCL and is capable of identifying thickening within the ligament or more obvious full thickness tears. MR arthrography enhanced with intra-articular gadolinium improves the diagnosis of partial undersurface tears.[7]

Patients who wish to continue throwing, have failed nonoperative treatment, have an accurate diagnosis, and are willing to participate in the lengthy rehabilitation are indicated for surgical reconstruction. Certain career and timing

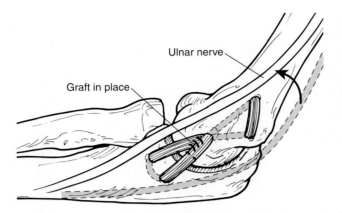

Fig 30-1. Original UCL reconstruction technique as described by Frank W. Jobe demonstrating detachment of the flexor-pronator mass, transposition of the ulnar nerve, and bone tunnels directed posterior on the humeral epicondyle.

situations may favor more immediate reconstruction without demonstrating failed nonoperative treatment. Relative contraindications include an inability to participate in lengthy rehabilitation and poor patient motivation.

Patients who present with valgus extension overload should also be thoroughly evaluated and considered for UCL reconstruction. In a report of professional baseball players who underwent olecranon debridement, 25% developed valgus instability and eventually required UCL reconstruction.[8] This important observation suggests that both the olecranon and the UCL contribute to valgus stability. Therefore, olecranon resection may increase the demand placed on the UCL in resisting valgus forces during throwing. A recent biomechanical study demonstrated that increasing amounts of olecranon resection result in increased elbow valgus angulation.[9] The authors of that study suggested that these kinematic alterations place the UCL at increased risk for injury. Ahmad et al. have demonstrated that UCL injury results in contact alterations in the posterior

compartment that leads to osteophyte formation (Ahmad et al., AOSSM Annual Meeting, Orlando, Fla, 2003). Based on these clinical and basic science studies, we advocate careful evaluation of the UCL in patients presenting with valgus extension overload. Consideration should be given to UCL reconstruction in combination with posterior debridement in these patients who fail nonoperative treatment and have combined posteromedial impingement and UCL injury.

■ SURGICAL TECHNIQUES

Jobe Technique

The patient is positioned supine and the arm is placed on an arm board. An examination under anesthesia is performed and a pneumatic tourniquet is placed on the upper arm. After prepping and draping, a consistent valgus stress is applied to the elbow using a small towel placed beneath the extended elbow with the forearm supinated. The arm is exsanguinated and the tourniquet inflated. A skin incision is centered over the medial epicondyle and extended 5 cm both proximally in the direction of the humerus and distally in the direction of the ulna. Dissection is carried down to the muscle fascia while identifying and protecting all sensory branches of the medial antebrachial cutaneous nerve **(Fig. 30-2)**. A longitudinal incision in the common flexor mass is made at its posterior third in line with a tendinous raphe of the flexor carpi ulnaris **(Fig. 30-3)**. A periosteal elevator is used to separate the flexor muscle mass from the UCL-capsular complex. Blunt retractors are placed and the ligament is inspected and palpated under valgus stress **(Fig. 30-4)**.

If a gross ligament tear is not obvious, a longitudinal split is made in the ligament to allow inspection of the joint for loose bodies, degenerative changes, and quality of the length tension of the ligament with valgus force. Valgus stress with the elbow at 30 degrees flexion will reveal any opening of the

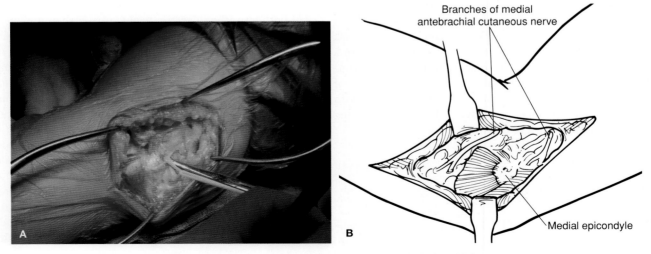

Fig 30-2. Identification and protection of branches of the medial antebrachial cutaneous nerve.

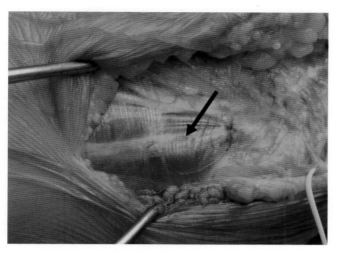

Fig 30-3. Flexor pronator mass with the tendinous raphe of the flexor carpi ulnaris indicated.

ulnohumeral articulation, with greater than 2 mm of gap indicating insufficiency of UCL **(Fig. 30-5)**.

If necessary, posterior olecranon osteophytes can be removed at this time through a vertically oriented, posterior arthrotomy. Care must be taken to protect the ulnar nerve while an osteotome and a rongeur are used to remove the tip of the olecranon or debride posterior loose bodies. The arthrotomy is closed with absorbable suture. An alternative for patients with posterior olecranon osteophytes or loose bodies is to perform elbow arthroscopy prior to ligament reconstruction.

The ulnar tunnel is created with converging 3.2-mm drill holes made just anterior and posterior to the sublime tubercle of the coronoid process that serves as the anterior bundle's insertion site. The drill holes are approximately 5 mm distal to the articular surface with at least a 5-mm bridge

between the holes **(Fig. 30-6)**. A curette is then used to connect the tunnels at their apex.

The initial humeral tunnel is created with a 4.5-mm drill hole made at the site of anatomic origin of the anterior bundle of UCL on the medial epicondyle directed superiorly. Care is taken to avoid penetration of the posterior cortex and injury to the ulnar nerve **(Fig. 30-7)**. To create the superior humeral tunnels, the medial supracondylar ridge is exposed with a second longitudinal split in the flexor-pronator mass. A 3.2-mm drill hole is placed just anterior to the epicondylar attachment of the medial intermuscular septum and directed to communicate with the 4.5-mm drill hole in the epicondyle. A second 3.2-mm drill hole is made in the anterosuperior surface of the epicondyle approximately 1 cm from the previous 3.2-mm hole and also communicating with the 4.5-mm epicondylar hole.

Attention is then turned to harvesting the palmaris longus tendon graft. With the forearm fully supinated, the tendon is identified just ulnar to the flexor carpi radialis. A 1-cm transverse incision is then made at the level of the distal flexor wrist crease directly over the tendon **(Fig. 30-8)**. A hemostat is used to develop the tendon from surrounding soft tissue. The tendon is palpated proximally and a second transverse incision is made approximately 8 cm from the distal incision. Serial transverse incisions are made more proximally as needed, in a fashion similar to the first and second incisions, until the level of the musculotendinous junction is identified. Usually three incisions are required. The tendon is transected distally and brought out through the proximal incision. The tendon is divided at the musculotendinous junction to give a length of 15 to 20 cm. The incisions are irrigated and closed routinely.

A 1-0 nonabsorbable braided suture is placed in one end of the graft using a locking stitch. The graft is then passed through the ulnar tunnel using a hooked suture passer or a

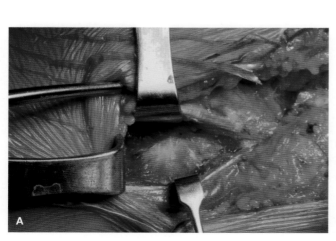
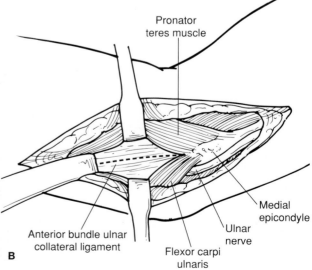

Fig 30-4. Muscle split approach with retractors in place and UCL well visualized.

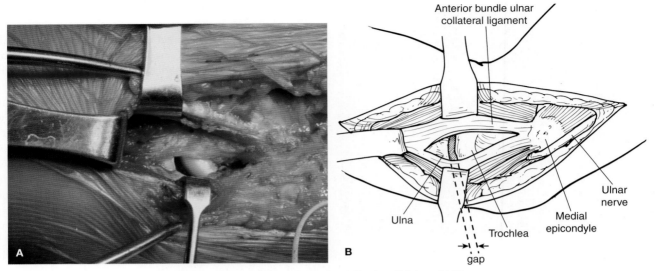

Fig 30-5. Ulnohumeral opening following division of UCL.

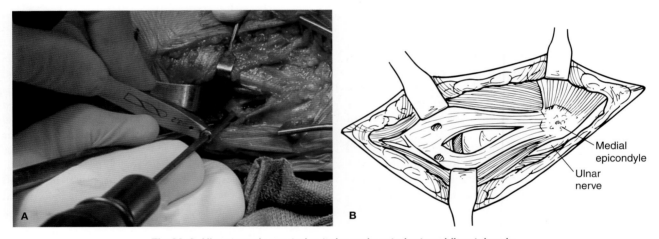

Fig 30-6. Ulnar tunnels created anterior and posterior to sublime tubercle.

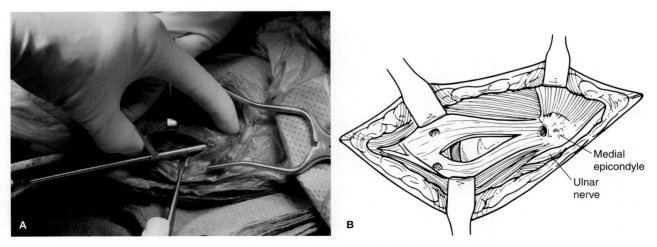

Fig 30-7. Inferior humeral tunnel created at anatomic UCL insertion.

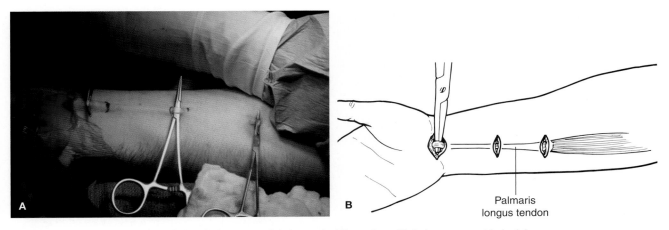

Fig 30-8. Palmaris longus graft is harvested through multiple transverse skin incisions.

curved free needle and weaved through the humeral tunnels in a figure-eight fashion across the joint. With a standard-length autogenous graft, an effort is made to pull the excess graft end back into the ulnar tunnel, creating a three-ply reconstruction **(Fig. 30-9)**.

The elbow is positioned with varus stress, 60 degrees of flexion, and the forearm in supination, while tension is applied to the graft. The ulnar side of the graft is sutured to the remnants of the ulnar collateral ligament adjacent to the sublime tubercle. The proximal limb of the graft is sutured to the tough tissue of the medial intermuscular septum outside the drill hole on the superior surface of the epicondyle. The elbow is then brought through a range of motion to verify isometry of the ligament reconstruction. Simple sutures are placed in the crossing limbs of the graft. The native ligament is sutured to the graft. The muscle fascia is repaired and the skin is closed. A sterile dressing is applied, followed by a posterior splint with the elbow in 90 degrees of flexion and neutral rotation, leaving the wrist and hand free.

■ TECHNICAL ALTERNATIVES AND PITFALLS

Graft Sources

The presence or absence of the palmaris longus tendon should be assessed prior to the procedure. When this tendon is available, it is the tissue of choice for reconstruction; however, absence of the palmaris longus occurs in approximately 6% to 25% of the general population.[10] When absent, the gracilis, plantaris, toe extensor tendons, a medial strip of the Achilles tendon, and allograft tendons are alternative options.

Ulnar Nerve

Also prior to surgery, the ulnar nerve should be palpated in elbow flexion and extension to confirm its location and to ensure that it does not subluxate anteriorly. Symptoms related to ulnar nerve irritation should be ascertained. We

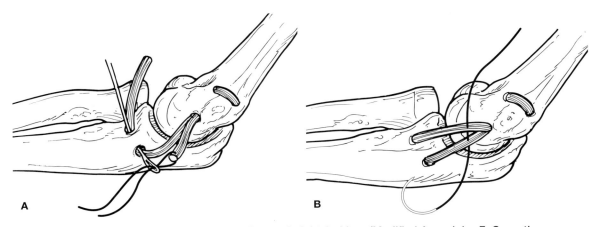

Fig 30-9. The graft is passed in a figure of eight fashion. (Modified from Jobe F. *Operative Techniques in Upper Extremity Sports Injuries*. Philadelphia: Mosby; 1996, with permission.)

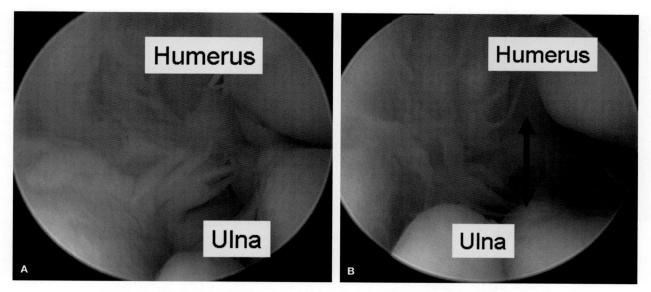

Fig 30-10. Arthroscopic visualization of ulnohumeral opening when valgus stress is applied.

reserve ulnar nerve transposition for patients with ulnar neuritis that involve compromised motor function or ulnar neuritis combined with ulnar nerve subluxation.

Arthroscopy Prior to Ligament Reconstruction

Arthroscopic evaluation of the elbow joint prior to ligament reconstruction has been advocated by some.[5,11] Arthroscopic assessment of valgus stability may be performed by placing valgus stress to the elbow while positioned at 90 degrees of flexion with the forearm maximally pronated. Normal elbows demonstrate a maximum of 1 to 2 mm of opening, while elbows with UCL insufficiency demonstrate greater than 2 to 3 mm of opening **(Fig. 30-10)**. Although ulno-humeral opening may be appreciated, a cadaveric study demonstrated that the anterior bundle of the UCL cannot be directly visualized arthroscopically. Arthroscopy does facilitate diagnostic examination of the anterior and poste-rior compartments, and associated procedures may be per-formed when necessary, such as removal of loose bodies and marginal osteophytes, anterior capsular release, and anterior, posterior, or lateral debridement.[12]

Docking Technique

The docking technique modification utilizes the muscle splitting approach with tunnel creation on the ulna similar to the Jobe technique **(Fig. 30-11)**. The inferior tunnel on the epicondyle is also created similar to the Jobe technique. This tunnel should be assessed for adequate length of 1.5 cm with-out violating the superior cortex. Small divergent drill holes are then connected to this tunnel from the superior humeral cortex for passage of the graft fixation sutures **(Fig. 30-12)**. The graft is passed through the ulnar tunnel and the free ends are brought into the proximal tunnel, creating a

double-stranded graft. The graft length must be accurately fashioned to allow proper tensioning and fixation **(Fig. 30-13)**. The graft is then tensioned and the sutures tied over the humeral bony bridge as shown in **Figure 30-14**. This tech-nique was developed to facilitate easier graft tensioning and decrease the number of bone tunnels required.[5]

Interference Screw Fixation Technique

A new technique of UCL reconstruction has been evaluated in the laboratory that reconstructs the central isometric fibers of the native ligament and achieves fixation in single bone tunnels in the ulna and humeral epicondyle using interference screw fixation **(Fig. 30-15)**. This technique is less technically demanding since the required number of drill holes necessary is reduced from five to two. Less dissection through a muscle-splitting approach is afforded since only a single central tunnel is required rather than two tunnels with

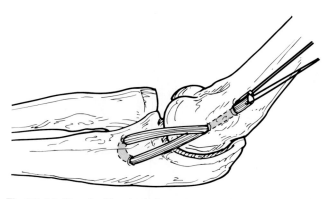

Fig 30-11. The docking technique creates a humeral tunnel that accepts both limbs of the graft with tensioning performed through superior exit holes.

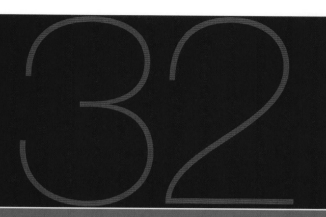

LACERTUS SYNDROME IN THROWING ATHLETES

■ STEVE E. JORDAN, MD

■ HISTORY OF THE TECHNIQUE

In 1959, George Bennett[1] summarized his experiences caring for throwing athletes. The following paragraph is excerpted in its entirety from that article.

> There is a lesion which produces a different syndrome. A pitcher in throwing a curve ball is compelled to supinate his wrist with a snap at the end of his delivery. This movement plus extension leads to the development of an irritation in front of and below the internal condyle of the humerus, which is extremely disabling. On examination, one will note distinct fullness over the pronator radii teres, beneath which are the tendinous attachments of the brachialis and the flexor sublimes digitorum. These are covered by a strong fascial band, a portion of which is the attachment of the biceps, which runs obliquely across the pronator muscle. A pitcher may be able to pitch for two or three innings but then the pain and swelling become so great that he has to retire. Roentgenograms in the majority of cases are entirely within normal limits, and my experience shows that exploration of the joint reveals no pathology and, therefore, is not advised. The muscle tissue generally is normal in appearance. A simple linear and transverse division of the fascia covering the muscles has relieved tension on many occasions and rehabilitated these men so that they were able to return to the game. I am at a loss to explain it except that tension develops from some unidentified irritation to the muscle tissue, or it is quite possible that this may be secondary to an irritation of the ulna at its articulation with the internal condyle.

This is the first known reference to a condition that has undoubtedly disabled many players and possibly ended careers of an untold number of throwing athletes. While Bennett did not fully understand the causes or even the mechanics involved (i.e., he thought the pitcher supinates instead of pronates upon release of the baseball), he did describe a simple operative treatment that has allowed us to prolong the careers of several throwing athletes. I have successfully treated 24 athletes diagnosed with a postexertional compartment syndrome of the medial elbow called the lacertus syndrome.

■ INDICATIONS AND CONTRAINDICATIONS

Athletes with the lacertus syndrome usually present with a vague history of slowly increasing discomfort in the flexor-pronator muscles after throwing. The discomfort is described as an achy painful tightness of the medial elbow, which develops in the first few hours after activity. Initially, the symptoms are minor and often ignored. A few hours rest leads to complete relief. As the condition progresses, the symptoms increase in severity and duration, and it requires a longer period of rest to relieve the discomfort and return to throwing. Just as Bennett described, these symptoms may progress to the point that the player cannot continue throwing. For position players in baseball, this problem is often not debilitating; however, for pitchers it may be. Quarterbacks complain most often during the repetition of practice. It is at this point, when the symptoms have progressed to a degree that they interfere with participation that the player usually presents to the trainer or doctor.

The duration of symptoms may vary markedly. In our series, symptoms ranged from eight hours to 4 days before resolving, only to begin again if the athlete threw too much. Duration of recurrent symptoms ranged from 6 months to 3 years. In all patients the symptoms were disabling if the throwing activity resumed before the acute symptoms had resolved.

The key feature of the history in patients with the lacertus syndrome is the delayed onset of symptoms, which is like

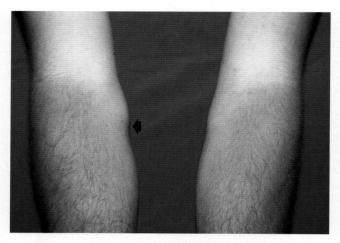

Fig. 32-1. Indentation caused by the tight lacertus fibrosus fascia of the affected right elbow *(arrow)*. Note the proximal fullness of the flexor pronator muscles. The asymptomatic left elbow exhibits a subtle indentation caused by the normal lacertus fascia.

that seen in exertional compartment syndromes of the legs in runners. This, together with the fact that a period of rest allows the athlete to resume throwing without discomfort, is diagnostic. Trauma to the elbow is usually not a factor in the etiology of the lacertus syndrome. The physician should take a careful history and perform a thorough physical exam of the elbow to help rule out more common abnormalities such as medial epicondylitis, ulnar collateral ligament injuries, and cubital tunnel syndrome or ulnar neuritis. Other conditions that can cause medial elbow pain in throwers are bicipital tendonitis and stress fractures. Pronator teres syndrome or intra-articular pathologies should also be considered and ruled out.

In patients who have a history of postexertional medial elbow pain and tightness and who have the lacertus syndrome as part of their differential diagnosis, it is essential to examine the player after a workout. The examination should begin with a careful inspection of the arm, looking for abnormal contours of the medial musculature just distal to the medial epicondyle. In players with severe or advanced cases, the proximal portions of the flexor pronator muscles appear grossly swollen and the distinct oblique band of the lacertus fibrosus is readily visible **(Fig. 32-1)**. The patient should be asked to flex and pronate the wrist, which further exaggerates any abnormality in the area of the lacertus fascia. Palpation of the area will likely reveal tenderness in the muscle directly beneath and just distal to the crossing fascial band.

Radiographs and magnetic resonance imaging exams are performed to help exclude other more common diagnoses. There are no findings on these studies to confirm the diagnosis of lacertus syndrome, but the tests are obviously helpful in ruling out other conditions. The diagnosis of lacertus syndrome can usually be made with a careful history and physical exam alone.

High-speed video of the pitching motion has revealed that pitches are released with a terminal pronation of the hand and forearm.[2] Although Bennett was incorrect in his assertion that curveball pitchers supinate upon release, he was correct in his belief that curveball pitchers are more prone to develop the lacertus syndrome. Sixty-six percent of the pitchers in our series listed the breaking ball as their prominent pitch. The curveball is held during the acceleration phase of pitching with greater supination of the hand, putting more stretch on the pronator teres than seen in a fastball or change-up, both of which are normally held in a forearm neutral position during acceleration. This may lead to more work for the pronator muscles in the release of a breaking ball and thus account for the greater propensity of breaking ball pitchers to develop the condition. Repetitive pronation of the forearm is the mechanism that leads to the symptoms.

The pathophysiology of the lacertus syndrome is similar to that of exertional compartment syndrome in the legs of runners.[3] The lacertus syndrome differs from compartment syndromes of the leg due to the peculiar anatomy of the lacertus fascia. The lacertus fibrosus fascia is not the primary muscle fascia for the flexor pronator group of muscles. It does not define an entire compartment; it merely invests a portion of the muscle compartment acting as an extrinsic constrictor and prevents normal tissue expansion during and after exercise. Postexercise compartmental pressure measurements taken in symptomatic patients revealed pressures 15 to 22 mm Hg greater under the area of the lacertus fascia than in the same muscles proximal to the crossing lacertus fascia. Therefore, the pathophysiology of the lacertus syndrome is that of a partial compartment syndrome. Only the tissue below the crossing fascia has elevated pressures, and it is here that the symptoms are generated.

The two syndromes are similar in their presentation. Both are conditions brought on by exertion and relieved by rest. The symptoms in both conditions usually peak 1 to 2 hours postexertion. These findings lead to the conclusion that the lacertus syndrome is a postexertional partial compartment syndrome in the flexor pronator muscles where they are bound down, not by their own fascia, but by the overlying lacertus fibrosus. The success of a simple fasciotomy in all cases has supported this conclusion.

■ NONOPERATIVE TREATMENT

The first priority of nonoperative treatment is to rule out more common causes of elbow pain in throwers and to make a definitive diagnosis. Once the diagnosis is made, patient education activity modification and treatment can be implemented. Two players in our series were treated nonoperatively. One was a collegiate catcher who had 3 months of competitive baseball to play before attending graduate school; the second was a major league relief pitcher who saw limited action as a situational left-handed pitcher. Both players were better able to manage their symptoms after they understood the etiology of their problem. With the support of his coaching staff the catcher avoided repetitive hard throwing whenever possible and was able to complete his collegiate career without incident or the need for surgery. The professional pitcher controlled his symptoms by limiting nonessential pitching and avoiding weight training, which involved repetitive pronation and wrist flexion. Resting the arm and avoiding repetitive pronation are the essentials of nonoperative treatment in the lacertus syndrome.

■ SURGICAL TECHNIQUE

The lacertus fibrosus fascia has been known by several names through the years. These include the more formal aponeurosis musculi bicipitis brachii and the simpler bicipital fascia or aponeurosis.[4] Henry[5] described it as a "sort of retinaculum" arising from the biceps tendon and extending over the median nerve and the distal end of the brachial artery, attaching or investing into the fascia of the medial muscles of the forearm. In the days of the barber surgeons this aponeurosis was called the "grace a Dieu" fascia (praise to God fascia) because it protected the artery and nerve during phlebotomy.[6] The fascia arises from the medial border of the bicipital tendon and the lower medial portion of the muscle; it has a thickened proximal edge, which, in some, can be seen and palpated. It passes distally and medially to fuse with the deep fascia of the flexor pronator muscles in the upper forearm until it ultimately reaches the ulna posteromedially.[7] During surgery the fibers of the lacertus fibrosus can be distinguished from the investing muscle fascia by the oblique orientation of its fibers wrapping down and around the musculature **(Fig. 32-2)**.

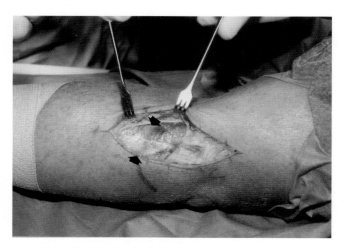

Fig. 32-2. The proximal edge of the lacertus fibrosus fascia is seen in line with the preoperative line drawn on the skin *(arrows)*. The investing fascia proximal to this point is thinner and less restrictive of the underlying muscle.

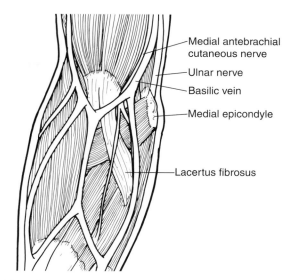

Fig. 32-3. Superficial medial anatomy: lacertus fibrosus, medial epicondyle, ulnar nerve, medial antebrachial cutaneous nerve, basilic vein. (Adapted from Jobe FW. *Operative Techniques in Upper Extremity Sports Injuries*. St. Louis: Mosby; 1996.)

The basilic vein and the anterior and ulnar branches of the medial antebrachial cutaneous nerve are the only structures of immediate significance when exposing the lacertus fibrosus **(Fig. 32-3)**. Each usually crosses the elbow anterior to the medial epicondyle. Typically, the dissection is well anterior to the cubital tunnel and the ulnar nerve is not at risk when releasing the fascia. However, one must be aware of the branches of the ulnar nerve, especially the first motor branch, which supplies the humeral head of the flexor carpi ulnaris. This branch can have a higher than normal origin within the cubital tunnel and it may encroach upon the field of surgery at the most medial aspect.[8]

The indication for surgery is failure of nonoperative treatment to allow the athlete to participate in sports. After ruling out other possible etiologies for the patient's pathology and exhausting conservative treatments measures, the patient is prepared for surgery. Patients are asked to throw 30 to 50 times the day before or the morning of surgery when possible. This makes the area of compression under the lacertus fascia more distinct.

The patient is positioned supine with the arm extended on a hand table. A tourniquet is used about the upper arm to control bleeding and improve visualization. A 4- to 6-cm longitudinal incision is made centered over the lacertus indentation in the flexor-pronator muscle group. The skin and subcutaneous tissue are carefully dissected away from the underlying muscle and fascial layers. Care is taken to protect the branches of the medial antebrachial cutaneous nerve.

Once the muscles are visualized, the lacertus fibers are identified (Fig. 32-2). The proximal edge is usually the easiest to see, and it is typically the area of the most prominent indentation of the muscles. One or two simple fasciotomies are made from proximal to distal, always under direct visualization.

Labels on Fig. 32-3:
- Medial antebrachial cutaneous nerve
- Ulnar nerve
- Basilic vein
- Medial epicondyle
- Lacertus fibrosus

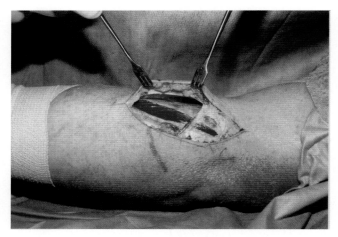

Fig. 32-4. Fasciotomy of the lacertus fibrosus. The normal contour of the flexor pronator muscle mass is restored.

These should restore the contour to the muscles and eliminate the indentation caused by the crossing lacertus fibrosus **(Fig. 32-4).** The distinctness and width (proximal to distal) of the lacertus fibrosus varies from patient to patient. In some patients the proximal fibers are thick and the area of compression is narrow. In others the fibers are less distinct and the fibers extend 3 to 4 cm from proximal to distal. The surgeon should feel that a releasing fasciotomy has been done over the proximal flexor pronator muscle group, restoring the normal muscle contour, prior to closing. In other words there have been no complications to overreleasing the fascia, whereas there may be recurrence if it is underreleased. Irrigation and a simple wound closure complete the case.

■ POSTOPERATIVE CARE

The patients are placed in a soft dressing and given a sling to wear for 2 weeks. Routine postoperative wound checks are performed. Gentle range of motion is begun as tolerated or needed for daily personal care. Players are encouraged to refrain from vigorous exercise with the affected arm for the first month and then they are released to progress as tolerated. Return to throwing is individualized and the decision is based on the patient's examination. If the player is pain free and the wounds are completely healed, there is no contraindication to begin tossing with advancement to throwing as tolerated. Players are told this usually begins at 4 weeks and return to hard throwing is normally expected at about 6 weeks. There have been no postoperative complications. The earliest any player has returned to throwing is 3 weeks. There have been no recurrences with minimum follow-up of 2 years and a maximum follow up of 12 years.

■ SUMMARY

The lacertus syndrome is a postexertional or overuse syndrome affecting the medial elbow of throwing athletes. The pathology is identical to that of a compartment syndrome caused by the constriction of active muscles by an overlying fascia. The lacertus fibrosus fascia constricts the flexor pronator muscles in predisposed athletes, causing pain and discomfort that can lead to an inability to throw regularly. The diagnosis can be made with a careful history and physical. The treatment is a simple release of the tight lacertus fibrosus.

■ ACKNOWLEDGMENT

The author wishes to thank Rick Williams ATC for his invaluable assistance throughout the course of this study.

■ SELECTED READINGS

Black KP, Schultz TK, Cheung NL. Compartment syndrome in athletes. Clin Sports Med. 1990 Apr;9:471.

Glousman RE, Barron J, Jobe FW, et al. An electromyography analysis of the elbow in normal and injured pitchers with medial collateral ligament insufficiency. Am J Sports Med. 1992;20(3):311.

Jobe FW, Stark H, Lombardo SJ. Reconstruction of the ulnar collateral ligament in athletes. J Bone Joint Surg Am. 1986;68:1158–1163.

Kan D. *Forearm Compartment Syndromes, Operative Techniques in Upper Extremity Sports Injuries.* St. Louis: Mosby; 1996.

Pappas AM, Zawacki RM, Sullivan TJ. Biomechanics of baseball pitching: a preliminary report. Am J Sports Med. 1985;13:216–222.

Rorabeck CH, Bourne RB, Fowler PJ. The surgical treatment of exertional compartment syndrome in athletes. J Bone Joint Surg Am. 1983;65:1245–1251.

Slocum DB. Classification of elbow injuries from baseball pitching. Tex Med. 1968;64:48.

■ REFERENCES

1. Bennett GE. Elbow and shoulder lesions of baseball players. Am J Surg. 1959;98,484.

2. Jobe FW, Nuber G. Throwing injuries of the elbow. Clin Sports Med. 1986;5(4):621.

3. Tulles HS, et al. Unusual lesions of the pitching arm. Clin Orthop. 1972;88:169.

4. Goss CM. *Gray's Anatomy*, 29th ed. Philadelphia: Lea and Febiger; 1973.

5. Henry A. *Extensile Exposure*, 2nd ed. Edinburgh: Churchill Livingstone; 1973.

6. Ellis H. *Clinical Anatomy*. London: Blackwell Scientific Publications; 1977.

7. Hollingshead WH. *Textbook of Anatomy*, 2nd ed. Hagerstown: Harper Row; 1967.

8. Jordan SE. *Surgical Anatomy of the Elbow, Operative Techniques in Upper Extremity Sports Injuries.* St. Louis: Mosby; 1996.

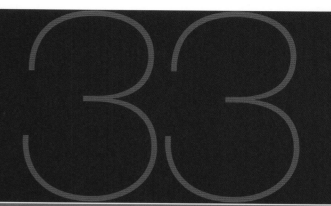

ULNAR NERVE INJURY IN THE THROWING ATHLETE

JEFFREY R. DUGAS, MD, E. LYLE CAIN, JR, MD

The overhead throwing motion generates significant forces in the shoulder and elbow articulations. These extreme forces subject the tissues in and around the joints of the upper extremity to stresses that, in many cases, are greater than the normal capacity of those tissues. At the elbow, valgus stress during the acceleration phase of throwing exceeds the maximum tensile strength of the ulnar collateral ligament (UCL). The excess stress is taken up by the surrounding tissues, including the ulnar nerve. The ulnar nerve courses from the medial aspect of the upper arm, around the medial epicondyle via the cubital tunnel, to the medial side of the forearm where it divides into its various branches. Ulnar neuritis is a common reason for pain and neurologic symptoms in the throwing elbow, but often represents a secondary condition caused by an underlying abnormality, especially valgus instability. Although medial elbow instability is a common cause of ulnar nerve symptoms, other conditions can lead to similar symptoms such as flexor-pronator strains/tendonitis/tears, medial epicondyle apophysitis or avulsion, valgus extension overload, stress fractures, and articular injuries. Also, the presence of cervical spine pathology can mimic ulnar neuritis via compression of one or more nerve roots at the cervical level. Compression of some or all of the brachial plexus can also cause focal elbow symptoms that can mimic more peripheral ulnar nerve compression.

The physician caring for overhead athletes must have a thorough understanding of the anatomy and physiology of the various structures in and around the elbow joint. An understanding of the biomechanics of the throwing motion and the pathomechanics that can lead to injury is also mandatory. The purpose of this chapter is to review the diagnosis and treatment of ulnar nerve problems in the overhead athlete.

■ HISTORY OF THE TECHNIQUE

When adequate conservative management fails to relieve symptoms, surgical treatment options in the throwing athlete include ulnar nerve neurolysis with or without transposition out of the cubital tunnel. There continues to be some differences of opinion in the printed literature regarding simple decompression versus submuscular or subcutaneous transposition.[1-3] Although medial epicondylectomy has been advocated for ulnar nerve decompression in the nonathlete, it is not recommended in the overhead-throwing athlete because of the threat of injury to the proximal attachment of the UCL and the possibility of nonunion.[4]

Anterior transposition of the ulnar nerve completely frees the nerve and places it in a healthy bed, as well as effectively lengthening the nerve and decreasing traction forces by rerouting it anterior to the medial epicondyle and anterior to the axis of motion of the elbow. This increased effective length is especially important to decrease ulnar nerve tension forces in the throwing athlete because of the valgus and flexion moments on the medial elbow during overhead throwing. Transposition anteriorly also removes the nerve from the position of greatest tension near the main valgus stabilizer of the elbow, the ulnar collateral ligament. For these reasons, anterior transposition is most often combined with neurolysis in the athlete.

In Situ Decompression (Neurolysis)

Proponents of simple decompression of the ulnar nerve suggest that this simple procedure preserves the native anatomy and vascular supply to the nerve and allows an easy rehabilitation. In this procedure, the cubital tunnel fascia (arcuate ligament) is released along a course beginning at the arcade of Struthers and ending well into the fibrous band at the flexor carpi ulnaris (FCU) origin. The nerve remains in its native bed, but is allowed to move freely without any direct compression or adhesions. The nerve is not removed from the cubital tunnel.

Although several authors have noted better outcomes with simple decompression compared to submuscular or subcutaneous transposition in the nonathletic population, simple decompression is generally not sufficient to relieve the traction forces caused by the act of overhead throwing.[1,3] Simple decompression has also been noted to result in a high recurrence rate and may worsen any ulnar nerve instability or subluxation.[5,6] We do not currently perform simple decompression or neurolysis except in the rare revision procedure in a patient with persistent symptoms after previous anterior transposition.

Submuscular Transposition

First described by Learmonth[7] in 1942, submuscular transposition has been widely utilized for the treatment of ulnar nerve symptoms in the throwing athlete, especially with associated UCL reconstruction using the technique pioneered by Jobe et al.[8] The nerve is released along the entire cubital tunnel region, from the arcade of Struthers well into the FCU, and is transposed under the detached flexor-pronator muscle mass. Submuscular transposition provides the nerve a straight path with a layer of muscular protection from the direct and indirect trauma that may occur during sports participation. Improved visualization of the underlying UCL is also an advantage of the submuscular technique. Although several authors have reported significant complication rates using the submuscular transposition, others have reported reasonable success.[4,9–11] Delpizzo et al.[12] reported the results of submuscular anterior transposition of the ulnar nerve in 19 high-level baseball players with symptoms of ulnar neuritis that failed adequate conservative treatment. Only nine of 15 (60%) patients evaluated at 3 to 58 months postoperatively were able to return to play. The authors reported that the technique allowed easy inspection of the UCL and easy arthrotomy to remove loose bodies or osteophytes, if present. They also believed that submuscular transposition provided stable fixation with protection from direct trauma.

Often ulnar nerve symptoms are present in the setting of medial elbow laxity due to an incompetent ulnar collateral ligament. Surgical management of the ulnar nerve symptoms with transposition is unlikely to succeed unless the underlying UCL pathology is addressed simultaneously.[4] Despite initial enthusiasm, several later reports by Jobe and Nuber[8] and Conway et al.[13] have shown that the ulnar nerve may be at risk with a submuscular transposition. These authors reported 31% and 21% incidence of postoperative ulnar nerve dysfunction, respectively, after UCL reconstruction with submuscular transposition of the ulnar nerve. Based on this experience, Jobe and Attrache[14]

have recommended performing submuscular ulnar nerve transfer with UCL reconstruction only in the setting of preoperative ulnar neuritis or the need for posterior compartment exploration.

Despite these authors' success, we currently do not performed submuscular ulnar nerve transposition in the throwing athlete because of concerns about the ultimate strength and healing of the flexor-pronator muscle mass and difficulty with nerve dissection in the case of revision elbow surgery.

Subcutaneous Transposition

Subcutaneous ulnar nerve transposition is our procedure of choice. This procedure is performed by executing a thorough neurolysis from the arcade of Struthers down to and within the FCU muscle mass. The nerve is then anteriorly transposed and loosely secured beneath a small leash of the flexor-pronator fascia. The cubital tunnel is then closed to obliterate the space and prevent relocation of the nerve if the leash fails. In our hands, subcutaneous nerve transposition stabilized with a fascial sling has provided good results with few surgical complications and low rates of recurrence.[15,16] Other benefits of the subcutaneous technique include the less invasive nature of the procedure, preservation of the flexor pronator muscle mass, and the ability to perform accelerated rehabilitation. Since Curtis[17] initially described subcutaneous ulnar nerve transfer in 1898, several authors have reported the surgical technique and results of various ways to perform subcutaneous transposition.[16,18,19] In series of 16 baseball players including 7 pitchers by Eaton et al.,[19] the subcutaneous technique was utilized, and all were able to return to competition without symptoms. No complications were reported in their series.

Rettig and Ebben[18] reported excellent results with anterior subcutaneous transfer of the ulnar nerve stabilized with a fascial sling in 20 athletes who had failed nonoperative management. At an average follow-up of 19 months (6 to 50 months), 95% (19 of 20) were able to compete, ten at the same level without limitations, and nine at a lower level with mild limitations. Average return to play was 12.6 weeks, and the authors recommended subcutaneous over submuscular transposition due to faster rehabilitation and decreased surgical morbidity.

From our institution, Andrews and Timmerman[15] reported on eight professional baseball players after anterior subcutaneous ulnar nerve transfer, including six patients who also had posteromedial olecranon osteophyte excision. Seven of eight (88%) returned to play for at least one season at the professional level. Azar et al.[16] reported that preoperative ulnar nerve symptoms resolved in nine of ten patients when subcutaneous ulnar nerve transfer was performed in conjunction with UCL reconstruction. Subcutaneous transposition may offer less morbidity compared to submuscular transfer in the setting of UCL reconstruction.

3

KNEE

R R

A

ANTERIOR CRUCIATE LIGAMENT RECONSTRUCTION

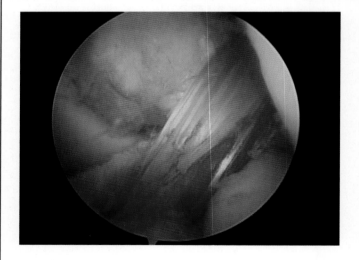

34

ANTERIOR CRUCIATE LIGAMENT RECONSTRUCTION: GENERAL CONSIDERATIONS

■ NATALIE A. SQUIRES, MD, ROBIN V. WEST, MD, CHRISTOPHER D. HARNER, MD

■ INTRODUCTION

The anterior cruciate ligament (ACL) is the primary restraint to anterior translation of the tibia and is the secondary restraint to tibial rotation, varus, and valgus stress.[1,2] ACL injury alters the kinematics and the stability of the knee. Acute tears may be associated with meniscal tears in 42% to 77% of cases,[3–8] and chondral injuries in 20% to 23% of the cases,[3,5] resulting in the "syndrome of the ACL deficient knee." Even an isolated ACL tear can result in subsequent meniscal or cartilage injury, leading to early degenerative changes. Age and activity level play an important role in the natural history of the ACL deficient knee. Older patients tend to be more sedentary, and a lower activity level places less stress on the knee; while younger, active patients place more stress on the knee. Chronic instability is common in ACL deficient knees. Marzo et al. found that many patients who were treated nonsurgically with an ACL injury had recurrent instability. Seventy-six percent of patients with an "unacceptable" result reported instability, and 45% of patients with an "acceptable" result had instability.[9]

Altered mechanics puts the knee at risk for degenerative changes. The focus of this chapter is on the general considerations of anterior cruciate ligament reconstruction surgery. ACL reconstruction is 90% successful in restoring knee stability and patient satisfaction.[10] Reconstruction, however, is not necessary in all patients who sustain an injury. The indications for surgery are not absolute. The most commonly accepted indications include a patient's inability to participate or function in his or her chosen athletic field, instability that affects activities of daily living, and an associated repairable meniscal injury or a multiple ligament knee injury with instability.

Although the relative indications may be widely agreed upon, there is little consensus on which reconstruction technique provides the most stable and functional outcome. Ideally the reconstruction should closely reproduce the ACL anatomy and biomechanical properties, and the graft should have structural properties similar to the ACL.

■ ANATOMY

The ligament's cross sectional area is 44 mm^2, with an ultimate tensile load of 2,160 N, a stiffness of 242 N/mm, and a strain of 20% before failure.[11,12] The forces in the intact ACL range from 100 N during passive knee extension to about 400 N with walking, and up to 1,700 N with cutting and acceleration-deceleration activities.[15,16] The ACL experiences loads that exceed its failure capacity only with unusual loading patterns on the knee. The goal of surgery is to restore stability and normal range motion. The success of anterior cruciate reconstruction is influenced by graft type, tunnel placement, graft tension, and fixation. Functional and clinical outcomes are also influenced by the rehabilitation regimen employed.

■ GRAFT SELECTION

Many factors, including the age of the patient, the activity level, the preoperative exam, and coexisting morbidities, should be considered when selecting a graft for an ACL reconstruction. Graft sources can be compared by many different criteria. The criteria that are most commonly used for graft comparison are the biomechanical properties, the biology of the healing, the ease of harvesting the graft, the fixation strength, the morbidity associated with the graft, and the "return to play" guidelines.

Many graft options exist, including synthetic ligaments, autograft, and allograft tissue. Autograft options include the

TABLE 34-1	Biomechanical Properties of Various ACL Graft Tissues[13,14]			
Tissue	Ultimate tensile load (N)	Stiffness (N/mm)	Cross sect area (mm²)	Reference no.
Intact ACL	2,160	242	44	11
BPTB (10 mm)	2,977	620	35	12
Quadruple HS	4,090	776	53	13
Quad tendon (10 mm)	2,352	463	62	14

patellar tendon, hamstrings, and quadriceps tendon. Allograft choices consist of the quadriceps tendon, patellar tendon, Achilles tendon, hamstrings, fascia lata, and anterior and posterior tibialis tendons. Patellar tendon autografts are historically the most popular graft choice because of their strength characteristics, ease of harvest, rigid fixation, bone-to-bone healing, and good clinical outcomes. However, donor site morbidity of patellar tendon autografts has led to the investigation and use of alternative graft sources.

Autografts and allografts undergo a similar process of incorporation including graft necrosis, cellular repopulation, revascularization, and collagen remodeling. However, allografts have been shown to have a slower biologic incorporation.[17] Healing of the site of the graft attachment may be responsible for most of the graft strength observed after transplantation. From a biologic standpoint, patellar tendon grafts, compared with soft-tissue grafts, have the advantage of bone-to-bone healing. Bone-to-bone healing is similar to fracture healing and is stronger and faster than soft tissue healing. The graft is usually incorporated into the host bone by 6 weeks during bone-to-bone healing. Soft tissue grafts usually take 8 to 12 weeks to incorporate into the host bone.[18] The biomechanical properties of ACL grafts (Table 34-1) can vary significantly depending on the donor's age, the size of the graft, and the testing methods.

Ease of Harvest

The goals of graft harvest should be to obtain an adequate graft specimen and to minimize donor site morbidity. The ease of graft harvest is surgeon dependent. Each graft represents a unique set of technical challenges and potential pitfalls that should be thoroughly understood prior to harvest.

Patellar tendon autografts require harvesting a tibial tubercle and a patellar bone plug. Large, deep cuts can increase the risk for a stress fracture in the proximal tibia or patella. Also, the patellar articular cartilage is at risk if the patellar cut is too deep. Trapezoidal bone cuts, instead of triangular ones, reduce the risk of articular cartilage penetration.

The quadriceps tendon is more difficult to harvest than the patellar tendon. The differences in the quadriceps tendon harvesting technique occur because the proximal patella has denser cortical bone than the distal pole, the surface is curved instead of flat, and the proximal patella has close adherence to the suprapatellar pouch. Fulkerson has described a technique to harvest the quadriceps tendon safely and efficiently.[19]

Hamstring harvest requires a thorough understanding of the anatomy of the gracilis and semitendinosus insertions. The sartorius is split to expose the underlying tendons. The hamstring tendons can either be left on their insertion or detached from the tibia during the harvest, and a closed or open tendon stripper is then used to retrieve the tendons. Care should be taken to harvest the entire tendon and not to amputate it prematurely.

Morbidity of the Graft

Anterior Knee Pain

Anterior knee pain is a common problem encountered after ACL reconstruction. Symptoms can occur anywhere along the extensor mechanism and typically involve the patellar or quadriceps tendons, patellofemoral joint, or the peripatellar soft tissues. It has been suggested that anterior knee pain may be related to the choice of graft material. The literature remains mixed on this subject, but most studies show a strong tendency for a decrease in anterior knee pain with the use of hamstring autografts compared with patellar tendon autografts.[20–25] However, no difference regarding anterior knee pain has been shown in the comparison of patellar tendon autografts and allografts.[26] It has been suggested that anterior knee pain is related to the loss of motion and poor rehabilitation techniques rather than to graft choice. Sachs et al.[27] demonstrated a correlation between the development of patellofemoral symptoms and the presence of a flexion contracture and quadriceps weakness. Shelbourne and Nitz[28] noted a decrease in patellofemoral symptoms following an accelerated rehabilitation protocol, which they attributed to early range of motion and restored quadriceps strength. In an ACL reconstruction meta-analysis of 21 studies of patellar tendon autografts and 13 studies of hamstring grafts, there was a 17.4% incidence of anterior knee pain in the patellar group and a 12% incidence in the hamstring group.[10]

Quadriceps and Hamstring Strength

Quadriceps and hamstring weakness is another concerning issue following graft harvest. Most studies have shown no significant difference between the various grafts with regards to quadriceps strength. However, Rosenberg et al.[29]

found a significant quadriceps deficit with isokinetic testing and a significant decrease in the quadriceps cross-sectional area on computed tomography scan when they compared 10 randomly selected patients who had undergone an ACL reconstruction with patellar autograft 12 to 24 months before testing.

When they compared athletes who had undergone either a patellar tendon allograft or autograft ACL reconstruction, Lephart et al.[30] found no significant difference between the two groups with regards to thigh circumference, quadriceps strength and power, and functional performance tests. The quadriceps index (involved leg/uninvolved leg at 60 degrees per second) had similar results between the allografts and autografts, with the indexes averaging 90% to 95%. The findings in this study indicate that harvesting the central third of the patellar tendon does not diminish quadriceps strength or functional capacity in highly active patients who have intense rehabilitation.

Carter and Edinger[31] compared the hamstring and quadriceps isokinetic results 6 months postoperatively in 106 randomly selected patients who had undergone ACL reconstruction using either patellar tendon or hamstring autografts. No statistically significant differences were found with regard to knee extension or flexion strength when evaluating the different graft sources. However, the majority of patients had not achieved adequate strength to safely return to unlimited activities at 6 months postoperatively.

Hamstring strength has been shown to be decreased at deep flexion angles following ACL reconstruction with hamstring autograft. Nakamura et al.[32] evaluated hamstring strength at 2 years postoperatively in 74 consecutive patients who had undergone hamstring ACL reconstruction. Similar to other studies, recovery of peak flexion torque was over 90%. However, the recovery was less at 90 degrees knee flexion. These results suggest that the loss of hamstring strength after harvesting may be more prominent at deep flexion angles.

Yasuda et al.[33] isolated the effect of hamstring harvest from morbidity secondary to ACL reconstruction. They were able to demonstrate that tendon harvest did not affect quadriceps function, but hamstring function was affected. Soreness that affected activity level usually resolved at 3 months. Isometric hamstring strength returned by 3 months and isokinetic strength returned within 12 months.

Donor Site Complications

Reported complications with patellar tendon autograft are rare and include patella infera, patella fractures, patellar tendon ruptures, tendonitis, and numbness.[34] Numbness can also occur with hamstring autograft, due to injury of the superficial branch of the saphenous nerve.[33,35]

Outcomes and Other Complications

Freedman et al.[10] performed a meta-analysis of 21 studies (1,348 patients) from 1966 to 2000, with a minimum follow up of 24 months, comparing patellar tendon and hamstring tendon autografts. The rate of graft failure was significantly lower in the patellar tendon group (1.9% versus 4.9%). Laxity was measured clinically with the KT-1000 arthrometer and with pivot-shift testing. The results showed that a significantly higher proportion of the patellar tendon group (79%) had a side-to-side difference of less than 3 mm compared to the hamstring group (73.8%). The patellar tendon group had a significantly higher rate of subjects requiring lysis of adhesions (6.3% versus 3.3%), and the patellar group also demonstrated a higher rate of anterior knee pain (17.4% versus 11.5%). The hamstring group had a higher rate of hardware removal following the reconstruction (5.5% versus 3.1%). Infection rates between the two groups were not significantly different (0.5% in the patellar group versus 0.4% in the hamstring group).

Allografts

The fear of disease transmission with allografts has largely been eliminated with the development of modern donor screening and testing procedures. The American Association of Tissue Banks (AATB) first printed its guidelines in 1986 to ensure sterility and quality during allograft processing. Since then, the guidelines have been revised and updated six times, most recently in 1996. A potential cadaveric donor must first pass through a detailed medical, social, and sexual history questionnaire completed by the next of kin or life partner. A physical examination is also performed to detect for hepatosplenomegaly, lymphadenopathy, cutaneous lesions, and other signs of infectious diseases. Laboratory tests, required by the Food and Drug Administration (FDA) and the AATB, are performed. These tests include blood cultures, harvested tissue cultures, antibodies to HIV types 1 and 2, hepatitis B surface antigen, hepatitis C, syphilis, and human T-cell lymphotrophic virus.[36–39]

Despite the extensive screening, there is still a window of vulnerability between the infection and the production of antibodies by the donor. To decrease this window, more than 50% of tissue banks use polymerase chain reaction (PCR) testing to directly detect the viral antigens. The use of PCR can dramatically increase the detection of HIV. PCR is very sensitive and can detect as few as 5 to 20 viral DNA copies per sample tested.[39]

To date, there have been three reported cases of disease transmission from bone-patellar tendon-bone allografts used to reconstruct the ACL.[37] The first reported case was HIV in 1985, and there were two reported cases in 1991 of hepatitis C.[39]

In the past, the high-dose radiation used for sterilization resulted in weakened structural properties of the graft tissue. The alternative use of ethylene oxide sterilization resulted in adverse surgical reactions, most commonly chronic effusions. Ethylene oxide does not alter the mechanical properties of the graft and can effectively remove micro-organisms. However, it leaves behind a chemical residue, which may result in chronic synovitis and subsequent graft failure.[38] The current sterilization techniques are gamma radiation and cryopreservation. Cryopreservation has been shown to have no effect on the structural properties of ligament, tendon, or meniscal tissue.

Gamma radiation is an effective method of sterilization, but doses above 3.0 Mrad are necessary to kill viruses. Unfortunately, this level of radiation has detrimental effects on the graft strength. The difficulties associated with the sterilization of a cleanly procured graft have led to the development of a technique of aseptic harvest and a special cleaning process. This process consists of antibiotic soaks, multiple cultures, and low-dose radiation (<3.0 Mrad). This sterilization technique is the most commonly used process for producing a sterile ACL graft.[38] New low-temperature chemical sterilization methods with good tissue penetration have been developed. These appear to be sporicidal and do not seem to adversely affect the biomechanical properties of tissue. Other sterilization techniques, such as supercritical CO_2 and the use of antioxidants in combination with gamma irradiation are being developed.[39]

Synthetics and Prosthetics

Synthetic ligaments have been shown to have an increased complication rate secondary to synovitis and poor post-op tensile strength when compared to allograft and autograft reconstructions.[40–42] Prosthetic implants have also had very limited success. They have been associated with recurrent instability, chronic effusions, and synovitis.

Authors' Preference

The patellar tendon autograft continues to have the largest reported outcomes in the literature and is the mostly widely used graft source.[37] The hamstring tendons are gaining increasing popularity, mainly due to the excellent stiffness and tensile load properties, improved fixation techniques, reduced harvest morbidity, and excellent outcome and patient satisfaction scores. However, there continues to be a reported higher degree of instrumented (KT-1000) tested laxity for hamstring reconstruction and a lower return to preinjury activity levels.[20–24]

Allografts have gained a recent resurgence in the literature. Improved sterilization techniques, along with a wide range of graft sources, have lead to increased safety and availability. The benefits of decreased surgical morbidity and easier rehabilitation must be weighed against the higher costs of the allografts and a slower incorporation period.[16]

In our practice, we tend to use patellar tendon autografts in high-demand individuals who participate in cutting, pivoting, or jumping sports. We also favor the patellar tendon autograft in athletes who desire a "quick return to play." Pre-existing anterior knee pain and certain lifestyle activities (kneeling for work, religion) are relative contraindications to the patellar tendon autograft. Quadruple hamstring autograft is our preference in "lower" demand patients, recreational athletes, younger patients with open growth plates, and for cosmesis. Contraindications to the hamstring autograft include generalized increased ligamentous laxity, competitive sprinters (terminal flexion weakness), and a previous hamstring injury. Our preference is not to use hamstring autografts in "high-demand athletes." We opt for the patellar tendon allograft in lower-demand patients, older patients who prefer an easier rehabilitation, and in the multiple-ligament injured knee. We prefer not to use allograft in younger patients and do not use synthetic grafts.

■ TUNNEL PLACEMENT

Tunnel placement is based on the anatomy of the innate ACL. The ACL is a collection of fibers that attach to the femur and tibia over a broad area. The tibial attachment is adjacent to the anterior horn of the lateral meniscus, and the femoral attachment is in the posterior aspect of the intercondylar notch on the medial wall of the lateral femoral condyle. The fibers of the ACL have been divided into two distinct bundles. The anteromedial bundle (AMB) originates from the proximal aspect of the femoral attachment and inserts on the anteromedial aspect of the tibial attachment. The posterolateral bundle (PLB) inserts onto the posterolateral aspect of the tibial attachment. When the knee is extended, the PLB is tight, while the AMB is moderately lax. With knee flexion, the AMB tightens and the PLB becomes loose.[43]

Good clinical results following ACL reconstruction have been associated with anatomic tibial and femoral tunnel placement on the lateral radiographs.[44–47] Good outcomes have been related to a femoral tunnel placed 60% or more posteriorly along the Blumensaat line and to a tibial tunnel placed 20% to 40% posteriorly along the plateau (behind the Blumensaat line on a lateral in full extension).

Tunnel placement should be based upon anatomy and not choice of graft or method of fixation. Several arthroscopic reference points have been proposed to assist in reproducibly placing the tibial tunnel. These anatomic landmarks include the PCL, the posterior aspect of the anterior horn of the lateral meniscus, the medial tibial spine, and the ACL footprint. There are fewer reference points described for establishing the femoral tunnel.

A cadaveric study at the University of Pittsburgh was performed using a robotic/universal force-moment sensor testing system to test anterior tibial and rotational loads following an ACL reconstruction.[48] The resulting data revealed that the reconstructions (patellar tendon and quadruple-loop hamstring autografts) were successful in limiting anterior tibial translation but were insufficient to control a combined rotatory load of internal and valgus torque.

To improve the combined rotatory instability following an ACL reconstruction, some physicians have modified the standard technique to produce a more anatomic reconstruction. Double bundle reconstructions and medial portal techniques have been described in biomechanical and outcome studies.[49–55]

Most ACL reconstructions focus on replacing only the anteromedial bundle. The posterolateral bundle has not received as much attention in the past. The double bundle technique focuses on reproducing both the anteromedial and posterolateral bundles. Yagi et al.[56] tested the biomechanical function of ACL-intact knees, ACL-deficient knees, single bundle and double bundle ACL reconstructed knees. They found that the normalized in situ force was 97% for the double bundle reconstructions and 89% for the single bundle reconstructions. With combined rotatory load, the normalized in situ force at 30 degrees of flexion in the double bundle was 91% and 66% in the single bundle reconstruction.

Using the medial portal technique, the femoral tunnel is drilled through the medial portal instead of through the tibial tunnel. This technique better reproduces the normal anatomy of the ACL by allowing for a more posterior and inferior femoral tunnel.[57] Posterior wall blowout can be more easily avoided with the medial portal technique since the knee can be hyperflexed. Since the interference screw is also placed through the medial portal, parallel placement of the screw to the graft is easier with this technique, and divergence can be more easily avoided.

Biomechanical studies have also supported the medial portal technique. Loh et al.[58] showed than the 10 o'clock femoral tunnel (more inferior) position improved rotatory stability when compared with the 11 o'clock position. Both tunnel positions were effective in stabilizing the knee under anterior tibial load, but the combined rotatory loads were better controlled by the 10 o'clock position. Neither tunnel position could restore the kinematics and the in situ forces to the level of the intact knee.

■ GRAFT TENSION

Although there is no substitute for perfect tibial and femoral attachments, a poor outcome can still result if the graft is poorly tensioned. Graft tension is an important factor in the restoration of normal knee stability and kinematics. However, the optimal initial tension remains unknown. As previously discussed, the native ACL has two distinct bundles. The tension in these bundles vary with knee flexion. None of the fibers are truly neutral or isotonic at any point in flexion.[59] ACL graft tension throughout knee range of motion cannot be exactly reproduced during reconstruction. Some tension in the construct is necessary to prevent anterior tibial translation and maintain joint stability.

A low initial tension may not provide enough restraint to anterior translation. Yasuda et al.[60] studied the effects of initial tension on clinical outcome. Loads of 20, 40, and 80 N were applied at 30 degrees of flexion. A significant difference was identified in post-operative laxity. At 2 years after reconstruction, AP translation was 2.1, 1.4, and 0.6 mm, respectively.

A high initial tension may result in less AP laxity but can also have other deleterious effects secondary to high stress on the graft. High graft tension can limit joint motion, alter

knee kinematics, and ultimately result in degenerative changes at the articular surface.[61,62] Graft elongation and potential disruption can occur.

How much tension is appropriate? There is currently no consensus. Yasuda et al.[60] recommend an initial tension of 80 N. Yoshiya et al.[61] pretensioned grafts with a load of 1 N and 39 N and were able to demonstrate poor vascularity and focal myxoid degeneration in the grafts tensioned at 39 N. These changes were not observed when the graft was tensioned at 1 N. Friederich and O'Brien[63] found that a preload of 67 N to 89 N consistently restored knee kinematics within 1 mm. They also stressed that an appropriate pretension will restore normal knee kinematics throughout range of motion. However, "nonphysiologic" pressures (either under or overconstrained) will lead to abnormal knee kinematics, regardless of the knee position. The balance between preventing excessive translation while maintaining range of motion and graft integrity is a delicate one that has not yet been perfected.

Knee angle at the time of tensioning also has an effect on graft tension and knee kinematics. High initial tension applied with the knee highly flexed will result in increased tension as the knee extends and possibly limit full extension. High tension applied with the knee extended may result in increased tension as the knee flexes and possibly limit flexion. Amis and Jakob[62] reported that graft failure was most imminent with a sudden rise in graft tension as the knee approaches full extension. One can then conclude that less flexion is better during graft fixation. However, excessive tightening in full extension can lead to limited flexion. Friederich and O'Brien[63] found normal kinematics is restored with appropriate tension regardless of the flexion angle. Woo et al.[64] showed less anterior translation with graft fixation at 30 degrees than in full extension. Yasuda et al.[60] also recommended a 30 degree flexion angle at the time of fixation. Bylski-Austrow et al.[65] found that 44 N at full extension best restrained anterior translation. They acknowledged that since AP translation is greatest at 30 degrees, tensioning at this angle would adequately tighten the knee. However, tensioning at this angle may overconstrain the knee. Amis and Jakob[62] recommended 10 degrees of flexion during fixation. Currently there is no consensus regarding the angle of knee flexion during graft fixation.

■ GRAFT FIXATION

Fixation of the graft is vitally important in the stability of the reconstruction. Full biologic incorporation of the graft into host bone may not occur for at least 6 months in patellar tendon autograft, and longer in allograft.[16] Thus, the initial stability depends on the ability of the fixation device to withstand normal cyclic loads as well as sudden loads. Multiple studies have shown that early instability following ACL reconstruction is often due to a failure of fixation.[66-69] Rodeo et al.,[18] in their study of tendon-to-bone healing, showed that although tendon-to-bone healing occurs most rapidly during the first 4 weeks, failure at the graft bone interface occurred up to 8 weeks. Failure between 12 to 24 weeks occurred at the graft midsubstance. They also demonstrated that tendon-to-bone healing occurs secondary to progressive organization and mineralization of the collagen at the tendon-to-bone interface and ultimately in-growth of bone into the tendon. The construct is morphologically similar to Sharpey fibers.

Bone-patellar tendon-bone (BPTB) healing is similar to fracture healing. It is stronger and faster than tendon-to-bone healing. During the first 6 to 12 weeks, while healing of the graft to host bone occurs, the fixation device must withstand normal cyclic loads that occur during rehabilitation, as well as sudden forces that can be as high as 450 to 500 N.[70]

Failure occurs most commonly at the tibial tunnel.[69,71] In fact, tibial fixation has been called the "weak link" in ACL reconstruction, with a lower ultimate load of failure.[71] This low ultimate load may be influenced by two factors: bone density and the angle between the tunnel and the intra-articular portion of the graft. Dual energy x-ray absorptiometry (DEXA) scans of the tibia and femur show less bone mineral density in the tibia compared with the femur. There appears to be a positive correlation between bone mineral density and mean load to failure.[72] Less dense bone provides less contact for the fixation device. Also, during weight bearing, the tibial tunnel and the graft are more colinear compared with the oblique orientation between the femoral tunnel and the graft. This allows for larger axial forces at the tibia-graft interface and may result in a lower failure load.[73] Improving contact or the interference in the tibial tunnel by compacting the cancellous bone and allowing a more precise match of the tunnel to the graft diameter can increase the pull out strength of the graft. Underreaming the tibial tunnel by 2 mm and then sequentially dilating the tunnel by 0.5 mm can help compact the bone and improve contact.[74]

Tunnel length may also play a role. Increasing the length of the tibial screw may improve interference.[74]

Historically fixation methods have been varied and include screws, staples, washers, or sutures over buttons. Multiple studies have been conducted to assess strength and stiffness of these devices.[66–86] It is difficult to compare fixation studies because of the wide variation in fixation and testing methods **(Table 34-2)**. In general, direct fixation devices such as screws and cross pins allow less longitudinal graft motion than indirect fixation.

Interference screw fixation has become the standard for BPTB reconstruction. Kurosaka et al.[66] demonstrated that interference screws provide the greatest strength and load failure when compared to staples or sutures over buttons. Factors that affect the fixation strength include screw diameter, gap size, and the divergence angle between the screw and the bone block.[66–68]

Care should be taken to insert the screw in a parallel alignment with the graft. Divergence greater than 15 degrees can result in a loss of fixation and bone plug pull out.[81] The size of the gap between the bone plug and the tunnel wall should also be assessed. Though Brown et al.[68] found no significant difference in femoral fixation strength between 9 mm (rear entry inserted) and 7 mm (arthroscopically inserted) screws, Butler et al.[67] found that there was a significant difference if the gap size was 3 to 4 mm. The 9 mm screws provided better fixation for a gap between the bone plug and the tunnel wall of 3 to 4 mm. No difference in fixation strength was found between the 7 and 9 mm screws for a gap of 1 to 2 mm. Butler et al. recommend using a 9 mm screw for a gap of 3 to 4 mm. Pitfalls of interference screws include inadvertent graft advancement with loss of tension, suture laceration with loss of fixation, and screw-plug length mismatch.[82]

TABLE 34-2	Failure Strength of Various Devices of Graft Fixation	
Fixation device	**Ultimate failure load (N)**	**Reference no.**
Patellar tendon		
Metal interference screw	558	74
Bioabsorbable interference screw	552	74
Hamstring—femoral		
Bone Mulch Screw	1,112	85
EndoButton	1,086	85
Rigidfix	868	85
SmartScrew ACL	794	85
BioScrew	589	85
RCI Screw	546	85
Hamstring—tibial		
Intrafix	1,332	86
WasherLoc	975	86
Tandem spiked washer	769	86
SmartScrew ACL	665	86
BioScrew	612	86
Soft Silk	471	86

Interference screw sizes include 7 mm, 8 mm, and 9 mm at varied lengths (20 mm, 25 mm, 30 mm). Femoral fixation is routinely accomplished with 7 mm and 8 mm screws. The tibia typically requires 9 mm screws. Bioabsorbable screws have been shown to be comparable to titanium screws at physiologic loads with the added advantage of computed tomography and magnetic resonance imaging compatibility, less risk to sutures, and no need for removal in revision surgery. The disadvantages of biodegradable screws include breakage and failure during insertion. Also, their effect on graft healing is not well documented.

Soft tissue fixation is stronger with screw and washer constructs and weakest with staple fixation.[83] Bioabsorbable interference screws may be used as the tendon and sutures are at less risk of injury than with metallic screws, but there is still concern about slippage. The diameter of the bioabsorbable screw should approximate that of the tunnel to help improve the pull out strength.[78] Femoral fixation can be accomplished with a bioscrew, cross-pin, an EndoButton, or a post. Kousa et al.[85,86] reviewed the fixation strength of six hamstring tendon graft fixation devices for the tibial and femoral side during ACL reconstruction. On the femoral side, they noted superior fixation with the Bone Mulch Screw (1112 N) when compared to the other techniques in the single-cycle load-to-failure test. The other devices that were evaluated were the EndoButton CL (1086 N), RigidFix (868 N), SmartScrew ACL (794 N), BioScrew (589 N), and the RCI Screw (546 N). The yield load of the Bone Mulch Screw was significantly greater than the BioScrew and the RCI Screw. The stiffness of the Bone Mulch Screw fixation (115 N/m) was significantly higher than the stiffness of the EndoButton CL (79 N/m), RigidFix (77 N/m), BioScrew (66 N/m), and the RCI Screw (68 N/m). The Bone Mulch Screw stiffness was not significantly greater than the SmartScrew (96 N/m).[84]

On the tibial side, Kousa et al.[86] showed that Intrafix (1332 N) was the strongest (statistically significant) in the single-cycle load-to-failure test, followed by the WasherLoc (975 N), spiked washer (769 N), SmartScrew ACL (665 N), BioScrew (612 N), and SoftSilk (471 N). The Intrafix also had a significantly higher stiffness (223 N) than the WasherLoc (87 N/m), the spiked washer (69 N/m), the SmartScrew ACL (115 N/m), the BioScrew (91 N/m), and the SoftSilk (61 N/m).

■ REHABILITATION

Rehabilitation of the ACL reconstructed knee is extremely important to the patient's overall functional outcome. The philosophy that has influenced rehabilitation protocols has undergone a drastic change in the past 15 years. The conservative approaches that emphasized healing of the graft and stability of the knee were based largely on concepts that both time and control of the forces across the knee were necessary for ligament healing and a good outcome.[87] Long periods of immobilization (3 to 12 weeks), followed by gradual weight bearing and progressive range of motion, with slow return to activities and strengthening, were the norm. Changes in the mid- to late 1980s allowed for less immobilization, but the trend was still toward protection of the knee.[88] Complications such as joint stiffness, arthrofibrosis, extensor lag, and quad weakness have been attributed to delayed joint motion and muscle strengthening.[28,89,90] Accelerated protocols, promoted since 1990, have been proven to improve patient functional outcomes and to result in less complications.[28,89,91] The goal of rehabilitation is to return the patient to preinjury joint motion and strength, without injuring or elongating the graft. Protocols are varied, but studies that analyze strain behavior of the native ACL during various exercises have provided some guidelines. Beynnon et al.[92] have shown increased ACL strain with quadriceps dominated exercises between 0 to 30 degrees, simultaneous quadriceps and hamstring exercises at 15 degrees, and unrestrained active range of motion with or without weights. They recommended immediate passive range of motion and low strain ACL exercises such as isometric hamstring exercises, simultaneous quad and hamstring contractions at 30 degrees, 60 degrees, 90 degrees, and active flexion and extension without weights at 35 degrees to 90 degrees. The rehabilitation process is slower for allografts than for autografts. A detailed rehabilitation protocol was recently published by Wilk et al.[93]

■ RETURN TO PLAY

Multiple criteria, including functional testing, clinical evaluation, and subjective assessment, should be used to determine when to allow a patient to return to full activity. These criteria evaluate different aspects of the recovery process.

A full range of motion is needed for return to sports. Regaining less than full motion will place the extremity at a mechanical disadvantage and increases the risk for reinjury. Muscle strength and balance must be achieved to provide the required dynamic stability.

What defines successful return to play? Is it based on an earlier return to play, level of competition, or stability and strength of the knee? Most of the data, which are surgeon and technique-dependent, support the patellar tendon autograft as the graft of choice for a "quicker" return to play.

O'Neill[94] performed a prospective randomized analysis of three ACL reconstruction techniques in 127 patients, including hamstring autograft, two-incision patellar tendon autograft, and a single-incision patellar tendon autograft. The return to preinjury level of activity was 88% in the hamstring group, 95% in the two-incision group, and 89% in the one-incision group.

In a prospective randomized comparison, Shaieb et al.[22] showed a significant reduction in activities following ACL reconstruction with both the patellar tendon and hamstring autografts. The reduction in activity was 45% in the patellar group and 37% in the hamstring group. Many patients reported a decrease in activity because they were no longer participating in high school or college sports.

Bach et al.[95] retrospectively reviewed 97 patients who had undergone ACL reconstruction with a two-incision technique, using patellar tendon autograft. Fifty-three patients (58%) returned to their preinjury sports level, and 18 (18%) indicated a decrease in activity level because of their knee. Fourteen patients (15%) had a decrease in activity unrelated to their knee. Three patients (3%) stated that they stopped all sports because of knee problems, and 4 (4%) stopped for problems unrelated to their knee.

A meta-analysis by Yunes et al.[96] compared patellar tendon and hamstring autografts. Four studies with at least a 2-year follow-up met the criteria for inclusion. The patellar tendon group had significantly better results regarding return to preinjury activity levels. The patellar group had a 75% return to preinjury activity level compared to a 64% return level with the hamstring reconstruction.

Shino et al.[97] reviewed 84 patients who had undergone ACL reconstruction with soft-tissue allografts. All but two of the patients had injured their knees during a sporting event. Seventy-nine patients (94%) returned to their desired activity level.

For patients whose priority is a quick return to sports, Shelbourne and Urch[98] recommend ACL reconstruction with a contralateral patellar tendon autograft. They reviewed patients who had undergone a primary ACL reconstruction with either the contralateral ($N = 434$) or ipsilateral ($N = 228$) patellar tendon to determine the difference between the groups with regards to range of motion, quadriceps strength, and return to sports. The patients were divided into three subgroups. The competitive subgroup consisted of 260 athletes who competed in twisting, pivoting, or jumping sports at either a high school, collegiate, or professional level. The recreational subgroup consisted of 172 patients, over 26 years old, who competed in similar activities at a recreational level. The third subgroup had 230 patients who were either participating in sports that did not involve jumping or pivoting, or who did not meet the age requirement for the recreational subgroup. The average time for the patients to return to sport participation at their full preinjury capacity was 4.9 and 6.1 months for the contralateral and ipsilateral groups, respectively. The competitive subgroup returned to sports at their full capability at 4.1 months for the contralateral group and 5.5 months for the ipsilateral group.

Return to play outcomes are variable depending on the study. Many of the reported ACL series do not address the preinjury or postinjury activity level. Following an ACL reconstruction, many patients do not return to their preinjury level. Various factors have been cited for this decrease in activity including lifestyle changes (out of school, no longer competing), fear of recurrent knee injury, instability, and pain. Return to play criteria should incorporate many factors such as agility, strength, clinical stability, and range of motion.

■ SUMMARY

The ideal graft for ACL reconstruction should have similar biomechanical properties as a native ACL, allow for stable initial fixation, and have rapid biological incorporation and low morbidity. The most appropriate graft depends on many factors, including the surgeon's philosophy and experience, tissue availability, and the patient's activity level.

Tunnel placement must be anatomically precise to reproduce the anatomy and isometry of the ACL. Until there is biologic incorporation of the graft into host bone, the fixation device has to withstand normal cyclic forces during rehabilitation without graft slippage or pullout. There has recently been a vast increase in the types of fixation devices that are available for ACL reconstruction and a significant improvement in the ultimate failure loads of these devices.

The graft must then be tensioned adequately to prevent anterior-posterior translation, but also to allow for full range of motion. High graft tension alters knee kinematics and can lead to loss of motion, failure, and degenerative change within the graft and at the articular surface. Low graft tension can result in persistent instability and subsequent meniscal or articular cartilage injury. The flexion angle of the knee during tibial fixation remains controversial. Aggressive rehabilitation helps to decrease complications and allows for a quicker return to play.

■ REFERENCES

1. Butler DL, Noyes FR, Grood ES. Ligamentous restraints to anterior-posterior drawer in the human knee. J Bone Joint Surg. 1980;62A:259–270.
2. Markolf KL, Mensch JS, Amstutz HC. Stiffness and laxity of the knee: the contributions of the supporting structures. J Bone Joint Surg. 1976;58A:583–593.
3. Indelicato PA, Bittar ES. A perspective of lesions associated with ACL deficiency of the knee. Clin Orthop. 1985;198:77–80.
4. Cerabona F, Sherman MF, Bonomo JR, et al. Patterns of meniscal injury with acute ACL tears. Am J Sports Med. 1988;16:603–609.
5. Noyes FR, Bassett RW, Grood ES, et al. Arthroscopy in acute traumatic hemarthrosis of the knee: incidence of anterior cruciate ligament tears and other injuries. J Bone Joint Surg. 1980;62A:687–695.
6. Noyes FR, McGinnis GH, Grood ES. The variable functional disability of the anterior cruciate-deficient knee. Orthop Clinic North Am. 1985;16:47–67.
7. DeHaven KE. Diagnosis of acute knee injuries with hemarthrosis. Am J Sports Med. 1980;8:9.
8. Warren RF, Levy IM. Meniscal lesions associated with anterior cruciate ligament injury. Clin Orthop. 1983;172:32–37.
9. Marzo JM, Waren RF. Results of treatment of anterior cruciate ligament injury: changing perspectives. Adv Orthop Surg. 1991; 15:59–69.
10. Freedman KB, D'Amato MJ, Nedeff DD, et al. Arthroscopic anterior cruciate ligament reconstruction: a meta-analysis comparing patellar tendon and hamstring tendon autografts. Am J Sports Med. 2003;31:2–11.
11. Woo SL-Y, Hollis JM, Adams DJ, et al. Tensile properties of the human femur-anterior cruciate ligament complex. Am J Sports Med. 1991;19:217–225.
12. Noyes FR, Butler DL, Grood ES, et al. Biomechanical analysis of human ligament grafts used in knee-ligament repairs and reconstruction. J Bone Joint Surg. 1984;66-A:344–352.

13. Hamner DL, Brown CH, Steiner ME, et al. Hamstring tendon grafts for reconstruction of the anterior cruciate ligament: biomechanical evaluation of the use of multiple strands and tensioning techniques. J Bone Joint Surg. 1999;81-A:549–557.

14. Staubli HU, Schatzmann L, Brunner P, et al. Mechanical tensile properties of the quadriceps tendon and patellar ligament in young adults. Am J Sports Med. 1999;27:27–34.

15. Butler DL, Grood ES, Noyes FR, et al. On the interpretation of our anterior cruciate ligament data. Clin Ortho. 1985;196:26–34.

16. Markholf KL, Burchfield DM, Shapiro MM, et al. Biomechanical consequences of replacement of the anterior cruciate ligament with a patellar ligament allograft. Part II: forces in the graft compared with forces in the intact ligament. J Bone Joint Surg. 1996;78A: 1728–1734.

17. Jackson DW, Grood ES, Goldstein, JD, et al. A comparison of patellar tendon autograft and allograft used for anterior cruciate ligament reconstruction in the goat model. Am J Sports Med. 1993;21:176–185.

18. Rodeo SA, Arnoczky SP, Torzilli PA, et al. Tendon-healing in a bone tunnel: a biomechanical and histological study in the dog. J Bone Joint Surg. 1993;75A:1795–1803.

19. Fulkerson JP, Langleland R. An alternative cruciate reconstruction graft: the quadriceps tendon. Arthroscopy. 1995;2:252–254.

20. Aune A, Holm I, Risberg MA, et al. Four-strand hamstring tendon autograft compared with patellar tendon-bone autograft for anterior cruciate ligament reconstruction: a randomized study with two-year follow-up. Am J Sports Med. 2001;29:722–728.

21. Ejerhed L, Kartus J, Sernet N, et al. Patellar tendon or semitendinosus tendon autografts for anterior cruciate ligament reconstruction? A prospective randomized study with a two-year follow-up. Am J Sports Med. 2003;31:19–25.

22. Shaieb MD, Kan DM, Chang SK, et al. A prospective randomized comparison of patellar tendon versus semitendinosus and gracilis tendon autografts for anterior cruciate ligament reconstruction. Am J Sports Med. 2002;30:214–220.

23. Jansson KA, Linko E, Sandelin J, et al. A prospective randomized study of patellar versus hamstring tendon autografts for anterior cruciate ligament reconstruction. Am J Sports Med. 2003;31:12–18.

24. Beynnon BD, Johnson RJ, Fleming BC. Anterior cruciate ligament replacement: comparison of bone-patellar tendon-bone grafts with two-strand hamstring grafts. J Bone Joint Surg. 2002; 84A:1503–1513.

25. Aglietti P, Buzzi R, D'Andria S, et al. Patellofemoral problems after intraarticular anterior cruciate ligament reconstruction. Clin Orthop Relat Res. 1993;288:195–204.

26. Shelton WR, Papendick L, Dukes AD. Autograft versus allograft anterior cruciate ligament reconstruction. Arthroscopy. 1997;13: 446–449.

27. Sachs RA, Daniel DM, Stone ML, et al. Patellofemoral problems after anterior cruciate ligament reconstruction. Am J Sports Med. 1989;17:760–765.

28. Shelbourne KD, Nitz P. Accelerated rehabilitation after anterior cruciate ligament reconstruction. Am J Sports Med. 1990;18: 292–299.

29. Rosenberg TD, Franklin JL, Baldwin GN, et al. Extensor mechanism function after patellar tendon graft harvest for anterior cruciate ligament reconstruction. Am J Sports Med. 1992;20:519–526.

30. Lephart SM, Kocher MS, Harner CD, et al. Quadriceps strength and functional capacity after anterior cruciate ligament reconstruction. Am J Sports Med. 1993;21:738–743.

31. Carter TR, Edinger S. Isokinetic evaluation of anterior cruciate ligament reconstruction: hamstring versus patellar tendon. Arthroscopy. 1999;15:169–172.

32. Nakamura N, Horibe S, Sasaki S, et al. Evaluation of active knee flexion and hamstring strength after anterior cruciate ligament reconstruction using hamstring tendons. Arthroscopy. 2002;18: 598–602.

33. Yasuda K, Tsujino S, Yasumitsu O, et al. Graft site morbidity with autogenous semitendinosus and gracilis tendons. Am J Sports Med. 1995;23:706–714.

34. Viola R, Vianello R. Three cases of patella fracture in 1,320 anterior cruciate ligament reconstructions with bone-patellar tendon-bone autograft. Arthroscopy. 1999;15:93–97.

35. Miller SL, Gladstone JN. Graft selection in anterior cruciate ligament reconstruction. Orthop Clin North Am. 2002;33:675–683.

36. Shelton WR. Allografts in knee reconstruction: basic science and current status. J Am Acad Orthop Surg. 1998;6(3):165–168.

37. Simonds RJ, Holmberg SD, Hurwitz RL, et al. Transmission of human immunodeficiency virus type 1 from a seronegative organ and tissue donor. N Engl J Med. 1992;326:726–732.

38. Jackson DW, Windler GE, Simon TM. Intraarticular reaction associated with the use of freeze-dried, ethylene oxide-sterilized bone-patellar tendon-bone allografts in the reconstruction of the anterior cruciate ligament. Am J Sports Med. 1990;18:1–10.

39. Vangsness CT, Garcia IA, Mills R, et al. Allograft transplantation in the knee: tissue regulation, procurement, processing, and sterilization. Am J Sports Med. 2003;31:474–481.

40. Zoltan DJ, Reinecke C, Indelicato PA. Synthetic and allograft anterior cruciate ligament reconstruction. Clin Sports Med. 1988;7:773–784.

41. Makisalo S, Skutnabb K, Holmstrom J, et al. Reconstruction of the anterior cruciate ligament with carbon fiber. Am J Sports Med. 1988;16:589–593.

42. Kumar K, Maffulli N. The ligament augmentation device: a historical perspective. Arthroscopy. 1999;15:422–432.

43. Arnoczky SP, Warren RF. Anatomy of the cruciate. In: Feagin JA, ed. *Crucial Ligaments*. New York: Churchill Livingstone; 1988:179–196.

44. Buzzi R, Zaccherotti G, Giron F, et al. The relationship between the intercondylar roof and the tibial plateau with the knee in extension: relevance for tibial tunnel placement in anterior cruciate ligament reconstruction. Arthroscopy. 1999;15:625–631.

45. Howell SM, Taylor MA. Failure of reconstruction of the anterior cruciate ligament due to impingement by the intercondylar roof. J Bone Joint Surg. 1993;75-A:1044–1055.

46. Jackson DW, Gasser SI. Tibial tunnel placement in ACL reconstruction. Arthroscopy. 1994;10:124–131.

47. Khalfayan EE, Sharkley PF, Alexander AH, et al. The relationship between tunnel placement and clinical results after anterior cruciate ligament reconstruction. Am J Sports Med. 1996;24:335–341.

48. Woo SL-Y, Kanamori A, Zeminski J, et al. The effectiveness of reconstruction of the anterior cruciate ligament with hamstrings and patellar tendon: a cadaveric study comparing anterior tibial and rotational loads. J Bone Joint Surg. 2002;84A:907–914.

49. Zaricznyj B. Reconstruction of the anterior cruciate ligament of the knee using a doubled tendon graft. Clin Orthop. 1987;220: 162–175.

50. Romano VM, Graf BK, Keene JS, et al. Anterior cruciate ligament reconstruction: the effect of tibial tunnel placement on range of motion. Am J Sports Med. 1993;21:415–418.

51. Tekeuchi R, Saito T, Mituhashi S, et al. Double-bundle anatomic anterior cruciate ligament reconstruction using bone-hamsting-bone composite graft. Arthroscopy. 2002;18:550–555.

52. Maracci M, Molgora AP, Zaffagnini S, et al. Anatomic double-bundle anterior cruciate ligament reconstruction with hamstrings. Arthroscopy. 2003;19:540–546.

53. Pederzini L, Adriani E, Botticella C, et al. Double tibial tunnel using quadriceps tendon in anterior cruciate ligament reconstruction. Arthroscopy. 2000;16:E9.

54. Hara K, Kubo T, Suginoshito T, et al. Reconstruction of the anterior cruciate ligament using a double bundle. Arthroscopy. 2000; 16:860–864.

55. Muneta T, Sekiya I, Yagishita K, et al. Two-bundle reconstruction of the anterior cruciate ligament using semitendinosis tendon with endobuttons: operative technique and preliminary results. Arthroscopy. 1999;15:618–624.

56. Yagi M, Wong, EK, Kanamori A, et al. Biomechanical analysis of an anatomic anterior cruciate ligament reconstruction. Am J Sports Med. 2002;30:660–666.

57. Giron F, Buzzi R, Aglietti P, et al. Femoral tunnel position in anterior cruciate ligament reconstruction using three techniques: a cadaver study. Arthroscopy. 1999;15:750–756.

58. Loh JC, Fukada Y, Tsuda E, et al. Knee stability and graft function following anterior cruciate ligament reconstruction: comparison between 11 o'clock and 10 o'clock femoral tunnel placement. Arthroscopy. 2003;19:297–304.

59. Amis AA, Dawkins GP. Functional anatomy of the anterior cruciate ligament: fiber bundle actions related to ligament replacements and injuries. J Bone Joint Surg Br. 1991;73(2):260–267.

60. Yasuda K, Tsujino J, Tanabe Y, et al. Effects of initial graft tension on clinical outcome after anterior cruciate ligament reconstruction: autogenous doubled hamstring tendons connected in series with polyester tapes. Am J Sports Med. 1997;25(1):99–106.

61. Yoshiya S, Andrish JT, Manley MT, et al. Graft tension in anterior cruciate ligament reconstruction: an in vivo study in dogs. Am J Sports Med. 1987;15:464–470.

62. Amis AA, Jakob RP. Anterior cruciate ligament graft positioning, tensioning and twisting. Knee Surg Sports Traumatol Arthrosc. 1998;6(suppl 1):S2–S12.

63. Friederich NF, O'Brien WR. Anterior cruciate ligament graft tensioning versus knee stability. Knee Surg Sports Traumatol Arthorsc. 1998;6(suppl 1):S38–S42.

64. Woo SL-Y, Hollis JM, Adams DJ, et al. Tensile properties of the human femur-anterior cruciate ligament complex. Am J Sports Med. 1991;19:217–225.

65. Bylski-Austrow DI, Grood ES, Hefzy MS, et al. Anterior cruciate ligament replacements: a mechanical study of femoral attachment location, flexion angle at tensioning, and initial tension. J Orthop Res. 1990;8:552–531.

66. Kurosaka M, Yoshiya A, Andrish JT. A biomechanical comparison of different surgical techniques of graft fixation in anterior cruciate ligament reconstruction. Am J Sports Med. 1987;15(3):225–229.

67. Butler JC, Branch TP, Hutton WC. Optimal graft fixation—the effect of gap size and screw size on bone plug fixation in ACL reconstruction. Arthroscopy. 1994;10:524–529.

68. Brown CH, Hecker AT, Hipp JA, et al. The biomechanics of interference screw fixation of patellar tendon anterior cruciate ligament grafts. Am J Sports Med. 1993;21(6):880–886.

69. Steiner ME, Hecker AT, Brown CH, et al. Anterior cruciate ligament graft fixation: comparison of hamstring and patellar tendon grafts. Am J Sports Med. 1994 Sept-Oct;22(5):659–666.

70. Frank CB, Jackson DW. The science of reconstruction of the anterior cruciate ligament. J Bone Joint Surg. 1997;79-A:1556–1576.

71. Kohn D, Rose C. Primary stability of interference screw fixation: influence of screw diameter and insertion torque. Am J Sports Med. 1994;22:334–338.

72. Brand J, Caborn D, Steenlage E, et al. Interference screw fixation strength of a quadrupled hamstring tendon is directly correlated to bone mineral density measured by dual photon absorptimetry (DEXA). Arthroscopy. 1999;15:S8–S9.

73. Brand J, Weiler A, Caborn DNM, et al. Graft fixation in cruciate ligament reconstruction. Am J Sports Med. 2000;28(5):761–774.

74. Caborn DNM, Urban WP Jr, Johnson DL, et al. Biomechanical comparison between bioscrew and titanium alloy interference screws for bone-patellar tendon-bone graft fixation in anterior cruciate ligament reconstruction. Arthroscopy. 1997;13:229–232.

75. Selby JB, Johnson DL, Hester P, et al. Effect of screw length on bioabsorbable interference screw fixation in a tibial bone tunnel. Am J Sports Med. 2001;29(5):614–619.

76. Steenlage E, Brand J, Caborn D, et al. Interference screw fixation of a quadrupled hamstring graft is improved with precise match of tunnel to graft diameter. Arthroscopy. 1999;15:S9–S10.

77. Kurosaka M, Yoshiya S, Andrish JT. A biomechanical comparison of different surgical techniques of graft fixation in the anterior cruciate ligament reconstruction. Am J Sports Med. 1987;15(3):225–229.

78. Gerich TG, Cassim A, Lattermann C, et al. Pullout strength of tibial graft fixation in anterior cruciate ligament replacement with a patellar tendon graft: interference screw versus staple fixation in human knees. Knee Surg Sports Traumatol Arthrosc. 1997;5:84–89.

79. Martin SD, Martin TL, Brown CH. Anterior cruciate ligament graft fixation. Orthop Clin North Am 2002;33:685–696.

80. Fu FH, Bennett CH, Lattermann C, et al. Current trends in anterior cruciate ligament reconstruction. Part 1: Biology and biomechanics of reconstruction. Am J Sports Med. 1999;27:821–830.

81. Lemos MJ, Douglas WJ, Lee TQ, et al. Assessment of initial fixation of endoscopic interference femoral screws with divergent and parallel placement. Arthroscopy. 1995;11:37–41.

82. Matthews LS, Soffer SR. Pitfalls in the use of interference screws for anterior cruciate ligament reconstruction: brief report. Arthroscopy. 1989;5:225–226.

83. Robertson DB, Daniel DM, Biden E. Soft tissue fixation in bone. Am J Sports Med. 1986;14:398–403.

84. Clark R, Olsen RE, Larson BJ, et al. Cross-pin femoral fixation: a new technique for hamstring anterior cruciate ligament reconstruction of the knee. Arthroscopy. 1998;14:258–267.

85. Kousa P, Jarvinen TL, Vihavainen M, et al. The fixation strength of six hamstring tendon graft fixation devices in anterior cruciate ligament reconstruction: part I: femoral site. Am J Sports Med. 2003;31:174–181.

86. Kousa P, Jarvinen TL, Vihavainen M, et al. The fixation strength of six hamstring tendon graft fixation devices in anterior cruciate ligament reconstruction: part II: tibial site. Am J Sports Med. 2003;31:182–188.

87. Paolos LE, Noyes FR, Grood ES. Knee rehabilitation after ACL reconstruction and repair. Am J Sports Med. 1981;9:140–149.

88. Huegel M, Indelicato P. Trends in rehab following ACL reconstruction. Clin Sports Med. 1988;7:801–811.

89. Shelborne KD, Wilckens JH, Mollabashy A, et al. Arthrofibrosis in acute anterior cruciate ligament reconstruction. The effect of timing of reconstruction and rehabilitation. Am J Sports Med. 1991;19:332–336.

90. Hughston JC. Complications of anterior cruciate ligament surgery. Orthop Clin North Am. 1985;16:237–240.

91. Wilk KE, Andrews JR. Current concepts in the treatment of anterior cruciate ligament disruption. J Orthop Sports Phys Ther. 1992;15:279–293.

92. Beynnon BD, Fleming BC, Johnson RL, et al. Anterior cruciate ligament strain behavior during rehabilitation exercises in vivo. Am J Sports Med. 1995;23:24–34.

93. Wilk KE, Reinold MM, Hooks TR. Recent advances in the rehabilitation of isolated and combined anterior cruciate ligament injuries. Orthop Clin North Am. 2003;34:107–137.

94. O'Neill DB. Arthroscopically assisted reconstruction of the anterior cruciate ligament: a prospective randomized analysis of three techniques. J Bone Joint Surg. 1996;78A:803–813.

95. Bach BR, Tradonsky S, Bojchuk J, et al. Arthroscopically assisted anterior cruciate ligament reconstruction using patellar tendon autograft: five- to nine-year follow-up. Am J Sports Med. 1998;26:20–29.

96. Yunes M, Richmond JC, Engels EA, et al. Patellar versus hamstring in anterior cruciate ligament reconstruction: a meta-analysis. Arthroscopy. 2001;17:248–257.

97. Shino K, Inque M, Horibe S, et al. Reconstruction of the anterior cruciate ligament using allogeneic tendon. Am J Sports Med. 1990;18:457–465.

98. Shelbourne KD, Urch SE. Primary anterior cruciate ligament reconstruction using the contralateral autogenous patellar tendon. Am J Sports Med. 2000;28:651–658.

ANTERIOR CRUCIATE LIGAMENT RECONSTRUCTION WITH PATELLAR TENDON AUTOGRAFT: SURGICAL TECHNIQUE

35

BRUCE S. MILLER, MD, EDWARD M. WOJTYS, MD

■ HISTORY OF THE TECHNIQUE

The natural history of anterior cruciate ligament (ACL) insufficiency in an active individual has been well described and includes recurrent functional instability, failure of secondary restraints, meniscal and chondral injuries, and the subsequent development of arthrosis.[1,2] Consequently, surgical treatment is frequently indicated in those who are physically active. Early efforts at anatomic repair of the injured ACL resulted in poor functional outcomes.[3] As a result, direct repair is presently reserved primarily for distal tibial avulsion fractures. Several factors have led to the emergence and popularity of modern techniques for reconstruction of the ACL.

Numerous extra-articular reconstructive procedures have been described for ACL insufficiency. Unlike present intra-articular anatomic ACL reconstructive techniques, these extra-articular procedures were intended to address instability by tightening secondary restraints, most commonly on the lateral side of the knee. Tenodesis of the iliotibial band in some fashion was the most common extra-articular procedure. Presently, extra-articular techniques are rarely employed and are reserved primarily for supplementation of intra-articular reconstructions in the presence of severe laxity of secondary restraints.

The goal of intra-articular ACL reconstruction is to anatomically replace the torn ligament with a biologic graft. Many graft types, including autograft, allograft, and occasionally synthetic devices, are currently implanted using a similar arthroscopically assisted surgical technique.

■ INDICATIONS AND CONTRAINDICATIONS

Anterior cruciate ligament reconstruction is indicated in those individuals with symptomatic instability of the knee who wish to return to sporting or occupational activities that require jumping, cutting, or pivoting activities. A patient's desired activity level, rather than chronologic age, should guide the decision-making process. Thus, ACL reconstruction is certainly a viable option in the older ACL-deficient individual who desires to remain active. ACL reconstruction in the skeletally immature patient is commonly performed safely but is beyond the scope of this chapter.

ACL reconstruction may be contraindicated in the acutely injured knee. In the acute setting, resolution of pain and effusion, return of full range of motion, and complete recovery of quadriceps function should be the goal prior to surgical intervention. Unfortunately, meniscal and chondral injuries can make the preoperative goals difficult or even unattainable, creating a dilemma for the surgeon. Although one procedure is usually the goal to address all pathology present, if preoperative range of motion and function has been severely compromised, thought should be given to addressing these chondral or meniscal issues prior to ACL reconstruction. ACL reconstruction requires a challenging postoperative rehabilitation regimen and should not be considered in an individual who is unwilling or unable to meet this challenge.

The patellar tendon autograft is an excellent graft option for most patients. However, a history of patellar tendonitis, chronic anterior knee pain, or the presence of significant patellofemoral degenerative disease in the injured extremity may be considered a relative contraindication to the use of this graft.

■ SURGICAL TECHNIQUE

Anesthesia and Positioning

The patient is placed supine on the operating table, and a thigh tourniquet is applied as proximal as possible on the operative extremity. The patient's pelvis should be moved toward the edge of the table to allow flexion of the knee off the side of the table during the operative procedure. A lateral post is applied to the table about the level of the junction between the middle and distal thirds to facilitate arthroscopic evaluation of the medial compartment.

General or regional anesthesia can be employed for ACL reconstruction. However, we do not routinely advocate the use of regional nerve blocks for postoperative pain control, as these are usually unnecessary and may interfere with the patient's ability to protect the knee against inadvertent injury in the immediate postoperative period. The combination of ketorolac tromethamine (pre- and postoperatively) along with intra-articular morphine and parenteral-local anesthetics appears to provide excellent pain relief when used in combination with oral analgesics.

A careful examination under anesthesia is a critical component of the surgical decision-making process. A side-to-side comparison of range of motion and ligamentous stability is imperative. Lachman, anterior and posterior drawer, varus-valgus stress maneuvers, rotation and patellar tests should be performed and recorded. The pivot shift test, which is often difficult to assess in the office setting, can be performed consistently in the operating room.

Surface Anatomy

Relevant anatomic landmarks include the patella, patellar tendon, tibial tubercle, and joint line. These landmarks can be marked at the beginning of the procedure to facilitate the graft harvest. In addition, sites of arthroscopic portals and incisions for possible meniscus repairs should be delineated.

Skin Incision

Use of the tourniquet is optional. Although its use may delay return of muscle function postoperatively, it can decrease operating time by facilitating visualization. The leg is exsanguinated and the tourniquet elevated prior to incision to facilitate visualization during graft harvest. The skin incision can be placed in several positions for patella tendon harvest. A medially based incision at the edge of the tendon may yield more cosmetic results. A central incision extending longitudinally from the inferior pole of the patella at midline to the medial aspect of the tibial tubercle is also acceptable **(Fig. 35-1)**. The obliquity of the incision allows for adequate exposure for both graft harvest and tibial tunnel placement. If the patient's occupation requires frequent kneeling, then the incision can be moved more medially to avoid potential irritation over the midline and tibial tubercle. The incision may disrupt fibers of the infrapatellar branch of the saphenous nerve. As a result, the patient must be counseled to expect a small area of numbness lateral to the incision, which usually diminishes with time.

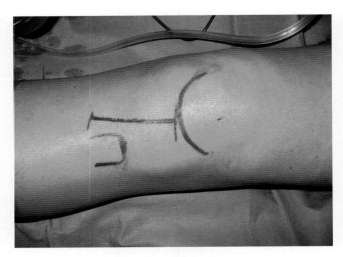

Fig. 35-1. Skin incision.

Graft Harvest and Preparation

The skin incision is carried sharply to the level of the peritenon. Transverse fibers can often be visualized in this layer and can help distinguish this layer from the longitudinal fibers of the patellar tendon below. The peritenon is divided longitudinally at midline and carefully dissected to reveal the medial and lateral aspects of the underlying patellar tendon. A ruler is then used to identify the central 10 mm of the tendon and a no. 11 scalpel is then employed to divide the tendon longitudinally in line with its fibers. A 10-mm wide by 20- to 30-mm bone plug (depending on patient size) is measured and marked at the tibial tubercle, with a similar plug marked on the distal pole of the patella. An oscillating saw is utilized with care to create the medial and lateral borders of a trapezoidal bone block from the tibial tubercle. The saw blade can be marked with tape at 10 mm to prevent deep cuts with the saw. The distal aspect of the bone block is also cut with the saw or prepared by multiple fenestrations with a drill bit. A straight, narrow osteotome is used to ensure completion of the osteotomy on all sides of the bone block, and the block is gently elevated off its tibial bed. With the knee in full extension to facilitate exposure of the patella, the oscillating saw is used to penetrate the dorsal cortex of the two sides of the proximal bone plug. The saw or drill is used to define the superior margin of the graft, and, with great care, an osteotome is used to complete the patellar harvest. Great care must always be taken in excising patellar tendon grafts. The fibers of the patella tendon frequently converge distally. Incisions across fibers render those fibers useless and decrease the functional width of the tendon. A poorly excised 10-mm graft can yield 6 or 7 mm of functional width. Narrowed grafts may leave the patient at risk for graft failure. Excess medial or lateral patella pressure, deep saw penetration, inappropriate use of osteotomes, and failure to bone graft defects can increase the likelihood of patella fracture. Most of these situations are avoidable and should be a central focus of each surgeon's technique.

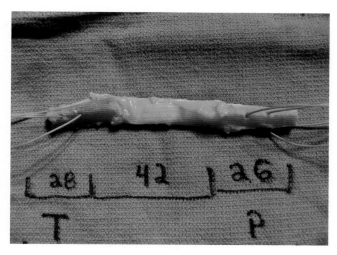

Fig. 35-2. Prepared graft.

The graft can be prepared near the surgical site or on the back table. Caution should be exercised in either preparation site to avoid accidental mishandling or contamination of the graft. The bone plugs are usually fashioned to fit through 10-mm spacers, and no. 5 nonabsorbable sutures are passed through drill holes in the bone plugs to facilitate later graft passage **(Fig. 35-2)**. The graft is wrapped in moistened sponges until implantation.

Arthroscopy

Standard arthroscopy portals are utilized for a thorough diagnostic evaluation of the knee. The menisci and chondral surfaces are inspected with great care, and all pathology is treated appropriately.

Excellent notch exposure is essential to proper graft placement. The tibial stump should be mostly, if not completely, removed. Stump remnants contain mechanoreceptors that may be of importance to the implanted graft. Consequently, efforts to preserve these fibers closest to the insertion may be worthwhile. The ACL remnant is cleared from the lateral intercondylar wall of the femur with a curette and shaving debrider to allow clear visualization of the over-the-top position. This position is identified by a veil of capsular tissue at the posterior aspect of the superior-lateral notch. This posterior position is often confused with a long ridge at the junction of the anterior two thirds and posterior one third referred to as the resident ridge. This ridge may function as a deflector for the ACL, providing a buttress to keep the ligament away from the lateral femoral condyle. Visualization posterior to the landmark is needed to properly position the graft, but complete removal of this ridge may be unwanted because of its suspected function. If the graft can be adequately positioned in this tunnel notch without bone resection, this approach is preferred. However, if there is evidence of notch stenosis, a formal notchplasty should be performed to improve visualization of the notch and protect the graft against

impingement against the lateral wall or roof of the intercondylar notch.

The tibial tunnel entrance is placed on the metaphyseal flare just anterior to the superficial medial collateral ligament. A periosteal flap measuring 2-cm long by 1-cm wide is raised prior to drilling. This flap will be sewn over the tunnel at the completion of the reconstruction. This medial site allows oblique positioning of the tibial and femoral tunnels and avoids locating the graft too centrally. A major shortcoming of the endoscopic approach that is increasingly popular today is the tendency to place the ACL graft too centrally. A centrally placed graft is nonanatomic. The central graft position can resist anterior translation, but does not provide adequate resistance to tibial rotation. If the femoral notch is pictured as the face of a clock, the preferred graft position for the right knee is 9:30 to 10:00 o'clock. In the left knee, the ideal position is between 2:00 and 2:30.

Prior to drilling the tibial tunnel, the tibial insertion of the ACL is cleared. Complete removal is usually not necessary. Care should be taken to avoid inadvertent injury to the underlying posterior cruciate ligament (PCL) or the intrameniscal ligament anteriorly. The tibial guide is introduced through the anteromedial portal. Anatomic landmarks to facilitate proper tibial tunnel placement include the native ACL footprint, the PCL, the anterior horn of the lateral meniscus, and the medial tibial eminence **(Fig. 35-3)**. The guide should be placed with enough obliquity in the coronal plane to allow for appropriate access to subsequent femoral tunnel placement. After the tibial guidewire is passed, it is overdrilled with a 10-mm reamer to create the tibial tunnel. Bone shavings from the tibial reamer are collected for later grafting of the patellar and tibial donor sites. The intra-articular aperture of the tunnel is cleared with a debrider.

The femoral guide is then introduced into the knee through the tibial tunnel and positioned as described above at the over-the-top position **(Fig. 35-4)**. For a planned 10-mm tunnel, a 6-mm posterior offset guide is used in order to

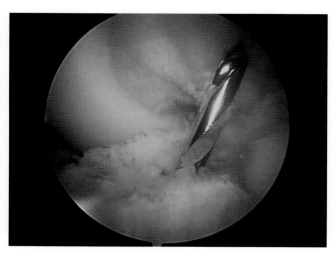

Fig. 35-3. Tibial guidewire placement.

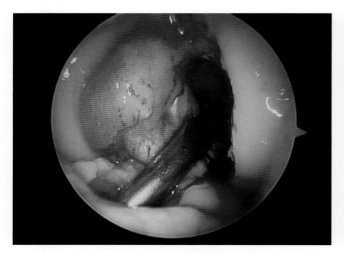

Fig. 35-4. Femoral guide placement.

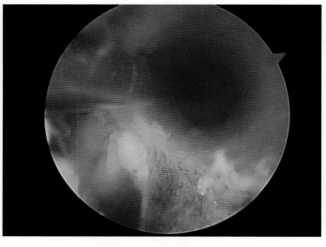

Fig. 35-5. Arthroscopic view of posterior wall of femoral tunnel.

maintain the integrity of the posterior femoral cortex. A 10-mm tunnel will have a 5-mm radius, which should leave a 1-mm thick posterior cortical wall. The femoral guidewire is passed through the femur and out the anterolateral thigh. This wire will serve as a guide for the femoral tunnel reaming as well as a device for passing the patellar tendon graft. A 10-mm reamer is placed through the tibial tunnel and advanced with care past the PCL. The femoral tunnel is created to a depth appropriate to accept the graft's tibial bone plug (usually 20 to 30 mm). At this point, the integrity of the back wall should be checked to determine if interference screw fixation is advisable **(Fig. 35-5)**. If the posterior cortex has been compromised, other forms of fixation, such as an EndoButton or a lateral cortex suture post, should be considered.

The leading sutures from the graft's tibial bone plug are then placed through the eyelet of the guidewire that traverses the knee. The wire is pulled through the thigh, and the sutures are grasped as they exit the anterolateral thigh. Under direct arthroscopic visualization, the graft is delivered

into the joint and positioned as desired. Compression of the cancellous surface of the graft against the bone tunnel may optimize healing potential. This approach requires the interference screw to be positioned carefully against the tendinous portion of the graft. The surgeon may prefer to place the screw against the cancellous side of the bone plug to avoid injury to the tendinous portion of the graft. This position may achieve a more posterior graft position as well as facilitate safe interference screw placement.

Proximal fixation of the graft is usually achieved with a cannulated metal interference screw. Hyperflexion of the knee may improve interference screw positioning on the femur. Interference screw placement is one of the hazardous portions of this procedure and demands adequate precautions. The anterior aspect of the femoral tunnel can be notched with a small curette to facilitate positioning of the screw's guidewire. A guidewire is carefully placed in the interval between the tibial bone plug and the anterior wall of the femoral tunnel. The interference screw, usually 7 by

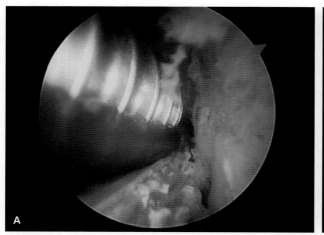

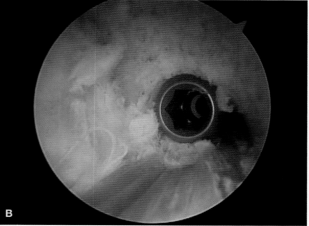

Fig. 35-6. **A:** Blue plastic sheath is protecting tendinous portion of graft from screw threads. **B:** Proximal end of graft after femoral screw fixation.

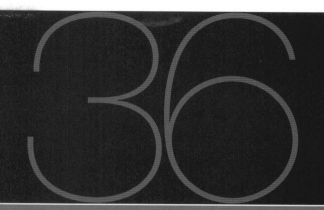

ANTERIOR CRUCIATE LIGAMENT RECONSTRUCTION: HAMSTRING AUTOGRAFT/ SINGLE AND DOUBLE BUNDLE TECHNIQUES

36

■ PETER S. CHA, MD, ROBIN V. WEST, MD, FREDDIE H. FU, MD

■ HISTORY OF THE TECHNIQUE

Complete anterior cruciate ligament (ACL) ruptures can lead to recurrent knee instability, meniscal tears, and articular cartilage degeneration. Reconstruction of the ACL has become a common procedure, and good-to-excellent clinical results have been reported.[1-4]

The ideal graft for the ACL during reconstruction should have similar structural and biomechanical properties as the native ACL, permit secure fixation, allow for rapid biological incorporation, and limit donor site morbidity. Patellar tendon autografts are historically the most popular graft choice because of their strength characteristics, ease of harvest, rigid fixation, bone-to-bone healing, and good clinical outcomes. However, donor site morbidity of patellar tendon autografts has led to the investigation and use of alternative graft sources.

Hamstring grafts have gained recent popularity due to their ease of harvest, avoidance of injury to the extensor mechanism, improved soft tissue fixation devices, and decreased incidence of anterior knee pain. Some concerns regarding the use of hamstring autografts include their strength, potential elongation, fixation methods, and a greater length of time required for incorporation into the bone tunnels.

Biomechanical data have shown that the quadrupled hamstring tendon graft has a higher ultimate tensile load and stiffness than a 10-mm patellar tendon graft.[5-7] The healing process of soft tissue grafts within the bone tunnels has been detailed.[8] Healing of the site of the graft attachment may be responsible for most of the strength observed after transplantation. From a biologic standpoint, patellar tendon grafts, compared with soft-tissue grafts, have the advantage of bone-to-bone healing. Bone-to-bone healing is similar to fracture healing and is stronger and faster than

soft tissue healing. The graft is usually incorporated into the host bone by 6 weeks during bone-to-bone healing. Soft tissue grafts usually take 8 to 12 weeks to incorporate into the host bone.

Histologic examination has demonstrated the formation of Sharpey-like fibers that extend between the bone and soft tissue graft between 4 and 12 weeks after reconstruction. Biomechanical testing has demonstrated a progressive increase in the strength of the tendon-to-bone interface over the first 12 weeks after implantation.[8]

Fixation of the graft is a crucial factor in ACL reconstruction. The fixation is the weak link during the initial 6- to 12-week period while healing of the graft to the host bone occurs. The graft must withstand the early aggressive rehabilitation that is recommended during this time period. It has been estimated that the forces during rehabilitation can be as high as 450 to 500 N.[9] If the fixation is poor, the graft may slip or the fixation may fail altogether, resulting in an unstable knee. Fixation failure usually occurs at the tibial side.[10]

Fixation methods for hamstring grafts have dramatically expanded. There are currently many fixation methods available, including absorbable and nonabsorbable implants. During biomechanical testing, these soft-tissue fixation devices have been shown to have a higher load to failure than the "gold standard" metal interference screw fixation for the patellar tendon grafts.[11,12]

■ INDICATIONS AND CONTRAINDICATIONS

Our indications for ACL reconstruction include ACL deficient young patients who want to continue athletic competition, have recurrent instability with activities of daily living, repairable meniscal tears, or multiligamentous knee injuries. We always review the graft options with the patient and have him or her select the graft of choice.

In our practice, we tend to use patellar tendon autografts in high-demand individuals who participate in cutting, pivoting, or jumping sports. We also favor the patellar tendon autograft in athletes who desire a "quick return to play." Preexisting anterior knee pain and certain lifestyle activities (kneeling for work, religion) are relative contraindications to the patellar tendon autograft. Quadruple hamstring autograft is our preference in "lower" demand patients, recreational athletes, younger patients with open growth plates, and for cosmesis. Contraindications to the hamstring autograft include generalized increased ligamentous laxity, competitive sprinters (terminal flexion weakness), and a previous hamstring injury. We opt for the patellar tendon allograft in lower demand patients, older patients who prefer an easier rehabilitation, and in the multiple-ligament injured knee.

Recently, we have switched to a double bundle, or anatomic, ACL reconstruction, using hamstring autografts. Cadaveric and biomechanical studies have shown that the standard ACL reconstruction is successful in limiting anterior tibial translation but insufficient in controlling a combined rotatory load of internal and valgus torque.[13] The anterior cruciate ligament is a collection of individual fascicles that attach to the femur and tibia over a broad area. The anteromedial bundle (AMB) originates from the proximal aspect of the femoral attachment and inserts on the anteromedial aspect of the tibial attachment. The posterolateral bundle (PLB) inserts onto the posterolateral aspect of the tibial attachment.[14] When the knee is extended, the PLB is tight, while the AMB is moderately lax. With knee flexion, the AMB tightens and the PLB becomes lax.

Most ACL reconstructions focus on replacing only the AMB. The PLB has not received sufficient attention. An anatomic ACL reconstruction, or double bundle technique, has been described in recent biomechanical and outcome studies.[15–23] The normalized in situ force of the double bundle reconstructions have been shown to be more similar to the intact ACL when compared to the single bundle reconstructions.[15,16]

With the biomechanical and clinical support for an anatomic ACL reconstruction, we recently started using a technique with the autogenous hamstrings to reproduce the two ACL bundles. We have been using this double bundle technique in our "high demand" athletes, ligamentously lax, and younger patients. The single bundle technique is reserved for lower-demand patients. We present our single bundle and double bundle (anatomic) ACL reconstruction techniques.

■ SURGICAL TECHNIQUE

Preoperative Visit

The surgeon reviews the indications, expectations, rehabilitation, and potential complications with the patient and his or her family. The operative consent is then obtained by the surgeon. A registered nurse reviews the preoperative plan with the patient, including where to go and what to bring on the day of surgery, and when to stop anti-inflammatory use. A physical therapist fits the patient for an ELS (extension lock splint) brace, explains the brace and Cryocuff usage, and reviews the postoperative exercises (quadriceps set, straight let raises, heel slides, calf pumps).

Anesthesia

The choice of anesthesia is at the discretion of the anesthesiology team based on the age of the patient, the patient's comorbid medical problems, and the previous anesthesia history of the patient. The anesthesia team typically chooses between a general anesthesia or a spinal anesthetic with concomitant intravenous (IV) sedation. If the anesthesiologist is at all concerned about airway management, then the general anesthesia is performed. At our center, there is an ongoing National Institutes of Health–funded grant that evaluates the effectiveness of preoperative femoral or sciatic nerve blocks for ACL reconstruction surgery. This prospective clinical trial randomizes the patients for femoral or sciatic nerve blocks and evaluates the pain scores postoperatively. The nerve blocks have not only been useful during the surgical procedure, but they offer 9 to 12 hours of postoperative pain relief. Prophylactic antibiotics are administered by the anesthesiologist.

Examination under Anesthesia

A thorough examination is performed to assess the range of motion, varus/valgus instability, posterolateral corner instability, posterior drawer, Lachman, and pivot-shift. If the history, radiographic studies, and examination correlate with an ACL tear, the graft is harvested prior to the arthroscopy. If there is any uncertainty in the diagnosis, an arthroscopy is performed first to assess the articular cartilage, menisci, and cruciate ligaments.

Positioning

The patient is positioned supine on the operating room table with the nonoperative extremity in a leg holder with the hip and the knee flexed to 90 degrees and the hip abducted and externally rotated. This extremity is well padded and loosely secured with a 6-inch elastic wrap. The foot of the table is dropped. A tourniquet is applied to the operative extremity and insufflated to 250 to 300 mmHg, depending on the patient's size and systolic blood pressure. Once the tourniquet is inflated, the thigh is placed into the leg holder **(Fig. 36-1)**.

Technique

The leg is prepped and draped with alcohol and Betadine. A skin marker is used to identify the surface anatomy around the

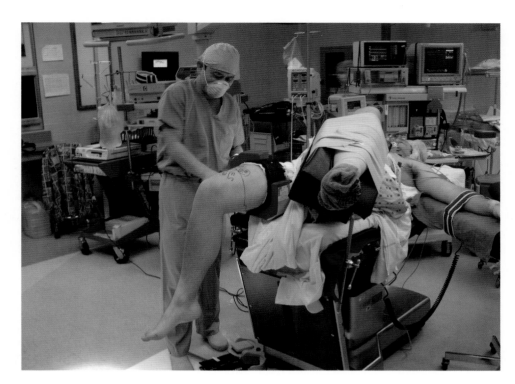

Fig. 36-1. Positioning of the patient.

knee **(Fig. 36-2)**. The tibial tubercle, the patella, the medial and lateral borders of the patellar tendon, and the medial and lateral joint lines are identified and marked. The portal sites are also marked. The preferred location of the anterolateral portal is adjacent to the lateral border of the patellar tendon at the level of the inferior border of the patella with the knee flexed to 90 degrees. The anteromedial portal for the single bundle reconstruction is just off the medial border of the patellar tendon, slightly inferior to the anterolateral portal.

The anteromedial portal for the double bundle ACL reconstruction is more inferior and medial than our tradi-

tional anteromedial portal. This portal is established under direct arthroscopic visualization with an 18 gauge spinal needle. Its placement is critical in obtaining the correct trajectory and entry point for the posterolateral femoral tunnel. A 3-cm longitudinal skin incision is marked on the anteromedial tibia at the midpoint between the anterior tibial crest and the posteromedial tibial border, just adjacent and distal to the tubercle. Through this single incision, the gracilis and semitendinosus tendons are easily harvested and the tibial tunnels are drilled and fixed.

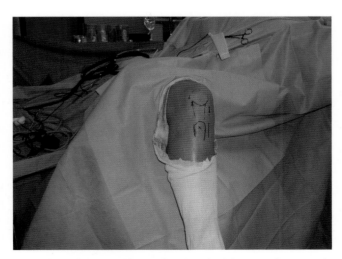

Fig. 36-2. Skin markings showing incisions and anatomic landmarks.

■ GRAFT HARVEST

The gracilis and semitendinosus tendons are identified an average of 2 cm distal and 2 cm medial to the tibial tubercle. The previously marked longitudinal incision over the anteromedial tibia is made, and dissection is carried through the subcutaneous tissue until the sartorial fascia is encountered. This fascia is then palpated to identify the underlying semitendinosus and gracilis tendons. The tendons blend together at their insertion on the tibia, and the interval between them is more distinct proximally and posteriorly. The sartorial fascia is then incised over this interval, in line with the tendons. A right-angled clamp is used to isolate the gracilis and the semitendinosus. Penrose drains are then passed around the tendons. The most prominent fascial bands of the medial gastrocnemius muscle that tether the semitendinosus must be released for an adequate harvest. A modified Krackow stitch, using no. 2 nonabsorbable suture,

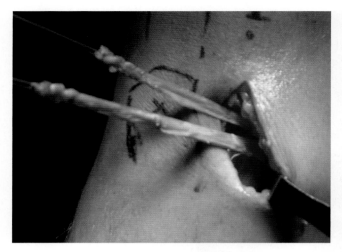

Fig. 36-3. Hamstring harvest.

is placed in the end of the tendons **(Fig. 36-3)**. The closed tendon stripper is then used to harvest the tendons.

During the single bundle technique, the tendons are doubled to make a single quadrupled graft. The tendons are quadrupled during the double bundle technique to make two quadrupled grafts. A tendon length of 10 cm is required for the single bundle technique, and a length of 30 to 35 cm is necessary for each tendon during the double bundle technique. The tendons are then taken to the back table and individually fashioned into two quadruple stranded grafts **(Fig. 36-4)**. Once the femoral tunnel lengths are determined, the corresponding EndoButton loop can be attached so that approximately 20 mm to 30 mm of graft is placed in the respective femoral tunnel. The larger semitendinosus tendon graft (~7 to 9 mm in cross-sectional diameter) is used to re-create the anteromedial bundle, and the smaller gracilis tendon graft (~6 to 8 mm in cross-sectional diameter) is used to re-create the posterolateral bundle during the double bundle reconstruction.

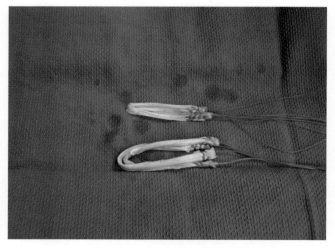

Fig. 36-4. Quadrupled gracilis and semitendinosus.

■ ARTHROSCOPY

The arthroscope is introduced into the standard anterolateral portal and the intra-articular knee joint is surveyed. If any intra-articular pathology exists (i.e., meniscal or chondral injury), then it is addressed at this point of the procedure. The ACL remnant is debrided to aid in visualization. A limited notchplasty is then done to identify the posterior cortex of the femur. We prefer to leave most of the ACL tibial footprint intact for its proprioceptive and vascular contributions. A small, curved curette is then used to elevate the posterior femoral periosteum and to confirm the "over-the-top" position.

■ GRAFT PREPARATION

Muscle and soft tissue remnants are removed from the tendon with the blunt side of a metal ruler. The various clamps on the graft preparation board are used to hold the tendons in place so that a stitch can be placed in the ends of the tendon. A modified Krakow stitch, using a no. 2 nonabsorbable suture, is placed in either end of the tendon. The tendons are then doubled over and attached to the EndoButton of appropriate length. This length is determined after the femoral tunnel has been drilled and measured. A 2-0 absorbable suture is then used to secure the four strands together just distal to the EndoButton. The graft is then placed through a sizer to determine its diameter. The graft is placed on tension on the preparation board and covered with a moist gauze.

The graft is prepared in a similar fashion for the double bundle technique. The only difference is that each tendon is divided in half and then doubled over to make a quadrupled graft **(Fig. 36-4)**.

■ SINGLE BUNDLE RECONSTRUCTION

Following the ACL debridement and limited notchplasty (if needed), the tibial tunnel is then addressed. The anatomic landmarks that are used to assist in proper tibial tunnel placement include the ACL stump, the anterior horn of the lateral meniscus, the posterior cruciate ligament (PCL), and the intercondylar roof. The guide wire is placed using a commercially available tibial guide set at 45 degrees to 50 degrees, depending on the length of the graft. The guide is placed through the anteromedial portal, and the incision that was used to harvest the hamstrings is used to drill the tibial tunnel. A cannulated reamer of appropriate diameter is then used to create the tibial tunnel. Due to the low bone density in the proximal tibia, we typically underdrill our tibial tunnel by 1 mm. Sequential dilation is then performed in 0.5-mm increments. The dilator is passed up the tibial tunnel and into the joint to perform the "impingement test." This test will confirm that full extension can be achieved with the dilator and subsequently with the graft. The arthroscopic shaver is used to remove the bone and soft tissue debris around the tunnel.

The appropriate femoral guide is then used to drill the femoral tunnel. We select a guide that will leave a 1 to 2 mm posterior wall after drilling and dilating. This guide is off-set either 5, 6, or 7 mm. For example, if the graft diameter is 8 mm, the radius of the graft is 4 mm. Therefore, if the 5 mm off-set guide is selected, a 1 mm posterior wall will remain.

The femoral guide is passed up the tibial tunnel and hooked over the posterior wall at about the 10 o'clock position for a right knee and the 2 o'clock position for a left knee. The knee is then flexed to 100 degrees, and the retrograde guide wire is inserted to a depth of about 20 mm. A cannulated acorn drill bit of appropriate diameter is used to drill the closed-ended femoral tunnel to a depth of about 30 mm. The femoral tunnel is drilled to the same size as the graft. Underdrilling is not performed, but the tunnel is dilated with the same size dilator as the acorn drill bit.

The femoral fixation is accomplished with the EndoButton, and the Mitek Rigidfix. For the EndoButton fixation, a 4.5-mm drill is passed up the tibial and femoral tunnel and used to drill out the anterolateral femoral cortex. Care is taken to keep the knee flexed to 100 degrees and to drill the hole in the center of the femoral tunnel. A calibrated depth gauge is then passed retrograde through the femoral tunnel to measure the entire length of the passing channel. With this measurement, the EndoButton length is selected. If the channel length is 50 mm, a 25 mm EndoButton will be selected to provide 25 mm of graft in the femoral tunnel.

The Rigidfix Cross Pin Guide, with the appropriate size femoral rod (to match the tunnel diameter), is inserted up the tibial and femoral tunnels. The Cross Pin Sleeve is then assembled over the Interlocking Trocar. Two small stab incisions are made to insert the Trocar and the Cross Pins. The Sleeve-Trocar assembly is then drilled until the hub meets the guide. The second hole is drilled in the top hole of the guide with the Sleeve-Trocar assembly. The guide is then detached from the Sleeves and removed. The Sleeves are left in the lateral femoral cortex to help guide the Cross Pins in place. A k-wire is then passed through both Sleeves to ensure that the drill holes have penetrated the femoral tunnel.

A Beath pin is passed up the tibial and femoral tunnels and out the hole in the anterolateral femoral cortex. This pin is used to pass the previously prepared graft. The EndoButton is flipped to sit on the anterolateral femoral cortex. After fixation has been confirmed by pulling on the graft in the tibial tunnel, the Cross Pins are inserted into the Sleeves using the Stepped Pin Insertion Rod and Mallet. The Sleeves are then removed.

The tibial fixation is accomplished with the Mitek Intrafix device. The knee is cycled 20 times to confirm range of motion and isometry of the graft. The knee is placed in full extension for the tibial fixation. A graft tensioner is available, but we do not routinely use it. The two ends of each tendon are tied together to allow for individual tensioning. The four strands are separated and tension is applied manually. The Intrafix dilator is inserted with a mallet between the strands to a depth of 30 mm. The sheath is then passed up the tibial tunnel between the strands, taking care to keep the hub of the sheath at the 12 o'clock position. Once the sheath is inserted, the Intrafix screw is advanced up the sheath. The screws come in variable sizes: 7 to 9 mm, 8 to 10 mm, and so forth. The size is chosen based on the diameter of the tibial tunnel. The middle number of the screw diameter should match the tibial tunnel size—i.e., a 7 to 9 mm screw would be used for an 8 mm tunnel.

■ DOUBLE BUNDLE TECHNIQUE

Following the minimal notchplasty (if needed) and ACL debridement, the posterolateral femoral tunnel is drilled through the modified medial portal. The 3.2 mm guide wire is passed into an anterior and inferior portion of the lateral notch of the femur **(Fig. 36-5)**. The guide wire should be placed close to the lateral femoral condyle articular surface and adjacent to the tibial plateau; however, adequate distance is needed so that the drill will not violate either of these surfaces. The guide wire should exit the lateral thigh in an anterior orientation so that the peroneal nerve is not injured. Once the pin is in an acceptable position, the tunnel is drilled over the guide wire to a depth of approximately 20 to 25 mm. The tunnel is drilled with a cannulated acorn drill bit to a diameter of 1 mm smaller than the actual diameter of the graft. Dilators are then used to expand the tunnel to the desired size in 0.5-mm increments. The far cortex is breeched with the EndoButton 4.5 mm drill, and the depth

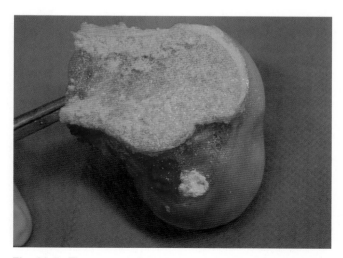

Fig. 36-5. The anatomic insertions of the anteromedial (red) and posterolateral (yellow) bundles of the ACL on the femur.

gauge is used to assess the distance to the far cortex (see single bundle technique). This tunnel typically requires a shorter EndoButton loop of approximately 15 to 20 mm to allow for 20 mm of graft in the tunnel.

Next, the posterolateral tibial tunnel is drilled with the tibial drill guide set at 45 degrees. The tip of the guide is placed in a more posterolateral position within the tibial footprint. This tunnel has a more medial starting point than the other tunnel, as it is placed just anterior to the superficial medial collateral ligament (MCL) fibers. Once acceptable placement of the posterolateral tibial pin is obtained, the anteromedial tibial guide wire is placed. The anteromedial guide wire is placed in a more anteromedial position on the tibial footprint using the tibial drill guide set at a 45-degree angle. The starting point of this anteromedial pin is more central relative to the posterolateral pin on the tibial cortex with an osseous bridge of approximately 2 cm. The posterolateral tunnel and then the anteromedial tunnel are underdrilled by 1 mm and then dilated to the desired diameter. The dilators are placed into the tibial footprint and observed within the joint to ensure that the grafts will pass concomitantly **(Fig. 36-6** and **Fig. 32-7).**

The femoral tunnel of the anteromedial bundle is now addressed. The transtibial technique is used in the similar manner as the single bundle reconstruction. The 6 or 7 mm off-set femoral guide is placed on the posterior cortex of the notch at the 10:30 or 11:00 o'clock position. The guide wire is then passed to a depth of approximately 10 to 15 mm. The acorn drill is then passed over the guide wire to a depth of approximately 25 to 30 mm. The tunnel is underdrilled by 1 mm, then dilated to the desired diameter. The far cortex is breeched with the 4.5-mm drill, and the depth gauge is used to assess the distance to the far cortex.

The posterolateral graft is passed first. A Beath pin with a long looped suture attached to the eyelet is passed via the

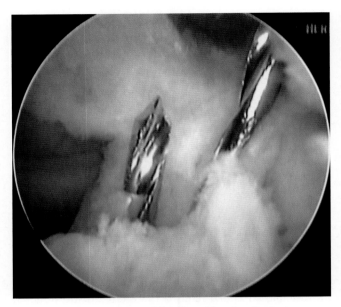

Fig. 36-7. The two tibial pin guide wires in place.

modified anteromedial tunnel. The suture is visualized in the joint and brought out the corresponding posterolateral tibial tunnel in a retrograde fashion. Arthroscopic graspers are used to retrieve the suture. The graft is then passed with the EndoButton loop and flipped in the usual manner. The anteromedial graft is then passed anterior to the posterolateral graft via the Beath pin. The EndoButton is flipped and the femoral fixation is completed for both grafts. The knee is cycled 30 times with tension on the grafts throughout a range of motion.

Tibial fixation is accomplished over a post with a single 4.5 mm fully threaded bicortical AO screw and a washer. The posterolateral bundle is tensioned and secured at 45 degrees

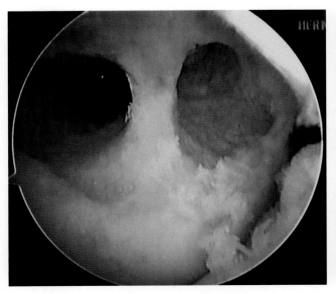

Fig. 36-6. The two femoral tunnels following dilation.

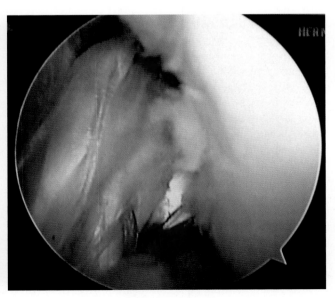

Fig. 36-8. Final picture of ACL reconstruction.

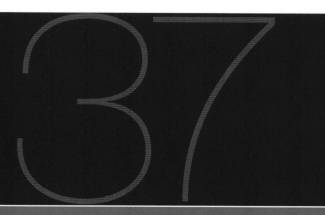

ANTERIOR CRUCIATE LIGAMENT RECONSTRUCTION: SOFT TISSUE GRAFTS

KEITH W. LAWHORN, MD, STEPHEN M. HOWELL, MD

■ HISTORY OF THE TECHNIQUE

Historically, the use of a soft tissue graft such as a hamstring or tibialis tendon as a graft source for a torn anterior cruciate ligament (ACL) has been limited by the poor biomechanical properties of fixation devices and inconsistent placement of the tunnels. The fixation devices for use with soft tissue grafts were not as strong or stiff and were more prone to slippage than interference screw fixation of bone plug grafts like the bone-patella tendon-bone grafts (BPTB). Furthermore, the healing of a tendon to a bone tunnel is slower than a bone plug, which means that the fixation devices for a soft tissue graft must be better than for a bone plug graft and should allow circumferential healing of the tendon to the tunnel wall.[1,2]

Over the past decade, improvements in fixation devices have increased the use of soft tissue autografts and allografts to reconstruct the torn ACL. Biomechanical studies support the use of high strength and high stiffness fixation devices that resist slippage and allow circumferential healing of the tendon.[3–9] Newer techniques that bone graft a soft tissue ACL graft in the femoral and tibial tunnel are now in use to promote graft-bone tunnel healing, fill voids, and further improve the stiffness at the time of implantation.[9]

A fixation technique, which uses the Bone Mulch Screw in the femur and WasherLoc in the tibia (Arthrotek, Warsaw, IN), was specifically developed for use with soft tissue grafts. The Bone Mulch Screw is a rigid crosspin placed through a stab incision on the lateral femur, and the WasherLoc is a multiple spiked washer that is compressed with a screw and countersunk in a recess in the tibia to avoid hardware symptoms. Both devices provide high strength and stiffness and resistance to slippage that is superior to interference screw fixation of BPTB grafts.[6,10] Bone graft is

used in conjunction with these two devices to promote circumferential tendon-tunnel healing, increase stiffness, and permit aggressive rehabilitation with soft tissue autografts and allografts.[7,8]

Over the past decade, improvements in the guidelines for placing the tibial and femoral tunnels in the sagittal and coronal plane has made the restoration of stability and motion of a knee reconstructed with a soft tissue graft better and more consistent. An error of a few millimeters in placement of the tibial and femoral tunnels causes impingement of a soft tissue graft against the roof in full extension, impingement against the posterior cruciate ligament (PCL) in flexion, and abnormal tension in the graft. Roof impingement causes extension loss and increased laxity, PCL impingement causes flexion loss and increased laxity, and abnormal graft tension overconstrains the knee. Impingement issues are more of a problem with the soft tissue grafts than with the bone plug grafts because the cross-sectional area of the soft tissue grafts is larger. Therefore, tunnel placement must be more precise with a soft tissue graft than a bone plug graft **(Fig. 37-1)**.

■ AUTOGRAFTS: SOFT TISSUE VERSUS BONE PLUG GRAFTS

The most commonly used soft tissue autograft is the double-looped semitendinosus and gracilis (DLSTG) graft. The DLSTG autograft has several advantages over bone plug autografts, such as the BPTB and quadriceps tendon-bone graft. The use of a DLSTG autograft avoids extensor mechanism problems such as anterior knee pain, kneeling pain, quadriceps weakness, patella tendon rupture, infrapatellar contracture syndrome, and patella fracture, which can occur with bone plug grafts. The morbidity of autogenous DLSTG graft is low with

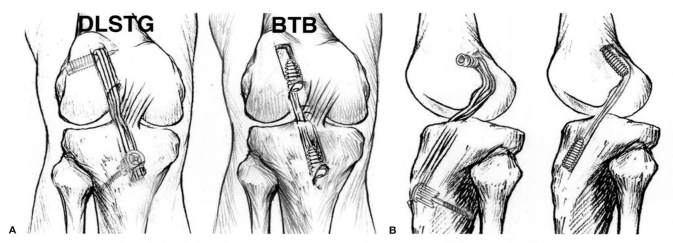

Fig. 37-1. A,B: Soft tissue grafts require more precise tunnel placement to avoid impingement due to their greater intra-articular cross-sectional diameter.

complete return of flexion strength and regeneration of the tendons following hamstring harvest.[11–16] The DLSTG is stronger (4,304 to 4,590 N) and stiffer (861 to 954 N/mm) than the bone plug grafts.[17,18] In contrast to the bone plug grafts, the biomechanical properties of a DLSTG do not deteriorate with age.[19,20] Mechanically, the four strand DLSTG fixed with the Bone Mulch Screw in a single femoral socket replicates the reciprocal-tensile behavior of the native ACL, which does not occur with the single strand bone plug graft.[9,18,21] The intra-articular biologic incorporation and remodeling of an autogenous DLSTG graft is more rapid than the bone plug grafts. The autogenous DLSTG graft does not die after transplantation,[22] and viability depends on readily available synovial diffusion and not on revascularization[23]; whereas bone plug grafts undergo central necrosis and require the development of a vascular supply.[24] Finally, clinical outcome studies support the use of autogenous DLSTG graft as they are as effective as an autogenous BPTB graft for restoring stability and function in the knee with a torn ACL.[25,26]

■ ALLOGRAFT SOFT TISSUE GRAFTS

The most commonly used soft tissue allograft is the single loop of tibialis tendon from either the anterior or posterior tibialis tendon. Soft tissue allografts are more readily available than bone plug allografts because one cadaver provides six soft tissue allografts (i.e., two DLSTG, two anterior tibialis, two posterior tibialis) and only four bone plug allografts (i.e., two bone patella tendon bone (BPTB), two Achilles tendon). Soft tissue allografts are ideal for use in revision ACL surgery and in reconstruction of the knee with multiple ligament injuries. Soft tissue allografts are also useful in primary ACL reconstruction because they avoid harvest morbidity, decrease surgical time, and surgical scars.[27] An allograft without a bone plug is quicker to thaw, easier to prepare, and has less disease transmission than an allograft with a bone plug.[28] The strength and

stiffness of a soft tissue allograft made from a single loop of tibialis tendon are greater than the bone plug grafts.[20]

The disadvantages of the use of soft tissue allograft center around cost, healing, and disease transmission. Soft tissue allografts generally cost a few hundred dollars less than the bone plug allografts. The added cost of the allograft may be offset to some degree by shortened operating time, less physical therapy, and quicker return to work. It is generally accepted that allografts require more time to incorporate and heal than an autograft.[29] The longer time for graft incorporation with the allograft places greater demand on the performance of fixation devices that need to provide sound fixation properties over a longer period of time. The use of allograft has an inherent possibility of transmitting an infectious disease from the donor to the recipient. Although the risk is low, HIV, hepatitis, and bacteria have been transmitted through the use of allograft tissue and there is also the theoretical possibility of transmitting slow viruses (prions).[30] Newer screening tests such as polymerase chain reaction (PCR) and nucleic acid testing (NAT) improve the detection of viral and bacterial DNA and RNA and may increase the accuracy of identifying infected donor tissue by minimizing the incidence of false-negatives and therefore the risk of disease transmission. Currently, tissue banks do not routinely perform PCR or NAT testing on allograft tissue. Irradiation of allograft tissue has been used to sterilize the tissue and lessen the risk of disease transmission. However, the high dose of irradiation (3 Mrad) required to sterilize allograft tissue also decreases the biomechanical properties of the allograft and does not prevent transmission of hepatitis when a bone plug allograft is used.[31] There are no studies showing that cryopreserved allograft performs better than a fresh-frozen allograft, which is not surprising since few donor cells survive the cryopreservation process and none survive the transplantation. The viability of a cryopreserved and fresh-frozen allograft depends solely on repopulation of the allograft with cells from the recipient.[32,33]

Although infection is rare, surgeons must counsel their patients on the risks and benefits of the use of allograft tissue. The use of a reputable tissue bank that follows state of the art procurement, testing, and preservation guidelines should improve the safety of allograft tissue. In our practices, we consider the use of allografts in patients requiring revision ACL surgery, treatment of unstable knees with multiple ligament injuries, and in patients that request allograft for a primary ACL reconstruction because they wish to avoid the morbidity of graft harvest.

■ FIXATION DEVICES

A variety of fixation devices for soft tissue grafts exist for ACL reconstruction. The principles of fixing a soft tissue graft include the use of fixation devices that have high strength, high stiffness, resist slippage under cyclic load, promote biologic incorporation of the soft tissue graft at the bone tunnel interface, and safely allow aggressive rehabilitation. In the femur, we use the Bone Mulch Screw femoral crosspin because of its high strength of 1,126 N, high stiffness of 225 N/mm, and resistance to slippage.[5,9] In the tibia, we use the WasherLoc because of its high strength of 905 N, high stiffness of 248 N/mm, and resistance to slippage.[5,6,9] The use of this combination of fixation devices and a DLSTG autograft or tibialis allograft allows the use of aggressive rehabilitation and a safe return to sports at 4 months.[7,34]

When choosing a fixation device the surgeon should consider whether the device enhances or retards the healing of a soft tissue graft to the bone tunnel. Tendons heal slower to a tunnel wall than a bone plug, and the healing isn't equivalent until 6 weeks after implantation.[1] Because healing of a soft tissue graft to a bone tunnel requires more time than healing of a bone plug to a bone tunnel, the fixation devices used with a soft tissue graft must be stronger, stiffer, and work for a longer period of time.[2,9]

Several controllable factors promote healing of a soft tissue graft to bone including lengthening the tunnel,[35] avoiding the insertion of fixation devices between the soft tissue graft and tunnel wall (i.e., interference screw),[3] increasing the tightness of fit,[35] and adding biologically active tissue (i.e., periosteum, bone).[36] Lengthening the tunnel and avoiding the insertion of an interference screw requires that the fixation device be placed at the end or outside the tunnel away from the joint line. Several studies have advocated fixation of a soft tissue ACL graft at the joint line with an interference screw to shorten the graft and increase stiffness.[37–39] A disadvantage of joint line fixation is that the rate of tendon graft-to-bone healing is slower than distal fixation because the interference screw blocks healing between the ACL graft and the tunnel wall.[3,40,41] Other studies have shown that distal fixation with the Bone Mulch Screw and WasherLoc provides even greater stiffness than joint line fixation with a wide variety of metal and bioabsorbable interference screws, even

though the graft is longer.[4–6,9] An advantage of distal fixation is that bone graft can be used as a supplementary fixation device. Bone graft in the form of drill reamings can be compacted into the femoral tunnel through a channel in the body of the Bone Mulch Screw, which increases stiffness 41 N/mm[9] and allows reciprocal tensile behavior in the graft.[21] A bone graft made from a dowel of cancellous bone harvested from the tibial tunnel with a coring device can be compacted back into the tibial tunnel in a space between the anterior surface of the soft tissue graft and WasherLoc and the tunnel wall, which increases stiffness 58 N/mm.[42] Tightening the fit by adding an autogenous bone graft or a biologically active tissue such as periosteum improves the rate of healing of a soft tissue graft to a bone tunnel.[35,36]

■ TIBIAL AND FEMORAL TUNNEL GUIDE SYSTEM

The success of a soft tissue graft with the Bone Mulch/WasherLoc technique relies on the use of a tibial and femoral guide system that consistently places the tibial and femoral tunnels in the sagittal plane and coronal plane so that roof impingement and PCL impingement is avoided and the tensile behavior in the graft matches the intact ACL. The strongest graft tissue, best fixation devices, or most carefully moderated rehabilitation protocol cannot overcome the complications from placing a tibial or femoral tunnel incorrectly in either the sagittal or coronal plane. The guideline for placing the tibial guide wire in the sagittal plane is to place the guide wire 5 mm posterior to the intercondylar roof in full extension, which avoids roof impingement. The tibial guide keys off the intercondylar roof. The guide wire is drilled with the knee in full extension, which customizes the position of the tibial tunnel in the sagittal plane for variation in knee extension and roof angle and avoids roof impingement without a roofplasty.[43–45] The guideline for placing the tibial guide wire in the coronal plane is to place the guide wire midway between the tibial spines at an angle of 65 degrees with respect to the medial joint line of the tibia, which avoids PCL impingement. An alignment rod is inserted into the handle of the tibial guide and the rod is aligned parallel to the joint line and perpendicular to the long axis of the tibia, which places the tibial tunnel at 65 degrees.[46] The tibial tunnel is used to select the placement of the femoral tunnel by inserting a femoral aimer with an offset that leaves a 1-mm thick back wall. Drilling a femoral tunnel through a tibial tunnel placed with these guidelines in the sagittal and coronal planes results in a tension pattern in the graft similar to the intact ACL and avoids roof and PCL impingement.[46]

Indication and Contraindications

We prefer to use the Bone Mulch Screw/WasherLoc ACL system in any patient requiring ACL reconstruction, including the knee with multiligament injuries. The DLSTG autograft is used in all patients who want to avoid the infectious complications of allograft tissue. The tibialis allograft is the preferred graft in patients who want to avoid the morbidity from graft harvest, in legs that are obese or large where harvesting autogenous hamstring tendons is technically challenging, and in the knee with a multiligament injury. Soft tissue grafts are preferred in the skeletally immature patient, and allografts are considered when the patient is small and the hamstring tendons are judged to be inadequate. In the patient with open physis, we recommend the use of fluoroscopy to be certain that the fixations devices do not cross the physis. In addition, bone graft is not used in the tibial and femoral tunnels in skeletally immature patients with significant growth remaining.

■ SURGICAL TECHNIQUE

Anesthesia

The Bone Mulch Screw/WasherLoc ACL procedure can be performed under general or regional anesthesia. We prefer general anesthesia because the duration of surgery is usually an hour or less. Acceptable regional techniques include spinal and epidural anesthesia.

Portal Placement

A modified anteromedial and anterolateral portal is used for the procedure. Position the modified anteromedial portal adjacent to and touching the medial border of the patellar tendon. Modifying the placement of the anteromedial portal so that the tibial guide touches the patellar tendon ensures that the tip of the guide can be centered inside the notch. Position the modified anterolateral portal adjacent to the lateral border of the patellar tendon at the level on the inferior pole of the patella. Alternatively, the lateral portal can be placed through the lateral one third of the patella tendon, which provides a better view of the femoral tunnel than the anterolateral portal. Use a standard superomedial portal if an outflow cannula is required so that the cannula does not interfere with the insertion of the Bone Mulch Screw on the lateral side of the knee.

Harvest the Autogenous DLSTG graft

To harvest the gracilis and semitendinosus tendons, make a 4 to 5 cm vertical or oblique incision centered three finger-breadths below the medial joint line. Position the incision so that the index finger of the surgeon can reach *past* the posteromedial edge of the tibia and well into the popliteal space. Adjusting the location of the incision to achieve this reach enables the identification, palpation, and release of all fascial attachments of the hamstring tendons to the medial gastrocnemius. Make the skin incision and expose the sartorius fascia, which overlies the gracilis and semitendinosus tendons. Palpate the gracilis tendon through the sartorius fascia and then incise the sartorius fascia along the inferior border of the gracilis tendon. Insert a gloved finger deep to

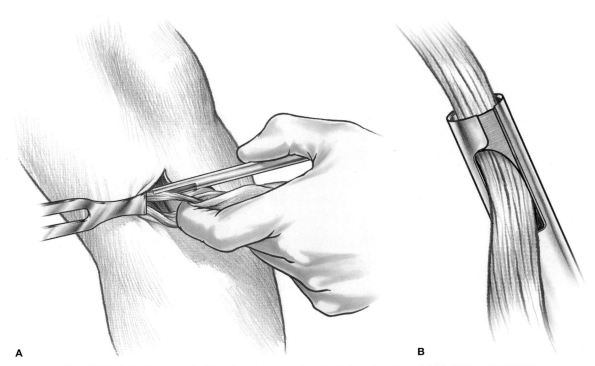

A   **B**

Fig. 37-2. A,B: Open-ended tendon stripper advanced along tendon while holding countertraction with finger and Penrose drain leaving the tendons attached to bone.

the sartorius fascia and bluntly dissect the gracilis tendon into the popliteal fossa. Hook the gracilis tendon with a right angle clamp and pass a 0.5 inch Penrose drain around the gracilis tendon. Use the Penrose drain to apply traction and manipulate the gracilis tendon and define any fascial attachments. Cut fascial attachments under direct view. Harvest the gracilis tendon with an open-ended tendon stripper and leave the tendon attached distally. Gently push the stripper proximally aiming toward the groin while applying a countertraction on the distal end of the tendon **(Fig. 37-2)**. Identify the semitendinosus, which is distal to the gracilis tendon and in the same tissue plane. Use the right angle clamp, Penrose drain, and open-ended tendon stripper to detach the semitendinosus and leave the tendon attached distally. Scrape the remaining muscle from each tendon with a curved Mayo scissors or periosteal elevator.

Prepare and Size the DLSTG Autograft and Allograft

The same technique is used to prepare and size the DLSTG autograft and allograft except that both ends of each allograft tendon are sewn, since the allograft is not attached to the tibia. Grasp the end of each tendon with an Allis clamp. Sew the end of each tendon using a whipstitch and a 36 inch no. 1 Vicryl suture. Loop each throw of the suture around four fifths of the cross section of the tendon spacing each throw 5 to 10 mm apart until 4 to 5 cm of tendon is sewn. Create the appearance of the thongs on a "Roman sandal" by continuing the throws in the same direction up and down the tendon **(Fig. 37-3)**. Later in the procedure, when traction is applied to the whipstitch to pass the graft, a "Chinese finger trap" tapers the tip of the tendon, which aids in graft passage around the Bone Mulch Screw. Size the DLSTG graft by looping the middle on both tendons over a suture or mersilene tape. Pass a series of sizing sleeves that differ in diameter by 1 mm over the double looped graft. The diameter of the sleeve that passes freely is used to select the diameter of the tibial and femoral tunnels.

Prepare the Tibialis Allograft

The tibialis allograft should be 24 cm or greater in length and at least 7 mm in diameter. Fold the tendon over a suture or mersilene tape and pass the graft through a series of sizing sleeves. Trim the width of the tibialis tendon until it freely passes through a 9 or 10 mm sleeve. Suture each end of the tendon using the previously described whipstitch. Tubulate the remaining unsewn section of the tibialis allograft with use of a 3-0 Vicryl suture. Pull the looped end of the graft into a sizing sleeve 1 mm smaller than the sized graft. Submerge the graft folded inside in the sizing sleeve in an antibiotic-laced basin of saline. Keeping the graft inside the sizing sleeve prevents the graft from swelling, which eases the passage of the graft later in the procedure **(Fig. 37-4)**.

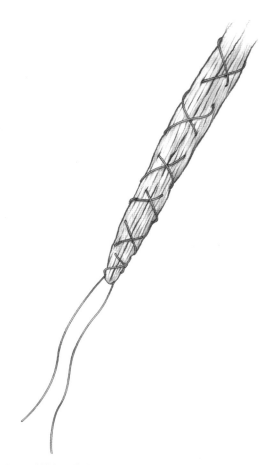

Fig. 37-3. Whip-stitch resembles a "Roman sandal" when completed. (Reprinted from Lawhorn KW, Howell SM. Scientific justification and technique for anterior cruciate ligament reconstruction using autogenous and allogeneic soft tissue grafts. Orthop Clin North Am. 2003;34:19–30. With permission from Elsevier.)

Place the Tibial Guide Wire

Excise the stump of the torn ACL. Insert the 9.5-mm wide tip of the Howell 65-degree tibial guide through the inferomedial portal. Attempt to pass the tip of the guide between the lateral femoral condyle and PCL, which is often too narrow to allow free passage of the tip of the guide. Perform a customized wallplasty with the angled osteotome and remove 2 to 3 mm of bone from the lateral femoral condyle until the tip of the guide freely passes into the notch without deforming the PCL **(Fig. 37-5)**. Widening the notch to 9.5 mm minimizes impingement of an 8-, 9-, and 10-mm wide graft against the lateral wall and PCL. Do not perform a roofplasty.

Position the tip of the tibial guide in the notch. Slowly extend the knee and arthroscopically visualize so that the tip on the guide remains inside the notch. Maintain the knee in hyperextension by placing the heel on a raised Mayo stand. Grasp the handle of the guide with the long and ring fingers and rest the hypothenar area of the hand on the patella. Seat the guide in the sagittal plane by gently

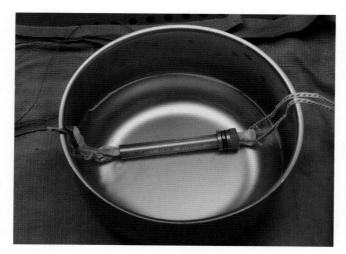

Fig. 37-4. Prepared allograft placed in sizing sleeve and stored in antibiotic saline.

lifting the handle of the guide toward the ceiling until the arm abuts the trochlear groove. Simultaneously press the patella toward the floor, hyperextending the knee. This maneuver customizes the angle and position of the guide in the sagittal plane to the roof angle and knee extension of the patient **(Fig. 37-6)**.

Adjust the angle of the tibial guide wire in the coronal plane. From the lateral side of the guide, insert the alignment rod into the proximal hole in the handle. Position the alignment rod parallel to the joint line and perpendicular to

the long axis of the tibia, which angles the tibial tunnel at 65 degrees with respect to the medial joint line (Fig. 37-6). If a DLSTG autograft is being used, then insert the drill sleeve through the harvest incision until it touches the portion of the superficial medial collateral ligament that overlies the posteromedial tibia. If a soft tissue allograft is being used, then make a 4 to 5 cm transverse incision so that the drill sleeve can be positioned on bone. Drill a 2.4 mm drill tip guide wire until it stops at the broad tip of the guide.

Assess the placement of tibial guide wire. Tap the K-wire into the notch. In the coronal plane, assess the placement of the K-wire with the knee in 90 degrees of flexion. In the sagittal plane, assess the placement of the K-wire with the knee in full extension. Use a nerve hook and confirm that there is 2 mm of space between the K-wire and intercondylar roof. The correct K-wire placement is lateral to the posterior cruciate ligament, pointing down the side wall of the notch and between the medial and lateral tibial spines **(Fig. 37-7)**.

Use intraoperative radiography or fluoroscopy when there is any uncertainty about the placement of the tibial guide wire. Obtain an AP and lateral roentgenogram or fluoroscopic image with the knee in full extension with the tibial guide, alignment rod, and tibial guide wire in place. In the coronal plane, the tibial guide wire is properly placed when it is centered between the tibial spines and the tibial guide wire forms an angle of 65 ± 3 degrees with the medial joint line. In the sagittal plane, the tibial guide wire is properly placed when the K-wire is 4 to 5 mm posterior and parallel to the intercondylar roof.

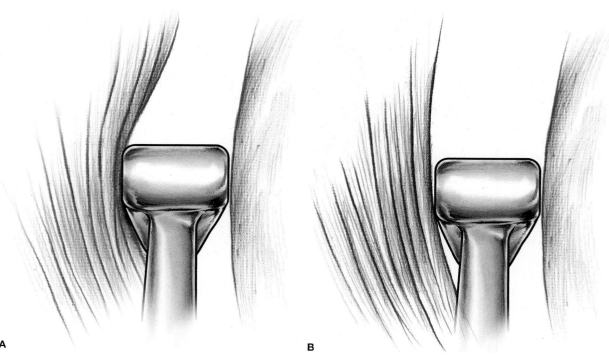

A   B

Fig. 37-5. A: Inadequate notch width for soft tissue graft indicated by deformation of PCL when passing guide tip into notch. **B:** Adequate notch width for soft tissue graft.

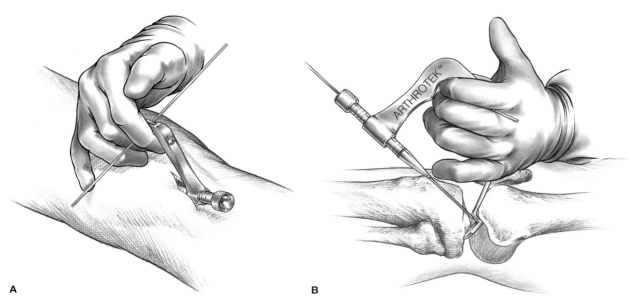

A   **B**

Fig. 37-6. **A,B:** AP and lateral views with tibial guide in place. (Reprinted from Lawhorn KW, Howell SM. Scientific justification and technique for anterior cruciate ligament reconstruction using autogenous and allogeneic soft tissue grafts. Orthop Clin North Am. 2003;34:19–30. With permission from Elsevier.)

Harvest the Bone Dowel and Drill the Tibial Tunnel

Choose a cannulated tibial reamer that matches the diameter of the soft tissue ACL graft. Drill the cannulated reamer over the guide wire a few millimeters until the distal tibial cortex is removed. Assemble the bone dowel harvester by locking an 8 mm harvester tube in the quick release handle. Insert the calibrated plunger up the harvester tube until the plunger is flush with the sharper cutting end. Impact the bone dowel harvester over the guide wire to the subchondral bone **(Fig. 37-8)**.

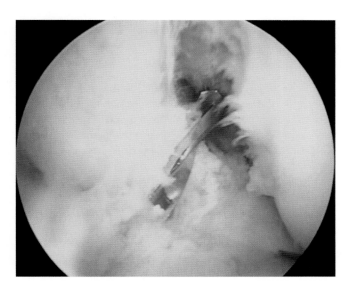

Fig. 37-7. Guide pin position should be lateral to the PCL, angle away from PCL and centered between the tibial spines.

Rotate the bone dowel harvester several times clockwise and counterclockwise to break off the cylindrical bone dowel and remove. Disengage the harvester tube from the handle. Read the calibrated plunger and determine whether the length of the bone plug is adequate (typically 25 to 35 mm) **(Fig. 37-9)**. If the tibial guide wire is removed with the harvester, then place an 8 mm femoral reamer into the tibial tunnel and reinsert the guide wire. Finish drilling the tibial tunnel.

Prepare the Counterbore for the WasherLoc

Use electrocautery and a rongeur to remove a 17 by 17 mm section of the superficial layer of the medial collateral ligament (MCL) from the cortical opening of the tibial tunnel. Because the majority of the superficial MCL fibers are retained and the deep fibers of the MCL are undisturbed, the medial stability of the knee is unaffected. Insert the counter bore guide into the tibial tunnel until the vertical sleeve is compressed against the distal end of the anterior edge of the tibial tunnel. Rotate the guide until the periscope on the counter bore is pointed toward the fibular head, which avoids damage to the posterior neurovascular structures **(Fig. 37-10)**. Impact the awl perpendicular to the back wall of the tibial tunnel through the sleeve until it is fully seated. Remove the counter bore guide and replace the awl in the pilot hole to maintain orientation. Memorize the orientation of the awl, remove it, and insert the tip of the counter bore into the pilot hole. Maintain the cutting surface of the counter bore parallel to the posterior wall of the tibial tunnel. Ream until the counter bore is flush with the posterior wall of the tibial tunnel (Fig. 37-10). Save the reamings.

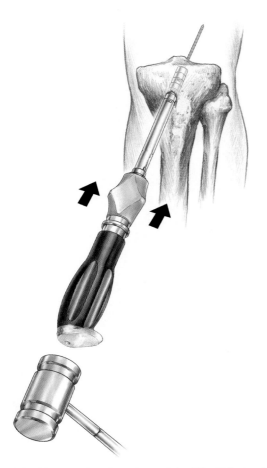

Fig. 37-8. After reaming the outer cortex of the tibia, tap the coring reamer over the guide wire until it reaches the subchondral bone.

Check for Roof Impingement and Remove the ACL Origin

Place the knee in maximum extension and insert an impingement rod the same diameter as the tibial tunnel through the tibial tunnel and into the notch. Free passage of the impingement rod indicates prevention of roof impingement **(Fig. 37-11)**. A roofplasty is rarely required with the Howell 65 degree Tibial Guide.

Insert the 70-degree angled curette through the medial portal and into the over-the-top position on the femur. Remove the remnant of the ACL origin down to bone. Removing the ACL origin allows the tip of the femoral aimer to rest on bone instead of soft tissue and prevents blowout of the posterior wall of the femoral tunnel.

Place the Femoral Tunnel

Select a femoral aimer the same diameter as the graft. Insert the femoral aimer through the tibial tunnel and hook the tip of the aimer into the over-the-top position on the femur. Allow the knee to flex until the femoral aimer locks in place. Rotate the femoral aimer a few degrees away from the PCL

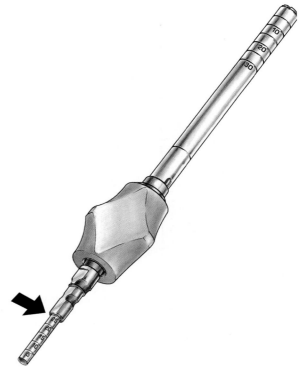

Fig. 37-9. The length of the cancellous bone dowel is indicated by calibrations on plunger.

to minimize PCL impingement. Drill a 2.4-mm drill-tipped guide wire into the femur and then drill a 30 mm in length femoral tunnel with an acorn reamer. The placement of the femoral tunnel is controlled by the angle and placement of the tibial tunnel in the coronal and sagittal plane since the femoral tunnel is drilled through the tibial tunnel. The use of the femoral aimer through a tibial tunnel placed with the previously discussed guidelines guarantees that the placement of the femoral tunnel prevents PCL impingement and that the tension pattern in the graft replicates the intact ACL.

Insert the Bone Mulch Screw

Insert the U-guide (Arthrotek, Inc.) with a tip that corresponds to the diameter of the tunnel through the tibial until it bottoms out at the end of the 30 mm femoral tunnel. Insert the drill sleeve and rotate the guide until it points medial. Make a 10 to 12 mm incision and advance the drill sleeve until the tip touches bone. Lock the drill sleeve into place. Determine the length of the Bone Mulch Screw by reading the screw sizes of the drill sleeve from inner edge of the U-guide. When the length is between sizes (17 mm, 20 mm, 25 mm, 30 mm) use a Bone Mulch Screw of shorter length.

Drill the guide wire into the lateral femur until it strikes the tip of the U-guide in the femoral tunnel **(Fig. 37-12)**. Remove the drill sleeve and U-guide. View the femoral tunnel by inserting the scope through either the modified anterolateral or anteromedial portal. Tap the guide wire

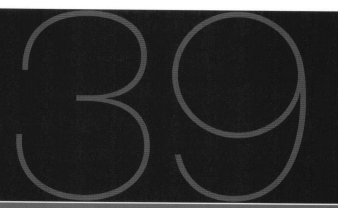

MEDIAL PORTAL TECHNIQUE FOR ANTERIOR CRUCIATE LIGAMENT RECONSTRUCTION

■ CHRISTOPHER A. RADKOWSKI, MD, CHRISTOPHER D. HARNER, MD

■ HISTORY OF THE TECHNIQUE

Several significant advances have been made in the realm of anterior cruciate ligament (ACL) reconstruction. Use of arthroscopy and the wide array of graft choices and fixation devices available to the surgeon offer a variety of means to obtain a successful ACL reconstruction.[1–5] Advances in early motion rehabilitation have also contributed to excellent clinical results.[6–8] Biomechanical and anatomic studies have enhanced our understanding of the ACL and its function.[9–12]

There are several potential causes of ACL reconstruction failure.[13–16] One of the most common preventable errors is in surgical technique, specifically errant femoral and tibial tunnel placement.[17,18] The desired position for femoral tunnel placement is posterior on the medial aspect of the lateral femoral condyle at the 10 or 2 o'clock position for right and left knees, respectively. This tunnel position has been shown to more effectively resist rotatory loads in a cadaveric study.[19] Use of a transtibial technique can make it more difficult to accurately place the femoral tunnel in the optimal position. In this manner, the femoral tunnel is limited to the confined space dictated by the position of the tibial tunnel.

The medial portal technique for femoral tunnel placement offers several advantages over the transtibial tunnel technique. First, use of the anteromedial portal facilitates accurate placement of the femoral tunnel that is not dependent on the tibial tunnel position. In addition to allowing the surgeon more freedom for anatomic placement of the femoral tunnel, this method provides an opportunity to better preserve any intact ACL fibers when performing anteromedial (AM) or posterolateral (PL) bundle augmentation. It can be used in the primary or revision ACL reconstruction setting and can be used regardless of the type of graft, instrumentation, or fixation.[20]

Another advantage of using the medial portal technique is in the placement of femoral interference screws. Because both the drill for the femoral tunnel and the screw are passed through the medial portal, the paths of the tunnel and the interference screw will be parallel. It has been shown that placement of the interference screw parallel with the tunnel provides stronger fixation than a divergent position.[21,22] In a series of 100 ACL reconstructions, O'Donnell and Scerpella[23] have shown that use of this technique leads to low divergence rates and angles between the femoral tunnel and interference screw.

Use of the medial portal technique may lead to a decrease in the number of errant femoral tunnels placed in ACL reconstruction. Yasuda et al.[24] recommended use of the medial portal to better visualize the anatomic insertion site of the PL bundle in ACL reconstruction. Other studies have shown successful results of ACL reconstruction using the medial portal technique.[23,25–31] In 1990, Harner et al.[32] progressed from the two-incision technique for ACL reconstruction to an all-arthroscopic technique. Because of concerns over lack of rotational stability in ACL reconstruction, the modification of lower femoral tunnel placement via the medial portal technique instead of a transtibial technique was implemented in 1999.

■ INDICATIONS AND CONTRAINDICATIONS

The medial portal technique may be used in any ACL reconstruction setting. This method may be utilized independent of the type of graft, the type of tunnel placement guide, and the type of fixation.[20] Establishing the femoral tunnel through the medial portal may be especially useful in AM or PL bundle augmentation cases. Another indication for this technique is in revision ACL reconstruction cases in which the tibial tunnel is well aligned but the femoral tunnel is not. Even in revision surgery, with well-placed femoral tunnels from a transtibial technique, use of the medial portal technique allows placement of a divergent femoral tunnel in native bone. In some cases with tunnel widening, this method may eliminate the need for a staged reconstruction procedure with bone grafting.

Because the knee must be flexed to 120 degrees, the medial portal technique cannot be used in cases in which a leg holder is placed circumferentially around the femur. There are no known relative or absolute contraindications for use of this technique.

■ SURGICAL TECHNIQUE

Preoperative Assessment

A thorough history and physical examination are obtained preoperatively in a clinic setting. Note is made of the active range of motion (ROM) of both knees and any positive findings that may suggest associated pathology. Magnetic resonance imaging (MRI) is frequently done to assess for meniscal pathology, which can be difficult to elucidate with a large effusion and a guarded physical examination. Informed consent is obtained in the clinic.

Anesthesia

The patient is identified in the preoperative holding area and the operative site is signed. Femoral nerve blocks are usually performed for postoperative pain management. The patient is taken to the operating room where spinal or general anesthesia is induced.

Patient Positioning

The patient is positioned supine on the operating room table. A padded bump is taped to the operating room table at the foot with the knee flexed to 90 degrees to hold the leg flexed during the case. A side post is placed on the operative side just distal to the greater trochanter to support the proximal leg with the knee in flexion. Padded cushions are placed under the nonoperative leg. A tourniquet and a leg holder are not used.

Examination under Anesthesia

An examination under anesthesia (EUA) is then performed. The non-operative knee is examined followed by the operative knee. The alignment and ROM is assessed with specific attention to terminal extension. A ligamentous exam is performed including a Lachman test, pivot shift test, anterior drawer test, posterior drawer test, and stability to varus and valgus stress at 0 and 30 degrees of flexion. This examination is critical for completing a thorough evaluation of the injured knee, which may often be obscured by guarding and effusion

in the office setting. Lower grades of Lachman and pivot shift tests may represent an intact AM or PL bundle of the ACL, whereas higher grades may signal a functional loss of the secondary stabilizers of the knee (i.e., medial meniscus).

Surface Anatomy and Skin Incisions

The knee is flexed to 90 degrees and the vertical arthroscopy portals are delineated. The anterolateral portal is placed just lateral to the lateral border of the patellar tendon and just inferior to the distal pole of the patella. The anteromedial portal is positioned approximately 1 cm medial to the medial border of the superior aspect of the patellar tendon. With the knee in extension, the superolateral outflow portal is placed between the extensor mechanism and iliotibial band, about the level of the superior pole of the patella, and oriented parallel to the Langer lines. The tibial tubercle is marked and the posteromedial aspect of the proximal tibia is palpated. If hamstring autograft is to be used, the tendons are palpated as well. A vertical line is drawn midway between the tibial tubercle and posteromedial aspect of the tibia approximately 2 cm distal to the top of the tibial tubercle and joint line, extending distally to the insertion of the hamstrings (Fig. 39-1). If meniscal repair or other surgical procedures are expected, these incisions are marked as well. The proposed incisions are then cleansed with sterile Betadine and then injected with a local anesthetic mixed with diluted epinephrine.

The leg is cleansed with an alcohol solution and gauze sponges with care taken to preserve the incision marks. Next the operative leg is prepped and draped using a sterile technique. After draping, the arthroscopy equipment is prepared and the fluoroscopy machine is placed in the room and later draped (Fig. 39-2).

Graft Selection and Harvest

Use of the medial portal technique does not limit the graft choice for ACL reconstruction. An extensive discourse on graft selection is beyond the scope of this chapter; for this reason, only use of hamstring tendon autograft will be discussed. Currently, the senior author (CDH) performs approximately 60% hamstring autograft, 30% soft tissue allograft, and 10% bone-patellar tendon-bone autograft for primary ACL reconstruction. In general, hamstring autograft is preferred in younger patients without a history of hamstring injury. Soft tissue allograft is recommended in older patients or patients with combined ligament injuries. If autograft tissue is to be used and the examination under anesthesia reveals significant laxity, the graft harvest is performed initially. If there is any question about the EUA, the diagnostic arthroscopy is performed first.

For hamstring tendon harvest, the hamstrings are palpated and a vertical incision is made through skin and subcutaneous tissue. A curved hemostat is used with Bovie electrocautery for meticulous hemostasis. The surgeon

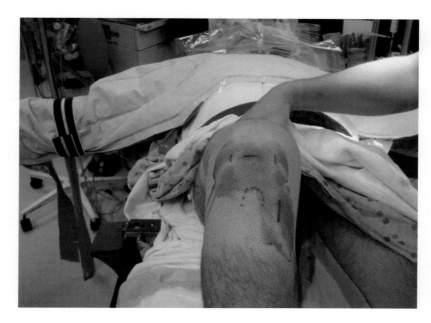

Fig. 39-1. Surface anatomy and skin incisions for a right knee ACL reconstruction with hamstring autograft. The proposed incisions were injected preoperatively under sterile conditions.

should be cognizant of the infrapatellar branch of the saphenous nerve during this dissection, but this is not routinely exposed. Metzenbaum scissors are used to cut down to sartorius fascia. Using a lap sponge, the fascia is bluntly cleared in all directions. The gracilis and semitendinosus tendons are again palpated. The sartorius fascia is split in line with its fibers between the two hamstring tendons horizontally. The tibial insertions of the tendons are then cut and right-angle clamps are placed on the distal ends of each tendon. The hamstrings are reflected medially to identify the individual tendons from their undersurface **(Fig. 39-3)**. The sartorius fascia is elevated from both tendons. A no. 2 Ethibond suture is placed in whipstitch fashion 2 cm along each tendon and used for traction. Blunt

manual dissection is performed to free any soft tissue attachments, and scissors are used with the tips pointed away from the hamstrings to cut the stout medial gastrocnemius attachment to the semitendinosus tendon. Each tendon is pulled distally by its tagging suture and palpated to review the orientation of the tendon. A closed tendon stripper is used to complete the harvest. Special care is taken to ensure that the stripper is placed in line with the posterior femur and directed toward the ischial tuberosity for the semitendinosus and toward the symphysis pubis for the gracilis. Constant traction is applied to the tendon while the stripper is advanced, and upon harvest the tendon is placed in a damp sponge soaked in sterile saline solution to await graft preparation.

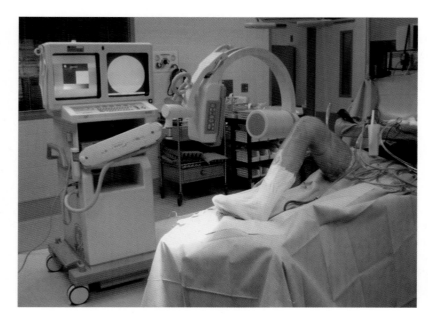

Fig. 39-2. A gel pad and post hold the right knee in position after sterile prep and drape of the leg. A fluoroscopic machine is placed in the room and later draped.

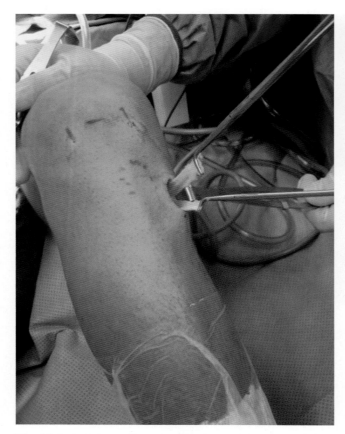

Fig. 39-3. Isolation of the gracilis and semitendinosus tendons in hamstring harvest for ACL reconstruction of the right knee.

Graft Preparation

The muscle is removed from the graft with the curved end of a metal ruler. A closed Endoloop is used without the EndoButton (Smith & Nephew Inc, Andover, Mass). With the standard EndoButton technique, a significant portion of the tunnel will contain only the Endoloop suture, with some graft left outside the tibial tunnel. The EndoButton is carefully removed using a wire cutter to avoid damage to the loop. This is done to minimize the amount of Endoloop and maximize the amount of graft within the femoral tunnel. In a recent study using a dog model for ACL reconstruction, increasing the length of tendon within the tunnel was shown to enhance pullout strength of the graft.[33]

The length of the Endoloop varies from 40 to 50 mm and the length of the graft is cut to 18 to 21 cm depending on the height of the patient. A whipstitch is placed in similar fashion to the free ends of each tendon. The hamstrings are passed through and doubled over the closed Endoloop. A no. 5 Ethibond suture is placed through the Endoloop and the graft is tensioned. The width of the graft is measured on the tibial and femoral ends. The graft is marked 27.5 mm from the femoral side of the graft for later reference during graft passage **(Fig. 39-4)**. A damp sponge is placed around the graft until it is passed.

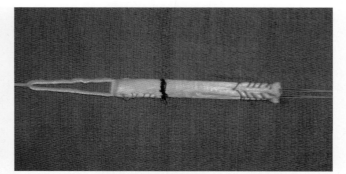

Fig. 39-4. A quadrupled hamstring autograft is placed under tension after preparation. The EndoButton has been cut from the Endoloop.

Arthroscopy

A diagnostic arthroscopy is performed to assess the ACL and evaluate for other knee derangements. The notch is examined for any remaining intact ACL fibers of the AM or PL bundles that are left for ACL augmentation. If specific fibers from either bundle are left, femoral tunnel placement should be adjusted to correspond with the femoral insertion of the bundle being reconstructed.[11] Ruptured ACL fibers are debrided, but those directly overlying the tibial footprint are left in place. The medial, lateral, and patellofemoral compartments are examined for any articular cartilage or meniscal damage. If there is any uncertainty or difficulty with visualization, a 70-degree arthroscope is used for the Gilquist view to assess the posterior horn of the medial meniscus.

A notchplasty is performed if necessary. In a majority of cases this is done to improve visualization and avoid crowding of the arthroscopic instruments. A curved curette is placed through the medial portal and passed along the medial wall of the lateral femoral condyle to elevate the periosteum and determine the over-the-top position **(Fig. 39-5)**. Next the

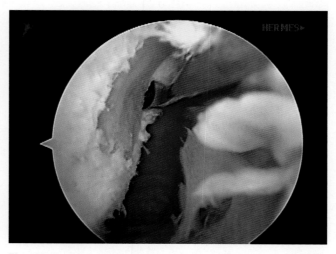

Fig. 39-5. A small curette is used to elevate the periosteum to identify the over-the-top position of the posterior wall in a right knee.

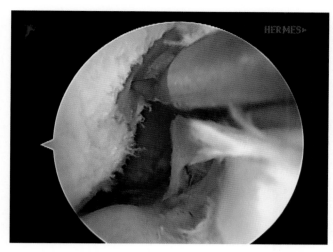

Fig. 39-6. An angled awl is used to create a starting hole at the 10 o'clock position in the right knee, approximately 4 to 6 mm anterior to the posterior wall.

anatomic femoral insertion site is identified in the 2 o'clock or 10 o'clock position for the left and right knees, respectively. A 30-degree angled awl is placed through the AM portal to establish a starting point. The awl is placed 4 to 6 mm anterior to the posterior wall of the femur, depending on the width of the graft **(Fig. 39-6)**.

Tibial Tunnel Preparation

The commercially available ACL tibial guide is set to 47.5 degrees and used to direct placement of the tibial tunnel. Several suggested landmarks have been recommended as reference points for placement of this guide, including the PCL, the medial and lateral tibial spines, and the ACL footprint. The guide should intersect the anterior horn insertions of the lateral and medial menisci. A 3/32–inch K-wire is passed once the guide is set in place along the anterior tibia. Once the wire is visible arthroscopically, the knee is brought into extension to check for impingement. The arthroscopic equipment is removed. Fluoroscopy is used to confirm appropriate tibial tunnel placement by obtaining a lateral view with the knee in full extension and the tibia is reduced **(Fig. 39-7)**. The wire should be placed adequately in the tibia, parallel to and 1 to 2 mm posterior to the Blumensaat line. A parallel drill guide may be used to correct the wire placement if necessary. Use of fluoroscopy can be very helpful to avoid incorrect tibial tunnel placement in primary and revision cases.[26]

The tibial periosteum is elevated medially and laterally. A cannulated compaction reamer is used over the guide wire to ream the tibial tunnel. The size of the reamer used is usually 0.5 to 1.0 mm smaller than the graft size. Serial dilators are used up to the size of the graft diameter. The last dilator remains in place while the knee is brought into full extension to inspect arthroscopically and clinically for impingement. If any additional notchplasty is required, it is performed at this time.

Femoral Tunnel Preparation

The knee is then placed in hyperflexion to 120 degrees, which allows for a more anterior-directed tunnel and avoids significant violation of the posterior wall.[23] A 3/32–inch K-wire is placed through the AM portal into the starting hole created by the awl on the medial wall of the lateral femoral condyle and impacted approximately 1.5 cm. A cannulated acorn reamer is passed over the guide wire through the AM portal **(Fig. 39-8)**. The reamer is started by hand to assess the bone quality and feel for any possible posterior cutout. Once firmly in bone, the reamer is passed under power to a depth of 30 mm. To avoid drilling through the

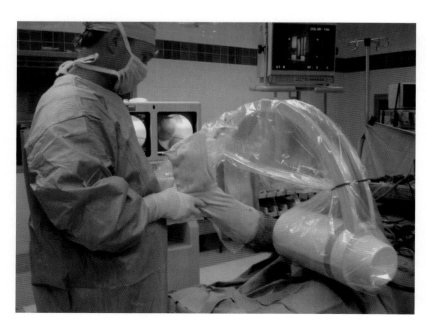

Fig. 39-7. Fluoroscopy is used to obtain a lateral view of the reduced tibia to ensure proper tibial tunnel placement.

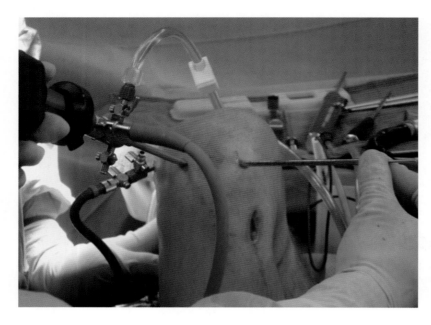

Fig. 39-8. The acorn reamer is passed over the guide wire through the anteromedial portal to drill the femoral tunnel.

outer cortex, remember that this distance may be shorter if the patient is of smaller stature.

The shaver is placed into the femoral tunnel to remove all debris. Next serial dilators are passed through the anteromedial portal into the femoral tunnel up to the graft size. The arthroscope is used to examine the tunnel **(Fig. 39-9)**. The EndoButton drill is passed through the superior aspect of the femoral tunnel and drilled through the lateral femoral cortex. A no. 5 Ethibond suture is passed through the eye of a Beath pin and tied to form a small loop. The Beath pin is passed through the medial portal into the femoral tunnel and out through the skin, with the loop still outside the AM portal, available for passage of the graft.

A pituitary rongeur is used to pass the leading suture from the graft through the tibial tunnel. Another pituitary is passed through the Ethibond loop of the Beath pin into the

anteromedial portal. This second rongeur retrieves the lead graft suture and pulls it out through the medial portal and the Beath pin loop. The Beath pin is pulled proximally with the lead graft suture out of the skin **(Fig. 39-10)**. A Kocher

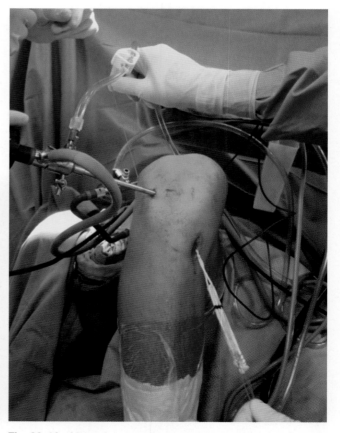

Fig. 39-10. After using rongeurs to pass the lead suture of the graft through the tibial tunnel and out the anteromedial portal, the Beath pin is pulled proximally with the lead suture for passage of the graft.

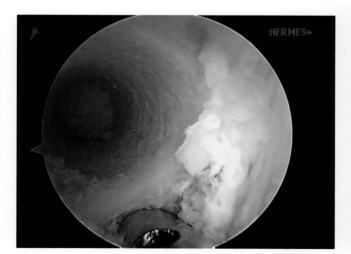

Fig. 39-9. The closed-end femoral tunnel is inspected after drilling and dilating. A smaller drill is later used to penetrate the outer cortex for graft passage.

clamp is used to pull the sutures, leading the graft into the tunnel. Under arthroscopic visualization, the marking on the graft entering the femoral tunnel is noted.

Graft Fixation: Hamstring Autograft or Soft Tissue Allograft

Once the graft is pulled into position, attention is turned to the superolateral portal. The knee is placed in 45 degrees flexion. The portal incision is extended along Langer lines to a length of 3 cm. Metzenbaum scissors are used to dissect the subcutaneous tissue down to fascia. The soft tissue is manually cleared from the fascia using a lap sponge. The interval between the vastus lateralis and the iliotibial band is easily identified and incised in line with their fibers. Next blunt finger dissection is performed just to the iliotibial band to clear soft tissue attachments posteriorly and distally. A finger is then swept underneath the vastus lateralis and creates a space between the vastus and the lateral femur. The lead graft suture is pulled taut and identified at its exit from the femur. These suture limbs are hooked with a finger and pulled out through the superolateral incision.

Next the lateral femur is exposed, retracting the vastus lateralis anterior and the iliotibial band posterior. The closed Endoloop is placed in position on the lateral femur with a tonsil to estimate its most proximal extent. The periosteum overlying the lateral femur is incised with Bovie electrocautery and elevated in the proximal and distal directions. The Endoloop is again checked and a 3.2-mm drill bit is used to drill a bicortical hole perpendicular to the long axis of the femur. After measuring the length, a commercially available 4.5-mm cortical screw and washer are placed through the Endoloop into the femur. As the screw catches the second cortex, the graft is pulled tight distally. The fixation is palpated to ensure the Endoloop limbs are tight on either side of the screw and washer.

The graft is cycled 20 times while tension is held on the distal graft sutures and isometry is assessed. The tibia is reduced posteriorly on the femur and the knee is placed in full extension for tibial fixation. Bovie electrocautery and the curved osteotome are used to expose the anteromedial tibia in the distal portion of the tibial incision, approximately 1.5 cm distal to the tibial tunnel. In similar fashion to the femoral side, a bicortical 4.5-mm screw and washer are placed from anteromedial to posterolateral within the proximal tibia. When the screw advances to the second cortex, the suture limbs from the tibial side of the graft are tied with tension over the post. The knee is fully extended and the screw is tightened. The arthroscope is inserted to confirm adequate position, tension, and fixation of the graft and to ensure no impingement **(Fig. 39-11)**.

Closure

The incisions are irrigated and Vicryl sutures are used to partially close the periosteum over the proximal tibia. The

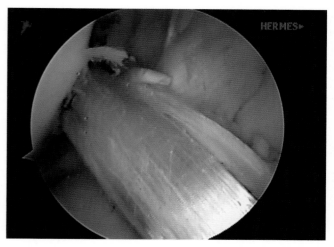

Fig. 39-11. A final arthroscopic view of the graft is obtained after fixation.

subcutaneous layer is approximated with interrupted, inverted 3-0 Vicryl suture and the skin is closed with a running 4-0 absorbable monofilament suture. The portals are closed with 3-0 nylon suture. The incisions are covered with Adaptic gauze and sterile gauze then wrapped in cast padding and bias wrap. A cryocuff device and a hinged knee brace locked in extension are placed on the knee. The patient is awakened and taken to the recovery room, where the anesthesiology staff assesses the patient's pain and will redose the catheter if required.

■ TECHNICAL ALTERNATIVES AND PITFALLS

For femoral tunnel placement, the primary technical alternatives to the medial portal technique are the two-incision technique and the standard transtibial endoscopic technique. Both have shown good clinical results.[32]

One potential pitfall of the medial portal technique is not hyperflexing the knee for placement of the femoral tunnel. Full flexion allows improved visualization of the anatomic position of the ACL bundle attachments, better access to the medial wall of the lateral femoral condyle, and a more anterior-directed tunnel to avoid significant disruption of the posterior wall. In addition, the medial portal incision should be made slightly larger than normal to accommodate the reamer for the femoral tunnel. Care must be used to guide the reamer past the articular surfaces of the medial femoral condyle and trochlea.

Another potential concern is catching anterior soft tissue during passage of the graft. This occurrence can be minimized by passing the pituitary in the medial portal directly against the Beath pin guidewire to avoid passing it through a portion of the infrapatellar fat pad or subcutaneous tissue. This is noted when the graft is passed and does not lie directly from tibial to femoral tunnel. Should this occur, the soft tissue can be removed with a pituitary rongeur or the graft can be pulled on both ends to release the soft tissue band.

■ REHABILITATION

Patients are given instructions for exercises (quad sets, straight-leg raises, calf pumps, and heel slides) and crutch use prior to discharge on the same day. Patients with isolated ACL reconstructions are weightbearing as tolerated with crutches upon discharge. They may unlock their brace to perform heel slides for the first week. Patients are re-examined in 1 week and have their sutures removed. Instructions are given then to unlock the brace for ambulation and remove the brace at night. Gait training with crutches and exercises are reviewed with emphasis on obtaining full extension. Patients return at 1 month and are generally allowed to discontinue their crutches and brace. Physical therapy is prescribed to follow an ACL rehabilitation protocol at 1 month or earlier if there are concerns about motion. Patients can begin running at 5 to 6 months and may return to sports at 9 to 12 months.

■ OUTCOMES AND FUTURE DIRECTIONS

Placement of the femoral tunnel through the medial portal technique may prove to be another important advancement in ACL reconstruction. In addition to the use of fluoroscopy, use of the medial portal technique can help reduce the number of avoidable errors in this procedure. Because errant tunnel placement remains one of the most common causes of ACL reconstruction graft failure, future prospective studies may show a potential decrease in the number of graft failures using the medial portal technique.

■ REFERENCES

1. Freedman KB, D'Amato MJ, Nedeff DD, et al. Arthroscopic anterior cruciate ligament reconstruction: a meta-analysis comparing patellar tendon and hamstring tendon autografts. Am J Sports Med. 2003;31(1):2–11.
2. Martin SD, Martin TL, Brown CH. Anterior cruciate ligament graft fixation. Orthop Clin North Am. 2002;33(4):685–696.
3. Miller SL, Gladstone JN. Graft selection in anterior cruciate ligament reconstruction. Orthop Clin North Am. 2002;33(4):675–683.
4. Sherman OH, Banffy MB. Anterior cruciate ligament reconstruction: which graft is best? Arthroscopy. 2004;20(9):974–980.
5. West RV, Harner CD. Graft selection in anterior cruciate ligament reconstruction. J Am Acad Orthop Surg. 2005;13(3):197–207.
6. Frndak PA, Berasi CC. Rehabilitation concerns following anterior cruciate ligament reconstruction. Sports Med. 1991;12(5):338–346.
7. Fu FH, Irrgang JJ, Harner CD. Loss of motion following anterior cruciate ligament reconstruction. In: Jackson DW, Arnoczky SP, Woo SLY, et al., eds. The Anterior Cruciate Ligament: Current and Future Concepts. New York: Raven Press; 1993:373–380.
8. Petsche TS, Hutchinson MR. Loss of extension after reconstruction of the anterior cruciate ligament. J Am Acad Orthop Surg. 1999;7:119–127.
9. Andersen HN, Amis AA. Review on tension in the natural and reconstructed anterior cruciate ligament. Knee Surg Sports Traumatol Arthrosc. 1994;2(4):192–202.
10. Beynnon BD, Fleming BC. Anterior cruciate ligament strain in-vivo: a review of previous work. J Biomech. 1998;31:519–525.
11. Harner CD, Baek GH, Vorgin TM, et al. Quantitative analysis of human cruciate ligament insertions. Arthroscopy. 1999;15(7):741–749.
12. Woo SL, Livesay GA, Engle C. Biomechanics of the human anterior cruciate ligament. ACL structure and role in knee motion. Orthop Rev. 1992;21(7):835–842.
13. Allen CR, Giffin JR, Harner CD. Revision anterior cruciate ligament reconstruction. Orthop Clin North Am. 2003;34(1):79–98.
14. Greis PE, Johnson DL, Fu FH. Revision anterior cruciate ligament surgery: causes of graft failure and technical considerations of revision surgery. Clin Sports Med. 1993;12(4):839–852.
15. Harner CD, Giffin JR, Dunteman RC, et al. Evaluation and treatment of recurrent instability after anterior cruciate ligament reconstruction. Instr Course Lect. 2001;50:463–474.
16. Vergis A, Gillquist J. Graft failure in intra-articular anterior cruciate ligament reconstructions: a review of the literature. Arthroscopy. 1995;11(3):312–321.
17. Getelman MH, Friedman MJ. Revision anterior cruciate ligament reconstruction surgery. J Am Acad Orthop Surg. 1999;7:189–198.
18. Johnson DL, Swenson TM, Irrgang JJ, et al. Revision anterior cruciate ligament surgery: experience from Pittsburgh. Clin Orthop. 1996;325:100–109.
19. Loh JC, Fukada Y, Tsuda E, et al. Knee stability and graft function following anterior cruciate ligament reconstruction: comparison between 11 o'clock and 10 o'clock femoral tunnel placement. Arthroscopy. 2003;19:297–304.
20. Cha PS, Chhabra A, Harner CD. Single-bundle anterior cruciate ligament reconstruction using the medial portal technique. Oper Tech Orthop. 2005;15(2):89–95.
21. Johma NM, Raso VJ, Leung P. Effect of varying angles on the pullout strength of interference screw fixation. Arthroscopy. 1993;9:154–158.
22. Lemos MJ, Douglas WJ, Lee TQ, et al. Assessment of initial fixation of endoscopic interference femoral screws with divergent and parallel placement. J Arthros Rel Res. 1995;11:37–41.
23. O'Donnell JB, Scerpella TA. Endoscopic anterior cruciate ligament reconstruction: modified technique and radiographic review. Arthroscopy. 1995;11(5):577–584.
24. Yasuda K, Kondo E, Ichiyama H, et al. Anatomic reconstruction of the anteromedial and posterolateral bundles of the anterior cruciate ligament using hamstring tendon grafts. Arthroscopy. 2004;20:1015–1025.
25. Deehan DJ, Salmon LJ, Webb VJ, et al. Endoscopic reconstruction of the anterior cruciate ligament with an ipsilateral patellar tendon autograft. A prospective longitudinal five-year study. J Bone Joint Surg Br. 2000;82(7):984–991.
26. Giron F, Aglietti P, Cuomo P, et al. Anterior cruciate ligament reconstruction with double-looped semitendinosus and gracilis tendon graft directly fixed to cortical bone: 5-year results. Knee Surg Sports Tramatol Arthrosc. 2005;13:81–91.
27. Otto D, Pinczewski LA, Clingeleffer A, et al. Five-year results of single-incision arthroscopic anterior cruciate ligament reconstruction with patellar tendon autograft. Am J Sports Med. 1998;26(2):181–188.

28. Pinczewski LA, Deehan DJ, Salmon LJ, et al. A five-year comparison of patellar tendon versus four-strand hamstring tendon autograft for arthroscopic reconstruction of the anterior cruciate ligament. Am J Sports Med. 2002;30(4):523–536.
29. Roe J, Pinczewski LA, Russell VJ, et al. A 7-year follow-up of patellar tendon and hamstring tendon grafts for arthroscopic anterior cruciate ligament reconstruction: differences and similarities. Am J Sports Med. 2005;33(9):1337–1345.
30. Scranton PE, Bagenstose JE, Lantz BA, et al. Quadruple hamstring anterior cruciate reconstruction: A multicenter study. Arthroscopy. 2002;18:715–724.
31. Webb JM, Corry IS, Clingeleffer AJ, et al. Endoscopic reconstruction for isolated anterior cruciate ligament rupture. J Bone Joint Surg Br. 1998;80(2):288–294.
32. Harner CD, Marks PH, Fu FH, et al. Anterior cruciate ligament reconstruction: endoscopic versus two-incision technique. Arthroscopy. 1994;10(5):502–512.
33. Greis PE, Burks RT, Bachus K, et al. The influence of tendon length and fit on the strength of a tendon-bone tunnel complex: A biomechanical and histologic study in the dog. Am J Sports Med. 2001;29(4):493–497.

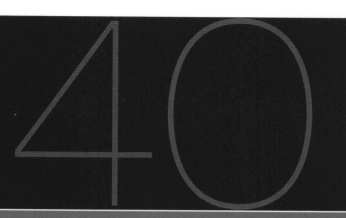

ALTERNATIVE ANTERIOR CRUCIATE LIGAMENT FIXATION TECHNIQUES: RETROSCREW

MELISSA D. KOENIG, MD, JAMES P. BRADLEY, MD

Since the first anterior cruciate ligament (ACL) reconstruction was performed, surgeons have continued to strive for ways to make the construct as anatomic as possible. This concept has led to developments in graft type, tunnel location, and graft fixation. The concept of aperture fixation, that is fixation at the intraarticular ends of the femoral and tibial tunnels, was popularized in the 1990s. Although early results were promising, this technique was technically demanding. The development of the Retroscrew (Arthrex, Inc, Naples, Fla), an interference screw placed retrograde in a standard tibial tunnel, has made this procedure more feasible.

Benefits of aperture fixation include increased graft pull-out strength, decreased graft "windshield wiper" motion, decreased tunnel widening, and a more stable construct throughout knee range of motion. The Retroscrew can be used to fix any graft including autogenous bone-patellar-tendon bone and hamstring grafts as well as all allograft options. The Retroscrew construct has been described for fixation of both single tunnel reconstructions and single femoral socket and double bundle constructs.

■ SURGICAL TECHNIQUE

The graft and tunnels are prepared using standard techniques. Both tunnels are notched with the Retro Tunnel Notcher (Arthrex, Inc, Naples, Fla). Before the graft is passed, a FiberStick (Arthrex, Inc, Naples, Fla) is passed into the tibial tunnel. The suture end is grasped and withdrawn through the anteromedial portal. The suture is kept anterior as the graft is passed into the joint and seated into the femoral tunnel.

To fix the graft using a femoral Retroscrew **(Fig. 40-1A, B,C,D,E),** the cannulated screwdriver is placed over the stiff end of the FiberStick. The driver is advanced through the tibial tunnel anterior to the graft. Outside of the knee, the

free end of the suture is passed through the head of the screw and out of the other end. A Mulberry knot is tied to secure the screw on the suture. The screw is secured into the plastic cannula and inserted into the joint through the anteromedial portal. An obturator is used to push the screw into the joint.

The suture exiting the screwdriver handle is pulled to guide the screw onto the tip of the driver. Any visible soft tissue must be removed to allow the screw to seat fully. The suture is removed with a grasper from the anteromedial portal and the screw is advanced to the opening of the femoral tunnel. The graft is tensioned and the screw is advanced into the tunnel. The screwdriver is disengaged from the screw and kept in the tibial tunnel.

To place the tibial Retroscrew **(Fig. 40-2A,B,C,D,E),** another FiberStick is advanced through the screwdriver. The suture is retrieved through the anteromedial portal as described above. The screw is secured to the suture with a Mulberry knot tied behind the head of the screw. The screw is passed into the joint as previously described. Pulling on the suture guides the screw tip onto the screwdriver. Once the screw is fully seated, the suture is secured around the grommets on the handle of the screwdriver. The graft is tensioned and the screw is inserted in a counterclockwise fashion until the head is flush with the tibial tunnel. The suture is grasped at the knot through the anteromedial portal and removed. Secondary tibial fixation can be performed, if desired, according to the surgeon's preference.

■ TECHNICAL ALTERNATIVES AND PITFALLS

Throughout the development and use of this technique, we have learned several "pearls" to make the screw insertion

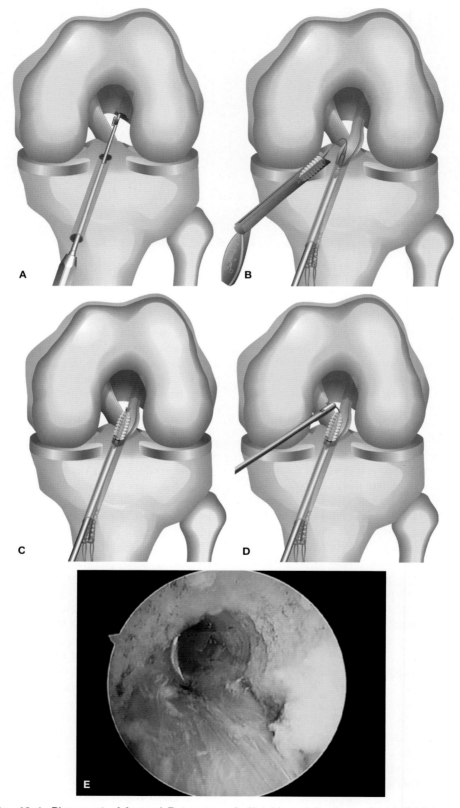

Fig. 40-1. Placement of femoral Retroscrew. **A:** Notching of the femoral and tibial tunnels. **B:** Passage of the screw into the joint. **C:** Seating the screw on the driver. **D:** Removal of the suture. **E:** Appearance after femoral fixation of the graft.

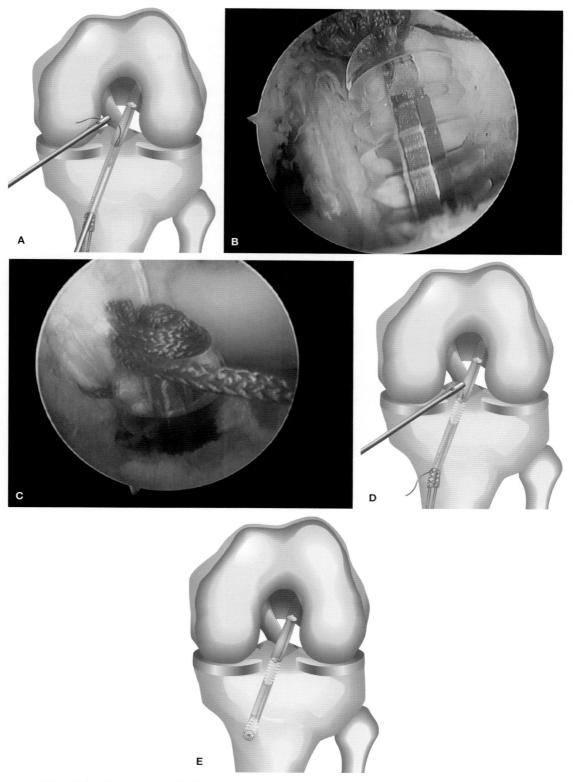

Fig. 40-2. Placement of tibial Retroscrew. **A:** Retrieval of suture from the joint. The suture is then passed through the screw and secured with a Mulberry knot behind the head. **B:** After seating the screw, it is placed retrograde into the tibial tunnel. **C:** The suture coils around the knot as the screw is advanced. **D:** After checking that the graft is fixed securely, the suture is removed through the anteromedial portal. **E:** The completed graft/Retroscrew construct. Supplement tibial fixation (shown here with an interference screw) can be added according to surgeon preference.

proceed smoothly. First, when using a bone-tendon-bone graft, make sure that the tibial bone plug and the screwdriver can pass through the tunnel sizer together. Next, notch the medial aspect of the tibial tunnel so that as the screw engages, it doesn't spin into the posterior cruciate ligament (PCL). In addition, we prefer to thread the suture through the screwdriver prior to placing the construct into the joint. The scrub assistant assembles the screwdriver-suture construct by passing the FiberStick through the screwdriver, grasping the suture at the screwdriver tip, and then withdrawing the FiberStick. The construct is then passed through the tibial tunnel and the suture is retrieved and drawn out of the anteromedial portal. Finally, once the tibial screw is placed, undo the suture from the grommets, remove the screwdriver from the tunnel, and clamp the suture with a hemostat at the base of the screwdriver. Do not remove the suture from the inside of the screwdriver until the stability of the fixation has been assessed. Should the screw require removal to re-tension the graft, the suture guides you easily to it.

■ SUMMARY

Recent developments have led to easier techniques for fixing ACL grafts anatomically. The advantages of aperture fixation include increased stability, as aperture fixation has been shown to be more stable than peripheral fixation. Additionally, placing the tibial screw retrograde maintains tension on the graft as the screw is advanced. When placed anterograde, the graft tension tends to decrease as the screw is advanced. Secondary tibial fixation of a bone-patellar-tendon graft with a posteriorly placed screw further increases the pullout strength. This combination has been termed the "Killer S" construct. Other studies have shown decreased tunnel expansion with aperture fixation. Finally, with anatomic fixation, graft motion in the tibial tunnel is decreased, which may result in better graft incorporation. Although long-term prospective randomized trials are needed to assess the clinical results, aperture fixation remains a biomechanically superior fixation option.

■ SUGGESTED READINGS

Benfield D, Otto DD, Bagnall KM, et al. Stiffness characteristics of hamstring tendon graft fixation methods at the femoral site. Inter Ortho. 2005;29:35–38.

Fauno P, Kaalund S. Tunnel widening after hamstring anterior cruciate ligament reconstruction is influenced by the type of graft fixation used: a prospective randomized study. Arthroscopy. 2005;21:1337–1341.

Ishibashi Y, Rudy TW, Livesay GA, et al. The effect of anterior cruciate ligament graft fixation site at the tibia on knee stability: evaluation using a robotic testing system. Arthroscopy. 1997;13:177–182.

Morgan CD, Caborn D. Anatomic graft fixation using a retrograde biointerference screw for endoscopic anterior cruciate ligament reconstruction: single-bundle and 2-bundle techniques. Tech Ortho. 2005;20:297–302.

Scheffler SU, Sudkamp NP, Gockenjan A, et al. Biomechanical comparison of hamstring and patellar tendon graft anterior cruciate ligament reconstruction techniques: the impact of fixation level and fixation method under cyclic loading. Arthroscopy. 2002;18:304–315.

41

REVISION ANTERIOR CRUCIATE LIGAMENT RECONSTRUCTION

NIKHIL N. VERMA, MD, RUSSELL F. WARREN, MD,
THOMAS L. WICKIEWICZ, MD

■ HISTORY OF THE TECHNIQUE

Anterior cruciate ligament (ACL) reconstruction continues to be one of the most common procedures performed in orthopedics.[1] Although primary reconstructions result in a satisfactory outcome more than 75% to 90% of the time, a significant number of patients may still require revision procedures.[2,3] The approach to revision surgery should follow the same principles as those applied to primary reconstruction. The etiology of failure should be initially identified, allowing the surgeon to plan a revision procedure to address deficiencies that lead to failure of the primary reconstruction. Results of revision surgery to date have been inferior to primary reconstruction. However, as experience with revision cases expands, and with continued improvement in arthroscopic techniques, we believe that good results can be achieved.

■ INDICATIONS AND CONTRAINDICATIONS

The indications for revision ACL reconstruction are based primarily on the etiology of failure, which can often be elicited from the patient history and the patient's symptoms. It is important to listen to the primary complaints of the patient, as this will help differentiate between recurrent instability, pain, or stiffness. The timing of failure can also provide an important clue in determining the etiology of failure. Early failure (within 6 months) is often due to a technical error such as failure of fixation, incorrect tunnel placement, or improper tensioning. Late failures (after 1 year) can be caused by failure of graft incorporation, traumatic rerupture, or progression of traumatic arthrosis.[4-6] The main indication for revision ACL reconstruction is recurrent instability that impairs quality of life.

A thorough physical examination should be performed on all patients who have failed a primary reconstruction. The patient should be examined standing and during gait to assess alignment and evaluate for varus or valgus thrust. Range of motion should be accurately evaluated, particularly to ensure full extension is present. Instability examination, including Lachman and pivot shift testing, should be performed. Finally, a thorough evaluation of the integrity of the medial structures and posterolateral corner should be performed as failure to address injuries to these structures has been reported as a cause of early failure after ACL reconstruction.[7,8] Correction of instability at the side of the knee is important in revision surgery as excess stresses are placed on the ACL graft with varus or valgus instability and particularly with increases of external rotation of more than 10 degrees to 15 degrees.

Plain radiographs should be obtained in all cases of failed ACL reconstruction. Specific views required include standing anteroposterior and lateral views, a merchant view, a notch view, and a weight-bearing anteroposterior 45-degree flexion view.[9] The tibial and femoral tunnels can be evaluated on both the AP and lateral views to evaluate for tunnel widening and position, as well as the presence of retained hardware **(Fig. 41-1A,B)**. The flexion weight-bearing view can be used to assess for early degenerative disease, which can affect prognosis.[9] Finally, if any malalignment is appreciated on physical examination, a full-length standing mechanical axis view should be obtained to determine if an alignment-correcting osteotomy is necessary in addition to or in place of ligament reconstruction.

In most cases, magnetic resonance imaging (MRI) should also be obtained as a routine preoperative study. MRI allows for direct evaluation of the integrity of the ligament graft[10] **(Fig. 41-2A,B,C)**. Tunnel position as well as tunnel

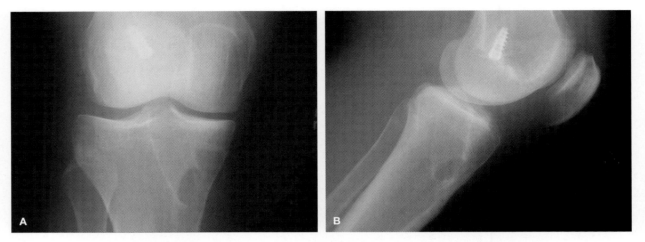

Fig. 41-1. (A) Anteroposterior and **(B)** lateral radiograph demonstrating significant tibial tunnel widening after primary ACL reconstruction.

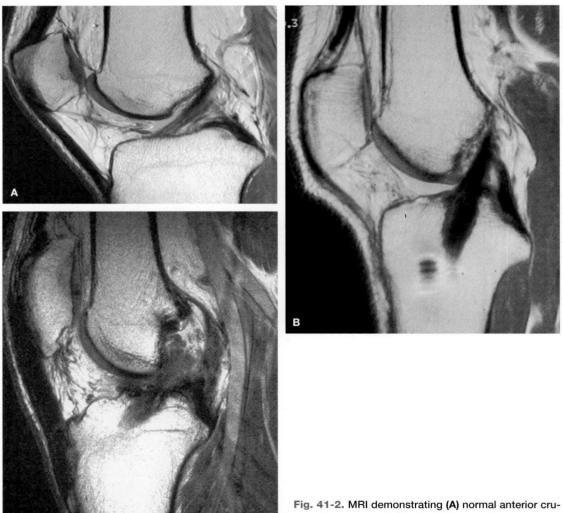

Fig. 41-2. MRI demonstrating **(A)** normal anterior cruciate ligament and **(B)** reconstructed ligament with bone-patellar tendon-bone autograft, and **(C)** traumatic graft rerupture.

widening can also be evaluated in both the sagittal and coronal planes. However, it should be noted that although the MRI may demonstrate graft integrity with a uniform low signal, the graft may be nonfunctional with persistent knee instability and a positive pivot shift test. The integrity of the menisci can be evaluated to allow for planning of alternate procedures that may be required at the time of revision surgery. The competency of the medial and lateral structures can be evaluated and correlated with the physical exam findings. Finally, with the development of newer cartilage sensitive MRI techniques, the integrity of the articular cartilage can be evaluated to help identify degenerative changes that can affect prognosis.[11]

Absolute or relative contraindications to revision reconstruction are relatively limited. Absolute contraindications include active local or systemic infection. Relative contraindications include significant degenerative changes. In these cases, care must be taken to assess whether the major complaint is pain or instability. If instability is present, revision reconstruction may still be indicated with the limited goal of restoring stability with activities of daily living. In cases in which pain and degenerative changes are accompanied by malalignment, consideration should be given to isolated osteotomy or combined osteotomy and revision ACL reconstruction. Previously we felt that patients with both degenerative disease and a positive pivot shift examination required both procedures. Subsequently, we have noted that the pivot shift examination will decrease or be eliminated by a closing wedge osteotomy that decreases the slope of the tibial plateau, thus eliminating the need for revision ACL reconstruction in some patients.

■ SURGICAL TECHNIQUE

Preoperative Planning

In order to understand the surgical techniques and principles associated with revision ACL reconstruction, one must first understand the potential etiologies of primary reconstruction failure. Proper identification of the etiology of failure is necessary to properly plan the approach to revision surgery. Although potential causes of failure also include loss of motion, persistent pain, and patient dissatisfaction, in this chapter we will focus on recurrent instability.

In our experience, return of instability after ACL reconstruction can be classified into three broad categories. Classification of patients into one of these three categories is based primarily on the patient history and physical examination. The first category is traumatic graft rerupture. This group of patients presents with a complaint of recurrent instability after a single event trauma in a previously stable knee. The mechanism of failure is the same as that which occurs in a native ACL rupture, and the primary reconstruction can be assumed to have been optimally placed. Important considerations in these cases include identification of the

graft used for the primary reconstruction, and appropriate graft selection for the revision procedure. The surgeon may choose to avoid grafts that have been associated with slightly higher failure rates such as four-strand hamstring tendon (publication pending, Wickiewicz TL, Williams RJ)[12] in favor of autograft patellar tendon or allograft tissue. Given that the primary reconstruction resulted in a stable knee, it is assumed that the primary procedure was technically well done and the same tunnels as those used for the primary surgery can be used for the revision.

The second category of recurrent instability is atraumatic graft failure. These patients present with a technically well-done reconstruction, but with progressive return of instability in the absence of trauma. Potential sources of failure in these cases include failure of graft biological integration, improper graft tension, failure of bone healing, or missed associated instabilities such as persistent medial laxity or posterolateral corner deficiency.[7,8,17] In these cases, the surgeon must again be cognizant of the graft used for primary reconstruction when choosing an appropriate graft for the revision procedure. Furthermore, a careful physical examination should be performed to assess for alternate instability patterns that can predispose an ACL reconstruction to early failure. These secondary instability patterns must also be corrected at the time of revision surgery in order to achieve a successful outcome.

If no coexisting pathology is identified, tunnels are assessed based on preoperative radiographs and MRI. In most cases, the tunnel position is optimal and the same tunnels may be used for the revision procedure. If tunnel widening is present, a decision should be made as to whether this can be addressed at the time of revision using techniques such as larger bone plugs, stacked interference screws, or single stage bone grafting, or if a two-stage procedure is required **(Fig. 41-3A,B,C)**. Careful attention should be paid to thorough graft removal, proper graft tensioning, and secure graft fixation.

The third category of recurrent instability is graft failure. This can occur due to a malpositioned graft or a failure of fixation. Loss of fixation can occur secondary to poor bone quality, screw breakage, screw divergence, or graft damage during screw insertion.[18,19] If recognized early (within the first week) it may be amenable to revision fixation. However, in most cases, revision reconstruction is necessary. If bone quality is poor, options include compaction drilling or bone grafting. Supplementary fixation such as EndoButton (Acufex, Mansfield, OH) fixation on the femoral side or soft tissue button fixation on the tibial side can also be used. Whenever possible, aperture fixation should be achieved. If graft injury has occurred during femoral screw placement, the graft can be reversed placing the tibial bone block on the femoral side and using soft tissue fixation techniques on the tibial side.

Graft malposition can occur on either the femoral or tibial tunnel. The most frequent cause of a need for revision surgery is incorrect tunnel placement on the femur. Tibial tunnel placement is important to avoid a vertical graft, but

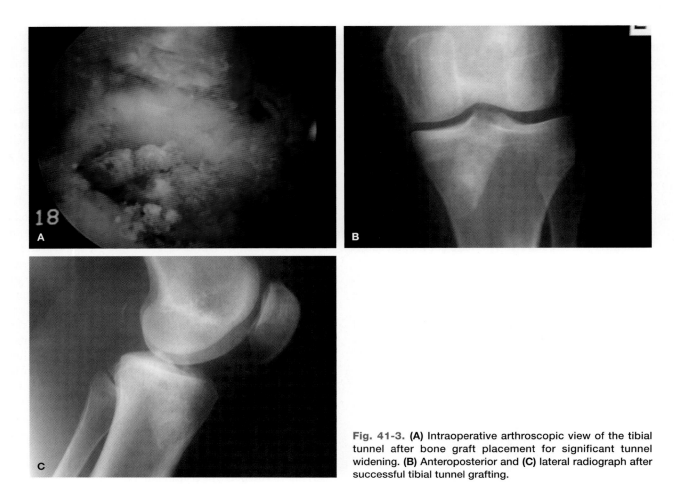

Fig. 41-3. (A) Intraoperative arthroscopic view of the tibial tunnel after bone graft placement for significant tunnel widening. **(B)** Anteroposterior and **(C)** lateral radiograph after successful tibial tunnel grafting.

malposition is much less frequent. Anterior femoral tunnel placement results in flexion deficits and early graft failure due to impingement in extension[20] **(Fig. 41-4A)**. In this case, a proper posterior tunnel may be placed posterior to the original anterior tunnel (Fig. 41-4B). If pre-existing hardware is not impeding proper tunnel placement, it should be left in place to avoid creating a larger defect. If sufficient room is not available to place a correct posterior tunnel, a two-stage procedure may be necessary with initial bone grafting followed by revision reconstruction in 12 weeks. Posterior femoral tunnel position with femoral cortical compromise can be revised using a two-incision technique to create divergent tunnels. If this is not possible, a two-stage revision should be considered. Central femoral tunnel position results in a vertical graft, which provides anteroposterior stability without rotation control **(Fig. 41-5A)**. This can be manifested on physical examination with a negative Lachman exam and a persistent pivot shift. If adequate bone stock remains, a proper femoral tunnel should be created using either an endoscopic or two-incision technique. (Fig. 41-4B) Otherwise, a two-stage revision should be considered.

Tibial tunnel malposition can also result in failure of primary ACL reconstruction.[21–24] An anteriorly placed tibial tunnel will result in graft impingement in extension and

early graft failure. A posterior position will result in tightness in extension and possible laxity. It is important to note that when using an endoscopic technique, the coronal plane obliquity of the tibial tunnel will affect femoral tunnel position. A tibial tunnel that is placed at less than 30 degrees to the sagittal axis will make it difficult to place the femoral tunnel in the appropriate lateral position. If the femoral tunnel is placed vertically, the resulting graft will not control rotation. In cases of tibial tunnel malposition, an attempt can be made to drill a properly oriented tibial tunnel if bone stock is present, but most cases require bone grafting in either a single or two-staged fashion.

Once the etiology of failure has been identified and the need for revision surgery confirmed, proper preoperative planning is essential for attaining a successful outcome. The first step is to identify the graft material to be used for the revision procedure. Current options include ipsilateral or contralateral patellar tendon, quadriceps tendon, hamstring tendon, or allograft tissue. At our institution, we prefer allograft tissue as our graft of choice for revision procedures. The main advantages of allograft tissue is the absence of morbidity associated with graft harvest and decreased operative time. Second, the large bone blocks with allograft tissue provide the surgeon with the flexibility to create bone blocks of a

42

ANTERIOR CRUCIATE LIGAMENT RECONSTRUCTION IN THE SKELETALLY IMMATURE PATIENT

■ MININDER S. KOCHER, MD, MPH

Anterior cruciate ligament (ACL) injuries in skeletally immature patients are being seen with increased frequency. Management of these injuries is controversial. Nonreconstructive treatment of complete tears typically results in recurrent functional instability with risk of injury to meniscal and articular cartilage. A variety of reconstructive techniques have been utilized, including physeal sparing, partial transphyseal, and transphyseal methods using various grafts. Conventional adult ACL reconstruction techniques risk potential iatrogenic growth disturbance due to physeal violation. Growth disturbances after ACL reconstruction in skeletally immature patients have been reported.

In this chapter, we discuss our approach to ACL reconstruction in the skeletally immature patient based on physiological age (Fig. 42-1). In prepubescent patients, we perform a physeal-sparing, combined intra-articular, and extra-articular reconstruction utilizing autogenous iliotibial band. In adolescent patients with significant growth remaining, we perform transphyseal ACL reconstruction with autogenous hamstrings tendons with fixation away from the physis. In older adolescent patients approaching skeletal maturity, we perform conventional adult ACL reconstruction with interference screw fixation using either autogenous central third patellar tendon or autogenous hamstrings.

■ HISTORY OF THE TECHNIQUE

Intrasubstance ACL injuries in children and adolescents were once considered rare, with tibial eminence avulsion fractures considered the pediatric ACL injury equivalent.[1–4] However, intrasubstance ACL injuries in children and adolescents are being seen with increased frequency and have received increased attention. ACL injury has been reported in 10% to 65% of pediatric knees with acute traumatic hemarthroses in series ranging from 35 to 138 patients.[5–10]

Controversy exists regarding the management of ACL injuries in patients with open physis. Nonoperative management of partial tears may be successful in some patients.[11] However, nonoperative management of complete tears in skeletally immature patients generally has a poor prognosis with recurrent instability leading to further meniscal and chondral injury, which has implications in terms of development of degenerative joint disease.[12–18] Graf et al.,[13] Mizuta et al.,[17] and Janarv et al.[14] have reported instability symptoms, subsequent meniscal tears, decreased activity level, and need for ACL reconstruction in the majority of skeletally immature patients treated nonoperatively in series of 8, 18, and 23 patients, respectively. Similarly, when comparing the results of operative versus nonoperative management of complete ACL injuries in adolescents, McCarroll et al.[15] and Pressman et al.[18] found that those managed by ACL reconstruction had less instability, higher activity and return to sport levels, and lower rates of subsequent reinjury and meniscal tears.

Conventional surgical reconstruction techniques risk potential iatrogenic growth disturbance due to physeal violation. Cases of growth disturbance have been reported in animal models[19–21] and clinical series.[22–24] Animal models have demonstrated mixed results regarding growth disturbances from soft tissue grafts across the physis. In a canine model with iliotibial band grafts through 5/32 inch tunnels, Stadelmaier et al.[25] found no evidence of growth arrest in the four animals with soft tissue graft across the physis, whereas the four animals with drill holes and no graft demonstrated physeal arrest. In a rabbit model using a semitendinosus graft through 2-mm tunnels, Guzzanti et al.[19] did have cases of growth disturbance; however, these were not common: 5% shortening (1/21) and 10% distal femoral

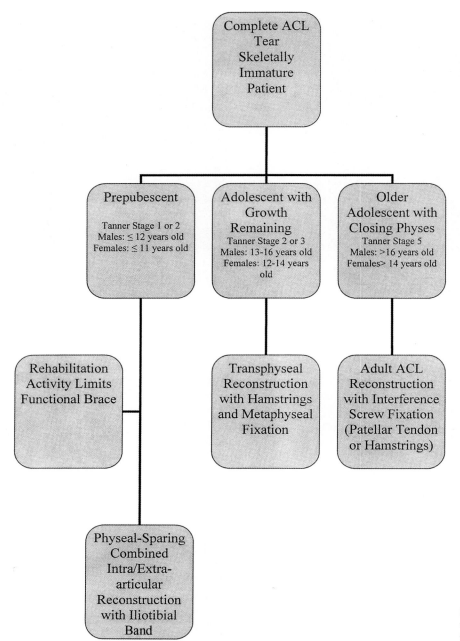

Fig. 42-1. Algorithm for management of complete ACL injuries in skeletally immature patients.

valgus deformity (2/21). Examining the effect of a tensioned soft-tissue graft across the physis, Edwards et al.[21] found a substantial rate of deformity. In a canine model with iliotibial band graft tensioned to 80 N, these investigators found significant increases, compared to the nonoperated control limb, in distal femoral valgus deformity and proximal tibial varus deformity despite no evidence of a bony bar. Similarly, Houle et al.[20] reported growth disturbance after a tensioned tendon graft in a bone tunnel across the rabbit physis.

Clinical reports of growth deformity after ACL reconstruction are unusual. Lipscomb and Anderson[22] reported one case of 20 mm shortening in a series of 24 skeletally immature patients reconstructed with transphyseal semitendinosus and

gracilis grafts. This was associated with staple graft fixation across the physis. Koman and Sanders[23] reported a case of distal femoral valgus deformity requiring osteotomy and contralateral epiphysiodesis after transphyseal reconstruction with a doubled semitendinosus graft. This case was also associated with fixation across the distal femoral physis. Kocher et al.[24] reported an additional 15 cases of growth disturbances gleaned from a questionnaire of expert experience, including eight cases of distal femoral valgus deformity with an arrest of the lateral distal femoral physis, three cases of tibial recurvatum with an arrest of the tibial tubercle apophysis, two cases of genu valgum without arrest due to a lateral extra-articular tether, and two cases of leg length discrepancy (one shortening and one overgrowth). Associated factors included fixation hardware across the lateral distal femoral physis in three cases, bone plugs of a patellar tendon graft across the distal femoral physis in three cases, large (12 mm) tunnels in two cases, lateral extra-articular tenodesis in two cases, fixation hardware across the tibial tubercle apophysis in two cases, over-the-top femoral position in one case, and suturing near the tibial tubercle apophysis in one case.

Surgical techniques to address ACL insufficiency in skeletally immature patients include primary repair, extra-articular tenodesis, transphyseal reconstruction, partial transphyseal reconstruction, and physeal sparing reconstruction. Primary ligament repair[26,27] and extra-articular tenodesis alone[13,15] have had poor results in children and adolescents, similar to adults. Transphyseal reconstructions with tunnels that violate both the distal femoral and proximal tibial physis have been performed with hamstring autograft, patellar tendon autograft, and allograft tissue.[12,15,28–37] Partial transphyseal reconstructions violate only one physis with a tunnel through the proximal tibial physis and over-the-top positioning on the femur or a tunnel through the distal femoral physis with an epiphyseal tunnel in the tibia.[38–40] A variety of physeal-sparing reconstructions have been described to avoid tunnels across either the distal femoral or proximal tibial physis.[7,41–47]

■ INDICATIONS AND CONTRAINDICATIONS

All skeletally immature patients are not the same. Some have a tremendous amount of growth remaining, while others are essentially done growing. The consequences of growth disturbance in the former group would be severe, requiring osteotomy or limb lengthening. However, the consequences of growth disturbance in the latter group would be minimal. When treating a skeletally immature athlete with an ACL injury, it is important to know his or her chronological age, skeletal age, and physiological age. Skeletal age can be determined from an anteroposterior radiograph of the left hand and wrist per the atlas of Greulich and Pyle.[48] Alternatively, skeletal age can be estimated from knee radiographs per the atlas of Pyle and Hoerr.[49] Physiological age is established using the Tanner staging system **(Table 42-1)**.[50] In the office, the patient can be informally staged by questioning. In the operating room, after the induction of anesthesia, Tanner staging can be confirmed.

The vast majority of ACL injuries in skeletally immature patients occur in adolescents. The management of these injuries in preadolescent children is particularly vexing, given the poor prognosis with nonoperative management, the substantial growth remaining, and the consequences of potential growth disturbance.

TABLE 42-1	Tanner Staging Classification of Secondary Sexual Characteristics		
Tanner Stage		**Male**	**Female**
Stage 1 (Prepubertal)	Growth	5–6 cm/y	5–6 cm/y
	Development	Testes <4 ml or <2.5 cm	No breast development
		No pubic hair	No pubic hair
Stage 2	Growth	5–6 cm/y	7–8 cm/y
	Development	Testes 4 ml or 2.5–3.2 cm	Breast buds
		Minimal pubic hair at base of penis	Minimal pubic hair on labia
Stage 3	Growth	7–8 cm/y	8 cm/y
	Development	Testes 12 ml or 3.6 cm	Elevation of breast; areolae enlarge
		Pubic hair over pubis	Pubic hair of mons pubis
		Voice changes	Axillary hair
		Muscle mass increases	Acne
Stage 4	Growth	10 cm/y	7 cm/y
	Development	Testes 4.1–4.5 cm	Areolae enlarge
		Pubic hair as adult	Pubic hair as adult
		Axillary hair	
		Acne	
Stage 5	Growth	No growth	No growth
	Development	Testes as adult	Adult breast contour
		Pubic hair as adult	Pubic hair as adult
		Facial hair as adult	
		Mature physique	
Other		Peak Height Velocity: 13.5 y	Adrenarche: 6–8 y
			Menarche 12.7 y
			Peak Height Velocity: 11.5 y

Our approach to ACL reconstruction in the skeletally immature patient is based on physiological age **(Fig. 42-1)**. In prepubescent patients, we perform a physeal-sparing, combined intra-articular and extra-articular reconstruction utilizing autogenous iliotibial band. In adolescent patients with significant growth remaining, we perform transphyseal ACL reconstruction with autogenous hamstrings tendons with fixation away from the physis. In older adolescent patients approaching skeletal maturity, we perform conventional adult ACL reconstruction with interference screw fixation using either autogenous central third patellar tendon or autogenous hamstrings.

In the prepubescent patient with a complete ACL tear without concurrent chondral or repairable meniscal injury, we first attempt nonreconstructive treatment with a program of rehabilitation, functional bracing, and return to non– high-risk activities. Although the results of nonreconstructive treatment are generally poor with subsequent functional instability and risk of injury to meniscal and articular cartilage, surgical reconstruction poses the risk of growth

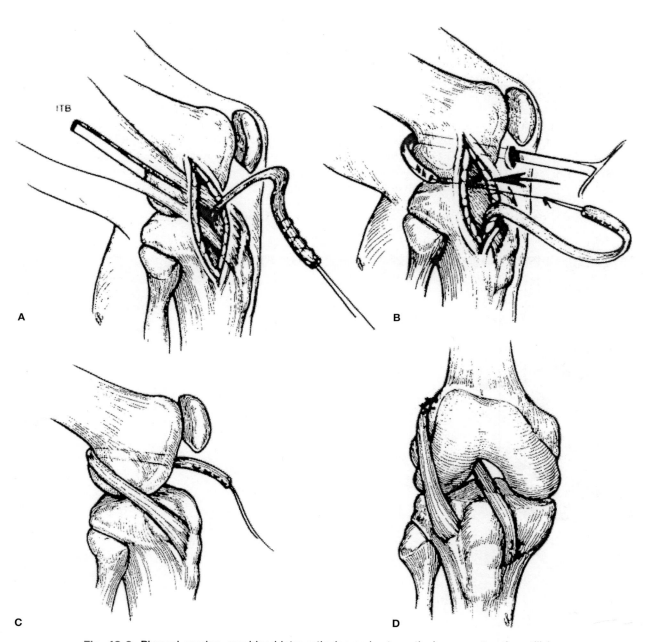

Fig. 42-2. Physeal-sparing, combined intra-articular, and extra-articular reconstruction utilizing autogenous iliotibial band for prepubescents. **A:** The iliotibial band graft is harvested free proximally and left attached to the Gerdy tubercle distally. **B:** The graft is brought through the knee in the over-the-top position posteriorly. **C:** The graft is brought through the knee and under the intermeniscal ligament anteriorly. **D:** Resulting intra-articular and extra-articular reconstruction.

disturbance. Furthermore, some patients are able to cope with their ACL insufficiency or modify their activities, allowing for further growth and aging such that an adolescent-type reconstruction can be performed with transphyseal hamstrings tendons in a more anatomic manner.

For those prepubescent patients with concurrent chondral or repairable meniscal injury, or those with functional instability after nonreconstructive treatment, we perform a physeal-sparing, combined intra-articular and extra-articular reconstruction utilizing autogenous iliotibial band. This procedure is a modification of the combined intra-articular and extra-articular reconstruction described by MacIntosh and Darby.[51] Our rationale for utilization of this technique is to provide knee stability and improve function in prepubescent skeletally immature patients with complete intrasubstance ACL injuries while avoiding the risk of iatrogenic growth disturbance by violating the distal femoral or proximal tibial physis. In our opinion, the consequences of potential iatrogenic growth disturbance caused by transphyseal reconstruction in these young patients are prohibitive. Recognizing that this reconstruction is nonanatomic, we counsel patients and families that they may require revision reconstruction if they develop recurrent instability, but that this procedure may temporize for further growth such that they may then undergo a more conventional reconstruction with drill holes.

For adolescent patients with growth remaining who have a complete ACL tear, we do not advocate initial nonreconstructive treatment since the risk of functional instability with injury to the meniscal and articular cartilage is high, the risk and consequences of growth disturbance from ACL reconstruction are less, and our transphyseal technique is an anatomic reconstruction. In these patients, we perform transphyseal ACL reconstruction with autogenous hamstrings tendons with fixation away from the physis.

For older adolescent patients who are approaching skeletal maturity who have a complete ACL tear, we perform conventional adult ACL reconstruction with interference screw fixation using either autogenous central third patellar tendon or autogenous hamstrings.

In skeletally immature patients, as in adult patients, acute ACL reconstruction is not performed within the first 3 weeks after injury to minimize the risk of arthrofibrosis. Prereconstructive rehabilitation is performed to regain range of motion, decrease swelling, and resolve the reflex inhibition of the quadriceps. ACL reconstruction may be staged in some cases if there is a displaced, bucket-handle tear of the meniscus that requires extensive repair in order to protect the meniscal repair from the early mobilization prescribed by ACL reconstruction. Skeletally immature patients must be emotionally mature enough to actively participate in the extensive rehabilitation required after ACL reconstruction.

■ SURGICAL TECHNIQUE

In older adolescent patients who are approaching skeletal maturity who have a complete ACL tear, we perform

conventional adult ACL reconstruction with interference screw fixation using either autogenous central third patellar tendon or autogenous hamstrings. This is a standard one-incision, arthroscopically assisted technique that is covered elsewhere in the text and will not be further detailed in this chapter.

Prepubescent Patients: Physeal-sparing, Combined Intra/Extra-articular Reconstruction with Autogenous Iliotibial Band

In prepubescent patients, we perform a physeal-sparing, combined intra-articular and extra-articular reconstruction utilizing autogenous iliotibial band **(Fig. 42.2)**. The procedure is performed under general anesthesia as an overnight observation procedure. Local anesthesia with sedation may not be reliable in prepubescent children with the potential for a paradoxical effect of sedation. The child is positioned supine on the operating table with a pneumatic tourniquet about the upper thigh, which is used routinely. Examination under anesthesia is performed to confirm ACL insufficiency.

First, the iliotibial band graft is obtained. An incision of approximately 6 cm is made obliquely from the lateral joint line to the superior border of the iliotibial band **(Fig. 42.3A)**. Proximally, the iliotibial band is separated from subcutaneous tissue using a periosteal elevator under the skin of the lateral thigh. The anterior and posterior borders of the iliotibial band are incised and the incisions carried proximally under the skin using curved meniscotomes (Fig. 42-3A). The iliotibial band is detached proximally under the skin using a curved meniscotome or an open tendon stripper. Alternatively, a counterincision can be made at the upper thigh to release the tendon. The iliotibial band is left attached distally at the Gerdy tubercle. Dissection is performed distally to separate the iliotibial band from the joint capsule and from the lateral patellar retinaculum (Fig. 42-3B). The free proximal end of the iliotibial band is then tubularized with a no. 5 Ethibond whipstitch.

Arthroscopy of the knee is then performed through standard anterolateral viewing and anteromedial working portals. Management of meniscal injury or chondral injury is performed if present. The ACL remnant is excised. The over-the-top position on the femur and the over-the front position under the intermeniscal ligament are identified. Minimal notchplasty is performed to avoid iatrogenic injury to the perichondrial ring of the distal femoral physis, which is in very close proximity to the over-the-top position.[52] The free end of the iliotibial band graft is brought through the over-the-top position using a full-length clamp (Fig. 42-2A, 42-3C) or a two-incision rear-entry guide (Fig. 42-2B) and out the anteromedial portal (Fig. 42-2C, Fig. 42-3D).

A second incision of approximately 4.5 cm is made over the proximal medial tibia in the region of the pes anserinus insertion. Dissection is carried through the subcutaneous tissue to the periosteum. A curved clamp is placed from this incision into the joint under the intermeniscal ligament (Fig. 42-3E). A small groove is made in the anteromedial

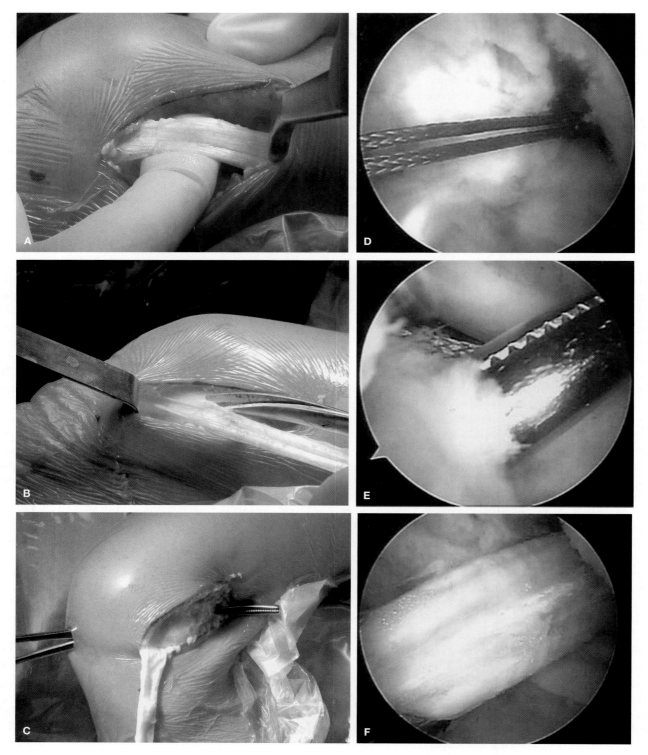

Fig. 42-3. Physeal-sparing, combined intra-articular, and extra-articular reconstruction utilizing autogenous iliotibial band for prepubescents. **A:** The graft is harvested through the lateral incision. **B:** The graft is left attached to the Gerdy tubercle distally. **C,D:** The graft is brought through the knee in the over-the-top position using a full length clamp. **E:** The graft is brought under the intermeniscal ligament. A groove can be made in the epiphysis in this region with a rasp. **F:** Intra-articular reconstruction component.

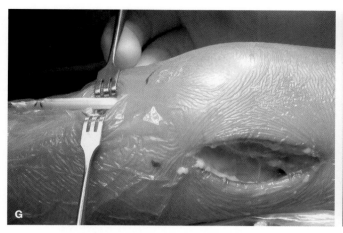
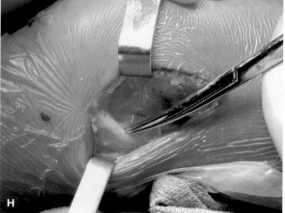

Fig. 42-3. *(Continued)* **G:** The graft is brought out the medial tibial incision and fixed here to a trough in the periosteum. **H:** Extra-articular reconstruction component.

proximal tibial epiphysis under the intermeniscal ligament using a curved rat-tail rasp to bring the tibial graft placement more posterior. The free end of the graft is then brought through the joint (Fig. 42-3F) under the intermeniscal ligament in the anteromedial epiphyseal groove, and out the medial tibial incision (Fig. 42-3G). The graft is fixed on the femoral side through the lateral incision with the knee at 90 degrees flexion and 15 degrees external rotation using mattress sutures to the lateral femoral condyle at the insertion of the lateral intermuscular septum to effect an extra-articular reconstruction (Fig. 42-3H). The tibial side is then fixed through the medial incision with the knee flexed 20 degrees and tension applied to the graft. A periosteal incision is made distal to the proximal tibial physis as checked with fluoroscopic imaging. A trough is made in the proximal tibial medial metaphyseal cortex and the graft is sutured to the periosteum at the rough margins with mattress sutures (Fig. 42-3D).

Postoperatively, the patient is maintained touch-down weight bearing for 6 weeks. Range of motion is limited from 0 degrees to 90 degrees for the first 2 weeks, followed by progressive full range of motion. A continuous passive motion (CPM) from 0 degrees to 90 degrees and cryotherapy are used for 2 weeks postoperatively. A protective postoperative brace is used for 6 weeks postoperatively.

Adolescent Patients with Growth Remaining: Transphyseal Reconstruction with Autogenous Hamstrings with Metaphyseal Fixation

In adolescents with growth remaining, we perform transphyseal ACL reconstruction with autogenous hamstrings tendons with metaphyseal fixation away from the physis. This is a fairly standard one-incision, arthroscopically assisted technique utilizing a four-stranded gracilis/semitendinosis graft with EndoButton fixation on the femur. On the tibial side, the graft is either fixed with a soft-tissue interference screw if there is adequate tunnel distance (at least 30 mm) below the

physis to ensure metaphyseal placement of the screw or with a post and spiked washer.

The procedure is performed under general anesthesia as an overnight observation procedure. Local anesthesia with sedation may be performed in the emotionally mature adolescent children. The patient is positioned supine on the operating table with a pneumatic tourniquet about the upper thigh, which is not used routinely. Examination under anesthesia is performed to confirm ACL insufficiency.

First, the hamstrings tendons are harvested. If the diagnosis is in doubt, arthroscopy can be performed first to confirm ACL tear. A 4-cm incision is made over the palpable pes anserinus tendons on the medial side of the upper tibia **(Fig. 42-4A)**. Dissection is carried through skin to the sartorius fascia. Care is taken to protect superficial sensory nerves. The sartorius tendon is incised longitudinally and the gracilis and semitendinosus tendons are identified. The tendons are dissected free distally and their free ends whipstitched with no. 2 or no. 5 Ethibond suture. They are dissected proximally using sharp and blunt dissection. Fibrous bands to the medial head of gastrocnemius should be sought and released. A closed tendon stripper is used to dissect the tendons free proximally. Alternatively, the tendons can be left attached distally and an open tendon stripper used to release the tendons proximally. The tendons are taken to the back table, where excess muscle is removed and the remaining ends are whipstitched with no. 2 or no. 5 Ethibond suture. The tendons are folded over a closed loop EndoButton. The graft diameter is sized and the graft is placed under tension.

Arthroscopy of the knee is then performed through standard anterolateral viewing and anteromedial working portals. Management of meniscal injury or chondral injury is performed if present. The ACL remnant is excised. The over-the-top position on the femur is identified. Minimal notchplasty is performed to avoid iatrogenic injury to the perichondral ring of the distal femoral physis, which is in very close proximity to the over-the-top position.[52]

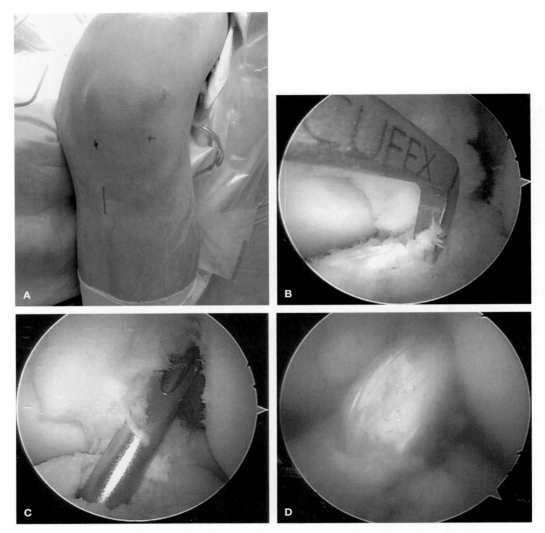

Fig. 42-4. Transphyseal reconstruction with autogenous hamstrings for adolescents with growth remaining. **A:** The gracilis and semitendinosus tendons are harvested through an incision over the proximal medial tibia. **B:** The tibial guide is used to drill the tibial tunnel. **C:** The transtibial over-the-top offset guide is used to drill the femoral tunnel. **D:** Hamstrings graft after fixation.

A tibial tunnel guide (set at 55 degrees) is used through the anteromedial portal (Fig. 42-4B). A guide wire is drilled through the hamstrings harvest incision into the posterior aspect of the ACL tibial footprint. The guidewire entry point on the tibia should be kept medial to avoid injury to the tibial tubercle apophysis. The guidewire is reamed with the appropriate diameter reamer. Excess soft tissue at the tibial tunnel is excised to avoid arthrofibrosis. The transtibial over-the-top guide of the appropriate offset to ensure a 1 or 2 mm back wall is used to pass the femoral guide pin (Fig. 42-4C). The femoral guide pin is overdrilled with the EndoButton reamer. Both are removed in order to use the depth gauge to measure the femoral tunnel length. The guide pin is replaced and brought through the distal lateral thigh. The femur is reamed to the appropriate depth (femoral tunnel length − EndoButton length + 6 to 7 mm to flip the EndoButton).

The no. 5 Ethibond sutures on the EndoButton are placed in the slot of the guidewire and pulled through the tibial tunnel, through the femoral tunnel, and out the lateral thigh. These are then pulled to bring the EndoButton and graft through the tibial tunnel and into the femoral tunnel. One set of sutures is used to "lead" the EndoButton, while the other set of sutures is used to "follow." Once the graft is fully seated in the femoral tunnel, the "follow" sutures are pulled to flip the EndoButton (Fig. 42-4D). The flip can be palpated in the thigh and tension is applied to the graft to endure no graft slippage. The knee is then extended to ensure no graft impingement. The knee is then cycled approximately ten times with tension applied to the graft. The graft is fixed on the tibial side with the knee in 20 degrees to 30 degrees of flexion, tension applied to the graft, and a posterior force placed on the tibia. On the tibial side,

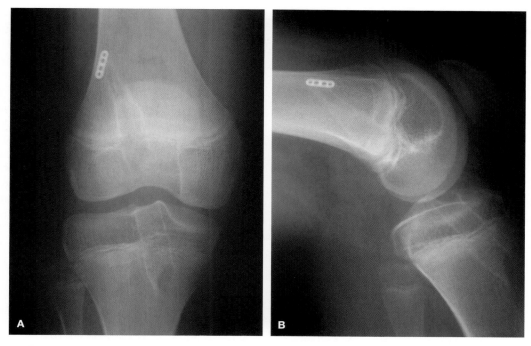

Fig. 42-5. Transphyseal reconstruction with autogenous hamstrings for adolescents with growth remaining. Postoperative anteroposterior (**A**) and lateral (**B**) radiographs.

the graft is either fixed with a soft-tissue interference screw if there is adequate tunnel distance (at least 30 mm) below the physis to ensure metaphyseal placement of the screw or with a post and spiked washer. Fluoroscopy can be used to ensure that the fixation is away from the physis. Postoperative radiographs are shown in **Figure 42-5**.

Postoperatively, the patient is maintained touch-down weight bearing for 2 weeks. Range of motion is limited from 0 degrees to 90 degrees for the first 2 weeks, followed by progressive full range of motion. A continuous passive motion (CPM) from 0 degrees to 90 degrees and cryotherapy are used for 2 weeks postoperatively. A protective postoperative brace is used for 6 weeks.

■ TECHNICAL ALTERNATIVES AND PITFALLS

Transphyseal reconstruction, partial transphyseal reconstruction, and physeal sparing reconstruction techniques have been described to address ACL insufficiency in skeletally immature patients.

In prepubescent patients, physeal sparing techniques have been described that utilize hamstrings tendons under the intermeniscal ligament and over-the-top on the femur, through all-epiphyseal femoral and tibial tunnels, and with a femoral epiphyseal staple.[7,41–47]

In adolescent patients with growth remaining, transphyseal reconstructions have been performed with hamstrings autograft, patellar tendon autograft, and allograft tissue.[12,15,28–37]

In addition, partial transphyseal reconstructions have been described with a tunnel through the proximal tibial physis and over-the-top positioning on the femur or a tunnel through the distal femoral physis with an epiphyseal tunnel in the tibia.[38–40,53]

Pitfalls to avoid with the physeal-sparing iliotibial band reconstruction in prepubescents include harvesting a short graft insufficient to reach the medial tibial incision, difficulty passing the graft through the posterior joint capsule, and difficulty passing the graft under the intermeniscal ligament.

Pitfalls to avoid with the transphyseal hamstrings reconstruction in adolescents with growth remaining include amputation of the hamstring grafts, poor tunnel placement, and graft impingement.

Based on the 15 cases of growth disturbance after ACL reconstruction in skeletally immature patients that we reported, we recommend careful attention to technical details during ACL reconstruction in skeletally immature patients, particularly the avoidance of fixation hardware across the lateral distal femoral epiphyseal plate.[24] Care should also be taken to avoid injury to the vulnerable tibial tubercle apophysis. Given the cases of growth disturbances associated with transphyseal placement of patellar tendon graft bone blocks, we recommend the use of soft tissue grafts. Large tunnels should likely be avoided as the likelihood of arrest is associated with greater violation of epiphyseal plate cross-sectional area. The two cases of genu valgum without arrest associated with lateral extra-articular tenodesis raise additional concerns about the effect of tension on physeal growth. Finally, care should be taken to avoid dissection or notching around the posterolateral aspect of the physis during over-the-top nonphyseal femoral placement to avoid potential injury to the perichondrial ring and subsequent deformity.

■ REHABILITATION

Rehabilitation after ACL reconstruction in skeletally immature patients is essential to ensure a good outcome, allow return to sports, and avoid reinjury. Rehabilitation in prepubescent children can be challenging. A therapist who is used to working with children who can make therapy interesting and fun is very helpful. Compliance with therapy and restrictions should be carefully monitored.

After physeal-sparing iliotibial band reconstruction in prepubescent patients, we restrict full weight bearing for 6 weeks to allow graft healing. After transphyseal hamstring reconstruction in adolescents with growth remaining, we restrict full weight bearing for 2 weeks. A CPM machine is used for 2 weeks postoperatively. A postoperative brace is used for 6 weeks.

Progressive rehabilitation consists of range-of-motion exercises, patellar mobilization, electrical stimulation, pool therapy if available, proprioception exercises, and closed chain strengthening, during the first 3 months postoperatively, followed by straight-line jogging, plyometric exercises, sport cord exercises, and sport-specific exercises.

Return to full activity, including cutting sports, is usually allowed at 6 months postoperatively. A functional knee brace is used routinely during cutting and pivoting activities for the first 2 years after return to sports.

■ OUTCOMES AND FUTURE DIRECTIONS

We have reviewed the results of physeal-sparing iliotibial band reconstruction in prepubescent patients in a preliminary series of 8 patients.[47] More recently, we have reviewed the minimum 2-year results in 44 prepubescent patients. Between 1980 to 2002, 44 skeletally immature preadolescent children who were Tanner stage one or two (mean chronological age: 10.3 years old; range: 3.6 to 14.0 years old) underwent physeal sparing combined intra-articular and extra-articular ACL reconstruction using autogenous iliotibial band. Twenty-four patients had additional meniscal surgery. Functional outcome, graft survival, radiographic outcome, and growth disturbance were evaluated at a mean of 5.3 years (range: 2.0 to 15.1 years) after surgery. Two patients underwent revision ACL reconstruction for graft failure at 4.7 and 8.3 years after initial surgery (revision rate: 4.5%). In the remaining 42 patients, the mean International Knee Documentation (IKDC) subjective knee score was 96.7 ± 6.0 (range: 88.5 to 100) and the mean Lysholm knee

score was 95.7 ± 6.7 (range: 74 to 100). Per IKDC criteria, Lachman examination was normal in 23 patients, nearly normal in 18 patients, and abnormal in 1 patient. Pivot-shift examination was normal in 31 patients and nearly normal in 11 patients. Four patients who underwent concurrent meniscus repair had repeat arthroscopic meniscal repair or partial meniscectomy. Mean growth in total height from the time of surgery to final follow-up was 21.5 cm (range: 9.5 to 118.5 cm). There were no cases of significant angular deformity measured radiographically or leg length discrepancy measured clinically. Thus, physeal sparing combined intra-articular and extra-articular ACL reconstruction using iliotibial band in preadolescent skeletally immature patients appears to provide for excellent functional outcome with a low revision rate and a minimal risk of growth disturbance.

■ REFERENCES

1. Rang M. *Children's Fractures*. 2nd ed. Philadelphia: Lippincott; 1983.
2. Kocher MS, Micheli LJ, Gerbino P, et al. Tibial eminence fractures in children: prevalence of meniscal entrapment. Am J Sports Med. 2003;31(3):404–407.
3. Kocher MS, Foreman ES, Micheli LJ. Laxity and functional outcome after arthroscopic reduction and internal fixation of displaced tibial spine fractures in children. Arthroscopy. 2003;19(10):1085–1090.
4. Kocher MS, Mandiga R, Klingele KE, et al. Anterior cruciate ligament injury versus tibial spine fracture in the skeletally immature knee: a comparison of skeletal maturation and notch width index. J Pediatr Orthop. 2004;24(2):185–188.
5. Eiskjaer S, Larsen ST, Schmidt MB. The significance of hemarthrosis of the knee in children. Arch Orthop Trauma Surg. 1988;107(2):96–98.
6. Kloeppel-Wirth S, Koltai JL, Dittmer H. Significance of arthroscopy in children with knee joint injuries. Eur J Pediatr Surg. 1992;2(3):169–172.
7. Vahasarja V, Kinnuen P, Serlo W. Arthroscopy of the acute traumatic knee in children. Prospective study of 138 cases. Acta Orthop Scand. 1993;64(5):580–582.
8. Stanitski CL, Harvell JC, Fu F. Observations on acute knee hemarthrosis in children and adolescents. J Pediatr Orthop. 1993;13(4):506–510.
9. Kocher MS, DiCanzio J, Zurakowski D, et al. Diagnostic performance of clinical examination and selective magnetic resonance imaging in the evaluation of intraarticular knee disorders in children and adolescents. Am J Sports Med. 2001;29(3):292–296.
10. Luhmann SJ. Acute traumatic knee effusions in children and adolescents. J Pediatr Orthop. 2003;23(2):199–202.
11. Kocher MS, Micheli LJ, Zurakowski D, et al. Partial tears of the anterior cruciate ligament in children and adolescents. Am J Sports Med. 2002;30(5):697–703.
12. Aichroth PM, Patel DV, Zorrilla P. The natural history and treatment of rupture of the anterior cruciate ligament in children and adolescents. A prospective review. J Bone Joint Surg Br. 2002;84(1):618–619.
13. Graf BK, Lange RH, Fujisaki CK, et al. Anterior cruciate ligament tears in skeletally immature patients: meniscal pathology at presentation and after attempted conservative treatment. Arthroscopy. 1992;8(2):229–233.
14. Janarv PM, Nystrom A, Werner S, et al. Anterior cruciate ligament injuries in skeletally immature patients. J Pediatr Orthop. 1996;16(5):673–677.

15. McCarroll JR, Rettig AC, Shelbourne KD. Anterior cruciate ligament injuries in the young athlete with open physes. Am J Sports Med. 1988;16(1):44–47.

16. Millett PJ, Willis AA, Warren RF. Associated injuries in pediatric and adolescent anterior cruciate ligament tears: does a delay in treatment increase the risk of meniscal tear? Arthroscopy. 2002;18(9):955–999.

17. Mizuta H, Kubota K, Shiraishi M, et al. The conservative treatment of complete tears of the anterior cruciate ligament in skeletally immature patients. J Bone Joint Surg Br. 1995;77(6):890–894.

18. Pressman AE, Letts RM, Jarvis JG. Anterior cruciate ligament tears in children: an analysis of operative versus nonoperative treatment. J Pediatr Orthop. 1997;17(4):505–511.

19. Guzzanti V, Falciglia F, Gigante A, et al. The effect of intra-articular ACL reconstruction on the growth plates of rabbits. J Bone Joint Surg Br. 1994;76(6):960–963.

20. Houle JB, Letts M, Yang J. Effects of a tensioned tendon graft in a bone tunnel across the rabbit physis. Clin Orthop. 2001(391):275–281.

21. Edwards TB, Greene CC, Baratta RV, et al. The effect of placing a tensioned graft across open growth plates: a gross and histologic analysis. J Bone Joint Surg Am. 2001;83-A(5):725–734.

22. Lipscomb AB, Anderson AF. Tears of the anterior cruciate ligament in adolescents. J Bone Joint Surg Am. 1986;68(1):19–28.

23. Koman JD, Sanders JO. Valgus deformity after reconstruction of the anterior cruciate ligament in a skeletally immature patient: a case report. J Bone Joint Surg Am. 1999;81:711–715.

24. Kocher MS, Saxon HS, Hovis WD, et al. Management and complications of anterior cruciate ligament injuries in skeletally immature patients: survey of the Herodicus Society and the ACL Study Group. J Pediatr Orthop. 2002;22(4):452–457.

25. Stadelmaier DM, Arnoczky SP, Dodds J, et al. The effect of drilling and soft tissue grafting across open growth plates: a histologic study. Am J Sports Med. 1995;23(4):431–435.

26. Clanton TO, DeLee JC, Sanders B, et al. Knee ligament injuries in children. J Bone Joint Surg Am. 1979;61:1195–1201.

27. Engebretsen L, Svenningsen S, Benum P. Poor results of anterior cruciate ligament repair in adolescents. Acta Orthop Scand. 1988;59:684–686.

28. Angel KR, Hall DJ. Anterior cruciate ligament injury in children and adolescents. Arthroscopy. 1989;5(3):197–200.

29. Aronowitz ER, Ganley TJ, Goode JR, et al. Anterior cruciate ligament reconstruction in adolescents with open physes. Am J Sports Med. 2000;28(2):168–175.

30. Fuchs R, Wheatley W, Uribe JW, et al. Intra-articular anterior cruciate ligament reconstruction using patellar tendon allograft in the skeletally immature patient. Arthroscopy. 2002;18(8):824–828.

31. Matava MJ, Siegel MG. Arthroscopic reconstruction of the ACL with semitendinosis-gracilis autograft in skeletally immature adolescent patients. Am J Knee Surg. 1997;10(2):60–69.

32. McCarroll JR, Shelbourne KD, Porter DA, et al. Patellar tendon graft reconstruction for midsubstance anterior cruciate ligament rupture in junior high school athletes: An algorithm for management. Am J Sports Med. 1994;22:478–484.

33. Shelbourne KD, Gray T, Wiley BV. Results of transphyseal anterior cruciate ligament reconstruction using patellar tendon autograft in Tanner stage 3 or 4 adolescents with clearly open growth plates. Am J Sports Med. 2004;32(5):1218–1222.

34. Simonian PT, Metcalf MH, Larson RV. Anterior cruciate ligament injuries in the skeletally immature patient. Am J Orthop. 1999;28(11):624–628.

35. Stanitski CL. Anterior cruciate ligament injury in the skeletally immature patient: diagnosis and treatment. J Am Acad Orthop Surg. 1995;3(3):146–158.

36. Volpi P, Galli M, Bait C, et al. Surgical treatment of anterior cruciate ligament injuries in adolescents using double-looped semitendinosis and gracilis tendons: supraepiphysary femoral and tibial fixation. Arthroscopy. 2004;20(4):447–449.

37. Edwards PH, Grana WA. Anterior cruciate ligament reconstruction in the immature athlete: long-term results of intra-articular reconstruction. Am J Knee Surg. 2001;14:232–237.

38. Andrews M, Noyes FR, Barber-Westin SD. Anterior cruciate ligament allograft reconstruction in the skeletally immature athlete. Am J Sports Med. 1994;22(1):48–54.

39. Bisson LJ, Wickiewicz T, Levinson M, et al. ACL reconstruction in children with open physes. Orthopedics. 1998;21(6):659–663.

40. Guzzanti V, Falciglia F, Stanitski CL. Preoperative evaluation and anterior cruciate ligament reconstruction technique for skeletally immature patients in Tanner stages 2 and 3. Am J Sports Med. 2003;31(6):941–948.

41. Brief LB. Anterior cruciate ligament reconstruction without drill holes. Arthroscopy. 1991;7:350–357.

42. DeLee J, Curtis R. Anterior cruciate ligament insufficiency in children. Clin Orthop. 1983;172:112–118.

43. Kim SH, Ha KI, Ahn JH, et al. Anterior cruciate ligament reconstruction in the young patient without violation of the epiphyseal plate. Arthroscopy. 1999;15(7):792–795.

44. Parker AW, Drez D, Cooper JL. Anterior cruciate ligament injuries in patients with open physes. Am J Sports Med. 1994;22(1):44–47.

45. Anderson AF. Transepiphyseal replacement of the anterior cruciate ligament in skeletally immature patients: a preliminary report. J Bone Joint Surg Am. 2003;85-A(7):1255–1263.

46. Guzzanti V, Falciglia F, Stanitski CL. Physeal-sparing intraarticular anterior cruciate ligament reconstruction in preadolescents. Am J Sports Med. 2003;31(6):949–953.

47. Micheli LJ, Rask B, Gerberg L. Anterior cruciate ligament reconstruction in patients who are prepubescent. Clin Orthop. 1999(364):40–47.

48. Greulich WW, Pysle SI. *Radiographic Atlas of Skeletal Development of the Hand and Wrist.* 2nd ed. Stanford, CA: Stanford University Press; 1959.

49. Pyle SI, Hoerr NL. *A Radiographic Standard of Reference the Growing Knee.* Springfield, IL: Charles Thomas; 1969.

50. Tanner JM, Whitehouse RH. Clinical longitudinal standards for height, weight, height velocity, and stages of puberty. Arch Dis Child. 1976;51:170–179.

51. MacIntosh DL, Darby DT. Lateral substitution reconstruction in proceedings and reports of universities, colleges, councils, and associations. J Bone Joint Surg Br. 1976;58:142.

52. Behr CT, Potter HG, Paletta GA Jr. The relationship of the femoral origin of the anterior cruciate ligament and the distal femoral physeal plate in the skeletally immature knee: an anatomic study. Am J Sports Med. 2001;29:781–787.

53. Lo IK, Kirkley A, Fowler PJ, et al. The outcome of operatively treated anterior cruciate ligament disruptions in the skeletally immature child. Arthroscopy. 1997;13(5):627–634.

Part

B

ISOLATED AND COMBINED POSTERIOR CRUCIATE LIGAMENT INJURIES

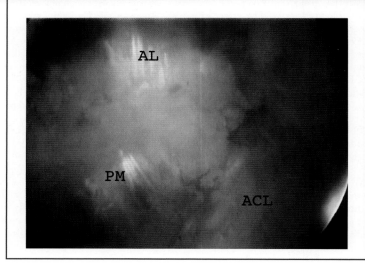

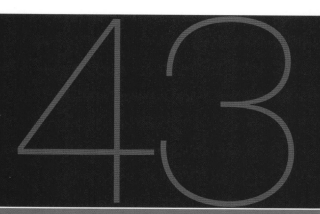

POSTERIOR CRUCIATE LIGAMENT RECONSTRUCTION USING THE TIBIAL INLAY

HANS P. OLSEN, MD, MARK D. MILLER, MD

■ HISTORY OF THE TECHNIQUE

The posterior cruciate ligament (PCL) is infrequently injured with an estimated incidence of 3 to 16% of all knee injuries.[1] There has been less investigation of the mechanics and function of the PCL when compared with the anterior cruciate ligament (ACL). In recent years a better understanding of the short- and long-term consequences of PCL deficiency has spurred research to find the optimal method for reconstructing this ligament. There have been several techniques of PCL reconstruction developed; however, no single operation has emerged as the gold standard to predictably restore posterior stability and PCL function. We believe that, as with other procedures in orthopedic surgery, the best results stem from procedures that re-create normal anatomy.

The PCL originates at the posterolateral aspect of the medial femoral condyle, inserting extra synovially in a central sulcus located 1 cm distal to the posterior edge of the tibial plateau. The ligament consists of a large anterolateral and smaller posteromedial portion, each of which has distinct and consistent insertions, in addition to variable meniscofemoral ligaments. These ligaments originate from the lateral meniscus and insert anterior and posterior to the PCL on the medial femoral condyle. The meniscofemoral ligaments (ligaments of Humphrey and Wrisberg) commonly remain intact following PCL rupture and provide some posterior stability to the knee. The smaller posteromedial portion of the PCL consists of shorter fibers that are taut in knee extension. The anterolateral bundle is the thickest in diameter, contains the longest fibers, and is taut with knee flexion. This is the portion of the PCL that provides the greatest tensile strength and resists posterior tibial translation beginning at 30 degrees of flexion.[2,3]

Historically, most PCL reconstructions have emphasized an anterior to posterior approach to re-create the anterolateral bundle. This has been performed through a long oblique interosseous tunnel that creates difficulty with graft passage. These reconstructions require the graft to bend around a large angle at the back of the tibia, which has been dubbed the "killer turn," and has been implicated as a cause of graft failure.[4]

The tibial inlay technique was originally developed in Europe and introduced to the United States by Berg[5] in 1995. This method produces a more anatomic reconstruction of the PCL by placing the distal portion of the graft directly in the PCL sulcus, in the posterior aspect of the tibia. Thus, the tibial inlay method avoids creating the "killer turn" of the graft associated with other reconstruction techniques.

This chapter describes the combined original concept of the tibial inlay with a posterior approach to the tibia as described by Burks and Schaffer.[6] Additional refinements have been added, leading to the technique discussed herein.

■ INDICATIONS AND CONTRAINDICATIONS

Diagnosis

A thorough history of the events of injury is needed to make the diagnosis of a PCL injury. Common mechanisms of PCL injury include "dashboard injuries" during motor vehicle accidents or overloading of the knee and quadriceps in hyperflexion during athletic events. Isolated PCL injuries are more likely to be associated with athletic injury than any other mechanism. Acute, isolated PCL rupture is often associated with a smaller hemarthrosis than with ACL injury. Problems with knee instability with cutting or rapid

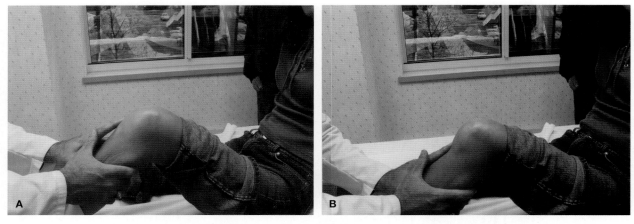

Fig. 43-1. Posterior drawer test. **A:** Image shows normal tibio-femoral relationship prior to test. **B:** Image showing abnormal posterior tibial translation with applied posterior stress force.

deceleration movements are less common than with ACL injured patients, although they may give a history of an instability sensation especially when on uneven ground. Many athletes will continue to play on a PCL injured knee and won't seek medical attention until they develop a pain or ache in the following days. Patients with PCL injuries may complain that the knee is just "not right" or have other subjective complaints such as a generalized "aching." Chronic PCL injured patients will report pain (medial and patellofemoral) with ambulation or descending stairs.

PCL tears frequently occur with concomitant ligamentous, bony, or capsular injuries to the knee. In the trauma setting, these associated injuries can occur up to 60% of the time.[7] Following medial or lateral collateral ligament damage, varus or valgus stress to the tibia may result in PCL injury. A hyperextension mechanism of PCL rupture can occur after the ACL is torn and is also associated with a posterior capsular injury. The most common combination is the combined PCL and posterolateral corner injury, which is reported to occur in up to 60% of all combined injuries.[7]

The physical exam is critical to making the correct diagnosis of PCL injury. The posterior drawer test is 90% sensitive and 99% specific for PCL pathology and should be considered the gold standard for diagnosis[8] **(Fig. 43-1A,B)**. The posterior sag test, the Godfrey test, the prone drawer, the quadriceps active test, and the dynamic posterior shift test may all be used to confirm a PCL injury. An isolated grade-III PCL injury is uncommon, thus other ligamentous injuries must be sought when looking for any additional instability. Knee dislocation must be ruled out any time there is the possibility of a multiligament injury. A careful hip and ankle exam as well as a neurovascular exam should be performed, especially if associated with high energy trauma or a potential knee dislocation. Posterolateral instability is commonly associated with PCL injury and may be diagnosed with external rotation asymmetry **(Fig. 43-2A,B)**, the external

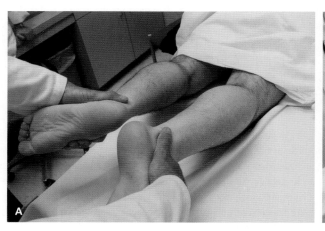
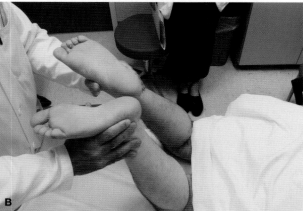

Fig. 43-2. External rotation asymmetry. **(A)** Excessive abnormal tibial external rotation of the patients left leg at 30 degrees of flexion and **(B)** 90 degrees of flexion, suggesting PCL and posterolateral corner injury.

rotation recurvatum test, posterolateral and posteromedial drawer test, or the reverse pivot shift test. External rotation asymmetry has been proven to be the most reliable indicator of posterolateral instability.

Radiographic studies, including plain films, stress radiography, and magnetic resonance imaging (MRI), are used to confirm clinical suspicion of a PCL injury. Plain films can be used to assess for any bony avulsion, tibial plateau fracture, or fibular head fracture suggesting possible posterolateral corner injury. Stress films are used to quantify posterior instability and can confirm clinical suspicions. It is noninvasive, reproducible, and a reliable method for determining the amount of posterior tibial translation **(Fig. 43-3A,B)**.

Historically, the management of PCL injuries has been nonoperative. Conservative management usually involves early brace treatment with progressive range of motion exercises, followed by a quadriceps strengthening program early in the postinjury period. Protecting the knee from posterior tibial translation is crucial. Patients are typically restricted from athletics until 90% of contralateral quadriceps and hamstring strength is obtained. Recently, the accepted management of complete PCL tears has become more aggressive, with a lower threshold for operative treatment. This is the result of long-term follow-up studies that demonstrate worse results with nonoperative treatment. These studies also show radiographic deterioration with time, especially in the medial and patellofemoral compartments.[9] The rate of arthrosis severity and progression depends upon the degree of posterior instability, quadriceps weakness, and the presence of additional ligamentous or meniscal damage. Nonoperative treatment is now reserved for asymptomatic, acute, isolated PCL tears with mild posterior laxity (grades I and II), or chronic isolated PCL injuries that are asymptomatic.

The development of pain and degenerative arthritis is more common in patients with combined PCL injuries.

Thus, patients who suffer PCL injuries in combination with bony avulsion injuries, posterolateral corner injuries, or concomitant ligamentous injuries (grade III medial collateral ligament [MCL] or ACL rupture) require operative reconstruction of the PCL. Combined MCL-PCL injuries often need both components fixed. Combined PCL and posterolateral corner injuries are an indication for operative treatment because the posterolateral corner is a secondary stabilizer to posterior displacement. Posterolateral corner injuries should be reconstructed within 2 weeks of injury. Isolated PCL injuries with grade-III posterior laxity/instability are also an indication for operative management. Finally, active, young patients who demonstrate less than 10 mm of posterior laxity on displacement testing (grade II) but with symptomatic complaints of instability or pain should also have the PCL reconstructed.

Another relative indication for the use of the tibial inlay technique involves the revision setting. The tibial inlay technique is useful when a previous nonanatomic reconstruction has been performed. This avoids complications associated with previous tibial tunnels that are too wide in diameter or too proximal on the tibia. Patients with tibial osteopenia, previous fracture, or previous osteotomy may benefit from the tibial inlay technique to prevent proximal graft migration.[10]

When operative management is indicated the type and site of injury is critical in choosing the correct surgical procedure. Bony avulsion injuries involving the PCL insertion at the posterior tibia are treated with primary repair using lag screws or suture fixation. Midsubstance tears of the PCL require ligament reconstruction, which attempts to reproduce normal anatomy. We believe that the tibial inlay technique produces the most anatomic PCL reconstruction.

The tibial inlay technique is contraindicated in patients who have had prior vascular procedures, especially those who have had remote vascular repairs.

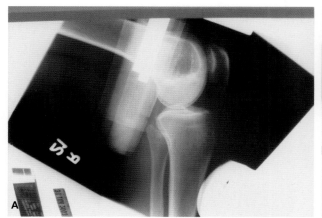
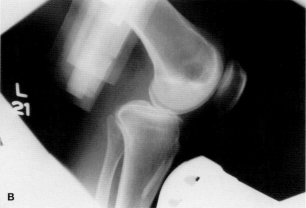

Fig. 43-3. Stress radiography. **A:** Normal stress radiograph. Note that there is no posterior displacement of the tibia as the drawer test is applied. **B:** Abnormal stress radiograph. Note the posterior displacement of the tibia suggesting PCL injury.

■ SURGICAL TECHNIQUE

Preoperative Planning

Prior to surgery, it is necessary to diagnose concomitant knee pathology and to quantify the degree of posterior instability. With the assistance of stress radiography (Fig. 43-3) or instrumented ligament testing using the KT-1000/2000 (MedMetric, San Diego, CA), PCL instability may be quantified.[11,12] Plain radiographs are used to exclude associated bony injury and to assess radiographic signs of arthrosis. Magnetic resonance imaging is also used as an adjunct to diagnosis and development of treatment plan. MRI is nearly 100% sensitive and specific for diagnosing PCL tears.[13] In addition, MRI may be used to diagnose meniscal injuries, which should be addressed at the time of surgery.

The arthroscopic exam is used as the final confirmation of intracapsular pathology.[14] At the time of surgery, arthroscopy provides direct visualization, looking for the presence of complete versus partial PCL tears, bony avulsions, ACL pseudolaxity, and degenerative changes.

Technique

Anesthesia, Positioning, and Setup

For anesthesia we prefer the use of a general anesthetic to allow for proper positioning and control during the procedure. Often we will employ the use of a femoral or sciatic nerve block that is placed prior to surgery for use in postoperative pain control. Epidural catheter placement is also an option for use in postoperative pain control.

Once adequate anesthesia is obtained, an exam under anesthesia is performed prior to final positioning and preparation of the patient. This is useful for confirmation of ligamentous laxity associated with PCL rupture and for ruling out previously unrecognized combined knee injuries. A broad-spectrum cephalosporin antibiotic or suitable alternative is given preoperatively. Following examination, the patient is placed in the lateral decubitus position with the injured leg up. The contralateral leg remains extended, with padding placed around the fibular head in order to protect the common peroneal nerve **(Fig. 43-4)**. The injured leg is abducted and externally rotated at the hip, flexed at the knee, and locked in place with a commercially available leg holder. From this position, graft harvest, arthroscopy, and drilling of the femoral tunnel are easily accomplished **(Fig. 43-5)**. The posterior approach and tibial inlay are performed with the leg positioned in extension, neutral rotation, and resting on a Mayo stand. Finally, a tourniquet is placed on the proximal thigh and the patient is prepped and draped in the usual sterile fashion.

Patellar Graft Harvest

Following preparation and draping, an 8-cm longitudinal incision is extended from the inferior pole of the patella to the tibial tubercle centered on the medial aspect of the patellar tendon. Care is taken to preserve saphenous nerve branches. The dissection is taken down to the paratenon and skin flaps are raised. The paratenon is carefully dissected off the patellar tendon both proximally and distally for use in later closure. A central third 11 to 12 mm patellar tendon graft with 20 mm bone-patellar tendon-bone blocks is harvested, taking special care to make parallel incisions. A shorter graft is typically obtained because it can better negotiate the needed angle for entry into the femoral tunnel.

The tibial bone plug is trimmed to achieve a trapezoidal shape with a flattened surface, and a 3.2 mm hole is drilled

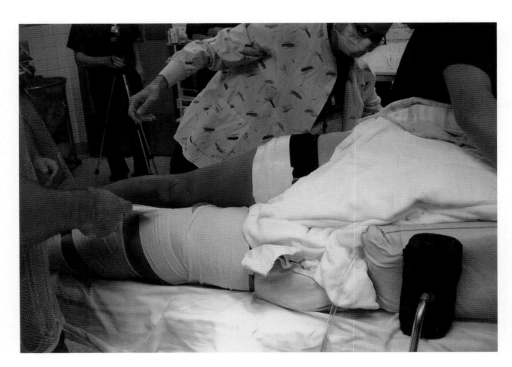

Fig. 43-4. Preoperative positioning. The patient is placed in the lateral decubitus position with the contralateral leg padded.

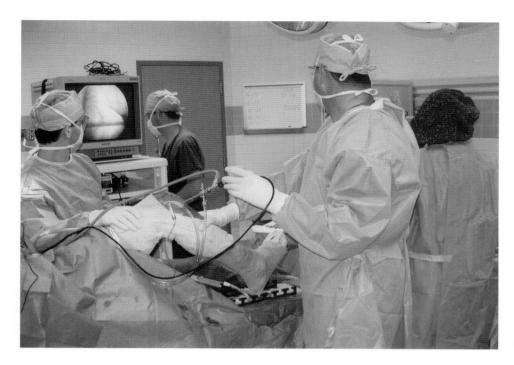

Fig. 43-5. External rotation and abduction of the leg allow for graft harvest and arthroscopy.

centrally. This hole is then tapped in preparation for tibial inlay fixation using a 4.5 mm bicortical screw **(Fig. 43-6)**. The patellar bone plug is sized so as to be able to fit through a 10 to 12 mm tunnel. The patellar bone plug is cylindrically contoured, tapering the leading edge such that it is bullet shaped for ease at insertion. Two perpendicularly oriented drill holes are placed approximately 5 mm and 10 mm from the distal tip of the patellar end of the graft. Two no. 5 non-absorbable sutures are placed through the leading edge of the bone plug at the drill hole sites. These sutures will later be used to manipulate the patellar bone plug into the femoral tunnel. A no. 2 Ethibond or Ticon suture is also placed at the patella-bone-tendon junction and will later be used to toggle the graft, permitting easier entry into the

femoral tunnel **(Fig. 43-7)**. Finally, all bone plug trimmings should be saved and used later as bone grafts.

Arthroscopy and Femoral Tunnel Placement

The affected limb is held in abduction, external rotation, and flexion by the leg holder. Standard anterolateral and medial arthroscopic portals are created. A thorough diagnostic arthroscopy is performed to confirm PCL deficiency, identify comorbid intra-articular pathology, and identify landmarks for reconstruction. Special attention should be directed to the lateral joint space of patients who have excessive opening with varus stress. These patients should be evaluated with a high index of suspicion for posterolateral corner injuries.[15] Following PCL debridement, all meniscal and cartilage work

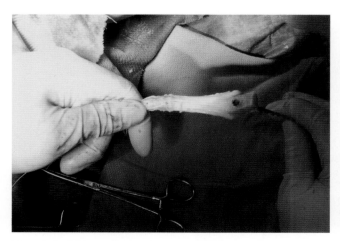

Fig. 43-6. PCL patellar tendon graft. Note the preparation of the tibial plug for passage of a 4.5 mm bicortical screw.

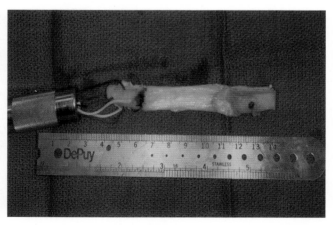

Fig. 43-7. Patellar tendon graft showing suture placement for femoral graft passage.

should be performed, and uninjured meniscofemoral ligaments should be left intact. After debridement of the PCL femoral footprint, a standard PCL femoral guide is placed into the knee via the anteromedial portal. This guide will be used to place the guide pin for the femoral tunnel. The drill guide is placed in the anterior portion of the PCL femoral insertion site, located 8 to 10 mm behind the medial femoral condyle articular surface at the 1 o'clock position in the notch for a right knee, and 11 o'clock for a left knee. A small 2 to 3 cm incision is made at the superior and medial borders of the patella. The vastus medialis oblique (VMO) muscle fibers are split or retracted and the external tunnel guide is positioned on the cortical surface of the femur away from the articular surface of the medial femoral condyle. A guide pin is inserted from outside in and identified on the intra-articular medial femoral condyle. After confirming the guide pin to be in the anterolateral PCL bundle footprint, the tunnel is overdrilled from outside in with a cannulated drill bit reamer sized appropriately for the graft. A small curette is placed into the joint to prevent the guide pin from injuring any intra-articular structures. Bone graft should be saved from the flutes of the drill bit for patellar and tibial tubercle bone grafting during closure. Following drilling, the posterior aspect of the tunnel is rasped, or smoothed, with a reverse cutting reamer to decrease abrasive forces on the graft. Once the femoral tunnel is fully prepared for graft placement, a looped 18-gauge wire is introduced into the tunnel from outside to inside. The guide wire is passed into the posterior aspect of the knee joint and will be used later to initiate and facilitate graft passage. At this time the pump/inflow is turned off and the arthroscope and equipment are removed from the knee. Attention is directed to the inlay portion of the case.

Posterior Approach and Inlay

The patient is repositioned, placing the injured leg on the padded Mayo stand in full extension and neutral rotation **(Fig. 43-8)**. A transverse incision is made in the flexion crease. The medial head of the gastrocnemius muscle is exposed by incising the medial aspect of the gastrocnemius fascia both transversely and distally on the medial side. Blunt dissection is used to develop an interval between the gastrocnemius and semimembranosus muscles. The medial sural cutaneous nerve must be kept in mind at this point, although it usually perforates the deep fascia distal to the incision. Once the interval is developed, the medial head of the gastrocnemius muscle is laterally retracted, exposing the posterior knee capsule. The middle and medial geniculate arteries may be encountered near the midposterior capsule and can be ligated if necessary. The medial head of the gastrocnemius is surprisingly mobile, but it is occasionally necessary to release a portion of its tendinous origin medially in order to gain adequate exposure. Slight knee flexion will also allow for greater lateral retraction of the medial head of the gastrocnemius and increase exposure. A cadaveric study previously demonstrated that the gastrocnemius muscle protects the popliteal artery during lateral retraction, and this exposure is safe, although one must be aware of anatomic variations.[10,16] Steinmann pins can be placed posteriorly into the tibia and bent laterally in order to assist with retraction of the medial head of the gastrocnemius.

Next, the PCL sulcus is palpated through the fibers of the popliteus muscle. The sulcus is defined by a large medial and smaller lateral bump. Electrocautery and an elevator are used to dissect the popliteus muscle from its origin, exposing the posterior tibial cortex. The position of the PCL sulcus is

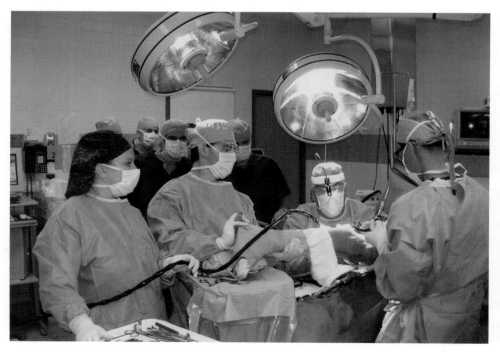

Fig. 43-8. Positioning for the posterior approach to the knee.

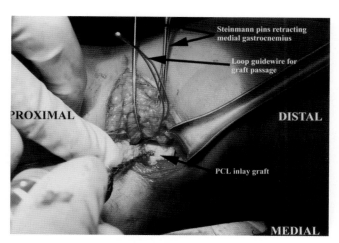

Fig. 43-9. Tibial inlay. Note the Steinmann pins used for lateral retraction of the gastrocnemius and the looped guide wire for passage of the graft into the femoral tunnel. The tibial portion of the patellar tendon graft is placed into the unicortical window and drilled from posterior to anterior.

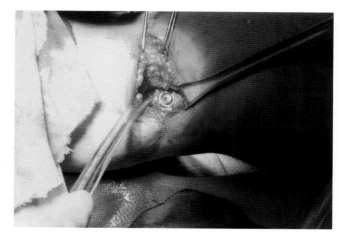

Fig. 43-10. Inlay fixation. Tibial inlay following placement of a 4.5 mm posterior to anterior bicortical screw.

reconfirmed at the central aspect of the posterior tibia. A generous capsular incision is made vertically, contiguous with the PCL sulcus. Any remaining scar tissue or PCL remnant is debrided at this time. At this point, the preplaced 18-guage passing wire may be retrieved through the new posterior arthrotomy site. The 18-guage wire will later be used to pass the no. 5 nonabsorbable sutures and graft through the femoral notch and into the femoral tunnel. A trough is developed at the PCL insertion site using an osteotome, burr, and tamp. The inlay site is fashioned such that it matches the size and shape of the tibial portion of the PCL graft. The graft is inlaid into the unicortical window. The graft/bone plug is carefully adjusted such that it fits snugly within the trough, flush with the posterior tibia. Before securing the graft, a second 18-guage looped guide wire is passed from the anteromedial arthroscopic portal and out the posterior arthrotomy **(Fig. 43-9)**. This looped guide wire is used to pull the no. 2 Ethibond suture out the antero-medial portal. The patellar end of the graft is then passed into the knee joint and femoral tunnel using the 18-gauge wire and no. 5 sutures.

After all necessary sutures and the patellar end of the bone-patellar tendon-bone graft are passed into the knee joint, the tibial bone plug is secured by lagging a 4.5-mm bicortical screw and washer through the predrilled tibial bone plug hole and into the anterior cortex of the tibia **(Fig. 43-10)**. Additional fixation with a second screw or a staple is sometimes beneficial.

Graft Passage and Fixation

Using the original looped 18-guage wire as a graft passer, the patellar end of the graft is passed through the posterior arthrotomy, into the notch, and then into the femoral tunnel. The knee is then passively taken through full range-of-motion (ROM) cycles while palpating the tibial inlay site in

order to ensure that there is no hang up at the posterior arthrotomy. The leg is then repositioned for arthroscopy and final graft placement. The no. 5 and no. 2 sutures should be pulled through the femoral tunnel and anteromedial arthro-scopic portal, respectively, if this has not been already per-formed. The no. 5 suture is used to pull the patellar bone plug into the femoral tunnel, while the no. 2 suture is used to toggle the graft for easier passage. The graft is optimally positioned with the patellar-bone plug-tendon junction located at the articular margin of the femoral tunnel. This graft/tunnel angle is sometimes referred to as the "critical corner" because poor positioning can contribute to excessive sheer stress and early graft failure.[17] While keeping moder-ate tension on the no. 5 suture, the knee is again passively cycled through full ROM cycles in order to rule out kinks in the graft and reconfirm a lack of impedance at the posterior arthrotomy site.

The graft is tensioned by placing an anterior drawer on a knee flexed to 70 degrees to 80 degrees while maintaining the desired intra-articular position of the patellar-bone plug-tendon junction. Proximal fixation is achieved with a 9 mm by 20 mm interference screw. Additional fixation with a plastic button tied with the no. 5 nonabsorbable sutures over the cortex at the tunnel entrance is also utilized. Intraoperative radiographs should be obtained to ensure proper graft and hardware placement **(Fig. 43-11A,B)**.

Wound Closure

Prior to wound closure, all bone grafts from femoral tunnel drilling and graft preparation should be packed into the patella and tibial tubercle harvest sites. Anteriorly, the paratenon is closed in an interrupted fashion using no. 0-Vicryl sutures over the patellar tendon and previous bone harvest sites. All subcutaneous tissues and skin layers are closed in standard fashion, and a sterile dressing is applied.

At the end of the procedure, the posterior capsule is closed and sutured with no. 0 absorbable suture. A one

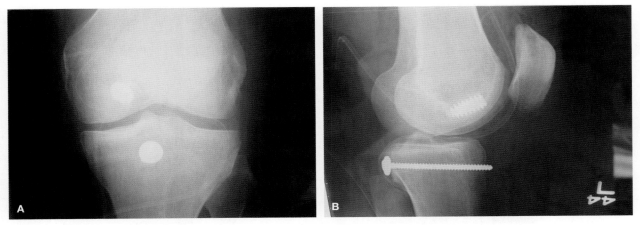

Fig. 43-11. Postoperative films **(A)** AP and **(B)** lateral radiograph of a patient's knee after PCL tibial inlay reconstruction.

eighth–inch closed drain is placed deep to the medial head of the gastrocnemius muscle for hematoma prevention. The medial gastrocnemius is allowed to fall into place, the subcutaneous layers are approximated, and the skin is closed in a routine fashion.

◼ TECHNICAL ALTERNATIVES AND PITFALLS

The surgeon should be particularly vigilant during certain periods of the PCL reconstruction in order to prevent operative complications. One potential pitfall is the failure to recognize an associated injury. Isolated PCL injury is uncommon, thus most injuries will involve another knee ligament or structure. This can lead to residual laxity on the posterior drawer test and present as recurrent symptomatic laxity following reconstruction.

Often avascular necrosis of the medial femoral condyle has been reported. Patients will usually present with medial knee pain and tenderness to palpation of the medial femoral condyle. To avoid this potential problem care must be taken to start the femoral tunnel 8 to 10 mm posterior to the articular margin as the etiology is secondary to femoral drilling too close to the articular surface or extensive soft tissue dissection over the medial femoral condyle. Avascular necrosis (AVN) of the medial femoral condyle can present months to years after surgery and is thought to be caused by local trauma to the subchondral bone blood supply causing increased pressure in the area. By using a more proximal entry site, maximal subchondral bone is preserved, thereby reducing the risk of AVN. It is also critical to ensure that the graft does not kink or hang up during passage from the posterior arthrotomy, through the femoral notch, and into the femoral tunnel. This complication decreases the stability of the reconstruction, causing persistent posterior laxity, but

can be easily avoided by palpating the PCL inlay site and using direct arthroscopic visualization of the graft while the knee is taken through passive, full ROM cycles. Persistent laxity can also be caused by overly aggressive rehabilitation, poor graft fixation or placement, and a previously stated failure to recognize any associated injuries. In addition, particular care should be taken to ensure that the patellar bone tendon junction is located at the intra-articular margin of the femoral tunnel in order to decrease graft degradation at this "critical corner." Finally, we previously used a hockey stick–shaped incision for the posterior approach to the knee. This approach was associated with an increased incidence of wound breakdown superiorly. By using a transverse incision at the flexion crease of the posterior knee, we nearly eliminated the problem of wound breakdown, while providing a better cosmetic result.

The most feared potential complication with any posterior exposure to the knee is vascular injury. Injury to vascular structures is always a risk during posterior knee exposure, especially in the revision setting where normal anatomy can be altered secondary to previous scar formation. The surgeon should be aware of potential vascular anomalies during the exposure as even the superficial dissection in the semimembranous–gastrocnemius interval can lead to inadvertent injury. Subperiosteal dissection of the popliteus provides additional soft tissue protection against any anatomic variants. The use of k-wires or Steinmann pins allows for continuous retraction during posterior dissection, thus avoiding repetitive repositioning of retractors and further potential for injury.

◼ REHABILITATION

In the immediate postoperative period, the extended leg is placed in a hinged knee brace. Special care is taken to support the tibia and prevent posterior translation. On postoperative day 1 the patient is permitted to bear weight as tolerated and ambulate with crutches. When bearing weight the patient is always in the brace locked at 0 degrees. Continuous passive motion, isometric quadriceps training, and straight leg raises should be implemented into the rehabilitation program as soon as the patient can tolerate such activity. Partner-assisted ROM exercises are also useful in the immediate postoperative period. These exercises are performed with the patient in the prone position in order to prevent posterior translation of the tibia. In the early postoperative period, weeks 0 to 4, gravity-assisted flexion exercises to 90 degrees and closed chain exercises for quadriceps strengthening are important. At 1 month post-op the patient is allowed to transition to unlocking the brace for ambulation and activities under supervision of the therapist. The patient may start to wean off crutches as tolerated. When the patient exhibits independent quadriceps control he or she may progress to open chain extension exercises, mini-squats, and isometric exercises. At 2 months the patient may add in stationary bike or stairmaster activities as well as leg presses within available ROM. From months 3 to 9 the patient may progress within his or her level of function and symptoms. The patient should ideally be allowed to return to normal activities 9 to 12 months postoperatively if the knee is stable, with full ROM and quadriceps strength equal to the contralateral leg.

■ OUTCOMES AND FUTURE DIRECTIONS

Even among experts PCL reconstruction is a relatively uncommon procedure, and there are a limited number of published reports in the literature. A growing body of data suggests that the tibial inlay technique is effective at decreasing posterior knee instability with good long-term results. A 2-year follow-up study performed by Jung et al.[18] in Korea demonstrated that the average posterior displacement on stress radiography decreased from 10.8 mm to 3.4 m, with 90% of patients reporting a satisfactory outcome. Likewise, Cooper[19,20] has presented two reports showing good results using the tibial inlay. The standard transtibial tunnel technique of PCL reconstruction has been popular, but biomechanical studies raise concern about the long-term outcomes of this method. A cadaveric, matched pair comparison of the tibial inlay versus tibial tunnel techniques found that the tibial tunnel group had greater anterior-posterior laxity postoperatively. Upon evaluation of the grafts, the tibial tunnel group revealed greater evidence of mechanical degradation at the acute angle.[21] These findings were confirmed by a second matched pair biomechanical comparison that demonstrated the tibial inlay method to be superior to the tibial tunnel technique with respect to graft failure, permanent graft lengthening, and graft thinning.[22]

Although research and experience have resulted in improved PCL injury management and reconstruction, even with the tibial inlay technique, the procedure is less successful than ACL reconstruction. Some researchers are experimenting with double bundle femoral reconstructions. We are not convinced that the theoretical improvement offered by two-bundle reconstruction justifies the additional technical difficulty and potential complications of this technique. Better grafts, improved techniques and instrumentation, and long-term results may change the way we perform PCL reconstructions in the future.

■ REFERENCES

1. Miyasaka KC, Daniel DM, Stone ML, et al. The incidence of knee ligament injuries in the general population. Am J Knee Surg. 1991;4:3–8.
2. Butler DL, Noyes FR, Grood ES. Ligamentous restraints to anterior-posterior drawer in the human knee: a biomechanical study. J Bone Joint Surg Am. 1980;63:259–270.
3. Gollehon DL, Torzilli PA, Warren RF. The role of the posterolateral and cruciate ligaments in the stability of the human knee: a biomechanical study. J Bone Joint Surg Am. 1987;69:233–242.
4. Miller MD, Bergfeld JA, Fowler PJ, et al. The posterior ligament injured knee: principles of evaluation and treatment. Instr Course Lect. 1999;48:199–207.
5. Berg EE. Posterior cruciate ligament tibial inlay reconstruction. Arthroscopy. 1995;11:69–76.
6. Burks RT, Schaffer JJ. A simplified approach to the tibial attachment of the posterior cruciate ligament. Clin Orthop. 1990;254: 216–219.
7. Fanelli GC, Edson CJ. Posterior cruciate ligament injuries in trauma patients: part II. Arthroscopy. 1995;11:526–529.
8. Miller MD, Johnson DL, Harner CD, et al. Posterior cruciate ligament injuries. Orthop Rev. 1993;22:1201–1210.
9. Dejour H, Walch G, Peyrot J, et al. The natural history of rupture of the posterior cruciate ligament. Fr J Orthop Surg. 1988;2: 112–120.
10. Noyes FR, Medvecky MJ, Bhargava M. Arthroscopically assisted quadriceps double-bundle tibial inlay posterior cruciate ligament reconstruction: an analysis of techniques and a safe operative approach to the popliteal fossa. Arthroscopy. 2003;19:894–905.
11. Puddu G. Radiographic view for PCL injuries: instructional course lecture. Paper presented at: Western Pacific Orthopaedic Association Meeting; November 1997; Taipei, Taiwan.
12. Hewett TE, Noyes FR, Lee MD. Diagnosis of complete and partial posterior cruciate ligament ruptures: stress radiography compared with KT-1000 arthrometer and posterior drawer testing. Am J Sports Med. 1997;25:648–655.
13. Gross ML, Grover JS, Bassett LW, et al. Magnetic resonance imaging of the posterior cruciate ligament: clinical use to improve diagnostic accuracy. Am J Sports Med. 1992;20:732–737.
14. Fanelli GC, Giannotti BF, Edson CJ. The posterior cruciate ligament arthroscopic evaluation and treatment: current concepts review. Arthroscopy. 1194;10:673–688.
15. LaPrade RF. Arthroscopic evaluation of the lateral compartment of knees with grade 3 posterolateral knee complex injuries. Am J Sports Med. 1997;25:596–602.
16. Miller MD, Kline AJ, Gonzales J, et al. Vascular risk associated with a posterior approach for posterior cruciate ligament reconstruction using the tibial inlay technique. J Knee Surg. 2002;15: 137–140.

17. Mariani PP, Adriani E, Bellelli A, et al. Magnetic resonance imaging of tunnel placement in posterior cruciate ligament reconstruction. Arthroscopy. 1999;15:733–740.

18. Jung Y-B, Tae S-K, Jin W-J, et al. Reconstruction of posterior cruciate ligament by the modified tibial inlay method. In: *Proceedings of the 2002 Annual Meeting of the American Academy of Orthopaedic Surgery*, vol. 3. Dallas, TX: AAOS; 2002:602.

19. Cooper DE. Revision PCL reconstruction with the tibial inlay technique. In: *AOSSM Proceedings*. Keystone, CO: AOSSM, 2001.

20. Cooper DE, Stewart D. Posterior cruciate ligament reconstruction using single-bundle patella tendon graft with tibial fixation. 2- to 10-year follow-up. Am J Sports Med. 2004;32:346–360.

21. Bergfeld JA, McAllister DK, Parker RD, et al. A biomechanical comparison of posterior cruciate ligament reconstruction techniques. Am J Sports Med. 2001;29:129–136.

22. Markolf KL, Zemanovic JR, McAllister DR. Cyclic loading of posterior cruciate ligament replacements fixed with tibial tunnel and tibial inlay methods. J Bone Joint Surg Am. 2002;84:518–524.

44

SINGLE-BUNDLE AUGMENTATION FOR POSTERIOR CRUCIATE LIGAMENT RECONSTRUCTION

CHRISTOPHER A. RADKOWSKI, MD, CHRISTOPHER D. HARNER, MD

■ HISTORY OF THE TECHNIQUE

Posterior cruciate ligament (PCL) injuries are relatively infrequent occurrences that present a challenge to the orthopedic surgeon. Traditionally, nonsurgical treatment has been recommended for lower-grade isolated PCL ruptures, while some surgical results have shown persistent posterior laxity of the knee.[1-6] However, other studies have shown degenerative changes and poor objective outcomes associated with conservative treatment of PCL injuries.[7-11] Advances in the understanding of the anatomy and biomechanics of the PCL have led to an increased interest in arthroscopic reconstruction of the PCL. Anatomic studies have delineated separate characteristics of the anterolateral (AL) and posteromedial (PM) bundles within the PCL.[12-15] The larger AL bundle has increased tension in flexion while the PM bundle has more tension in extension. The smaller meniscofemoral ligaments also contribute to the overall strength of the PCL.[14]

Other investigations have shown different biomechanical properties of the different PCL bundles, with the AL bundle possessing increased stiffness and ultimate strength.[14,16,17] Single-bundle PCL reconstruction may not completely restore normal knee kinematics.[18-21] Biomechanical and clinical studies revealed encouraging results with double-bundle PCL reconstruction.[18,19,22-26] Despite the increased understanding of the PCL and improving techniques for reconstruction, clinical results remain suboptimal and lag behind its ACL reconstruction counterpart.

■ RATIONALE

PCL reconstruction with augmentation of a single bundle offers advantages over other techniques in the treatment of PCL injuries. In addition to the intact AL or PM bundle, reconstruction of the injured bundle provides the equivalent of a double-bundle reconstruction, which has been shown to more closely restore normal knee laxity.[14,26] Preservation of the intact native tissue can promote healing of the single bundle reconstruction. Magnetic resonance imaging (MRI) studies have demonstrated the capacity of the PCL to spontaneously heal and regain continuity.[27,28] In addition, some surgeons have favored preservation of native tissue as well. Wang et al.[29] recommend saving the PCL remnants and the surrounding synovium to benefit ligament reconstruction healing. Yoon et al.[30] describe their technique of preserving PCL remnant tissue during arthroscopic double-bundle augmentation of PCL with a split Achilles tendon allograft. We believe that although this technique can be time consuming and difficult, preservation of PCL tissue can provide enhanced posterior stability of the knee and promote graft healing. Preservation of the entire remnant PCL bundle is recommended by Ahn et al.[22,31] for the same reasons.

Due to the reasons above and concerns over removing intact AL or PM bundle tissue in PCL reconstruction, the senior author (CDH) began single-bundle PCL augmentation with preservation of intact PCL tissue in 2000.

■ INDICATIONS AND CONTRAINDICATIONS

Single-bundle augmentation for PCL reconstruction is indicated in patients with an intact AL or PM bundle undergoing PCL reconstruction, usually for persistent posterior instability symptoms or a multiple ligament injury to the knee.

This technique is not recommended if there is complete rupture of both PCL bundles, although remnant tissue is preserved whenever possible. Single bundles with intact fibers that appear lax upon arthroscopic evaluation are also preserved unless located directly at the insertion site of the target bundle.

■ SURGICAL TECHNIQUE

Preoperative Assessment

A thorough history and physical examination are obtained preoperatively in a clinic setting. It is important to determine the chronicity of the injury. Note is made of the active range of motion (ROM) of both knees and any positive findings that may suggest associated pathology. An MRI is frequently obtained to determine the location of the PCL injury **(Fig. 44-1)** and to assess for meniscal pathology, which can be difficult to elucidate with a large effusion and a guarded physical examination. The lower extremity neurovascular examination is documented.

Anesthesia

The patient is identified in the preoperative holding area and the operative site is signed. The anesthesiology staff performs sciatic and femoral nerve blocks for postoperative pain management. The patient is taken to the operating room where spinal or general anesthesia is induced.

Patient Positioning

The patient is positioned supine on the operating room table. A padded bump is taped to the operating room table at the foot with the knee flexed to 90 degrees to hold the leg flexed during the case. A side post is placed on the operative

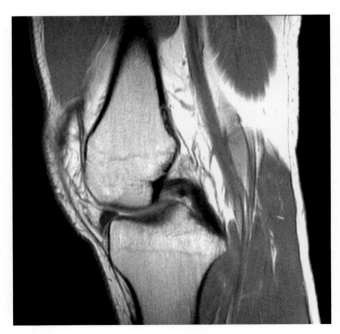

Fig. 44-1. A sagittal proton density MRI image of a knee demonstrate a partial proximal PCL injury.

side just distal to the greater trochanter to support the proximal leg with the knee in flexion. Padded cushions are placed under the nonoperative leg. A tourniquet is placed on the proximal thigh but is not routinely used.

Examination under Anesthesia

An examination under anesthesia (EUA) is then performed. The nonoperative knee is examined followed by the operative knee. The alignment and ROM are assessed with specific attention to terminal extension and flexion. A ligamentous examination is performed, specifically with the Lachman test, anterior drawer test, posterior drawer test, Godfrey test, pivot shift test, and reverse pivot shift test. A thorough evaluation also includes assessment of posteromedial rotatory instability, the Dial test, and stability to varus and valgus stress at 0 degrees and 30 degrees of flexion. Lower grades of posterior drawer and reverse pivot shift tests may represent an intact AL or PM bundle of the PCL. Fluoroscopy is used after the EUA. Lateral views are obtained with the tibia displaced posteriorly and then reduced with an anterior force. The sloped posterior tibial fossa is identified for later tibial tunnel placement.

Surface Anatomy and Skin Incisions

The knee is flexed to 90 degrees and the vertical arthroscopy portals are delineated. The anterolateral portal is placed just lateral to the lateral border of the patellar tendon and adjacent to the inferior pole of the patella. The anteromedial portal is positioned approximately 1 cm medial to the medial border of the superior aspect of the patellar tendon. An accessory posteromedial portal is created just proximal to the joint line and posterior to the MCL. If meniscal repair or other surgical procedures are expected, these incisions are marked as well. The proposed incisions are then cleansed with sterile Betadine paint and then injected with a local anesthetic and epinephrine.

The leg is cleansed with an alcohol solution and gauze sponges with care taken to preserve the incision marks. Next the operative leg is prepped and draped using a sterile technique. A hole is cut in the stockinette for access to the dorsalis pedis pulse throughout the case **(Fig. 44-2)**. After draping, the arthroscopy equipment is prepared and the fluoroscopy machine is later draped.

Graft Preparation

The diagnostic arthroscopy is conducted to determine the extent of injury and the nature of treatment. A discourse on graft choice is beyond the scope of this chapter. In general, a long (24 to 28 cm in length) tibialis anterior allograft is preferred. If a PCL augmentation is to be performed, soft tissue allograft is thawed in sterile saline solution. A whipstitch is placed in each of the free ends of the graft. A closed Endoloop of 25 to 40 mm in length is used without the EndoButton (Smith & Nephew Inc, Andover, Mass). With the standard EndoButton technique, a significant portion of the tunnel will contain only the Endoloop suture, with some

Exposure of the posterior tibia is essential for the success of this technique. This can be tedious but the surgeon should be careful and patient. Both aggressive debridement and inadequate exposure can lead to neurovascular injury. It is also important to assess for concomitant posterolateral corner (PLC) injury on the EUA and following PCL reconstruction. Deficiency of these structures may lead to graft failure.[35] Fluid extravasation during arthroscopy is also a concern. Lower extremity compartments should be monitored throughout the procedure.

■ REHABILITATION

Patients are given instructions for exercises (quad sets, straight-leg raises, and calf pumps) and crutch use prior to discharge the next day. Patients with isolated PCL bundle augmentation reconstructions are weightbearing as tolerated with crutches upon discharge. All dressing changes are performed with an anterior tibial force applied.

The knee is locked in extension for the first week. Mini-squats are performed from 0 to 60 degrees after the first week, which is increased to 90 degrees for weeks 3 and 4. The brace is unlocked at 4 weeks and usually discontinued at 8 weeks. Closed chain terminal knee extension exercises may begin at 8 weeks. Once full, pain-free ROM is achieved, strengthening is addressed.

■ OUTCOMES AND FUTURE DIRECTIONS

PCL reconstruction has been associated with persistent laxity postoperatively. Preserving an intact AL or PM bundle with single-bundle PCL augmentation may lead to decreased laxity and improved clinical results. Although the groups may represent a different severity of injury, future studies comparing single- or double-bundle reconstruction with single-bundle augmentation with preservation of the AL or PM bundle may provide further insight.

■ REFERENCES

1. Dandy DJ, Pusey RJ. The long-term results of unrepaired tears of the posterior cruciate ligament. J Bone Joint Surg Br. 1982;64(1): 92–94.
2. Fowler PJ, Messieh SS. Isolated posterior cruciate ligament injuries in athletes. Am J Sports Med. 1987;15(6):553–557.
3. Lipscomb AB Jr, Anderson AF, Norwig ED, et al. Isolated posterior cruciate ligament reconstruction: long-term results. Am J Sports Med. 1993;21(4):490–496.
4. Parolie JM, Bergfeld JA. Long-term results of nonoperative treatment of isolated posterior cruciate ligament injuries in the athlete. Am J Sports Med. 1986;14(1):35–38.
5. Pournaras J, Symeonides PP. The results of surgical repair of acute tears of the posterior cruciate ligament. Clin Orthop Relat Res. 1991;(267):103–107.

6. Torg JS, Barton TM, Pavlov H, et al. Natural history of the posterior cruciate ligament-deficient knee. Clin Orthop Relat Res. 1989;(246):208–216.
7. Cross MJ, Powell JF. Long-term follow-up of posterior cruciate ligament rupture: a study of 116 cases. Am J Sports Med. 1984; 12:292–297.
8. Keller PM, Shelbourne KD, McCarroll JR, et al. Nonoperatively treated isolated posterior cruciate ligament injuries. Am J Sports Med. 1993;21(1):132–136.
9. Shelbourne KD, Davis TJ, Patel DV. The natural history of acute, isolated, nonoperatively treated posterior cruciate ligament injuries: a prospective study. Am J Sports Med. 1999;27:276–283.
10. Shelbourne KD, Gray T. Natural history of acute posterior cruciate ligament tears. J Knee Surg. 2002;15(2):103–107.
11. Wang CJ, Chen HH, Chen HS, et al. Effects of knee position, graft tension, and mode of fixation in posterior cruciate ligament reconstruction: a cadaveric knee study. Arthroscopy. 2002;18: 496–501.
12. Amis AA, Gupte CM, Bull AM, et al. Anatomy of the posterior cruciate ligament and the meniscofemoral ligaments. Knee Surg Sports Traumatol Arthrosc. 2006;14(3):257–263.
13. Harner CD, Baek GH, Vogrin TM, et al. Quantitative analysis of human cruciate ligament insertions. Arthroscopy. 1999;15(7): 741–749.
14. Harner CD, Hoher J. Evaluation and treatment of posterior cruciate ligament injuries. Am J Sports Med. 1998;26(3):471–482.
15. Morgan CD, Kalman VR, Grawl DM. The anatomic origin of the posterior cruciate ligament: where is it? Reference landmarks for PCL reconstruction. Arthroscopy. 1997;13;325–331.
16. Race A, Amis A. The mechanical properties of the two bundles of the human posterior cruciate ligament. J Biomech. 1994;27(1): 13–24.
17. Race A, Amis A. Loading of the two bundles of the posterior cruciate ligament: an analysis of bundle function in A-P drawer. J Biomech. 1996;29(7):873–879.
18. Giffin JR, Haemmerle MJ, Vogrin TM, et al. Single- versus double-bundle PCL reconstruction: a biomechanical analysis. J Knee Surg. 2002;15(2):114–120.
19. Harner CD, Janaushek MA, Kanamori A, et al. Biomechanical analysis of a double-bundle posterior ligament reconstruction. Am J Sports Med. 2000;28:144–151.
20. Lenschow S, Zantop T, Weimann A, et al. Joint kinematics and in situ forces after single bundle PCL reconstruction: a graft placed at the center of the femoral attachment does not restore normal posterior laxity. Arch Orthop Trauma Surg. 2006;126(4):253–259.
21. Wang CJ, Chen SH, Huang TW. Outcome of arthroscopic single bundle reconstruction for complete posterior cruciate ligament tear. Injury. 2003;34:747–751.
22. Ahn JH, Yoo JC, Wang JH. Posterior cruciate ligament reconstruction: double-loop hamstring tendon autograft versus Achilles tendon allograft—clinical results of a minimum 2-year follow-up. Arthroscopy. 2005;21(8):965–969.
23. Borden PS, Nyland JA, Caborn DN. Posterior cruciate ligament reconstruction (double bundle) using anterior tibialis tendon allograft. Arthroscopy. 2001;17(4):E14.
24. Mannor DA, Shearn JT, Grood ES, et al. Two-bundle posterior cruciate ligament reconstruction: an in vitro analysis of graft placement and tension. Am J Sports Med. 2000;28(6):833–845.
25. Nyland J, Hester P, Caborn DN. Double-bundle posterior cruciate ligament reconstruction with allograft tissue: 2-year postoperative outcomes. Knee Surg Sports Traumatol Arthrosc. 2002;10:274–279.
26. Race A, Amis A. PCL reconstruction: in vitro biomechanical comparison of "isometric" versus single and double-bundled "anatomic" grafts. J Bone Joint Surg Br. 1998;80(1):173–179.
27. Shelbourne KD, Jennings RW, Vahey TN. Magnetic resonance imaging of posterior cruciate ligament injuries: assessment of healing. Am J Knee Surg. 1999;12:209–213.

28. Tewes DP, Fritts HM, Fields RD, et al. Chronically injured posterior cruciate ligament: magnetic resonance imaging. Clin Orthop Relat Res. 1997;(335):224–232.

29. Wang CJ, Chan YS, Weng LH. Posterior cruciate ligament reconstruction using hamstring tendon graft with remnant augmentation. Arthroscopy. 2005;21(11):1401.e1–1401.e3.

30. Yoon KH, Bae DK, Song SJ, et al. Arthroscopic double-bundle augmentation of posterior cruciate ligament using split Achilles allograft. Arthroscopy. 2005;21(12):1436–1442.

31. Ahn JH, Chung YS, Oh I. Arthroscopic posterior cruciate ligament reconstruction using the posterior trans-septal portal. Arthroscopy. 2003;19(1):101–107.

32. Greis PE, Burks RT, Bachus K, et al. The influence of tendon length and fit on the strength of a tendon-bone tunnel complex: a biomechanical and histologic study in the dog. Am J Sports Med. 2001;29(4):493–497.

33. Ahn JH, Ha CW. Posterior trans-septal portal for arthroscopic surgery of the knee joint. Arthroscopy. 2000;16(7):774–779.

34. Dennis MG, Fox JA, Alford JW, et al. Posterior cruciate ligament reconstruction: current trends. J Knee Surg. 2004;17(3):133–139.

35. Harner CD, Vogrin TM, Hoher J, et al. Biomechanical analysis of a double-bundle posterior cruciate ligament reconstruction: deficiency of the posterolateral structures as a cause of graft failure. Am J Sports Med. 2000;28(1):32–39.

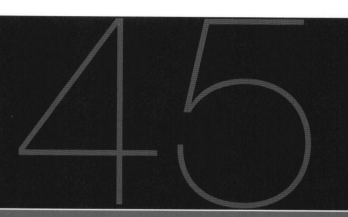

ARTHROSCOPIC POSTERIOR CRUCIATE LIGAMENT RECONSTRUCTION: TRANSTIBIAL TUNNEL TECHNIQUE

GREGORY C. FANELLI, MD

The incidence of posterior cruciate ligament (PCL) injuries is reported to be from 1% to 40% of acute knee injuries. This range is dependent upon the patient population reported and is approximately 3% in the general population and 38% in reports from regional trauma centers.[1-3] Our practice at a regional trauma center has a 38.3% incidence of PCL tears in acute knee injuries, and 56.5% of these PCL injuries occur in multiple trauma patients. Of these PCL injuries 45.9% are combined ACL/PCL tears, while 41.2% are PCL/posterolateral corner tears. Only 3% of acute PCL injuries seen in the trauma center are isolated.

This chapter illustrates my surgical technique of the arthroscopic single bundle/single femoral tunnel transtibial (SB/SFT TTT) PCL reconstruction surgical procedure and presents the Fanelli Sports Injury Clinic 2- to 10-year results of PCL reconstruction using this surgical technique. The information presented in this chapter has also been presented elsewhere, and the reader is referred to these sources for additional information regarding this topic.[4-19]

■ SURGICAL INDICATIONS

The SB/SFT TTT PCL reconstruction is an anatomic reconstruction of the anterolateral bundle of the PCL. The anterolateral bundle tightens in flexion, and this reconstruction reproduces that biomechanical function. While the SB/SFT TTT PCL reconstruction does not reproduce the broad anatomic insertion site of the normal PCL, there are certain factors that lead to success with this surgical technique:

1 Identify and treat all pathology (especially posterolateral instability).
2 Accurate tunnel placement.
3 Anatomic graft insertion sites.

4 Strong graft material.
5 Minimize graft bending.
6 Final tensioning at 70 degrees to 90 degrees of knee flexion.
7 Graft tensioning.
  a Arthrotek mechanical tensioning device.
8 Primary and back-up fixation.
9 Appropriate rehabilitation program.

■ SURGICAL INDICATIONS

Our indications for surgical treatment of acute PCL injuries include insertion site avulsions, tibial step off decreased 10 mm or greater, and PCL tears combined with other structural injuries. Our indications for surgical treatment of chronic PCL injuries are when an isolated PCL tear becomes symptomatic, or when progressive functional instability develops.

■ SURGICAL TECHNIQUE

Patient Positioning and Initial Set Up

The patient is positioned on the operating table in the supine position, and the surgical and nonsurgical knees are examined under general anesthesia. A tourniquet is applied to the operative extremity, and the surgical leg prepped and draped in a sterile fashion. Allograft tissue is prepared prior to beginning the surgical procedure, and autograft tissue is harvested prior to beginning the arthroscopic portion of the procedure. The arthroscopic instruments are inserted with the inflow through the superior lateral patellar portal, the arthroscope in the inferior lateral patellar portal, and the instruments in the inferior medial patellar portal. The portals are interchanged as necessary. The joint is thoroughly evaluated arthroscopically, and the PCL evaluated using the three-zone arthroscopic technique.[5] The PCL tear is identified, and the residual stump of the PCL is debrided with hand tools and the synovial shaver.

Initial Incision

An extra capsular posteromedial safety incision approximately 1.5 to 2.0 cm long is created **(Fig. 45-1)**. The crural fascia is incised longitudinally, taking precautions to protect the neurovascular structures. The interval is developed between the medial head of the gastrocnemius muscle and the posterior capsule of the knee joint, which is anterior. The surgeon's gloved finger is able to have the neurovascular structures posterior to the finger, and the posterior aspect of the joint capsule anterior to the surgeon's finger. This technique enables the surgeon to monitor surgical instruments such as the over-the-top PCL instruments and the PCL and anterior cruciate ligament (ACL) drill guides as they are positioned in the posterior aspect of the knee. The surgeon's finger in the posteromedial safety incision also confirms accurate placement of the guide wire prior to tibial tunnel drilling in the medial-lateral and proximal-distal directions **(Fig. 45-2)**.

Elevating the Posterior Capsule

The curved over-the-top PCL instruments are used to carefully lyse adhesions in the posterior aspect of the knee and to elevate the posterior knee joint capsule away from the tibial

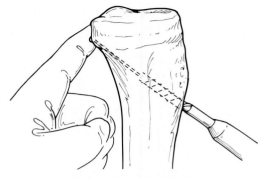

Fig. 45-2. The surgeon is able to palpate the posterior aspect of the tibia through the extracapsular extra articular posteromedial safety incision. This enables the surgeon to accurately position guide wires, create the tibial tunnel, and protect the neurovascular structures. (Adapted with permission from Arthrotek, Inc., Warsaw, Ind.)

ridge on the posterior aspect of the tibia. This capsular elevation enhances correct drill guide and tibial tunnel placement **(Fig. 45-3)**.

Drill Guide Positioning

The arm of the Arthrotek Fanelli PCL-ACL Drill Guide is inserted into the knee through the inferior medial patellar portal and positioned in the PCL fossa on the posterior tibia **(Fig. 45-4)**. The bullet portion of the drill guide contacts the anterior medial aspect of the proximal tibia approximately 1 cm below the tibial tubercle, at a point midway between the tibial crest anteriorly and the posterior medial border of the tibia. This drill guide positioning creates a tibial tunnel that is relatively vertically oriented and has its posterior

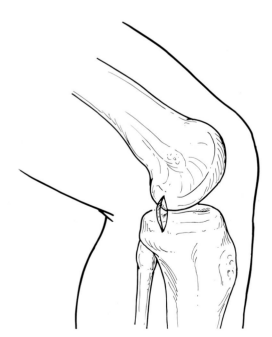

Fig. 45-1. Posteromedial extra-articular extracapsular safety incision. (Adapted with permission from Arthrotek, Inc., Warsaw, Ind.)

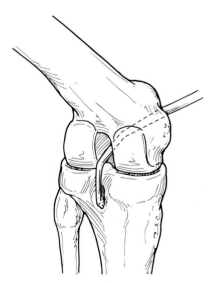

Fig. 45-3. Posterior capsular elevation using the Arthrotek PCL instruments. (Adapted with permission from Arthrotek, Inc., Warsaw, Ind.)

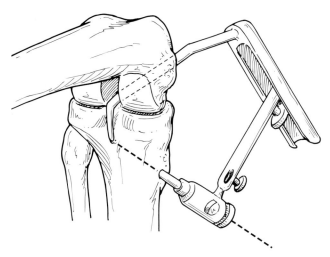

Fig. 45-4. Arthrotek Fanelli PCL-ACL drill guide positioned to place guide wire in preparation for creation of the transtibial PCL tibial tunnel. (Adapted with permission from Arthrotek, Inc., Warsaw, Ind.)

exit point in the inferior and lateral aspects of the PCL tibial anatomic insertion site. This positioning creates an angle of graft orientation such that the graft will turn two very smooth 45-degree angles on the posterior aspect of the tibia, eliminating the "killer turn" of 90-degree graft angle bending **(Fig. 45-5).**

The tip of the guide in the posterior aspect of the tibia is confirmed with the surgeon's finger through the extra capsular posteromedial safety incision. Intraoperative AP and lateral x-ray may also be used, as well as arthroscopic visualization to confirm drill guide and guide pin placement. A blunt spade-tipped guide wire is drilled from anterior to posterior and can be visualized with the arthroscope, in addition to being palpated with the finger in the posteromedial safety incision. We consider the finger in the posteromedial safety incision the most important step for accuracy and safety.

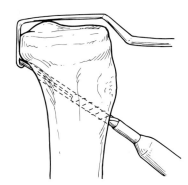

Fig. 45-6. The Arthrotek PCL closed curette is used to cap the guide wire during tibial tunnel drilling. (Adapted with permission from Arthrotek, Inc., Warsaw, Ind.)

Tibial Tunnel Drilling

The appropriately sized standard cannulated reamer is used to create the tibial tunnel. The closed curved PCL curette may be positioned to cup the tip of the guide wire **(Fig. 45-6).** The arthroscope, when positioned in the posteromedial portal, visualizes the guide wire being captured by the curette and protects the neurovascular structures, in addition to the surgeon's finger in the posteromedial safety incision. The surgeon's finger in the posteromedial safety incision is monitoring the position of the guide wire. The standard cannulated drill is advanced to the posterior cortex of the tibia. The drill chuck is then disengaged from the drill, and completion of the tibial tunnel reaming is performed by hand. This gives an additional margin of safety for completion of the tibial tunnel. The tunnel edges are chamfered and rasped with the PCL/ACL system rasp **(Fig. 45-7).**

Drilling of the Femoral Tunnel

The Arthrotek Fanelli PCL-ACL Drill Guide is positioned to create the femoral tunnel **(Fig. 45-8).** The arm of the guide is introduced into the knee through the inferior medial patellar portal and is positioned such that the guide wire will exit through the center of the stump of the anterolateral bundle

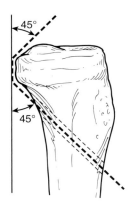

Fig. 45-5. Drawing demonstrating the desired turning angles the PCL graft will make after the creation of the tibial tunnel. (Adapted with permission from Arthrotek, Inc., Warsaw, Ind.)

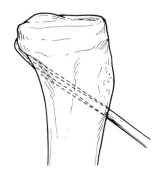

Fig. 45-7. The tunnel edges are chamfered after drilling to smooth any rough edges. (Adapted with permission from Arthrotek, Inc., Warsaw, Ind.)

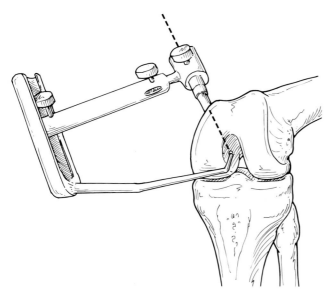

Fig. 45-8. The Arthrotek Fanelli PCL-ACL drill guide is positioned to drill the guide wire from outside in. The guide wire begins at a point halfway between the medial femoral epicondyle and the medial femoral condyle trochlea articular margin, approximately 2 to 3 cm proximal to the medial femoral condyle distal articular margin, and exits through the center of the stump of the anterolateral bundle of the PCL stump. (Adapted with permission from Arthrotek, Inc., Warsaw, Ind.)

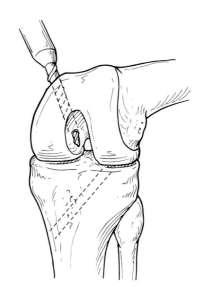

Fig. 45-9. Completion of femoral tunnel reaming by hand for an additional margin of safety. (Adapted with permission from Arthrotek, Inc., Warsaw, Ind.)

of the PCL. The blunt spade-tipped guide wire is drilled through the guide, and just as it begins to emerge through the center of the stump of the anterolateral bundle of the PCL, the drill guide is disengaged. The accuracy of the guide wire position is confirmed arthroscopically by probing and direct visualization. Care must be taken to ensure the patellofemoral joint has not been violated by arthroscopically examining the patellofemoral joint prior to drilling the femoral tunnel.

The appropriately sized standard cannulated reamer is used to create the femoral tunnel. A curette is used to cap the tip of the guide so there is no inadvertent advancement of the guide wire causing damage to the articular surface, the ACL, or other intra-articular structures. As the reamer is about to penetrate the wall of the intercondylar notch, it is disengaged from the drill, and the final femoral tunnel reaming is completed by hand for an additional margin of safety **(Fig. 45-9)**. The reaming debris is evacuated with a synovial shaver to minimize fat pad inflammatory response with subsequent risk of arthrofibrosis. The tunnel edges are chamfered and rasped.

Tunnel Preparation and Graft Passage

The Arthrotek Magellan suture-passing device is introduced through the tibial tunnel and into the knee joint and is retrieved through the femoral tunnel with an arthroscopic grasping tool **(Fig. 45-10)**. A 7.9 mm GoreTex Smoother (WL Gore, Inc., Flagstaff, Ariz.) flexible rasp may be used, and when used is attached to the Magellan suture-passing

device, and the GoreTex Smoother is pulled into the femoral tunnel, into the joint, and into and out of the tibial tunnel opening **(Fig. 45-11)**. The tunnel edges are chamfered and rasped at 0 degrees, 30 degrees, 60 degrees, and 90 degrees of knee flexion. Care must be taken to avoid excessive pressure using the GoreTex Smoother or the tunnel configuration could be altered or the bone destroyed. The traction sutures of the graft material are attached to the loop of the flexible rasp, and the PCL graft material is pulled into position.

Graft Tensioning and Fixation

Fixation of the PCL substitute is accomplished with primary and backup fixation on both the femoral and tibial

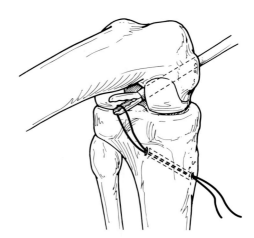

Fig. 45-10. Retrieval of suture passing wire. (Adapted with permission from Arthrotek, Inc., Warsaw, Ind.)

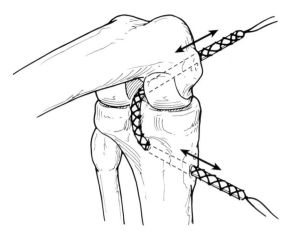

Fig. 45-11. The Arthrotek knee ligament graft tensioning boot. This mechanical tensioning device uses a ratcheted torque wrench device to assist the surgeon during graft tensioning. (Adapted with permission from Arthrotek, Inc., Warsaw, Ind.)

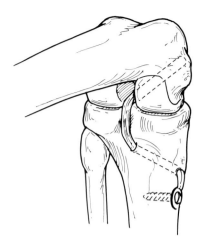

Fig. 45-13. Final graft fixation using primary and backup fixation. (Adapted with permission from Arthrotek, Inc., Warsaw, Ind.)

sides. Our preferred graft source for PCL reconstruction is the Achilles tendon allograft. Femoral fixation is accomplished with press fit fixation of a wedge-shaped calcaneal bone plug and aperture opening fixation using the Arthrotek Gentle Thread bioabsorbable interference screw, or with primary aperture opening fixation using the Arthrotek Gentle Thread bioabsorbable interference screw, and backup fixation with a ligament fixation button, or screw and spiked ligament washer, or screw and post assembly. The Arthrotek Tensioning Boot is applied to the traction sutures of the graft material on its distal end, set for 20 pounds, and the knee cycled through 25 full flexion-extension cycles for graft pretensioning and settling **(Fig. 45-12)**. The knee is placed in approximately 70 degrees of knee flexion, and tibial fixation of the Achilles tendon allograft is achieved with primary aperture opening fixation using the Arthrotek Gentle Thread bioabsorbable interference screw, and backup fixation with a ligament fixation button, or screw and post or screw and spiked ligament washer assembly **(Fig. 45-13)**.

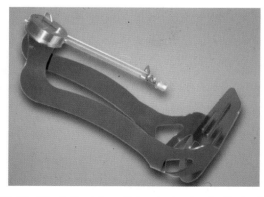

Fig. 45-12. The Arthrotek graft tensioning boot attached to the traction sutures of the PCL graft. (Adapted with permission from Arthrotek, Inc., Warsaw, Ind.)

■ ADDITIONAL SURGERY

When multiple ligament surgeries are performed at the same operative session, the PCL reconstruction is performed first, followed by the ACL reconstruction, followed by the collateral ligament surgery. The reader is referred to other sections of this textbook for descriptions of multiple ligament surgeries of the knee. At the completion of the procedure, the tourniquet is deflated, and the wounds are copiously irrigated. The incisions are closed in the standard fashion.

■ POSTOPERATIVE REHABILITATION AND RETURN TO PLAY RECOMMENDATIONS

The knee is kept locked in a long leg brace in full extension for 6 weeks, with nonweight bearing using crutches. Progressive range of motion occurs during weeks 4 through 6. The brace is unlocked at the end of 6 weeks, with progressive weight bearing at 25% body weight per week during postoperative weeks 7 through 10. The crutches are discontinued at the end of postoperative week 10. Progressive closed kinetic chain strength training and continued motion exercises are performed. Return to sports and heavy labor occurs after the sixth to ninth postoperative month, when sufficient strength, range of motion, and proprioceptive skills have returned.

■ FANELLI SPORTS INJURY CLINIC RESULTS

We have previously published the results of our arthroscopically assisted combined ACL/PCL and PCL/posterolateral complex reconstructions using the reconstructive technique described in this chapter.[6,10,18,19] Our most recently published 2- to 10-year results of combined ACL-PCL reconstructions are presented here.[10]

This study presented the 2- to 10-year (24 to 120 months) results of 35 arthroscopically assisted combined ACL/PCL reconstructions evaluated pre- and postoperatively using Lysholm, Tegner, and the Hospital for Special Surgery knee ligament rating scales, KT-1000 arthrometer testing, stress radiography, and physical examination.

This study population included 26 males and 9 females, with 19 acute and 16 chronic knee injuries. Ligament injuries included 19 ACL/PCL/posterolateral instabilities, 9 ACL/PCL/MCL (medial collateral ligament) instabilities, 6 ACL/PCL/posterolateral/MCL instabilities, and 1 ACL/PCL instability. All knees had grade-III preoperative ACL/PCL laxity and were assessed pre- and postoperatively with arthrometer testing, three different knee ligament rating scales, stress radiography, and physical examination. Arthroscopically assisted combined ACL/PCL reconstructions were performed using the single incision endoscopic ACL technique, and the SB/SFT TTT PCL technique. PCLs were reconstructed with allograft Achilles tendon (26), autograft BTB (7), and autograft semitendinosus/gracilis (2). ACL's were reconstructed with autograft BTB (16), allograft BTB (12), Achilles tendon allograft (6), and autograft semitendinosus/gracilis (1). MCL injuries were treated with bracing or open reconstruction. Posterolateral instability was treated with biceps femoris tendon transfer, with or without primary repair, and posterolateral capsular shift procedures as indicated.

Postoperative physical examination results revealed normal posterior drawer/tibial step off in 16 of 35 (46%) knees. Normal Lachman and pivot shift tests were found in 33 of 35 (94%) knees. Posterolateral stability was restored to normal in 6 of 25 (24%) knees, and tighter than the normal knee in 19 of 25 (76%) knees evaluated with the external rotation thigh foot angle test. Thirty degrees varus stress testing was normal in 22 of 25 (88%) knees, and grade I laxity in 3 of 25 (12%) knees. Thirty degree valgus stress testing was normal in 7 of 7 (100%) of surgically treated MCL tears, and normal in 7 of 8 (87.5%) brace-treated knees. Postoperative KT-1000 arthrometer testing mean side-to-side difference measurements were 2.7 mm (PCL screen), 2.6 mm (corrected posterior), and 1.0 mm (corrected anterior) measurements, a statistically significant improvement from preoperative status ($p = 0.001$). Postoperative stress radiographic side-to-side difference measurements measured at 90 degrees of knee flexion, and 32 pounds of posteriorly directed proximal force were 0 to 3 mm in 11 of 21 (52.3%), 4 to 5 mm in 5 of 21 (23.8%), and 6 to 10 mm in 4 of 21 (19%) knees. Postoperative Lysholm, Tegner, and HSS knee ligament rating scale mean values were 91.2, 5.3, and 86.8, respectively, demonstrating a statistically significant improvement from preoperative status ($p = 0.001$).

The conclusions drawn from the study were that combined ACL/PCL instabilities could be successfully treated with arthroscopic reconstruction and the appropriate collateral ligament surgery. Statistically significant improvement was noted from the preoperative condition at 2- to 10-year follow-up using objective parameters of knee ligament rating scales, arthrometer testing, stress radiography, and physical examination. Postoperatively, these knees are not normal, but they are functionally stable. Continuing technical improvements will most likely improve future results.

Another group of multiple ligament reconstructions that warrant attention are our 2- to 10-year results of combined PCL-posterolateral reconstruction.[18] This study presented the 2- to 10-year (24 to 120 months) results of 41 chronic arthroscopically assisted combined PCL/posterolateral reconstructions evaluated pre- and postoperatively using Lysholm, Tegner, and the Hospital for Special Surgery knee ligament rating scales, KT-1000 arthrometer testing, stress radiography, and physical examination.

This study population included 31 males and 10 females, with 24 left and 17 right chronic PCL/posterolateral knee injuries with functional instability. The knees were assessed pre- and postoperatively with arthrometer testing, three different knee ligament rating scales, stress radiography, and physical examination. PCL reconstructions were performed using the arthroscopically assisted SB/SFT TTT PCL reconstruction technique using fresh frozen Achilles tendon allografts in all 41 cases. In all 41 cases, posterolateral instability reconstruction was performed with combined biceps femoris tendon tenodesis and posterolateral capsular shift procedures. The paired t test and power analysis were the statistical tests used. Ninety-five percent confidence intervals were used throughout the analysis.

Postoperative physical exam revealed normal posterior drawer/tibial step off in 29 of 41 (70%) knees for the overall group, and 11 of 12 (91.7%) normal posterior drawer and tibial step off in the knees tensioned with the Arthrotek tensioning boot. Posterolateral stability was restored to normal in 11 of 41 (27%) knees, and tighter than the normal knee in 29 of 41 (71%) knees evaluated with the external rotation thigh foot angle test. Thirty degree varus stress testing was normal in 40 of 41 (97%) knees, and grade-I laxity in 1 of 41 (3%) knees. Postoperative KT-1000 arthrometer testing mean side-to-side difference measurements were 1.80 mm (PCL screen), 2.11 mm (corrected posterior), and 0.63 mm (corrected anterior) measurements. This is a statistically significant improvement from preoperative status for the PCL screen and the corrected posterior measurements ($p = 0.001$). The postoperative stress radiographic mean side-to-side difference measurement measured at 90 degrees of knee flexion, and 32 pounds of posterior directed force applied to the proximal tibia using the Telos device was 2.26 mm. This is a statistically significant improvement from preoperative measurements ($p = 0.001$). Postoperative Lysholm, Tegner, and the Hospital for Special Surgery knee ligament rating scale mean values were 91.7, 4.92, and 88.7, respectively, demonstrating a statistically significant improvement from preoperative status ($p = 0.001$).

Conclusions drawn from this study were that chronic combined PCL/posterolateral instabilities could be successfully treated with arthroscopic PCL reconstruction using fresh frozen Achilles tendon allograft combined with posterolateral corner reconstruction using biceps tendon transfer combined with posterolateral capsular shift procedure. Statistically significant improvement is noted ($p = 0.001$) from the preoperative condition at 2- to 10-year follow-up using objective parameters of knee ligament rating scales, arthrometer testing, stress radiography, and physical examination.

■ CONCLUSIONS

The arthroscopically assisted single bundle transtibial PCL reconstruction technique is a reproducible surgical procedure. There are documented results demonstrating statistically significant improvements from preoperative to postoperative status evaluated by physical examination, knee ligament rating scales, arthrometer measurements, and stress radiography. Factors contributing to the success of this surgical technique include identification and treatment of all pathology (especially posterolateral instability), accurate tunnel placement, placement of strong graft material at anatomic graft insertion sites, minimize graft bending, performing final graft tensioning at 70 degrees to 90 degrees of knee flexion using the Arthrotek graft tensioning boot, utilizing primary and backup fixation, and the appropriate postoperative rehabilitation program.

■ REFERENCES

1. Fanelli GC. PCL injuries in trauma patients. Arthroscopy. 1993;9;3:291–294.
2. Fanelli GC, Edson CJ. PCL injuries in trauma patients. Part II. Arthroscopy. 1995;11:526–529.
3. Daniel DM, Akeson W, O'Conner J, eds. *Knee Ligaments—Structure, Function, Injury, and Repair.* New York: Raven Press; 1990.
4. Malek M, Fanelli GC. Technique of arthroscopically PCL reconstruction. Orthopaedics. 1993;16(9):961–966.
5. Fanelli GC, Bradley G, Edson C. Current concepts review: the posterior cruciate ligament: arthroscopic evaluation and treatment. Arthroscopy. 1994;10(6):673–688.
6. Fanelli GC, Giannotti B, Edson CJ. Arthroscopically assisted PCL/posterior lateral complex reconstruction. Arthroscopy. 1996;12(5):521–530.
7. Fanelli GC, Monahan TJ. Complications of posterior cruciate ligament reconstruction. Sports Med Arthroscopy Rev. 1999;7(4):296–302.
8. Fanelli GC. Point counter point: arthroscopic posterior cruciate ligament reconstruction: single bundle/single femoral tunnel. Arthroscopy. 2000;16(7):725–731.
9. Fanelli GC, Monahan TJ. Complications in posterior cruciate ligament and posterolateral complex surgery. Operative Techniques Sports Med. 2001:9(2);96–99.
10. Fanelli GC, Edson CJ. Arthroscopically assisted combined ACL/PCL reconstruction. 2–10 year follow-up. Arthroscopy. 2002;18(7):703–714.
11. Fanelli GC, Edson CJ. Management of posterior cruciate ligament and posterolateral instability of the knee. In: Chow J, ed. *Advanced Arthroplasty.* New York: Springer-Verlag; 2001.
12. Fanelli GC, Monahan TJ. Complications and pitfalls in posterior cruciate ligament reconstruction. In: Malek MM, ed. *Knee Surgery: Complications, Pitfalls, and Salvage.* New York: Springer-Verlag; 2001.
13. Fanelli GC. Arthroscopic evaluation of the PCL. In: Fanelli GC, ed. *Posterior Cruciate Ligament Injuries. A Guide to Practical Management.* New York: Springer-Verlag; 2001.
14. Fanelli GC. Arthroscopic PCL reconstruction: transtibial technique. In: Fanelli GC, ed. *Posterior Cruciate Ligament Injuries. A Guide to Practical Management.* New York: Springer-Verlag; 2001.
15. Fanelli GC. Complications in PCL surgery. In: Fanelli GC, ed. *Posterior Cruciate Ligament Injuries. A Guide to Practical Management.* New York: Springer-Verlag; 2001.
16. Miller MD, Cooper DE, Ganelli GC, et al. Posterior cruciate ligament: current concepts. In: Beaty JH, ed. *American Academy of Orthopaedic Surgeons Instructional Course Lectures,* vol. 51. Rosemont, Ill.: 2005;51:347–351.
17. Arthrotek PCL Reconstruction Surgical Technique Guide. Fanelli PCL-ACL Drill Guide System. Arthrotek, Inc., Warsaw, Ind. 1998.
18. Fanelli GC, Edson CJ. Combined posterior cruciate ligament–posterolateral reconstruction with Achilles tendon allograft and biceps femoris tendon tenodesis: 2–10 year follow-up. Arthroscopy. 2004;20(4):339–345.
19. Fanelli GC, Giannotti BF, Edson CJ. Arthroscopically assisted combined anterior and posterior cruciate ligament reconstruction. Arthroscopy. 1996;12(1):5–14.

study, Miller et al.[22] found the fixation screw to be on average over 2 cm from the popliteal artery. Although this study demonstrates the safety of this approach relative to the seated screw, it does not allay the concerns of vascular injury during the approach itself, during retractor placement, or while drilling, tapping, and inserting the screw. In addition, in our hands, the tibial inlay procedure is technically more demanding than the transtibial tunnel technique and takes longer to perform.

Other technical alternatives involve the choice of graft tissue. Multiple grafts have been reported including Achilles tendon, hamstrings, patellar tendon, tibialis anterior, and quadriceps tendon. The choice of graft can limit your reconstructive options. For example, the Achilles/hamstring reconstruction as described could not be utilized for an inlay technique. A split Achilles or quadriceps tendon may be used with either technique; however, they have other potential disadvantages. These grafts have bony fixation on only one end and may lack the necessary bulk to fully recreate both bundles.[18,23,24] The bifid patellar tendon may be used with either the transtibial tunnel or tibial inlay, has bony fixation on both ends, and can reapproximate the normal PCL bulk[25]; however, passage of the graft can be difficult and whole patellar tendon availability may be a problem. In short, each graft has its own set of advantages and disadvantages. It is advisable that the sports medicine PCL surgeon be facile with several options to best fit the individual scenario for each patient.

■ REHABILITATION

Initially, the patient is kept locked in extension and partial weight bearing, with passive flexion exercises performed several times a day. An emphasis is placed on quadriceps muscle contraction and regaining full extension symmetrical to the contralateral, uninjured side. At 6 weeks, the brace is unlocked and weight bearing is slowly advanced to full. We also begin active flexion exercises in addition to passive. Isometric and light resistive exercises are continued at this point through a protected range of motion. At 3 months, physical therapy is advanced to a muscle-strengthening program with an emphasis on quadriceps muscle rehabilitation. At 6 months, straight running can be started on even ground without any cutting or pivoting movements. By 8 to 10 months, sports specific exercises can be performed in anticipation of a full return to sporting activities by 1 year postoperatively.

■ OUTCOMES AND FUTURE DIRECTIONS

Early clinical outcomes of double bundle PCL reconstructions are starting to emerge. Preliminary results are promising, but as of yet no long-term evaluations are available. Future studies comparing techniques will help resolve issues of tunnel number, graft type, and tibial fixation options. Other future directions will include investigating the questions of acute versus chronic repair, the utility and indications of sagittal plane tibial osteotomies in the PCL deficient knee, and finally the role of biological manipulation in ligament reconstruction.

Nyland et al.[26] published their results of doublebundle PCL reconstruction with a minimum 2-year follow-up. They used tibialis anterior allograft in 19 patients with a transtibial technique. Eighty-nine percent of patients were rated as normal or near normal, and posterior translation averaged only 2.4 mm. They concluded that their double bundle reconstruction reestablished PCL function to a greater extent than single bundle techniques.

Stannard et al.[18] investigated the use of a split Achilles allograft using the tibial inlay technique and two femoral tunnels. They followed 30 reconstructed PCLs in 29 patients. At an average of 25 months follow-up, 23 patients had no instability on examination and 7 had 1+ laxity. KT-2000 data measured average side-to-side differences in posterior tibial translation to be less than 0.5 mm. Clinical outcomes were overall very promising and did not deteriorate over the 2-year follow-up period.

Double bundle reconstruction of the PCL is still in its developmental stages with many questions yet to be answered. Future studies may help answer many of the lingering concerns that the increase in technical difficulty does not outweigh the clinical benefit when compared to traditional single bundle reconstructions. In addition, the debate surrounding tibial inlay versus transtibial tunnel techniques is far from settled. In all likelihood, both tibial fixation options will have a place in the knee surgeon's armamentarium.

Beyond the technical details of the reconstruction itself, other future considerations are at play with regard to PCL reconstruction. Principal among these is surgical timing. Several studies have reported that early reconstruction yields better functional outcomes. As early as 1994, Noyes and Barber-Westin[27] found that reconstructions performed acutely had decreased posterior laxity and better functional results. Other studies have supported the idea of early intervention.[9,11] In contrast, some authors report no deleterious effects from delaying reconstruction.[17,28] In general, however, the current trend is toward early reconstruction of acute injuries.

Although timing of surgery appears to be important in and of itself, it may be the sequelae of surgical delay that is the real culprit. In the chronic PCL deficient knee, the joint may develop an increasing and potentially static posterior sag with attenuation of secondary stabilizers such as the posterolateral corner. This fixed deformity may in part explain the poorer results with chronic PCL reconstruction. Realignment of the proximal tibia in the sagittal plane is a potential solution. Giffin et al.[29] evaluated the effect of an anterior opening wedge osteotomy on the resting position of the tibia relative to the femur. By increasing the tibial slope with an opening wedge osteotomy, they were able to shift the tibial resting position anterior under an axial load. The potential clinical application of this concept would be for the persistent tibial sag in the chronic PCL deficient knee. Correction of sagittal plane joint incongruity may eliminate one potential source of PCL reconstruction failure in the chronic setting and is a prime area for future study.

Finally, the future of all orthopedics will likely involve biological manipulation of surgical techniques. These interventions may aid not only in the reconstruction setting, but also as adjuncts for primary healing following acute injuries. The mode of delivery of these critical growth factors may be via direct application of individual factors, by introduction of pluripotential stromal cells, or by gene transfer.[30] The possibilities are endless and clinical use of tissue engineering during ligament reconstruction of the knee is within sight.

■ REFERENCES

1. Girgis FG, Marshall JL, Al Monajem ARS. The cruciate ligaments of the knee joint. Anatomical, functional, and experimental analysis. Clin Orthop. 1975;106:216–231.
2. Harner CD, Xerogeanes JW, Livesay GA, et al. The human posterior cruciate ligament complex: an interdisciplinary study—ligament morphology and biomechanical evaluation. Am J Sports Med. 1995;23:736–745.
3. Covey DC, Sapega AA, Sherman GM. Testing for isometry during reconstruction of the posterior cruciate ligament: anatomic and biomechanical considerations. Am J Sports Med. 1996;24:740–746.
4. Fox RJ, Harner CD, Sakane M, et al. Determination of in situ forces in the human posterior cruciate ligament using robotic technology. A cadaveric study. Am J Sports Med. 1998;26:395–401.
5. Mejia EA, Noyes FR, Grood ES. Posterior cruciate ligament femoral insertion site characteristics: importance for reconstructive procedures. Am J Sports Med. 2002;30:643–651.
6. Ahmad CS, Cohen ZA, Levine WN, et al. Codominance of the individual posterior cruciate ligament bundles: an analysis of bundle lengths and orientation. Am J Sports Med. 2003;31:221–225.
7. Race A, Amis AA. PCL reconstruction: in vitro biomechanical comparison of "isometric" versus single and double-bundled anatomic grafts. J Bone Joint Surg Br. 1998; 80:173–179.
8. Harner CD, Janaushek MA, Kanamori A, et al. Biomechanical analysis of a double-bundle posterior cruciate ligament reconstruction. Am J Sports Med. 2000;28:144–151.
9. Sekiya JK, West R, Ong BC, et al. Clinical outcomes after isolated arthroscopic single-bundle posterior cruciate ligament reconstruction. Arthroscopy. 2005;21:1042–1050.
10. Harner CD, Höher J. Evaluation and treatment of posterior cruciate ligament injuries. Am J Sports Med. 1998;26:471–482.
11. Harner CD, Waltrip RL, Bennett CH, et al. Surgical management of knee dislocations. J Bone Joint Surg Am. 2004;86:262–273.
12. Sekiya JK, Giffin JR, Harner CD. Posterior cruciate ligament injuries: isolated and combined patterns. In: Schenck RC, ed. *Multiple Ligamentous Injuries of the Knee in the Athlete*. Rosemont, IL: AAOS; 2002:73–90.
13. Sekiya JK, Haemmerle MJ, Stabile KJ, et al. Biomechanical analysis of a combined double-bundle posterior cruciate ligament and posterolateral corner reconstruction. Am J Sports Med. 2005;33:360–369.
14. Torg JS, Barton TM, Pavlov H, et al. Natural history of the posterior cruciate ligament-deficient knee. Clin Orthop. 1989;246:208–216.
15. Keller PM, Shelbourne KD, McCarroll JR, et al. Nonoperatively treated posterior cruciate ligament injuries: a prospective study. Am J Sports Med. 1999;27:276–283.
16. Boynton MD, Tietjens BR. Long-term follow-up of the untreated isolated posterior cruciate ligament-deficient knee. Am J Sports Med. 1996;24:306–310.
17. Fanelli GC, Edson CJ. Arthroscopically assisted combined anterior and posterior cruciate ligament reconstruction in the multiple ligament injured knee: 2- to 10-year follow-up. Arthroscopy. 2002;18:703–714.
18. Stannard JP, Riley RS, Sheils TM, et al. Anatomic reconstruction of the posterior cruciate ligament after multiligamentous knee injuries. Am J Sports Med. 2003;31:196–202.
19. Bergfeld JA, McAllister DR, Parker RD, et al. A biomechanical comparison of posterior cruciate ligament reconstruction techniques. Am J Sports Med. 2001;29:129–136.
20. Margheritini F, Mauro CS, Rihn JA, et al. Biomechanical comparison of tibial inlay versus transtibial techniques for posterior cruciate ligament reconstruction: analysis of knee kinematics and graft in situ forces. Am J Sports Med. 2004;32:587–593.
21. McAllister DR, Markolf KL, Oakes DA, et al. A biomechanical comparison of tibial inlay and tibial tunnel posterior cruciate ligament reconstruction. Am J Sports Med. 2002;30:312–317.
22. Miller MD, Kline AJ, Gonzales J, et al. Vascular risk associated with a posterior approach for posterior cruciate ligament reconstruction using the tibial inlay technique. J Knee Surg. 2002;15:137–140.
23. Richards RS, Moorman III, CT. Use of autograft quadriceps tendon for double-bundle posterior cruciate ligament reconstruction. Arthroscopy. 2003;19:906–916.
24. Noyes FR, Medvecky MJ, Bhargava M. Arthroscopically assisted quadriceps double-bundle tibial inlay posterior cruciate ligament reconstruction: an analysis of techniques and a safe operative approach to the popliteal fossa. Arthroscopy. 2003;19:894–905.
25. Sekiya JK, Kurtz CA, Carr DR. Transtibial and tibial inlay double-bundle posterior cruciate ligament reconstruction: surgical technique using a bifid bone-patellar tendon-bone allograft. Arthroscopy. 2004;20:1095–1100.
26. Nyland J, Hester P, Caborn DN. Double-bundle posterior cruciate ligament reconstruction with allograft tissue: 2-year postoperative outcomes. Knee Surge Sports Trauma Arthrosc. 2002;10:274–279.
27. Noyes FR, Barber-Westin SD. Posterior cruciate ligament allograft reconstruction with and without a ligament augmentation device. Arthroscopy. 1994;10:371–382.
28. Shelbourne KD, Porter DA, Clingman JA, et al. Low-velocity knee dislocation. Orthop Rev. 1991;20:995–1004.
29. Giffin JR, Vogrin TM, Zantop T, et al. Effects of increasing tibial slope on the biomechanics of the knee. Am J Sports Med. 2004;32:376–382.
30. Woo SL, Hildebrand K, Watanabe N, et al. Tissue engineering of ligament and tendon healing. Clin Orthop. 1999;367:312–232.

slight valgus moment in the anteroposterior plane. Patients should wear this brace locked in extension for all activities except physical therapy exercises and continuous passive motion (CPM) use for 4 weeks postoperatively. The weight bearing status is dependent on osteotomy fixation, but usually includes partial weight bearing with crutches. Patients should begin quad sets, straight leg raises, heel slides, and CPM use from 0- to 90-degree knee flexion over the first 4 weeks. At 4 weeks the brace may be unlocked for ambulation, and the patient may begin weight bearing as tolerated with crutches. The brace and crutches may be discontinued at 6 weeks if the patient has full extension, good quadriceps control with no extension lag on straight leg raise, and a non-antalgic gait pattern. Range of motion and gentle strengthening exercises continue, with more aggressive strengthening beginning at 3 months postoperatively.

Rehab Protocol for Posterior Cruciate Ligament Reconstruction

Following PCL reconstruction, the brace is locked in full extension for 1 week. The patient may be weight bearing as tolerated with crutches. At 1 week postoperatively the brace is unlocked for passive range of motion, with care taken by the therapist to protect against posterior tibial sagging. Patients should be counseled on the placement of a pillow under the proximal posterior tibia at rest to prevent posterior sag. Quadricep sets and hamstring and calf stretching may be initiated. At 1 month the patient should have full extension and flexion to 60 degrees with good quadriceps control. At this stage the brace may be unlocked for controlled supervised gait training, and the patient may begin active squats and wall slides with supervision (0 degrees to 45 degrees) to promote anterior tibial translation.[9] The brace may be discontinued at approximately 8 weeks. The complete protocol for rehabilitation in these patients is available in the article by Irrgang and Fitzgerald.[24]

■ OUTCOMES AND FUTURE DIRECTIONS

For PCL reconstruction failures, it is essential to perform a thorough assessment, determine the etiology of failure, and formulate a preoperative plan for each patient. It is important to consider not only intra-articular causes of failure, but also the secondary knee restraints such as bone, articular cartilage, menisci, and collateral ligaments. The PCL revision reconstruction may be performed as part of a one- or two-stage procedure. General principles of management of failed PCL surgery therefore include the correction of bony malalignment, the treatment of any combined elements of instability, reconstruction and not repair of the PCL, and compliance with an adequate postoperative rehabilitation protocol. With attention to these details one can expect adequate clinical results in this challenging patient population, but these are challenging complex procedures with expected results inferior to those in the primary PCL reconstruction setting.

■ REFERENCES

1. Mavrodontidis AN, Papadonikolakis A, Moebius UG, et al. Posterior tibial subluxation and short-term arthritis resulting from failed posterior cruciate ligament reconstruction. Arthroscopy. 2003;19(5):E43.
2. Allen CR, Kaplan LD, Fluhme DJ, et al. Posterior cruciate ligament injuries. Curr Opin Rheumatol. 2002;14(2):142–149.
3. Noyes FR, Barber-Weinstein SD. PCL revision with double-bundle quadriceps tendon autograft: analysis of failure mechanisms. Presented at American Academy of Orthopaedic Surgeons February 2003 Annual Meeting Proceedings in New Orleans, LA.
4. Freeman RT, Duri ZA, Dowd GS. Combined chronic posterior cruciate and posterolateral corner ligamentous injuries: a comparison of posterior cruciate ligament reconstruction with and without reconstruction of the posterolateral corner. Knee. 2002;9(4):309–312.
5. Vogrin TM, Hoher J, Aroen A, et al. Effects of sectioning the posterolateral structures on knee kinematics and in situ forces in the posterior cruciate ligament. Knee Surg Sports Traumatol Arthrosc. 2000;8(2):93–98.
6. Harner CD, Vogrin TM, Hoher J, et al. Biomechanical analysis of a posterior cruciate ligament reconstruction: deficiency of the posterolateral structures as a cause of graft failure. Am J Sports Med. 2000;28(1):32–39.
7. Johnson DH, Fanelli GC, Miller MD. PCL 2002: indications, double-bundle versus inlay technique and revision surgery. Arthroscopy. 2002;18(9 suppl 2):40–52.
8. Christel P. Basic principles for surgical reconstruction of the PCL in chronic posterior knee instability. Knee Surg Sports Traumatol Arthrosc. 2003;11(5):289–296.
9. Giffin JR, Vogrin TM, Zantop T, et al. Effects of increasing tibial slope on the biomechanics of the knee. Am J Sports Med. 2004;32(2):376–382.
10. Giffin JR, Haemmerle MJ, Vogrin TM, et al. Single- versus double-bundle PCL reconstruction: a biomechanical analysis. J Knee Surg. 2002;15(2):114–120.
11. Harner CD, Janaushek MA, Kanamori A, et al. Biomechanical analysis of a double-bundle posterior cruciate ligament reconstruction. Am J Sports Med. 2000;28:144–151.
12. Mannor DA, Shearn JT, Grood ES, et al. Two-bundle posterior cruciate ligament reconstruction: an in vitro analysis of graft placement and tension. Am J Sports Med. 2000;28(6):833–845.
13. Race A, Amis AA. PCL reconstruction. In vitro biomechanical comparison of "isometric" versus single and double-bundled "anatomic" grafts. J Bone Joint Surg Br. 1998;80(1):173–179.
14. Harner CD, Baek GH, Vogrin TM, et al. Quantitative analysis of human cruciate ligament insertions. Arthroscopy. 1999;15(7):741–749.
15. Bergfeld JA, McAllister DR, Packer RD, et al. A biomechanical comparison of posterior cruciate ligament reconstruction techniques. Am J Sports Med. 2001;29:129–136.
16. Cooper DE, Stewart D. Posterior cruciate ligament reconstruction using single-bundle patella tendon graft with tibial inlay fixation: 2- to 10-year follow-up. Am J Sports Med. 2004;32(2):346–360.
17. Mariani PP, Margheritini F, Camillieri G. One-stage arthroscopically assisted anterior and posterior cruciate ligament reconstruction. Arthroscopy. 2001;17(7):700–707.
18. Fanelli GC, Edson CJ. Arthroscopically assisted combined anterior and posterior cruciate ligament reconstruction in the multiple ligament injured knee: 2- to 10-year follow-up. Arthroscopy. 2002;18(7):703–714.

19. Nyland J, Hester P, Caborn DN. Double-bundle posterior cruciate ligament reconstruction with allograft tissue: 2-year postoperative outcomes. Knee Surg Sports Traumatol Arthrosc. 2002;10(5): 274–279. (E-pub 2002 Jun 28.)

20. Christel P, Djian P, Charon PH. Arthroscopic PCL reconstruction with 2-bundle bone-tendon-bone patellar autograft. Arthroscopy. 1999;15:S42.

21. Chen CH, Chen WJ, Shih CH. Arthroscopic double-bundled posterior cruciate ligament reconstruction with quadriceps tendon-patellar bone autograft. Arthroscopy. 2001;16:780–782.

22. Miller MD, Kline AJ, Gonzales J, et al. Vascular risk associated with a posterior approach for posterior cruciate ligament reconstruction using the tibial inlay technique. J Knee Surg. 2002;15(3): 137–140.

23. Matava MJ, Sethi NS, Totty WG. Proximity of the posterior cruciate ligament insertion to the popliteal artery as a function of the knee flexion angle: implications for posterior cruciate ligament reconstruction. Arthroscopy. 2000;16(8):796–804.

24. Irrgang JJ, Fitzgerald GK. Rehabilitation of the multiple-ligament-injured knee. Clin Sports Med. 2000;19(3):545–571.

SURGICAL TREATMENT OF POSTEROLATERAL CORNER INJURIES

48

■ BRYAN T. HANYPSIAK, MD, RICHARD D. PARKER, MD

■ HISTORICAL REVIEW

The history of the posterolateral corner (PLC) can be traced back to 1884.[1] The lateral collateral ligament (LCL) was identified and labeled as the "external lateral ligament," an extension of the peroneus longus. The work of defining and updating the anatomy of the posterolateral corner, however, did not begin in earnest until the late 1950s.[2-4]

It was, however, only after unrecognized injuries to the posterolateral corner were associated with the early failure of cruciate reconstructions that these injuries gained clinical significance.[5-11] In 1994 Veltri and Warren[12] determined that the LCL, popliteus, and popliteofibular ligament (PFL) were the major contributors to the stability of the posterolateral corner. It is these structures that must be addressed by surgeons seeking a successful anatomic reconstruction of the posterolateral corner.

Despite our increased understanding of the pathomechanics of the posterolateral corner, the diagnosis and treatment of these injuries has remained difficult. Posterolateral corner tears, which frequently occur in combination with injuries to other ligamentous structures,[13] are often undiagnosed, misdiagnosed, or untreated on initial presentation.[8] The orthopedic surgeon, therefore, must be prepared to diagnose and treat patients who present with chronic posterolateral corner injuries.

This chapter will address the relevant anatomy, history, physical examination, and repair or reconstructive technique of both acute and chronic posterolateral corner tears.

■ INDICATIONS AND CONTRAINDICATIONS

Understanding the anatomy of the posterolateral corner and clearly defining the injured structures are the keys to performing a successful repair or reconstruction. The anatomy of the posterolateral corner is complex. The terminology used in the literature is not universal, and with many authors using multiple names for the same structures, it is, at best, confusing. To add to the challenge, the ligaments involved are difficult to identify intraoperatively, and many are not present in all individuals.

An example of the significant anatomic variability of the key elements of the posterolateral corner, the arcuate ligament, and fabellofibular ligaments are both present in only 67% of patients.[14] The fabellofibular ligament is present alone in 20% of patients, while the arcuate ligament occurs alone in the remaining 13%. The presence or absence of the fabella on radiographs offers a hint to the anatomic configuration present. An absent fabella suggests an absent fabellofibular ligament, while a large fabella suggests an absent arcuate ligament.[15]

In preparing for a repair or reconstruction of the posterolateral corner, its complex anatomy warrants a brief review of the key components and their function as it relates to the our preferred technique.

In 1982 Seebacher et al.[15] divided the lateral structures of the knee into three layers. Layer I is composed of the iliotibial tract and the superficial biceps femoris. Layer II contains the quadriceps retinaculum anteriorly and patellofemoral ligaments posteriorly. Finally, layer III is made up by the lateral aspect of the capsule, coronary ligament, popliteus, LCL, and the fabellofibular and arcuate ligaments (Fig. 48-1A,B). The anatomy of the posterolateral corner is best understood when organized and reviewed by layer.

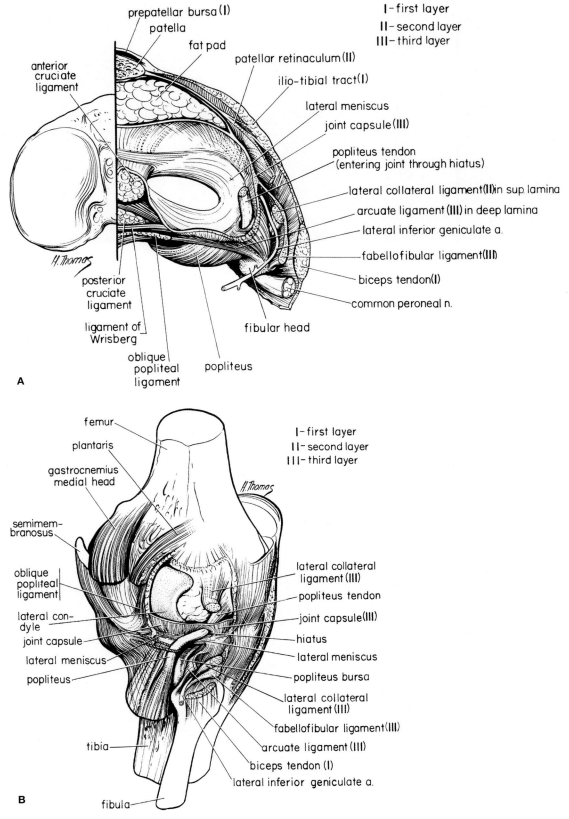

Fig. 48-1. A: Cross section artist depiction of the posterolateral corner. **B:** Lateral view artist depiction of the posterolateral corner.

■ POSTEROLATERAL CORNER ANATOMY

Layer I

Iliotibial Band

The iliotibial band (ITB) runs from the femoral supracondylar tubercle to Gerdy's tubercle of the tibia. The ITB acts as an accessory LCL and is a critical lateral compartment stabilizer. Clinically, it is the ITB that reduces a posteriorly subluxed tibia when a reverse pivot shift test is performed.

In flexion, the ITB externally rotates the tibia and pulls it posteriorly. Because the ITB moves anteriorly with extension, it is often spared in posterolateral corner injuries that result from a varus load to the knee.

Biceps Femoris Tendon

Divided into a short and long heads, the biceps runs posterior to the ITB and inserts primarily on the fibular styloid. A strong lateral stabilizer of the knee, the biceps also acts as an external rotator of the tibia in conjunction with the ITB.[16] Unlike the ITB, the biceps is frequently torn in posterolateral corner injuries, eliminating surgical options that describe its use as part of the reconstruction.

Layer II

Both the patellar and quadriceps retinaculum lie anterior to the midline of the knee and play little role in the stability of the posterolateral corner.

Layer III

Lateral Collateral Ligament

The LCL reinforces the posterior third of the joint capsule and is the most important stabilizer of the knee to varus stress. It is dynamically controlled by its attachments to the biceps femoris and acts secondarily to limit external rotation. Isolated injuries to the LCL are uncommon.

Popliteus

The popliteus originates from the posterior tibia, passes through a hole in the coronary ligament, attaches to the lateral meniscus, and inserts on the lateral femoral condyle. It is a dynamic and static stabilizer of the tibia on the femur, a weak knee flexor, and serves as reinforcement to the posterior third of the capsule. The popliteus unlocks the extended knee by rotating the femur on a fixed tibia, or equivalently, by internally rotating the tibia around a fixed femur. The popliteus acts to restrict posterior translation and external and varus rotation of the knee. Injuries to the popliteus cannot occur without weakening the surrounding structures.[14,17]

Popliteofibular Ligament

Present in 91% of cadaveric specimens,[18] the PFL runs from the anterior aspect of the lateral femoral condyle to the posterior aspect of the fibular head. Its anterior and posterior divisions give it the anatomic appearance of an inverted Y.[18,19] It provides a direct static attachment of the femur to the tibia and shares the resistance to posterior tibial translation and external and varus rotation.

Arcuate Ligament

It is important to differentiate in the arcuate complex, which Hughston et al.[20] defined as the LCL, arcuate ligament, popliteus muscle and tendon, and the lateral gastrocnemius muscle, from the arcuate ligament,[13,21] a confluence of capsular structures connecting the lateral femoral condyle to the fibular styloid process. When present, it is always posterior to the fabellofibular ligament and may be indistinguishable from it. The arcuate ligament has been divided into medial and lateral limbs with varying attachments, both limbs act as capsular reinforcements.

Fabellofibular Ligament

The fabellofibular ligament is the distal termination of the capsular arm of the short head of the biceps. It runs between the fabella, an osseous or cartilaginous sesamoid structure in the tendon of the lateral gastrocnemius muscle, and the lateral tip of the fibular styloid, medial to the direct arm of the short head of the biceps femoris. The fabellofibular ligament becomes tight in extension and serves as a capsular reinforcement.

Other Structures

Several other structures act to increase the overall stability of the lateral side of the knee. The lateral meniscus increases the concavity of the tibial plateau; the coronary ligament is a capsular attachment to the outer edge of the lateral meniscus; and the lateral gastrocnemius tendon blends with the arcuate ligament, a lateral capsular thickening. Finally, the popliteomeniscal fascicles connect the inferior surface of the lateral meniscus to the articular cartilage border of the lateral tibial plateau.

■ BIOMECHANICAL ANALYSIS

In an effort to identify an ideal reconstruction, a number of biomechanical studies were undertaken to define the significance of each discrete anatomic structure.[22–27] Through a series of selective sectionings, the exact contribution of each component of the posterolateral corner has been defined, and the major contributors to posterolateral stability have been identified. Only recently has there been a consensus among authors.

An intact posterolateral corner reduces anteroposterior (AP) translation of the tibia in extension and decreases external and varus rotation forces across the cruciates. The increased loads experienced by grafts placed in a PLC deficient knee led to early failure of both anterior cruciate ligament (ACL) and posterior cruciate ligament (PCL) reconstructions.[5–11] The following is a brief summary of the role of the PLC in controlling force across the knee:

AP translation is restrained by a dynamic interplay between the PCL and PLC. The role of the PLC in stabilizing posterior translation of the tibia decreases as knee flexion increases. Beyond 90 degrees of flexion, the PLC becomes lax and the PCL becomes primarily responsible for controlling posterior translation of the tibia on the femur. Several studies have demonstrated that sectioning of the PLC increases posterior translation of the lateral tibial plateau at 30 degrees, but less so at 90 degrees.[14,28,29] Cutting both the PCL and PLC increases the translation of both the medial and lateral tibial plateaus at all flexion angles. To summarize, the PLC is primarily responsible for limiting tibial translation in extension, while the PCL is primarily responsible for limiting translation in flexion.

Varus rotation is restrained by the LCL and secondarily by the popliteus. Sectioning of the LCL results in increased varus rotation from 0 degrees to 30 degrees. Maximum displacement occurs at 30 degrees with an intact PCL.[29] Sectioning both the LCL and PCL increases varus rotation at all angles of flexion, with the maximum displacement occurring at 60 degrees.[12,29] In summary, the PLC is predominantly responsible for controlling varus rotation near full extension, whereas the PCL has its greatest effect in flexion.

External rotation is restrained by the posterior joint capsule, popliteus, PFL, and secondarily by the LCL. Sectioning of these components of the posterolateral corner leads to increased external rotation in extension. The maximum effect occurs at 30 degrees, the minimum at 90 degrees. Combined cutting of both the PLC and PCL leads to increased external rotation in all flexion angles, with the maximum effect at 90 degrees.[12,29] Sectioning the PCL alone has no effect on external rotation at any flexion angle. Again, based on biomechanical studies, the posterolateral corner has its greatest effect near full extension, while the PCL provides secondary stabilization to external rotation in flexion.

Finally, intra-articular pressure in all three compartments is increased by combined sectioning of the PCL and PLC.[30] This may form the basis for the development of early osteoarthritis in patients with chronic deficiencies.

PATIENT HISTORY

Patients with an acute or chronically deficient posterolateral corner will often complain of lateral or posterolateral joint pain, difficulty with stairs, ramps, or cutting activities, and a sense of instability with knee extension, such as during the toe off phase of gait. Periodically, a foot drop is associated and may be either transient or permanent. Forty percent of these injuries occur as a result of a sports injury. The most common mechanism is a posterolateral blow to the anteromedial knee in extension or a hyperextension injury with a varus and rotatory force. Both contact and noncontact injuries have been

described. Less commonly, a varus load to a flexed knee may result in an injury to the posterolateral corner.[31]

Athletes with anatomic variations that place additional stress across the posterolateral corner, such as generalized ligamentous laxity, genu varum, recurvatum, or epiphyseal dysplasia, are predisposed to developing this injury.[32]

PHYSICAL EXAM

All patients presenting with ACL or PCL injuries must have their posterolateral corners carefully evaluated prior to proceeding with a reconstruction. A missed PLC injury will result in early graft failure. Although isolated injury to the PLC is uncommon, comprising only 2% of all acute ligamentous knee injuries,[33] there is a relatively high incidence of combined injury. LaPrade et al.,[34] in a series of 100 consecutive acute ACL tears, reported an 11% incidence of posterolateral rotatory instability. For patients with chronic posterolateral rotatory instability (PLRI), an estimated 43% to 80% have combined ligamentous injuries.

The physical exam of the PLC begins with visual inspection. The patient's alignment is documented as straight, valgus, or varus. Patients with PLC injuries will often demonstrate hyperextension of the knee in stance phase and a varus thrust during gait. Patients may compensate for a varus thrust by internally rotating their foot and walking with a flexed knee. A varus thrust can be exaggerated by asking patients to walk backward or with their foot externally rotated.

A complete ligamentous exam should be performed on both the ipsilateral and contralateral knee. Examiners should consider a knee dislocation in patients whose exam demonstrates multiple ligamentous deficiencies.

Varus joint line opening should be examined in full extension and 30 degrees of flexion. A comparison should always be made with the contralateral side. The PLC can be stressed by performing the test in internal rotation.

The external rotation recurvatum test **(Fig. 48-2)** is performed by lifting the extended leg by the great toe with the patient lying supine. The test is considered positive if the tibia falls into hyperextension and external rotation or the varus deformity increases. This test is generally positive in combined injuries.

The Dial test can be performed with the patient in the supine or prone position, though the supine position eliminates hip rotation. An external rotation force is applied to the foot at 30 degrees of knee flexion and the patient is examined for increased posterolateral tibial rotation. An increase of 10 to 15 degrees from the contralateral side denotes a positive test.[5] The test is then repeated at 90 degrees. A further increase in rotation is indicative of a cruciate injury, while a decrease in rotation indicates an intact PCL.

The posterolateral drawer test is performed with the patient positioned supine with the hip flexed 45 degrees and the knee flexed 90 degrees. The foot is externally rotated 15 degrees and a posterolateral rotation force is applied to the

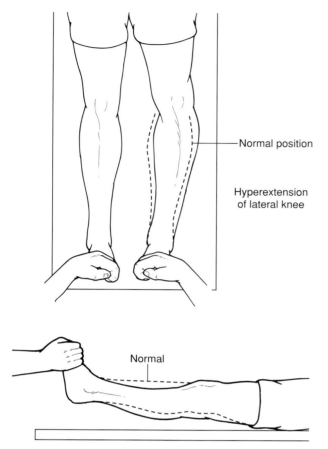

Fig. 48-2. External recurvatum test: By grasping the great toe of each foot, the examiner lifts both feet off the table. If asymmetric recurvatum on the lateral aspect of the knee occurs and the tibia externally rotates, the test is considered positive.

knee. A positive test demonstrates increased lateral tibial external rotation and posterior translation when compared to the opposite side.

The reverse pivot shift test **(Fig. 48-3)** is carried out with the patient's knee flexed to 60 degrees and the foot externally

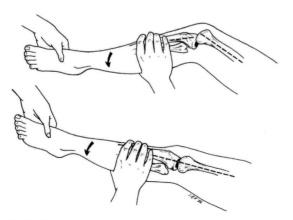

Fig. 48-3. Reverse pivot shift test: The tibia is externally rotated in a flexed position and the tibia subluxates posterior. With knee extension the tibia reduces.

rotated. In this position, a lax PLC will allow posterolateral rotation and subluxation of the tibia on the femur. A valgus force is applied to the knee as it is brought into extension. The ITB reduces the subluxation at 30 to 40 degrees of flexion, resulting in a clunk.[35] It is important to perform this test on both knees, as 35% of normal individuals will have a positive reverse pivot shift under general anesthesia.[36]

Finally, a careful neurological exam should be performed. The peroneal nerve is susceptible to adduction and rotatory stresses and is injured in 15% to 30% of grade III tears of the PLC.[32] Patients should be examined for foot drop, weak ankle dorsiflexion, and numbness on the dorsum of the foot.

■ IMAGING

Although typically unremarkable, radiographs of the knee in a suspected PLC injury should include a weightbearing AP film in full extension, a weightbearing posterior-anterior (PA) film in 45 degrees of flexion, a lateral and a Merchant view.[37] Full-length standing x-rays and varus stress radiographs to look for genu varus should be obtained in chronic injuries. Varus deformity must be corrected prior to performing a reconstruction; otherwise the repair will stretch out with time.

Three major avulsion fractures may occur in association with a PLC injury, and these are often ignored or misdiagnosed. An avulsion of the fibular head or styloid, referred to as an arcuate fracture,[38] represents a detachment of the insertion sights of the LCL, PFL, and biceps femoris. The presence of an arcuate fracture on x-ray signals a major lateral ligamentous injury until proven otherwise. Disruption of Gerdy's tubercle signals an ITB avulsion, while a Segond fracture, an avulsion of the meniscotibial portion of the midthird capsular ligament and the anterior arm of the short head of the biceps femoris from the anterolateral tibia, is often associated with a torn ACL[38] **(Fig. 48-4).**

Magnetic resonance imaging (MRI) with 1 to 2 mm cuts featuring coronal oblique views of the fibular head and styloid aligned along the course of the popliteus tendon should be obtained. This configuration allows for evaluation of the LCL, coronary ligament, popliteus complex, superficial and deep ITB, and the direct and anterior arms of the short and long heads of the biceps. Additionally, the cruciates, medial collateral ligament (MCL), articular cartilage and subchondral bone can be easily inspected. A bone bruise of the anteromedial femoral condyle is associated with injury to the PLC.

■ TREATMENT

Nonoperative Treatment

Most authors agree that grade I and II injuries of the PLC should be treated nonoperatively.[31] The significance of a

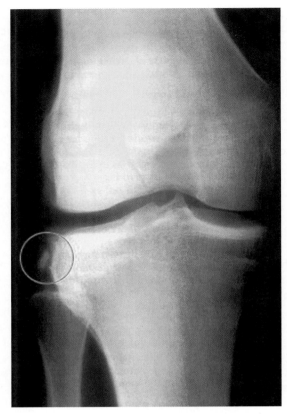

Fig. 48-4. Segund fracture: Avulsion fracture of the posterolateral capsule indicative of an anterior cruciate ligament tear.

partial injury has not been defined, and most patients do well, at least initially. An association between a partial injury and the development of early osteoarthritis is not known.

Patients presenting with an acute grade I or II tear should have their knee immobilized in full extension for 3 weeks. Toe touch weightbearing is allowed, and heel lifts should be prescribed to prevent ankle equinus and knee hyperextension.

Following initial immobilization, a progressive functional rehabilitation program, beginning with range of motion exercises and a stationary bicycle, should be instituted. A valgus unloader brace is often employed to further unload the PLC. Nonresponders should be re-evaluated for lateral meniscal hypermobility, resulting from the loss of the capsular attachments of the lateral meniscus or tearing of the popliteomeniscal fascicles. These patients will present with pain along the lateral joint line, which can be accentuated by placing the knee in the figure-four position. Patients with meniscal hypermobility can be treated by repairing the lateral meniscus to the popliteomeniscal fascicles.

Surgical Treatment: Acute Repair

Surgical repair is recommended for patients presenting with acute grade III PLC injuries.[31] These patients do poorly with nonoperative treatment. Functional instability will require a downgrading of activities, and cruciate reconstructions will stretch over time and fail.

An anatomic repair within the first 2 to 3 weeks after initial injury is recommended, as injured tissues retract and lose their integrity and ability to hold suture. Also, at this point, anatomic structures are relatively easy to identify. Beyond 6 weeks postinjury, repair becomes more difficult, as critical structures, such as the peroneal nerve, become encased in scar tissue.

Surgical Approach

The surgical approach of the PLC begins with proper patient positioning. The patient is placed supine on the table, with a leg holder placed at midthigh. A tourniquet is applied so that it lies within the leg holder. The foot of the bed is dropped, and a bump is placed under the contralateral hip to protect the femoral nerve from stretching.

A diagnostic arthroscopy is then conducted through standard portals. This should be done with the arthroscopic pump set to low pressure and high flow, with careful attention paid to the patient's leg swelling. Pressurized water flow from the scope may lead to extravasation of fluid into the leg and could theoretically trigger a compartment syndrome. Care should be taken to regularly assess the knee for fluid extravasation during the procedure.

Once the scope has entered the knee, the lateral compartment should be carefully inspected, with the arthroscopist careful to note the condition of the popliteus tendon, popliteomeniscal fascicles, meniscofemoral posterior capsule, coronary ligament, and midthird lateral capsular ligament. A positive drive through sign, or opening of the lateral compartment greater than 1 cm, is almost always present in grade III injuries[39] **(Fig. 48-5)**. In the case of multiple ligament injuries, in which an ACL or PCL reconstruction is performed concurrently with the PLC procedure, all arthroscopic work required for these procedures should be

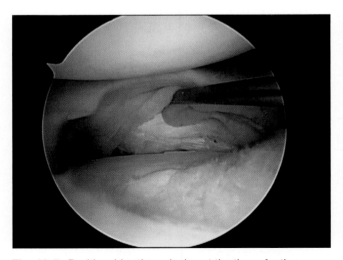

Fig. 48-5. Positive drive through sign at the time of arthroscopy. Note that the popliteus appears to have torn fibers, yet the popliteofibular ligament appears intact.

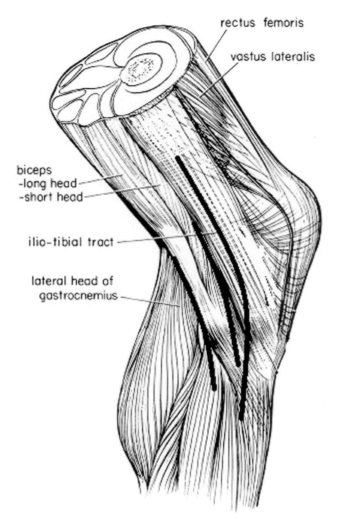

rectus femoris

vastus lateralis

biceps
-long head
-short head

ilio-tibial tract

lateral head of
gastrocnemius

Fig. 48-6. Artist depiction of the lateral side of the knee: the three incisions (black thick line) as described by LaPrade. First incision bisects the iliotibial band, the second is along the posterior aspect of the long head of the biceps tendon, and the third is between the iliotibial band and the short head of the biceps.

completed prior to undertaking the open portion of the PLC procedure.

The open portion of the procedure begins with a lateral incision, centered midway between the patella and fibular head, beginning 10 cm proximal to the joint line and extending 4 to 5 cm beyond it to Gerdy's tubercle.[40] The ITB and the short and long heads of the bicep femoris should be identified and exposed.

Terry and LaPrade[13] described a series of three fascial splitting incisions to adequately expose the entire PLC **(Fig. 48-6)**. The first incision bisects the ITB in line with its fibers. It runs from Gerdy's tubercle to the supracondylar process of the femur. The surgeon should expose both anteriorly and posteriorly to reveal the LCL, popliteus, lateral gastrocnemius, and midthird lateral capsular ligament. An arthrotomy can be made through the meniscofemoral portion of the midthird lateral capsular ligament (the capsular

thickening just anterior to the LCL) approximately 1 cm anterior to an imaginary line extended parallel to the anterior aspect of the fibular shaft. This will allow access to the lateral meniscus, popliteus origin, and popliteomeniscal fascicles.

The second longitudinal incision should be made in the fascia just posterior to the long head of the biceps femoris. It is through this interval that the common peroneal nerve should be identified and exposed. A vessel loop is passed around the nerve and a neurolysis should be performed prior to initiating the repair. Blunt dissection between the biceps and the peroneal nerve will create an interval anterior to the lateral gastrocnemius tendon and posterior to the soleus muscle belly. This space gives access to the posterior tibia, popliteus sulcus and musculotendinous junction, and the posteromedial aspect of the fibular styloid.

The third and final fascial incision should be located between the posterior border of the iliotibial tract and the anterior aspect of the short head of the biceps. This allows inspection of the normal attachment site of the PFL on the posteromedial fibular styloid. The fibular tunnel is drilled through this incision. Structures at risk for injury during this approach include the peroneal nerve, popliteal artery and vein, and the tibial nerve.

■ TREATMENT OF ACUTE INJURIES

Direct primary anatomic repair of the posterolateral corner structures is recommended when possible.[31] For acute tears, it may be possible to restore the normal anatomy by reattaching or reinforcing avulsed structures. To maximize the healing potential of an acute repair, the injury must be identified and brought to the operating room within 6 weeks of the initial injury, prior to formation of scar tissue. Direct repair requires the presence of good quality tissue that will hold suture and may not be possible in high-energy injuries **(Fig. 48-7)**. A few general guidelines should be observed:

1 Arcuate avulsion fractures of the fibular head: repair with suture cerclage or, if sufficiently large, open reduction internal fixation (ORIF) with a cortical screw.
2 Popliteus avulsions: reattach with suture or cancellous screws (Jakob and Warner procedure).[41]
3 LCL femoral avulsion: repair into 1 cm deep tunnel with transcondylar sutures tied over a button (Recess procedure).
4 LCL fibular styloid avulsion: repair directly to bone with sutures passed through transosseous drill holes or suture anchors.
5 Lateral meniscal hypermobility: repair popliteomeniscal fascicles.
6 PFL avulsions: repair directly to bone with sutures or anchors.
7 Short and long head of biceps femoris avulsions: repair directly to bone with sutures or anchors.

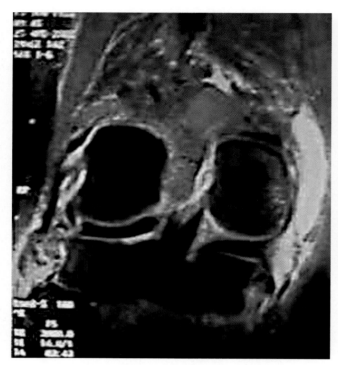

Fig. 48-7. MRI of a multiligament injured patient. Note the avulsion of the fibular portion of the lateral collateral ligament and biceps tendon. At surgery a portion of the tibial capsule was avulsed too.

8 Lateral gastrocnemius avulsion: repair directly to bone with anchors.
9 Deep ITB avulsions: suture to lateral intermuscular septum and the short head of the biceps.
10 Capsular/periosteal avulsion from tibia: repair with suture anchors.

Before tying any sutures, the leg should be positioned in 60 degrees of flexion and internally rotated to minimize the stress on the PLC during the repair. Depending upon the quality of the repaired tissues, augmentation using the biceps, ITB, hamstring, or allograft can be considered. The popliteus and PFL can be augmented with a central slip of the ITB or biceps tendon respectively. The LCL can be reinforced with a bone-patellar tendon-bone or Achilles allograft.

■ TREATMENT OF CHRONIC INJURIES

Patients presenting with chronic grade III posterolateral corner injuries should be examined for a varus thrust and genu valgum. These patients are prone to early failure and should undergo an opening wedge proximal tibial osteotomy prior to an attempted reconstruction to tighten the posterior capsule and popliteus complex and return the mechanical axis to the lateral compartment **(Fig. 48-8)**.

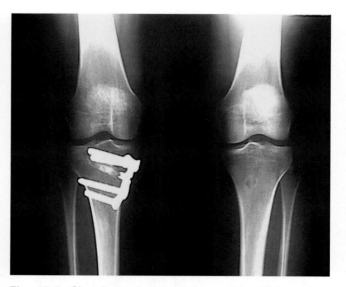

Fig. 48-8. Chronic posterolateral ligament insufficiency in a patient with a varus knee and a varus thrust. This patient was treated with an opening wedge high tibial osteotomy. Consideration for posterolateral corner reconstruction will be made at a later time and will be based on instability symptoms.

Our preferred technique is a modified version of one described by LaPrade et al.[34] It provides for an anatomic reconstruction of the LCL, PFL, and popliteus tendon. It should be used for chronic injuries or acute injuries in which adequate tissue is unavailable.

The modified LaPrade technique uses a double bundle Achilles allograft to restore static stability to the posterolateral corner. The surgical approach is the same as for acute repairs. The procedure begins by fashioning the bony end of an Achilles allograft into a 9 to 12 mm by 20 to 25 mm bone block. Consideration can be made to remove the bone completely and have a soft tissue graft. The tendinous portion of the graft is then split equally in two, beginning at the bony end of the tendon and continuing to the free end **(Fig. 48-9)**. The bone block will act as

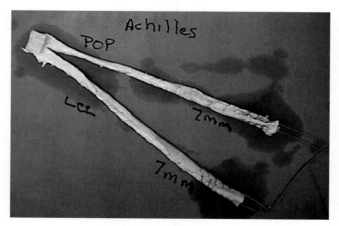

Fig. 48-9. An Achilles tendon graft split longitudinally for the two components of the reconstruction.

the femoral attachment site for both the popliteus and LCL.[42] To ensure adequate length of the graft prior to thawing the tendon, use only tendons 23 cm or longer. A small K-wire is then used to drill two parallel holes in the bone block and Ethibond suture is passed through these holes.

The femoral attachment site of the LCL and popliteus is viewed through the split in the ITB. It should be located proximal and posterior to the lateral epicondyle at respective isometric points. A bone tunnel corresponding to the Achilles bone block is then drilled to a depth of 20 mm at the attachment site.

The sutures are passed through the femur with cannulated eyelet tipped guide pins. The pins are drilled so they exit the distal femur proximal and medial to the medial epicondyle and adductor tubercle. This will prevent inadvertent passage through the notch. The pins are then brought out the medial aspect of the femur, and the sutures are used to pull the bone plug into the femoral tunnel. Once fully recessed into the tunnel, the bone block is fixed in position with an interference screw, and the sutures can be trimmed, or tied over a button through a small incision over the posteromedial cortex.

Tibial and fibular bone tunnels should be drilled using a cannulated tunnel-aiming device, such as an ACL guide. The first tunnel, used to reconstruct the popliteus, is drilled from the distal medial aspect of Gerdy's tubercle proximally to the popliteus tibial sulcus. Tunnel preparation begins by placing the tip of the ACL guide on the bony margin just under the articular cartilage at the posterior popliteus sulcus at the level of the musculotendinous junction. A K-wire is passed through the guide in the AP direction, with care taken to protect the posterior neurovascular structures. A 9-mm tunnel is created by reaming over the K-wire.

Looking through the incision between the iliotibial band and the biceps, a second tunnel is drilled through the fibular head from the attachment of the LCL to the PFL attachment on the posteromedial down slope of the radial styloid. Begin by placing the ACL guide laterally at the fibular insertion of the LCL and drilling a 9-mm tunnel through the fibula in an anterolateral to posteromedial fashion.

A Bunnell-type suture should be used to secure each of the grafts' free ends. The anterior graft is used to reconstruct the popliteus, and it is passed under the posterior limb and through the tibial drill hole in the popliteal hiatus to reach the anterior aspect of the lateral tibial plateau. The graft is pulled through the tibial tunnel from posterior to anterior. It emerges just medial and distal to Gerdy's tubercle.

The posterior graft is used to reconstruct the PFL and LCL. It is passed deep to the superficial layer of the ITB and the anterior arm of long head of the biceps. It is then brought through the fibular head and styloid from lateral to posteromedial and pulled through the tibial tunnel from

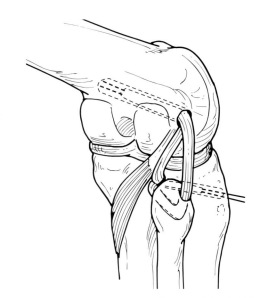

Fig. 48-10. Note the common attachment of the Achilles tendon to the region of the lateral epicondyle. One arm of the graft reproduces the lateral collateral ligament coursing through the fibular head and then proximal posterior and into the posterior tibia to reproduce the popliteofibular ligament. The other arm of the graft passes under the lateral collateral ligament and courses posterior to the tibia at the level of the popliteus muscle tendon junction and courses through a tunnel in the tibial with the popliteofibular ligament reconstruction.

posterior to anterior. The graft is fixed in the fibular head with an interference screw with the knee flexed 30 degrees and a slight valgus force. This completes the LCL reconstruction. The remainder of graft, running from the posteromedial fibula to the posterolateral tibia, reconstructs the PFL. Once in the popliteal hiatus, the remaining graft enters the previously drilled tibial tunnel and runs anteriorly alongside the popliteal graft. Both grafts are secured with a 9-mm soft tissue interference screw placed in the tunnel, or a staple, placed on the anterior cortex of the tibia. Before tightening the fixation, the sutures should be pulled taught, and the leg internally rotated and flexed 60 degrees **(Fig. 48-10)**.

Fascial closure is routine with Vicryl sutures, and the skin is closed with a running pullout Monocryl. Adhesive strips, petroleum gauze, four by fours, and an army battlefield dressing (ABD) are applied over the wounds, and the knee is placed in an immobilizer locked in extension.

■ COMBINED INJURIES

In combined injuries that involve the posterolateral corner, all other ligamentous injuries should be repaired or reconstructed concurrently **(Fig. 48-11A,B)**. This will reduce the risk of early graft failure and prevent increased graft stress. A period of brief immobilization should be followed by an attempt at early range of motion.

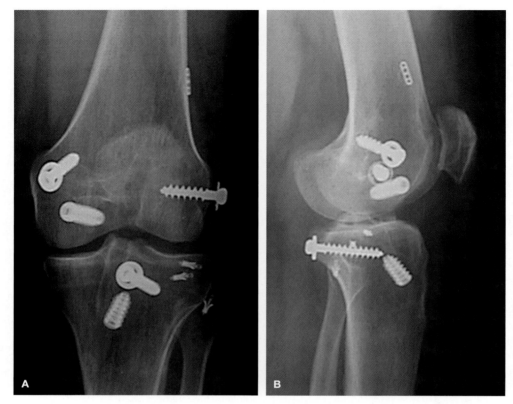

Fig. 48-11. Radiographic anteroposterior **(A)** and lateral **(B)** views of a knee that has undergone reconstruction of the ACL and PCL and repair of the posterolateral corner.

■ SURGICAL COMPLICATIONS

Surgical complications include infection, arthrofibrosis, common peroneal nerve palsy, and loosening and eventual failure of the graft. Retained hardware may become symptomatic.

■ OTHER TECHNIQUES

Proximal Bone Block Advancement

Described by Fleming et al.[6] in 1981, this procedure tightens the femoral components of a lax PLC by transferring them proximally. It requires intact LCL and popliteus attachments, as well as a structurally sound LCL and PFL. Good functional results were reported in 63% to 73% of patients.[8,33,43]

Noyes and Barber-Westin[43] described a modification of the original technique in which he recessed the bone block rather than advancing it, while Hughston and Jacobson[8] advocated moving the femoral attachment site anteriorly and distally.

Biceps Tenodesis

Clancy[44] used an intact biceps femoris tendon to tighten the posterolateral corner by transferring it anteriorly to the lateral femoral epicondyle. The tendon is freed from the lateral gastrocnemius and passed through a slit in the ITB and over a fixation point just anterior to the epicondyle. This technique is only recommended with an intact capsular arm and capsule-osseous confluence of the short head of the biceps. However, 75% of grade III tears have these structures disrupted. This technique has been shown to lead to permanent hamstring weakness and to overconstrain the knee in external rotation at 60 degrees and 90 degrees of flexion. There is no salvage procedure for a failed biceps tenodesis.

Split Patellar or Achilles Tendon Allograft

Described by Bowen et al.,[45] this reconstruction is based on an allograft split to make two free ends. One end, consisting of a single bone block, is recessed into the isometric point of the femur and held with a soft tissue interference screw. The two free ends are run distally, with the first anchored into the fibular head to reconstruct the LCL. The other end is passed through a tunnel originating in the popliteus remnant and exiting the anterior tibia to reconstruct the popliteus.

Lateral Collateral Ligament Allograft/Autograft

A bone-tendon-bone allograft or soft tissue graft alone (semitendinosus) is run from the superior fibula to the isometric point of the femur. Two tunnels are drilled, a 6-mm

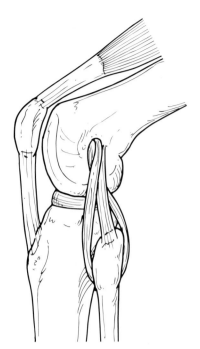

Fig. 48-12. Autograft semitendinosus can be used to reconstruct or augment the lateral collateral ligament.

tunnel is drilled 10 mm deep at the native LCL attachment on the femur, and a 6-mm tunnel is drilled anterior to posterior in the center of the fibular head/neck junction. Alternatively, a split Achilles allograft can be passed through tunnels anterior and posterior to the LCL remnant. This graft alone will decrease varus opening at 30 degrees and, to a lesser extent, decrease excessive external rotation **(Fig. 48-12).** It can be combined with a capsular plication, through a vertical incision posterior to the LCL. A pants-over-vest closure of the posterolateral structures is performed, and the LCL graft is then plicated to tighten the posterolateral corner.

Lateral Collateral Ligament Augmentation

The central two thirds of an uninjured biceps is harvested, while the distal insertion is left intact. The tendon is cut proximally at 12 cm and the ends are sutured with Bunnell or Thompson stitches. The tendon is secured at an isometric point with an interference screw or a button on the opposite cortex.

Popliteus Tendon Augmentation

A central slip of the ITB is harvested, left attached to the Gerdy tubercle, and passed through an anterior to posterior tunnel in the tibia to the popliteus insertion on the femur. It is held in place proximally with suture fixation.

Popliteus Recess Procedure

A bone block containing the popliteus tendon insertion is harvested and advanced anteriorly and proximally to tighten

the popliteus. Alternatively, the popliteus tendon can be wound around the bone block and reinserted into the harvest site.

Popliteus Tendon Reconstruction

An Achilles or patellar tendon allograft is passed through a tibial tunnel near the musculotendinous junction of the popliteus from posterior to anterior. It is fixed on the tibia with a button or screw and washer. The graft is anchored at the femoral isometric point with an interference screw or a button on the opposite cortex.

■ REHABILITATION

The rehabilitation program should be tailored to fit the intraoperative quality of the repair.[5] It is important for the surgeon to determine the range of motion (ROM) of the knee that does not strain the repair. A continuous passive motion (CPM) machine should be implemented immediately post-op. The patient should be kept toe touch weightbearing in a hinged knee brace. ROM for both the CPM and brace should be limited to the safe ROM defined intraoperatively. At 3 weeks, ROM should be increased as tolerated, with a goal of 120 degrees of flexion and full extension at 6 weeks. Reconstructed tissues can be advanced more quickly than repaired. Weightbearing is allowed at 6 to 8 weeks with the knee braced in full extension. Active hamstring exercises and external rotation should be avoided for 12 weeks.

■ OUTCOMES AND FUTURE DIRECTIONS: A SUMMARY

Only recently have we understood the clinical importance of a posterolateral corner injury. Reconstruction of the posterolateral corner is challenged by anatomy. The lateral structures are stronger, more substantial than the medial and are subjected to greater forces during gait. The normal mechanical axis passes just medial to the center of the knee, so during normal gait, the medial structures are compressed, while the lateral structures are placed under tension. A reconstruction of the lateral structures, therefore, is challenged at every step.

Despite our increased understanding, outcome data are sparse. The literature lacks randomized controlled studies, and those that are available are limited by a small number of subjects. These injuries frequently go unrecognized or are misdiagnosed, leading patients to miss out on a narrow window for anatomic repair.

Although multiple techniques for reconstruction of chronic injuries have been described, the ideal procedure remains elusive. Our hope for the future is that we will develop universally accepted terminology and operative techniques and conduct large, multicenter randomized trials with meaningful outcome data. Ultimately, we hope that the general practice orthopedic surgeon will be able to diagnose and treat acute posterolateral corner injuries as is currently done for cruciate injuries, reducing the number of chronic deficiencies and avoiding future reconstructive dilemmas.

■ REFERENCES

1. Sutton JB. On the nature of certain ligaments. J Anat Physiol. 1884;18:225–238.
2. Sneath RS. The insertion of the biceps femoris. J Anat. 1955;89:550–553.
3. Kaplan EB. The iliotibial tract: clinical and morphological significance. J Bone Joint Surg Am. 1958;40:817–832.
4. Kaplan EB. The fabellofibular and short lateral ligaments of the knee joint. J Bone Joint Surg Am. 1961;43:169–179.
5. Schenck RC Jr., ed. *Multiple Ligamentous Injuries of the Knee.* Rosemont, IL: American Academy of Orthopaedic Surgeons; 2002.
6. Fleming RE Jr., Blatz DJ, McCarroll JR. Posterior problems in the knee: posterior cruciate insufficiency and the posterolateral rotatory insufficiency. Am J Sports Med. 1981;9:107–113.
7. Hughston JC, Norwood LA Jr. The posterolateral drawer test and external rotational recurvatum test for posterolateral rotatory instability of the knee. Clin Orthop. 1980;147:82–87.
8. Hughston JC, Jacobson KE. Chronic posterolateral rotatory instability of the knee. J Bone Joint Surg Am. 1985;67:351–359.
9. LaPrade RF, Resig S, Wentorf F, et al. The effects of grade III posterolateral knee complex injuries on anterior cruciate ligament graft force: a biomechanical analysis. Am J Sports Med. 1999;27:469–475.
10. LaPrade RF, Muench C, Wentorf F, et al. The effect of injury to the posterolateral structures of the knee on force in a posterior cruciate ligament graft: a biomechanical study. Am J Sports Med. 2002;30:233–238.
11. O'Brien SJ, Warren RF, Pavlov H, et al. Reconstruction of the chronically insufficient anterior cruciate ligament with the central third of the patellar ligament. J Bone Joint Surg Am. 1991;73:278–286.
12. Veltri DM, Warren RF. Anatomy, biomechanics, and physical findings in posterolateral knee instability. Clin Sports Med. 1994;13:599–614.
13. Terry GC, LaPrade RF. The posterolateral aspect of the knee: anatomy and surgical approach. Am J Sports Med. 1996;24:732–739.
14. Chen FS, Rokitko AS, Pitman MI. Acute and chronic posterolateral rotatory instability of the knee. J Am Acad Orthop Surg. 2000;8:97–110.
15. Seebacher JR, Inglis AE, Marshall JL, et al. The structure of the posterolateral aspect of the knee. J Bone Joint Surg Am. 1982;64:536–541.
16. Terry GC, LaPrade RF. The biceps femoris muscle complex at the knee: its anatomy and injury patterns associated with acute anterolateral-anteromedial rotatory instability. Am J Sports Med. 1996;24:2–8.
17. Tencer AF, Johnson KD, Kyle RF, et al. Biomechanics of fractures and fracture fixation. Instr Course Lect. 1993;42:19–34.
18. Staubli HU, Birrer S. The popliteus tendon and its fascicles at the popliteal hiatus: gross anatomy and functional arthroscopic evaluation with and without anterior cruciate deficiency. Arthroscopy. 1990;6:209–220.
19. LaPrade RF, Ly T, Wentorf FA, et al. The posterolateral attachments of the knee: a qualitative and quantitative morphologic analysis of the fibular collateral ligament, popliteus tendon, popliteofibular ligament, and lateral gastrocnemius tendon. Am J Sports Med. November 2003;31:854–860.
20. Hughston JC, Andrew JR, Cross MJ, et al. Classification of knee ligament instabilities: Part II: the lateral compartment. J Bone Joint Surg Am. 1976;58:173–179.
21. Maynard MJ, Deng X, Wickiewicz TL, et al. The popliteofibular ligament: rediscovery of a key element in posterolateral instability. Am J Sports Med. 1996;24:311–316.
22. Watanabe Y, Moriya H, Takahasi K, et al. Functional anatomy of the posterolateral structures of the knee. Arthroscopy. 1993;9:57–62.
23. Markolf KL, Wawscher DC, Finerman GA. Direct in vitro measurement of forces in the cruciate ligaments: Part II: the effect of section of the posterolateral structures. J Bone Joint Surg Am. 1993;75:387–394.
24. Nielsen S, Helmig P. The static stabilizing function of the popliteal tendon in the knee: an experimental study. Arch Orthop Trauma Surg. 1986;104:357–362.
25. Veltri DM, Deng XH, Torzilli PA, et al. The role of the popliteofibular ligament in stability of the human knee: a biomechanical study. Am J Sports Med. 1996;24:19–27.
26. Vogren TM, Hoher J, Aroen A, et al. Effects of sectioning the posterolateral structures on knee kinematics and in situ forces in the posterior cruciate ligament. Knee Surg Sports Traumatol Arthrosc. 2000;8:93–98.
27. Nielsen S, Oveson J, Rasmussen O. The posterior cruciate ligament and rotatory knee instability: an experimental study. Arch Orthop Trauma Surg. 1985;104:53–56.
28. Noyes FR, Stowers SF, Grood ES, et al. Posterior subluxations of the medial and lateral tibiofemoral compartments: an in vitro ligament sectioning study in cadaveric knees. Am J Sports Med. 1993;21:407–414.
29. Grood ES, Stowers SF, Noyes FR. Limits of movement in the human knee: effect of sectioning the posterior cruciate ligament and posterolateral structures. J Bone Joint Surg Am. 1988;70:88–97.
30. Skyhr MJ, Warren RF, Ortiz GJ, et al. The effects of sectioning of the posterior cruciate ligament and the posterolateral complex on the articular contact pressures within the knee. J Bone Joint Surg Am. 1993;75:694–699.
31. Arendt, EA, ed. *Orthopeadic Knowledge Update: Sports Medicine 2.* Rosemont, Ill: American Academy of Orthopaedic Surgeons; 1999.
32. Jakob RP, Warner JP. Lateral and posterolateral rotatory instability of the knee. In: Delee JC, Drez D Jr., eds. *Orthopaedic Sports Medicine: Principles and Practice*, Vol. 2. Philadelphia: WB Saunders; 1974:1275–1312.
33. Delee JC, Riley MB, Rockwood CA Jr. Acute posterolateral rotatory instability of the knee. Am J Sports Med. 1983;11:199–207.
34. Laprade RF, Hamilton CD, Engebretsen L. Treatment of acute and chronic combined anterior cruciate ligament and posterolateral knee ligament injuries. Sports Med Arthrosc Rev. 1997;5:91–99.
35. LaPrade RF, Terry GC. Injuries to the posterolateral aspect of the knee: Association of anatomic injury patterns with clinical instability. Am J Sports Med. 1997;25:433–438.
36. Cooper DE. Tests for posterolateral instability of the knee in normal subjects: Results of examination under anesthesia. J Bone Joint Surg Am. 1991;73:30–36.
37. Rosenberg TD, Paulos LE, Parker RD, et al. The forty-five-degree posteroanterior flexion weight-bearing radiograph of the knee. J Bone Joint Surg Am. 1988;10:1479–1483.
38. Shindell R, Walsh WM, Connolly JF. Avulsion fracture of the fibula: the "arcuate sign" of posterolateral knee instability. Nebr Med J. 1984;69:369–371.

39. Laprade RF. Arthroscopic evaluation of the lateral compartment of knees with grade 3 posterolateral knee complex injuries. Am J Sports Med. 1997;25:596–602.

40. Miller MD, Howard RF, Plancher KD. *Surgical Atlas of Sports Medicine*. Philadelphia: Saunders; 2003.

41. Jakob RP, Staubli HU, eds. *The Knee and Cruciate Ligaments: Anatomy, Biomechanics, Clinical Aspects, Reconstruction, Complications, Rehabilitation*. Berlin: Springer-Verlag; 1992.

42. Harner CD, Vince KG, Fu FH. *Techniques in Knee Surgery*. Philadelphia: Lippincott, Williams & Wilkins; 2000.

43. Noyes FR, Barber-Westin SD. Surgical reconstruction of severe chronic posterolateral complex injuries of the knee using allograft tissues. Am J Sports Med. 2000;28:282–296.

44. Clancy WG Jr. Repair and reconstruction of the posterior cruciate ligament. In: Chapman MW, Madison M, eds. *Operative Orthopaedics*, Vol. 3. Philadelphia: JB Lippincott; 1988: 1651–1655.

45. Bowen MK, Warren RF, Cooper DE. Posterior cruciate ligament and related injuries. In: Insall JN, ed. *Surgery of the Knee*, 2nd ed. New York: Churchill Livingstone; 1993: 197–206.

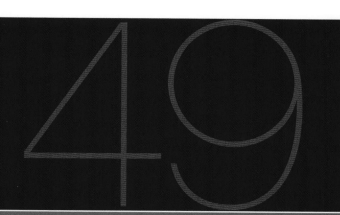

MULTIPLE LIGAMENT KNEE RECONSTRUCTION

■ PETER S. CHA, MD, JEFFREY A. RIHN, MD, CHRISTOPHER D. HARNER, MD

■ HISTORY OF THE TECHNIQUE

Traumatic knee dislocation has long been recognized as a serious injury. Injury to the cruciate and collateral ligaments, menisci, articular cartilage, and neurovascular structures complicate the evaluation and management of traumatic knee dislocation. The potentially disastrous consequences of mismanagement are known well, particularly in knee dislocation that involves limb-threatening vascular injury. The multiple-ligament-injured knee is a difficult problem that requires thorough evaluation and treatment by an experienced knee surgeon.

Treatment of multiligament knee injury has evolved over the past century. In the early to mid-1900s, traumatic knee dislocation was treated with cast immobilization. The majority of patients treated conservatively experienced a poor outcome. Surgical repair became a viable treatment option in the mid-1900s. Primary repair of the injured ligaments in the dislocated knee was reported by O'Donoghue[1] in 1955 with good results; the best results were obtained in those patients treated within 2 weeks of their initial injury. Several reports in the literature from the 1960s to the 1980s supported primary ligamentous repair as the recommended form of treatment of knee dislocation and multiple ligament injury.[2–6] Because of the limited potential for primary healing of the cruciate ligaments, cruciate ligament reconstruction has been the preferred method of treatment since the 1980s. Except in cases of osseous avulsion, primary repair of the cruciate ligaments has fallen out of favor. Most experienced knee surgeons currently approach the surgical management of acute knee dislocations with a goal of anatomic repair and reconstruction of all associated ligamentous and meniscal injuries.[7–10] This involves combined, arthroscopically assisted anterior cruciate ligament (ACL) and posterior cruciate ligament (PCL) reconstruction, meniscal repair or resection, and either primary repair or reconstruction of posterolateral corner (PLC) injuries, depending on the timing of the treatment and condition of the soft tissues. This chapter will review, in detail, our preferred method for surgical management of the multiple-ligament-injured knee with emphasis on the technical considerations.

■ INDICATIONS AND CONTRAINDICATIONS

Knee dislocation is a severe injury with potentially devastating consequences. Whereas surgical treatment of the majority of knee dislocations can be delayed 2 to 3 weeks from the time of initial injury, certain cases require immediate surgical intervention. Evaluation and initial management must be performed expeditiously to prevent limb-threatening complications and to identify indications for emergent intervention. Initial assessment includes a brief history, a directed physical examination, thorough neurovascular evaluation, and plain radiographs of the injured knee. Knee dislocation can be either a high-energy (e.g., motor vehicle accident), or low-energy (e.g., twisting injury during sports activity) injury. Up to 50% of knee dislocations spontaneously reduce prior to evaluation. Therefore, if the exam reveals substantial laxity of two or more of the major ligaments of the knee, then a presumptive diagnosis of knee dislocation should be made. In cases of gross knee dislocation, the knee should be reduced immediately through gentle traction-countertraction under conscious sedation and the limb should be stabilized in a long leg splint. A postreduction neurovascular exam should be performed, and reduction should be confirmed with anteroposterior and lateral radiographs.

Popliteal artery injury and peroneal nerve injury are reported to occur in up to 45% and 40% of knee dislocations, respectively.[5,11] The presence of these associated injuries will affect the surgical treatment plan and must be detected promptly. Some authors recommend the use of selective popliteal artery angiography in the setting of acute knee dislocation, performing angiography only in the presence of asymmetric distal pulses or an abnormal ankle brachial index (ABI).[12–15] Unfortunately, normal pulses, a warm foot, and brisk capillary refill can exist in the face of an intimal tear of the popliteal artery, which may not manifest itself for several days after the initial injury.[11,16] We currently perform popliteal artery angiography or CT angiography on all cases of suspected knee dislocation to rule out such an injury. The routine use of angiography in this setting is justified by the relatively low morbidity of the test, the high incidence of popliteal artery injury, and the potentially devastating consequences of any delay in diagnosis.

Emergent surgery is indicated in open or irreducible dislocations of the knee and in those cases of knee dislocation with associated vascular injury or compartment syndrome. In cases of open knee dislocation, the standard principles of wound management prevail. These include serial irrigation and debridement, intravenous antibiotics, and adequate soft tissue coverage. Ligament reconstruction should not be performed acutely in open knee dislocations. In some cases, soft tissue coverage problems may force ligament reconstruction to be delayed for several months. Irreducible dislocations are not common. When encountered, they require prompt surgical reduction to avoid prolonged traction on the neurovascular structures. Although ligament reconstruction can be done at the time of the reduction, we prefer to delay the definitive reconstruction to allow for more complete knee imaging, planning, and resource mobilization. Popliteal artery injuries require emergent intervention by a vascular surgeon. An orthopedic surgeon's input as to the location of incisions is often helpful for future reconstructive efforts. Saphenous vein grafting is often required, as are fasciotomies, following revascularization. Compartment syndrome is an orthopedic emergency. The presence of a knee dislocation does not change its management. Prompt diagnosis and fasciotomies are necessary for a successful outcome. During emergent surgery on a dislocated knee, it is acceptable to perform simple primary repair of injured soft tissue structures as they are encountered during the surgical exposure. Excessive foreign material, including suture, is avoided in open injuries. Additional incisions are avoided in the emergent setting. Definitive ligament reconstruction should be delayed several days to allow for recovery of the soft tissues and decreased swelling. In cases of vascular injury, additional time is required to ensure that the vascular repair is adequate and to allow limb swelling to subside.

The majority of multiple-ligament-injured knees are currently treated surgically, with the goal of anatomic repair and reconstruction of all associated ligamentous and meniscal injuries. This approach has been reported to provide adequate knee stability and motion and allow the patient to return to normal daily activities.[7–10,17] Closed reduction and cast immobilization of knee dislocation currently has few relative indications, including elderly or sedentary patients and patients who have debilitating medical or posttraumatic comorbidities. Patients who initially undergo a trial of conservative management often require surgery at a later date due to problems with knee function, including loss of motion and persistent instability. Prior to surgical treatment, additional evaluation is necessary to characterize the pattern of injury (i.e., which structures are injured) and determine an appropriate surgical plan. In addition to disruption of the cruciate ligaments, the majority of knee dislocations involve injury to the collateral ligaments, the posterolateral structures of the knee, or the menisci. The key components of this evaluation are physical examination, magnetic resonance imaging (MRI), and arthroscopy. A thorough ligamentous exam is performed after survival of the limb is ensured and the patient is stabilized. Because guarding can obscure the examination in an awake patient, examination under anesthesia should be performed prior to operative treatment. MRI is used to characterize soft tissue and occult osseous injuries only after the patient has been acutely stabilized. MRI results are helpful in determining which structures are reparable and which must be reconstructed. Arthroscopic examination at the start of the definitive operative procedure is necessary to confirm the preoperative diagnosis and detect additional injuries not detected during the preoperative workup.

■ SURGICAL TECHNIQUES

Anesthesia

The choice of anesthesia is made in conjunction with the surgeon, the anesthesiologist, and the patient. The factors influencing the preferred anesthesia technique include the age of the patient, the patient's comorbid medical problems, and the previous anesthesia history of the patient. The anesthesia team typically chooses between a general anesthesia or an epidural anesthetic with concomitant intravenous (IV) sedation. If the anesthesiologist is at all concerned about airway management, then general anesthesia is used. At our center, preoperative femoral or sciatic nerve blocks are routinely performed. The nerve blocks have not only been useful during the surgical procedure, but they offer 9 to 12 hours of postoperative pain relief. A Foley catheter is placed to help monitor the fluid status during the case. We recommend that a vascular surgeon be on call during the procedure as unexpected injuries to the vessels may occur.

Surface Anatomy and Skin Incision

The patient is seen in the preoperative holding area and the correct extremity is identified by both the surgeon and the patient. The correctly selected extremity should correlate with the written consent. Using an indelible marker, the surgeon then places his or her initials on the correct extremity

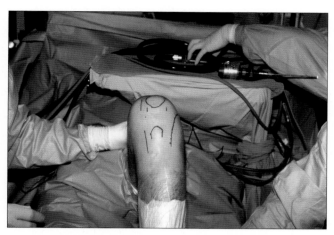

Fig. 49-1. Overview of the surface anatomy, skin incisions, and setup.

with the word *yes*; this should be strategically placed so that the signature is within the operative field.

A marker is used to identify the surface anatomy and the incisions that will be utilized during the procedure **(Fig. 49-1)**. The important osseous landmarks that include the patella, the tibial tubercle, Gerdy tubercle, and the fibular head are identified. The peroneal nerve is palpated and marked superficial to the fibular neck. The medial and lateral joint lines are identified. The potential skin incisions are then drawn. The anterolateral arthroscopy portal is placed adjacent to the lateral border of the patella above the joint line. The anteromedial arthroscopy portal is placed approximately 1 cm medial to the patellar tendon at the same level. A superolateral outflow portal is placed proximal to the superior border of the patella and posterior to the quadriceps tendon. The posteromedial portal is established if needed from an inside-out technique and thus is not initially marked. A longitudinal 3-cm incision that originates approximately 2 cm distal to the joint line and 2 cm medial to the tibial tubercle is drawn on the anteromedial proximal tibia for the ACL and PCL tibial tunnels. Also, a 2-cm incision is placed just medial to the medial trochlea articular surface and along the subvastus interval for the PCL femoral tunnel. If there is a medial ligament injury, then the distal incision for the tibial tunnels is traced proximally to the medial epicondyle and extended to the level of the vastus medialis in a curvilinear fashion. The incision for the lateral and posterolateral injuries is a curvilinear 12-cm incision that is drawn midway between the Gerdy tubercle and the fibular head and traced proximally just inferior to the lateral epicondyle while the knee is flexed 90 degrees.[18] The proximal extent of this incision parallels the plane between the biceps femoris tendon and the iliotibial band **(Fig. 49-2)**. We prefer the medial and lateral incisions as previously described and avoid the used of a midline incision as this could potentially be complicated by skin breakdown over the patella and often can limit access to the collateral ligaments. Finally, the dorsalis pedis pulse is palpated and marked.

Specifics of the Procedure

The patient is evaluated in the preoperative area for a detailed neurovascular examination with documentation of the status of the popliteal, dorsalis pedis, and posterior tibial pulses and the function of the tibial and peroneal nerves. After successful induction of anesthesia in the operating room suite, a thorough examination under anesthesia is performed and correlated with the preoperative impression from the office notes. It is of utmost importance to examine the opposite extremity and use it as a reference. The examination begins by taking the knee through a range of motion and noting any deficits. The anterior drawer, Lachman, and pivot shift tests reveal any deficits to the ACL. The PCL is examined by appreciating any posterior sag with associated step-off and by testing a posterior drawer at 90 degrees of flexion. The lateral collateral ligament (LCL) is palpated in the figure-four position and tested with a varus stress at 0 degrees and 30 degrees. The PLC is tested at 30 degrees and by holding the proximal tibia and externally rotating the leg; also, the PLC is tested by applying an external rotation force on the proximal tibia and fibula while the knee is flexed 90 degrees to feel for lateral dropout. The medial collateral ligament (MCL) is examined with a valgus stress at 0 degrees and 30 degrees. Once a thorough exam is completed, the extent of the ligamentous injuries is better understood, which helps guide the surgical procedure.

The two most common combined injury patterns with knee dislocations include the ACL, PCL, and MCL and the ACL, PCL, LCL, and PLC. Less commonly, the PCL is intact or only partially torn and does not require a reconstruction.[19,20] At our institution we are recognizing injury patterns with PCL injuries that preserve specific bundles of the PCL. Most commonly, we are observing that the anterolateral bundle is ruptured; however, the meniscofemoral ligament (MFL) and the posteromedial bundle may remain

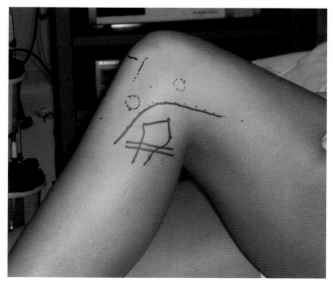

Fig. 49-2. Lateral curvilinear incision with landmarks.

intact. If we see this injury pattern, an attempt is made to preserve the intact portion of the PCL and MFL and to simply reconstruct the ruptured portion via a single bundle technique. Our approach is to reconstruct or repair all injured structures. The intrasubstance tears for the ACL, PCL, LCL, and PLC typically require reconstruction, while intrasubstance tears of the MCL and avulsed ligaments are usually repaired. Also, concomitant injuries to the articular cartilage and menisci are operatively addressed at the time of surgery.

Patient Positioning

The supine patient is properly positioned on the operating room table. Our goal is to have a full free range of motion of the involved extremity during the procedure with the ability to have the knee statically flexed at 80 degrees to 90 degrees without any manual assistance. We accomplish this by placing a small gel pad bump under the ipsilateral hip with a post placed on the side of the bed just distal to the greater trochanter; a sterile bump of towels or drapes is wedged between the post and the thigh. The heel rests on a 10 lb sandbag that is taped to the bed during the initial positioning (Fig. 49-1). A well-padded tourniquet is placed on the proximal thigh; however, it is not inflated unless necessary and thus rarely used. Intravenous antibiotics are administered prior to the skin incision. The previously described skin incisions are drawn and the pulses are once again palpated and marked. The extremity is prepped with alcohol and Betadine solution and draped in a meticulous fashion. The skin incisions are injected with 0.25% Marcaine with 1:100,000 epinephrine. The mini C-arm fluoroscopy machine is in the operating suite and draped.

Repair versus Reconstruction

With knee dislocations, the decision to repair or reconstruct the injured structures depends on numerous factors. Concerning cruciate injuries, the majority of injuries are intrasubstance tears that are not amenable to surgical repair but are best treated with ligament reconstruction. However, we do recommend a primary repair of the ACL or PCL if a large bony fragment remains on their respective tibial insertions.[21,22] The primary repair can be accomplished by passing large nonabsorbable sutures (no. 5) into the bony fragment and through bone tunnels in the tibia. Also, a primary repair of the PCL insertion may be advocated in the case of a "peel off" or a soft tissue avulsion of the PCL at its femoral insertion by a similar technique.[23] Concerning the MCL, LCL, and PLC, it is our experience that a primary repair may have successful results if operatively addressed within 3 weeks of injury. If the injury is chronic, scar formation and soft tissue contracture usually limit the success of a primary ligamentous repair and a ligament reconstruction is often necessary. The MCL can be directly repaired with intrasubstance sutures or with suture anchors if avulsed off the bone.

Repair of the posterolateral corner structures and the LCL can be accomplished with direct suture repair or by repair to bone via drill-holes versus suture anchors. If direct repair is not possible due to the quality of the tissue, then the involved structures should be augmented with hamstring tendons, biceps femoris, iliotibial band, or allograft; otherwise the involved structures should be reconstructed.[24]

Diagnostic Arthroscopy

The arthroscope is introduced into the anterolateral portal and the intra-articular findings are correlated with the preoperative MRI and exam under anesthesia. An arthroscopic approach is advocated to assist in the planning in the potential skin incisions (medial or lateral) needed for the procedure based on the pattern of injury. Gravity inflow is used with a superolateral outflow. Care must be taken to avoid a compartment syndrome, and the posterior leg and calf region must be palpated intermittently during the procedure. Factors that influence a potential compartment syndrome include an acute reconstruction (less than 2 weeks from the time of injury) in which the capsular healing was insufficient to maintain joint distension or if the capsule has been breeched iatrogenically during the procedure. If extravasation is noted and a potential compartment syndrome is suspected, then the arthroscopic technique is abandoned and the remainder of the procedure is performed via an open technique. However, the arthroscope can still be a valuable tool when used in a dry field by improving the visualization and magnification during the open procedure.

All compartments are assessed within the knee. The MCL is visualized in the medial compartment and the meniscal attachment to the deep MCL is assessed to determine if a femoral, midsubstance, or tibial-sided injury has occurred. The popliteus tendon is visualized and probed in the lateral compartment to determine where the injury occurred or if there is any functional compromise. The PCL is examined at both its femoral and tibial insertions. The PCL most often undergoes an interstitial tear of the ligament. A posteromedial portal is needed to completely visualize the tibial insertion of the ligament. This is established under direct visualization by placing the 70-degree arthroscope into the anterolateral portal and through the intercondylar notch adjacent to the posterior aspect of the medial femoral condyle. The spinal needle and trocar is delivered just anterior to the saphenous nerve and vein.

Once the intra-articular pathology is confirmed, any concomitant articular cartilage or meniscal injury is addressed. Every effort is made to preserve the meniscal tissue. Peripheral meniscal tears are repaired via the inside-out technique, whereas central or irreparable meniscal tears are debrided to a stable rim. Should the meniscus necessitate a repair, the sutures are tied down directly onto the capsule at 30 degrees of flexion at the end of the procedure after the grafts are passed and secured.

The necessary debridement is accomplished with a basket forceps and a 4.5-mm full radius shaver. This includes a debridement of the notch with preservation of any remaining intact PCL tissue, as previously described. The tibial insertion of the PCL is removed by introducing a shaver or a curette into the posteromedial portal and gently developing the plane between the PCL and the posterior capsule while looking through the anterolateral portal with a 70-degree arthroscope. Alternatively, the 30-degree arthroscope may be introduced through the posteromedial portal, and a PCL curette and rasp may be introduced through the anterolateral or anteromedial portals. Every attempt is made to debride the distal-most aspect of the tibial insertion of the PCL as this will help with the eventual placement of the guide wire for the tibial tunnel. We perform a limited notchplasty for the placement of the ACL femoral tunnel. We also try to preserve the very tibial insertion of the ACL for its proprioceptive and vascular factors. Every attempt is made to preserve the fat pad, and we only debride the fat that obscures our arthroscopic visualization.

Graft Selection and Preparation

There are many options for graft selection for the multiple ligament knee injury. The decision to choose a graft is multifactorial based on the extent of the injury, timing of the surgery (acute versus chronic), and experience of the surgeon. Autograft tissue may be harvested from the ipsilateral or contralateral extremity and has the advantage of better graft incorporation and remodeling. At our institution, we recommend the use of allograft over autograft in multiple ligament reconstruction surgery. The advantages of using allograft tissue include: decreased operative time, decreased skin incisions in a knee that has been severely traumatized, and no donor site morbidity.[7] We have also shown that the use of allograft decreases pain and stiffness postoperatively.[25] However, one must be willing to assume the risks of using allograft tissue, which include an increase in cost, a delay in the incorporation of the graft, and a risk of disease transmission.[26] Once the grafts are fashioned, they are wrapped in a sponge and bathed in warm saline.

ACL

We prefer to use an allograft bone-patellar tendon-bone (BPTB) for our ACL reconstructions. The BPTB allograft provides adequate biomechanical strength with rigid bony fixation at both the femoral and tibial attachment sites. We split the graft in half down the longitudinal axis; this is done so that we have an additional graft should something happen to the initial graft. We prefer 11-mm by 25-mm cylindrical bone plugs with an 11-mm tendon width. The patellar bone plug is usually fixed in the femoral tunnel and is fashioned to have a slightly tapered leading edge to facilitate easy graft passage. Two no. 5 nonabsorbable sutures are placed in both the patellar and tibial plugs through drill holes **(Fig. 49-3A,B)**.

PCL

We recommend the use of Achilles tendon allograft for PCL reconstruction. If a double bundle technique is indicated, then an ipsilateral hamstring tendon (semitendinosus) autograft is harvested in addition. The allograft Achilles tendon is an attractive choice for reconstruction of the PCL because it is a long graft, it has a significant cross-sectional area, and it has a calcaneal bone plug that provides rigid fixation in the femoral tunnel. The central portion of the calcaneal bone plug is fashioned such that it has a diameter of 11 mm and a length of 25 mm using compaction pliers and a rongeur. Two no. 5 nonabsorbable sutures are placed within the bone plug. Additionally, the tendon end is tubularized using a double-armed no. 5 nonabsorbable suture. This is passed along the long axis of the tendinous portion in a "Chinese finger trap" configuration so that the graft will not "ball up" during the graft passage **(Fig. 49-4)**.

LCL

The LCL is reconstructed with an Achilles tendon allograft with a 7-mm or 8-mm calcaneal bone plug. The bone plug can be fixed into the LCL insertion at the fibula through a bone tunnel. We do not tubularize the tendon as it is often reinforced to the native LCL tissue. Alternatively, the remaining bone-patellar tendon allograft may be used for the LCL reconstruction.

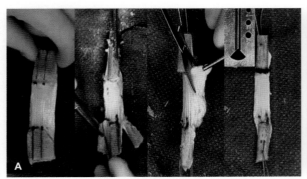
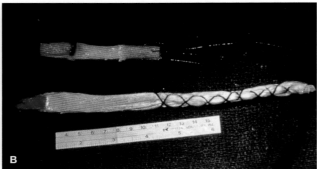

Fig. 49-3. A: Preparation of bone-patellar tendon-bone allograft for ACL reconstruction. **B:** Prepared bone-patellar tendon-bone (*top*) and Achilles (*bottom*) allografts.

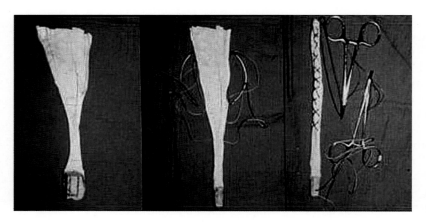

Fig. 49-4. Achilles tendon allograft for PCL reconstruction.

PLC

Our graft choice for reconstructing the popliteofibular ligament is a tibialis anterior soft tissue allograft or an ipsilateral hamstring (semitendinosus) autograft. These are fashioned with a whipstitch on both ends using a no. 2 braided nonabsorbable suture and usually fit into a 7-mm bone tunnel.

Cruciate Tunnel Preparation

We prefer to address the PCL tibial tunnel initially as this is the most dangerous and challenging portion of the procedure. We introduce a 15-mm offset PCL guide set at 50 degrees to 55 degrees via the anteromedial portal and place the tip of the guide at the distal and lateral third of the insertion site of the PCL on the tibia. The 3- to 4-cm medial proximal tibia skin incision is made, and the periosteum is sharply dissected from the bone. The starting point of the K-wire is approximately 3 to 4 cm distal to the joint line. The trajectory of the tibial PCL tunnel roughly parallels the angle of the proximal tibiofibular joint. We then pass a 3/32 mm Kirschner wire into the desired position and perforate the far cortex of the tibia at the PCL insertion; this is done under direct arthroscopic visualization. Caution must be taken when passing the guide wire through the cortex of the tibial insertion of the PCL because of the close proximity of the neurovascular structures. Oftentimes, the PCL tibial insertion site has a cancellous feel when the far cortex is breeched and no hard cortex can be felt while the K-wire is advanced. The location of this pin placement is then confirmed with the mini C-arm fluoroscopy machine on the true lateral projection of the knee (medial and lateral condyles of the femur are overlapping). Occasionally, the wire is too proximal on the PCL tibial insertion site and a 3-mm or 5-mm parallel pin guide will be used to obtain the ideal placement of the PCL tibial tunnel. The K-wire for the PCL tibial tunnel is left in place and attention is paid to the ACL tibial tunnel. The ACL tibial guide set at 47.5 degrees is introduced into the anteromedial portal and a 3/32-mm guide wire is placed in the center of the ACL tibial footprint. This position should rest approximately 7 mm anterior to the PCL and should coincide with the posterior

extent of the anterior horn of the lateral meniscus. The location of the ACL tibial tunnel is also confirmed on the full extension lateral projection with the mini C-arm fluoroscopic machine. The guide wire should rest posterior to the Blumenstaat line on the full extension lateral projection to ensure proper placement of the ACL tibial tunnel. The ACL tibial tunnel is proximal and anterior to the PCL tibial tunnel **(Fig. 49-5A,B)**.

After acceptable placement of the ACL and PCL tibial tunnel guide wires is confirmed, the PCL tunnel is drilled. A curette is placed directly on top of the guide wire over the area of the drill site. The 10-mm compaction drill bit is passed under direct arthroscopic visualization with a 30-degree arthroscope that is introduced through the posteromedial portal. This is initially passed through the tibia on power then completed by hand. The PCL tibial tunnel is then

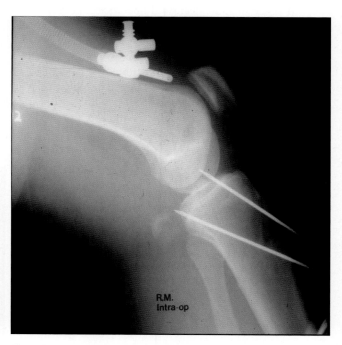

Fig. 49-5. Radiographic confirmation of the ACL and PCL guide wire placement.

Part C

MENISCAL PATHOLOGY AND THE POST-MENISCECTOMY KNEE

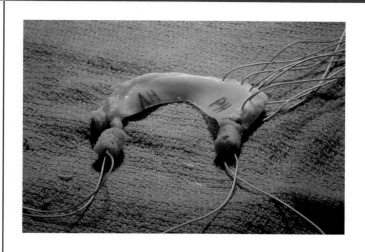

50

ARTHROSCOPIC MENISCUS REPAIR

HUSSEIN A. ELKOUSY, MD, FREDDIE H. FU, MD, DSC, DPS (HON)

■ HISTORY OF THE TECHNIQUE

Thomas Annandale performed the first meniscus repair in 1883. However, the technique was ignored mostly due to the perceived minor role that the meniscus plays in normal knee function. Several studies have subsequently proven the importance of the meniscus in normal knee function and documented the adverse sequelae of meniscectomy over time.[1-4] The menisci are now known to play important roles in joint lubrication, shock absorption, proprioception, articular cartilage nutrition, secondary stabilization, and load transmission.[1,5] As a result, several techniques were developed to repair, rather than to excise, a torn meniscus. An open technique was reported by DeHaven et al.[6] to have successful results, but arthroscopic techniques have become the standard. The first arthroscopic meniscus repair was done in Japan in 1969 by Ikeuchi.[7,8]

Arthroscopic meniscus repair can be broadly divided into three different techniques: inside-out, outside-in, and all-inside. Inside-out techniques use specially designed cannulae to pass sutures through the meniscus from the inside to the outside of the joint. This technique was introduced in North America in 1980 by Charles Henning.[7] The outside-in technique uses spinal needles or cannulae to pass sutures through the meniscus from outside the joint to the inside. This technique was popularized by Russell Warren in the 1980s.[9] The all-inside technique does not require any external incisions and all fixation is performed arthroscopically. This technique has changed significantly since its original descriptions in the early 1990s.[1,10]

This chapter will primarily discuss inside-out and outside-in techniques. We prefer the inside-out technique and will focus on this technique, but both are useful for successful repair of a torn meniscus. All-inside techniques vary due to the large number of devices manufactured by different vendors, but a short summary of all-inside techniques will be included.

■ INDICATIONS AND CONTRAINDICATIONS

Meniscus repair has two goals. First, it should relieve pain and allow the patient to return to his or her previous level of activity. Second, it theoretically preserves the function of the meniscus and minimizes future degenerative changes. The first goal can equally be achieved with partial meniscectomy.[11] However, it is the second goal that holds promise for meniscus repair. Several studies have been done to evaluate meniscus repair, but only a few have shown that it prevents future degenerative changes.[6,12,13]

Not every torn meniscus is amenable to repair. Certain parameters have been defined that help predict which tears can be repaired with a reasonable expectation for a successful result.[5,14] First, the tear should be in a well-vascularized area. Arnoczky and Warren[15,16] defined the zones of the meniscus based upon vascularity (Fig. 50-1). The peripheral 10% to 25%, termed the red-red zone, is supplied by a perimeniscal capillary plexus. The middle third is the red-white zone, and the central third is the white-white zone. The poor blood supply of these more central zones limits the healing potential of more central meniscus tears. Second, longitudinal tears have a higher rate of healing than radial, horizontal cleavage, or other complex tears. Bucket handle tears are a subset of longitudinal tears. Third, the knee must be stable. Meniscus repairs tend to fare poorly in anterior cruciate ligament–deficient knees, and improved outcomes are seen with concomitant anterior cruciate ligament (ACL) reconstruction.[16-18] Fourth, most candidates for repair are below the age of 40.[5,14] Some studies have demonstrated successful

467

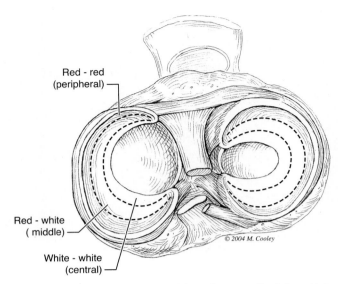

Fig. 50-1. Illustration of the medial meniscus on the left and lateral meniscus on the right. Each meniscus is divided by the dashed line into the three zones as defined by Arnoczky and Warren.

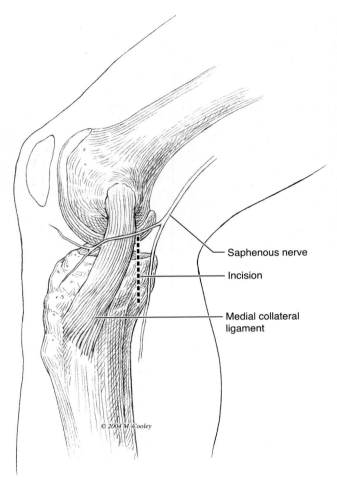

Fig. 50-2. Illustration depicting the site of the incision for inside-out medial meniscus repair.

outcomes in older populations.[18,19] However, the potentially limited benefit over partial meniscectomy should be carefully weighed in this older population considering the likely presence of articular cartilage changes, the hardships of rehabilitation, and the poorer quality of tissue and inferior blood supply. Finally, acute tears have a higher rate of healing than chronic tears.[14]

■ INSIDE-OUT MENISCUS REPAIR

Anesthesia

We generally use general endotracheal anesthesia. The patients who are candidates for meniscus repair are otherwise young and healthy; therefore, they generally have few risk factors that preclude this. A lower extremity regional nerve or plexus block is not unreasonable, but we cannot see any particular advantage to this at the present time, unless the ACL is reconstructed at the same sitting. Postoperative pain is generally adequately controlled with oral narcotics. In addition, some surgeons may infiltrate a local anesthetic such as Marcaine perioperatively to augment analgesia. We tend to avoid postoperative injections that may disrupt the internal milieu of the joint, particularly if fibrin clot is used.

Surface Anatomy and Skin Incision

The skin incision is marked at the beginning of the case prior to placing the arthroscope. The skin incision for a medial meniscus repair is placed just posterior to the medial collateral ligament **(Fig. 50-2)**. This site is approximated on

the skin by first placing the knee in 90 degrees of flexion. The medial joint line is marked by identifying and marking the lateral joint line and extrapolating this line medially. The medial joint line can sometimes be difficult to identify directly. As this line is directed posteriorly, care should be taken to re-create a small amount of posterior slope that is most certainly present. Next, the posteromedial border of the tibial diaphysis is palpated. A line is projected proximally and in-line with the diaphysis. This is the vertical line defining the anteroposterior position of the incision. A 3-cm to 4-cm incision is marked with one third of the incision proximal to the joint line and two thirds distal to the joint line.

The lateral incision is marked by placing the knee in 90 degrees of flexion and marking the joint line as for the medial side. The lateral collateral ligament and the fibular head are palpated and a vertical incision is marked along the posterior border of the lateral collateral ligament **(Fig. 50-3)**. The incision does not extend further distal than the tip of the fibular head. It is also placed one-third above and two-thirds below the joint line.

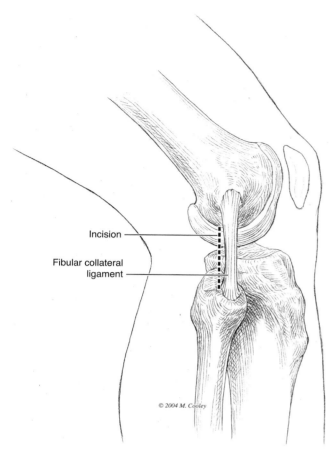

Fig. 50-3. Illustration of the deep anatomy on the medial aspect of the knee.

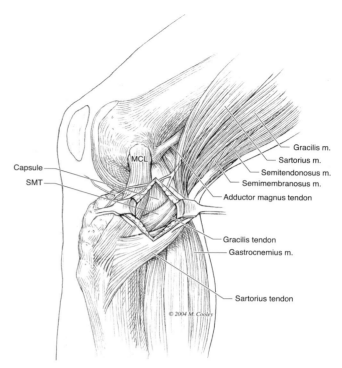

Fig. 50-4. Illustration depicting the site of the incision for inside-out lateral meniscus repair.

Deep Anatomy

The medial and lateral approaches require dissection through two layers of tissue. The superficial layer includes the skin, fat, and superficial fascia. The second layer on the medial side includes the pes anserine fascia proximal to the sartorius fascia **(Fig. 50-4)**. The superficial medial collateral ligament should be anterior to the plane of dissection. The retractor is placed superficial to the deep medial collateral ligament and the capsule **(Fig. 50-5)**. The structure at risk with this approach is the infrapatellar branch of the saphenous nerve **(Fig. 50-6)**.

Once the skin and superficial fascia are incised on the lateral approach, the iliotibial (IT) band and biceps femoris are identified **(Fig. 50-7)**. The plane of dissection remains anterior to the biceps femoris and extends to the lateral head of the gastrocnemius muscle. The retractor is placed between the lateral head of the gastrocnemius and the capsule. The structure most at risk with this approach is the peroneal nerve. However, this should not be an issue as long as the dissection remains anterior to the biceps femoris.

Surgical Details

Once the patient is asleep, the knee is examined. If there is any question of stability, this should be evaluated with a

thorough exam under anesthesia. Additional procedures such as ACL reconstruction should have been discussed with the patient preoperatively. If an ACL reconstruction is to be performed, the meniscus repair sutures are passed prior to ACL reconstruction, but they are not tied until after the ACL reconstruction is complete.

Potential medial and lateral incisions are marked as described in the section on superficial anatomy. This can be done after the knee is cleaned with Betadine solution and

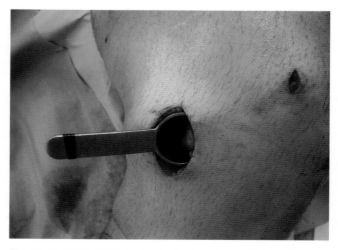

Fig. 50-5. The popliteal retractor is placed superficial to the capsule.

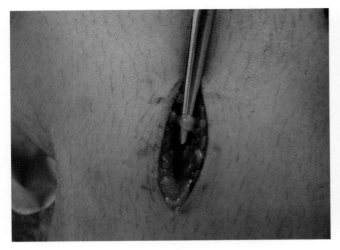

Fig. 50-6. Infrapatellar branch of the saphenous nerve.

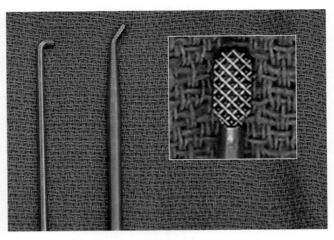

Fig. 50-8. Ninety- and 30-degree arthroscopic rasps.

draped, but we prefer to do this initially. The knee is then prepared and draped in sterile fashion.

A superolateral portal is established for outflow. Anterolateral and anteromedial portals are then established. The 70-degree arthroscope is placed first and a Gilquist maneuver is performed. The posteromedial joint is examined to identify a peripheral medial meniscus tear if present.

Once this is done, the camera is switched to a 30-degree arthroscope.

Once a tear is identified and deemed to be repairable, a rasp is placed in the working portal to prepare the tear site. This may be done through the ipsilateral, contralateral, or both portals with the camera moved appropriately. Several rasps are commercially available **(Fig. 50-8)**. Both sides of the tear should be abraded and a shaver may also be used judiciously with the suction off **(Fig. 50-9)**.

Once the tear is prepared, the arthroscope is switched to the ipsilateral portal. A probe or cannula is placed in the contralateral portal to assess the approach to the tear. Several systems exist for inside-out repair. We prefer to approach with the cannula in the contralateral portal, although some systems allow for an approach from the ipsilateral portal. Once the approach is deemed adequate, all instruments are removed from the knee and the appropriate incision is

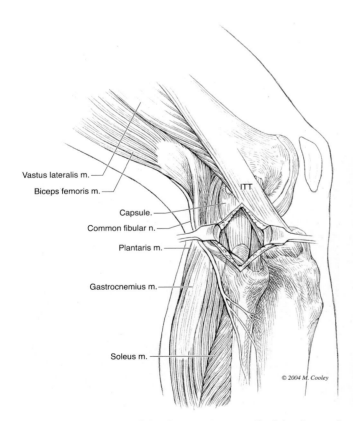

Vastus lateralis m.

Biceps femoris m.

Capsule.

Common fibular n.

Plantaris m.

Gastrocnemius m.

Soleus m.

ITT

© 2004 M. Cooley

Fig. 50-7. Illustration of the deep anatomy on the lateral aspect of the knee.

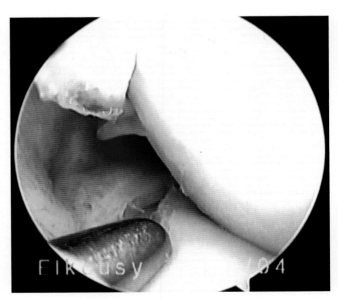

Fig. 50-9. Shaver with suction off used to prepare tear site.

made. The tourniquet is inflated prior to making the skin incision.

Medial Meniscus Repair

The knee is placed in 90 degrees of flexion. After the incision is made on the medial side, a Metzenbaum scissors is used to carefully dissect bluntly and sharply through the subcutaneous fat and superficial fascia. A sponge may be used to clear off any tissue adherent to the pes anserine fascia. This fascia is identified by the oblique/transverse orientation of its fibers. The infrapatellar branch of the saphenous nerve should be identified at this time if it is present in the incision. Generally it passes transversely across the superior aspect of the incision (Fig. 50-6). While protecting the nerve, a knife is used to vertically incise the fascia. A scissors is used to extend the incision proximally and distally. The capsule, deep medial collateral ligament, and posterior oblique ligament are beneath this layer (Fig. 50-4). A finger or blunt instrument is used to develop the plane between the capsule and the medial head of the gastrocnemius muscle posteriorly to allow placement of a popliteal retractor or a spoon (Fig. 50-5). The popliteal retractor works well with a small incision because the skin holds its position.

At this point, the surgical team must be appropriately positioned. Inside-out meniscus repair can be done with only a surgeon and an assistant; however, it is best done with two assistants. One assistant (passer) passes the suture through the cannula and the second assistant (catcher) retrieves the suture from the open incision. Some vendors have manufactured guns that allow the surgeon to perform the role of the passer as well **(Fig. 50-10)**. For medial meniscus repairs, the knee is placed in a small degree of flexion (less than 20 degrees) to allow access to the medial compartment. The catcher is generally seated across the operating room table or just to the right of the surgeon in a right knee or to the left of the surgeon in a left knee. Light is directed into the wound to allow the catcher to promptly identify the passing needles.

We use a zone-specific set in which the cannulas are pre-contoured to allow safe placement of sutures in the three different regions of the meniscus **(Fig. 50-11)**. The three regions are divided into posterior, middle, and anterior thirds. We generally start with the first suture posteriorly and place sequential stitches from posterior to anterior.

We prefer to place vertical mattress sutures, but this occasionally is not possible and a horizontal mattress suture may be placed **(Fig. 50-12A,B)**. Sutures are placed on the superior or inferior surface of the meniscus **(Fig. 50-13A,B)**. We tend to balance the superior sutures with inferiorly placed sutures in order to avoid placing an asymmetric force on the meniscus that may result in poor apposition on the inferior surface. All sutures are prepackaged 2-0 braided nonabsorbable sutures on double armed straight flexible needles. Reusable needles with eyelets are also available.

The surgeon positions the cannula so that the proximal flat portion of the cannula is either parallel to the joint line or is directed slightly inferior **(Fig. 50-14)**. Once the cannula has been positioned, the passer loads the needle into the cannula. A needle driver works well to advance the needles. The needle driver is positioned on the needle 2 to 4 mm from its entry into the cannula and advances are made in these small increments. The tip of the needle is pushed out the end of the cannula into the joint. This tip is used to pierce the meniscus to define the site of entry of the needle. Once this is done, the surgeon indicates to the passer to start advancing the needle in the short increments. After two or three advances, the needle should be visible in the medial incision. The passer does not pass it any further until signaled

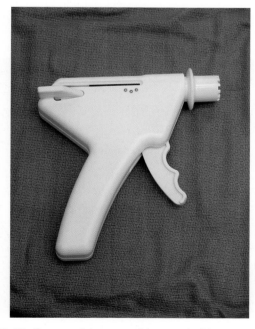

Fig. 50-10. Commercial gun used to pass inside-out sutures in small increments.

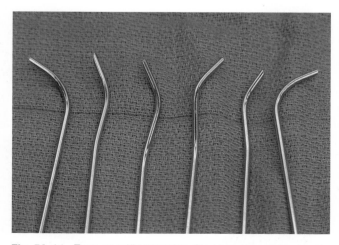

Fig. 50-11. Zone-specific cannulas. Six cannulae can be used to address the posterior, middle, and anterior thirds of each meniscus.

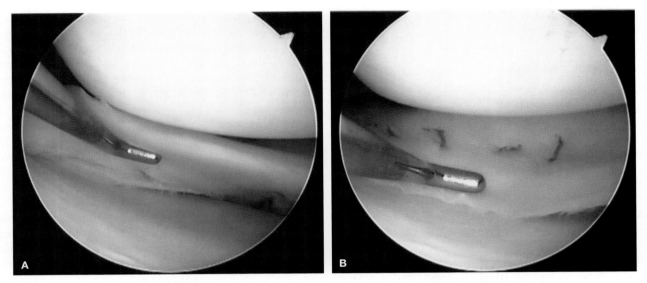

Fig. 50-12. A: Near full thickness 3 cm undersurface tear in a 15-year-old male. **B:** Horizontal and vertical mattress sutures have been placed.

by the catcher. The catcher locates the needle in the wound and uses a needle driver to grasp it and pull it through. If the needle is visible but the catcher cannot retrieve it because it is pressed against the retractor, the catcher may signal to the passer to continue passing the needle. The passer should not advance the needle further if it is not visible in the wound.

After the first arm of the stitch is passed and retrieved, the needle is removed and a small clamp is placed on the passed end. The cannula is now repositioned to allow placement of the second limb of the suture. Tension is maintained on the limb that has already been passed while the needle of the second limb is passed into the cannula. This tension is

necessary to prevent the second needle from lacerating the suture in the cannula. The same procedure is repeated for passing this limb. Once this second limb of the suture is passed and the needle is removed, it is clamped to the first limb. As all subsequent stitches are placed, care is taken to keep them organized on an Allis clamp to avoid confusing or tangling the sutures.

After all of the sutures have been passed, tension is placed on them to ensure adequacy of the repair. The sutures are sequentially tied from posterior to anterior. The knee is placed in full extension while tying the sutures. Care should be taken while tying to place adequate tension to repair the meniscus, but not so much that the suture breaks or pulls

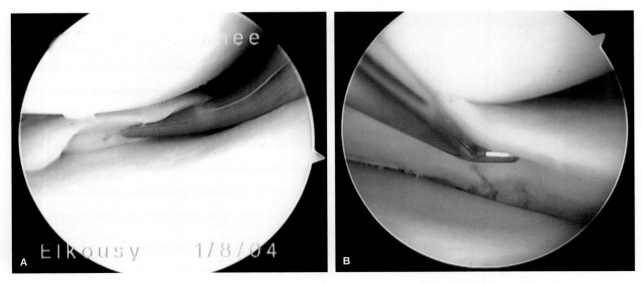

Fig. 50-13. A: Suture being placed on undersurface of meniscus. **B:** Vertical mattress suture on undersurface of meniscus.

51

MENISCAL ALLOGRAFT TRANSPLANTATION

CHRISTOPHER I. ELLINGSON, MD, JON K. SEKIYA, MD, CHRISTOPHER D. HARNER, MD

■ HISTORY OF THE TECHNIQUE

The menisci's role in load transmission and stability in the knee has been well documented since Fairbank's important work in 1948.[1-7] Meniscal injuries that result in damage or loss of the meniscus alter knee biomechanics and lead to degenerative changes of the knee.[7-11] Situations in which a partial or total meniscectomy are required have posed a difficult management issue, especially in young active patients. While meniscal allograft transplantation has emerged over the past 20 years as a viable treatment option for these patients, the surgical techniques continue to be refined.

Milachowski performed the first isolated meniscal allograft transplant in 1984 and reported his results in 22 patients with second look arthroscopy performed at 14 months.[12] Garrett[13] used an early open technique for meniscal transplantation with takedown of the MCL with a piece of bone off the femur. Secondary to the soft tissue trauma associated with open techniques, the use of mini-arthrotomies and arthroscopic methods are now the procedures of choice for meniscal allograft transplantation.

Meniscal allografts are available fresh, cryopreserved, fresh-frozen, or freeze-dried. Most meniscal allografts implanted today are fresh-frozen or cryopreserved. The use of fresh grafts is logistically difficult as they can be stored for only 7 days, allowing inadequate time for serological testing and sizing of grafts. The use of freeze-dried grafts is not recommended secondary to alterations in the biomechanical properties and size of these grafts. Cryopreservation of grafts maintains cell viability between 10% to 40%, but donor cell viability has not shown any clinical advantage and these cells are quickly replaced by host cells.[14] Fresh-frozen allograft preservation is simpler and more inexpensive than cryopreservation. The lack of cell viability in fresh-frozen grafts has not appeared to affect allograft survival and meniscal transplantation outcomes. Meniscal allograft sizing can be performed utilizing computed tomography (CT), magnetic resonance imaging (MRI), plain radiographs, or direct measurement. Most surgeons and tissue banks use the consistent relationship between plain radiographic landmarks and meniscal size for sizing allografts.[15] Shaffer et al.[16] evaluated MRI for allograft sizing and found only 35% measured to within 2 mm and there was not a significant difference when compared to plain radiographs.

■ INDICATIONS AND CONTRAINDICATIONS

Meniscal transplant in the meniscus-deficient knee should be considered only after nonoperative treatment modalities have failed to relieve symptoms or prevent progression of joint space narrowing. These nonoperative modalities include unloading braces, nonimpact activity modification, and pharmacological measures. An exception to this guideline is in patients with combined anterior cruciate ligament (ACL) and medial meniscus deficient knees who exhibit significant anteromedial rotatory instability (AMRI). In these select patients earlier intervention with a combined ACL reconstruction and medial meniscal transplantation may improve stability, ACL graft survival, and clinical outcome.[4,7,17-20]

Indications for meniscal transplant are patients under age 40 (upper limits of 50 in select cases) with an absent or nonfunctioning meniscus. These patients should have pain localized to the involved compartment associated with activities of daily living or sports. Mechanical alignment of the involved extremity must be normal and articular cartilage changes limited to Outerbridge grade I or II in the involved compartment.

Contraindications include age >50, Outerbridge grade IV articular cartilage changes, bony architectural changes (osteophytes), and significant varus/valgus malalignment or knee instability (unless addressed concurrently with an additional procedure).

Preoperative evaluation includes inspection of stance and gait, knee range of motion, joint line palpation, muscle strength, presence or absence of effusion, and ligamentous stability. Radiographs should be obtained using radiographic markers to include weight bearing posterior-anterior 45-degree flexion, merchant, and non–weight bearing lateral knee films. Long leg alignment films allow objective evaluation for varus/valgus malalignment. MRI can be used as an adjunct to provide information regarding the hyaline cartilage, subchondral bone, and menisci. Finally, a diagnostic arthroscopy can define the extent of the meniscal deficiency and arthrosis, but this adds the morbidity of an additional surgical procedure.

■ SURGICAL TECHNIQUES

Medial Meniscal Transplantation

The patient is positioned supine on a radiolucent table. After induction of general anesthesia via endotracheal tube, an exam under anesthesia is performed to document knee stability and range of motion. A nonsterile tourniquet is then placed about the patient's proximal thigh. A sandbag is taped to the table on the ipsilateral side transversely so as to allow the foot of the surgical leg to rest against it and hold the knee flexed. Additionally, a post is placed along the lateral aspect of the affected thigh, thereby allowing hands-free knee flexion and positioning during the case. After sterile prepping and draping, the medial and lateral borders of the patellar tendon are identified and marked along with standard arthroscopy portals. The incision for a posteromedial approach to the knee is drawn with a skin marker. Diagnostic arthroscopy is then performed to document the degree of meniscus deficiency and condition of the articular cartilage in the involved compartment. Once the diagnostic arthroscopy confirms the appropriateness of meniscal transplant the allograft is thawed and reconstituted in antibiotic solution according to standard protocol. We may use a femoral distractor positioned across the knee joint to provide valgus stress in order to open the medial compartment for meniscal debridement and graft passage. Arthroscopic debridement of the remaining native meniscus is performed to expose a remaining bleeding rim of 1 to 2 mm. This bleeding rim of native meniscus is left as a vascular source to aid in graft healing.

A posteromedial approach to the knee is performed in the interval between the medial collateral ligament and the posterior oblique ligament. The infrapatellar branch of the saphenous nerve should be carefully identified and protected in the proximal portion of this incision. The interval between the MCL and the posterior oblique ligament is incised, creating a posteromedial arthrotomy used for graft passage.

Medial meniscus allograft fixation is obtained using bone plugs through transosseous tunnels placed at the native medial meniscus insertion sites (Fig. 51-1A,B,C). A medial parapatellar arthrotomy is utilized for this, with extension distal enough to allow for placement of these tunnels using an ACL guide and a 7-mm drill. The allograft medial meniscus is prepared by debriding soft tissue from its rim and shaping the bone plugs to 7 mm in diameter. The posterior plug is often most difficult to pass and a shorter bone plug aids in its insertion. A no. 5 nonabsorbable suture (Ethibond) or no. 2 fiber wire is secured to each of the bone plugs to aid in graft passage and for fixation of the graft.

The graft is passed through the medial parapatellar arthrotomy with the knee in slight flexion (10 degrees to 20 degrees) and a valgus force. A Hewson suture passer is placed through the transosseous tunnels into the knee to pass the anterior and posterior bone plug sutures through their respective tunnels (Fig. 51-1B). Once this is accomplished and the graft is reduced, the sutures are tied together over the bone bridge between the tunnels to secure the anterior and posterior horns in the tunnels (Fig. 51-1C). The meniscal allograft is then secured to the remaining rim of bleeding native meniscal tissue using an inside-out technique with a monofilament absorbable suture beginning in the posteromedial corner.

The meniscal allograft is inspected arthroscopically to ensure proper positioning and fixation. All wounds are copiously irrigated and closed using an absorbable braided 2-0 suture for subcutaneous reapproximation followed by staples or nylon suture for the skin. A sterile dressing is placed with an elastic wrap from toes to thigh.

Lateral Meniscal Transplantation

The positioning, draping, evaluation under anesthesia, and arthroscopy are performed as described above. An incision for a posterolateral approach to the knee is drawn with a skin marker. Again, after confirmation by arthroscopy the graft is thawed in antibiotic solution. We may use a femoral distractor positioned across the knee joint to provide varus stress in order to open the lateral compartment for meniscal debridement and graft passage. The lateral meniscus is debrided back to a 1- to 2-mm rim of bleeding remnant. A small lateral parapatellar arthrotomy is made which will be used for graft passage. A small posterolateral approach is made through an incision over the posterior border of the lateral collateral ligament. The interval between the iliotibial band and the biceps femoris is incised in line with the fibers toward the Gerdy tubercle. Deeper dissection is then made between the lateral collateral ligament and the lateral gastrocnemius tendon to expose the posterolateral joint capsule. This will be used later for meniscal allograft suturing using an inside-out technique.

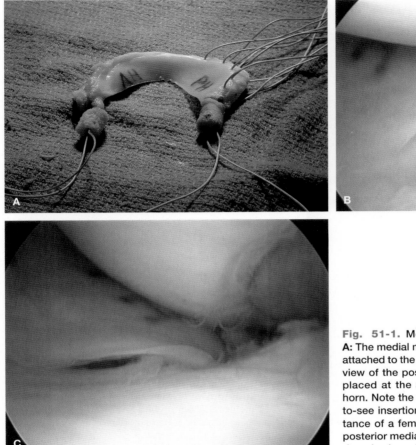

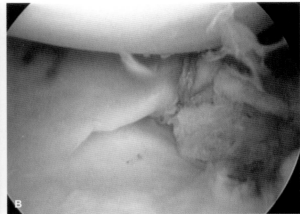

Fig. 51-1. Medial meniscal allograft transplantation. **A:** The medial meniscal allograft fashioned with bone plugs attached to the anterior and posterior horns. **B:** Arthroscopic view of the posterior horn pulled into the posterior tunnel placed at the anatomic insertion of the native posterior horn. Note the excellent visualization of this often difficult-to-see insertion site—this is accomplished with the assistance of a femoral distractor. **C:** Arthroscopic view of the posterior medial meniscal insertion site anatomically reproduced using a bone plug.

The shape of the lateral meniscus is more semicircular than the medial meniscus, which places the anterior and posterior horn insertion sites within 10 mm of each other.[21] Because of this close proximity of the horns, lateral meniscal allografts are fashioned and fixed using a bone bridge trough. A small quarter-inch curved osteotome or chisel is used to create a trough in the medial aspect of the lateral tibial plateau from the anterior to posterior horn insertion sites of the lateral meniscus. The osteotome can be placed through the anteromedial portal with the curve facing medially toward the ACL tibial insertion. A second cut is made approximately one-fourth inch lateral to the first, taking care to keep both in the sagittal plane and parallel to each other. The bone between these cuts can then be removed to create the preliminary bone trough. Bone trough gouges of known sizes (usually 7 to 9 mm) are used to finish the creation of the tibial trough to a specific size. The trough size is verified with a trough sizer to ensure the depth and width are sufficient.

Two transosseous tunnels are placed using the ACL drill guide and two guide pins from the anteromedial tibial cortex through the tibial plateau bone trough. These tunnels should be spaced at least 10 mm apart. Hewson suture passers are placed through these tunnels for later graft passage and fixation. The bone bridge for the meniscal allograft is fashioned to match the size of the tibial plateau trough and two no. 5 braided nonabsorbable (or no. 2 FiberWire) sutures are placed through two drill holes to match the distance between the transosseous tibial trough tunnels. Additionally, a no. 2 braided nonabsorbable suture is placed in the posterolateral corner of the allograft to act as a passing suture.

The anterior and posterior bone bridge sutures are passed through their respective transosseous tibial tunnels using the Hewson suture passers. The posterolateral passing suture is passed through the posterolateral joint capsule using a hemostat. The meniscus allograft is then placed through the arthrotomy and reduced in the lateral compartment by pulling on the 3 passing sutures **(Fig. 51-2A)**. Care must be taken to keep the graft properly oriented and the sutures untangled. Passage is aided by use of the femoral distractor or by placing the knee in the figure-four position. After reduction is verified by arthroscopy and palpation the transosseous sutures are tied to each other over the bone bridge between the two tunnels, thereby securing the anterior and posterior horns of the meniscus allograft. The meniscus allograft is then secured using an inside-out technique with a nonabsorbable 2-0 suture (Figs. 51-2B, 51-2C).

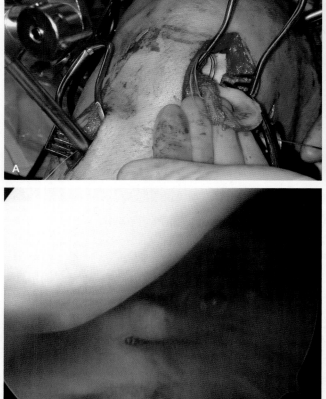
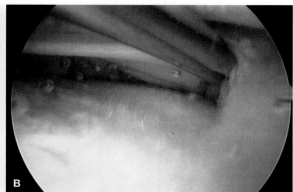

Fig. 51-2. Lateral meniscal allograft transplantation. **A:** The lateral meniscal allograft with the bone bridge securing the anterior and posterior horns is passed through a lateral parapatellar arthrotomy. **B:** Arthroscopically placed inside-out vertical mattress sutures secure the lateral meniscal allograft to the periphery. **C:** Second-look arthroscopy at 6 weeks postsurgery showing the healed meniscal allograft with a red-red peripheral rim encroaching upon the repair sutures.

The meniscal allograft is inspected arthroscopically to ensure proper positioning and fixation. All wounds are copiously irrigated and closed using an absorbable braided 2-0 suture for subcutaneous reapproximation followed by staples or nylon suture for the skin. A sterile dressing is placed with an elastic wrap from toes to thigh.

Meniscus Transplantation Combined with ACL Reconstruction

Meniscus transplantation with ACL reconstruction can be performed concomitantly in combined injuries, particularly in cases of failed ACL surgery secondary to subtotal medial meniscectomy with subsequent development of AMRI.[22] We utilize standard femoral and tibial tunnels, and our preferred graft choice is allograft patellar tendon, in order to decrease the added morbidity from this already complex surgical procedure. ACL graft passage and fixation is usually performed after the meniscus transplantation has been performed. ACL reconstruction combined with lateral meniscus transplantation requires special care as the tibial tunnel often encroaches on the bone trough for the meniscal allograft. We caution the use of a trough technique for medial meniscal allografts, as the anterior and posterior horns of the native medial meniscus are often in line with the ACL,

thereby risking damage to the ACL or encouraging potential medializing of the horn attachments.

■ TECHNICAL ALTERNATIVES AND PITFALLS

For the arthroscopically placed meniscal repair sutures, we strongly recommend an inside-out technique utilizing vertical mattress sutures. While several other techniques have become popular, including meniscal arrows and other devices, none have compared to the superior strength of the vertical mattress suture. Given the importance of a secure repair for meniscal allograft healing and function, we recommend the technique that has proven to remain the gold standard for meniscal fixation over time.

In addition, significant controversy exists regarding the type of fixation for the meniscal allograft anterior and posterior horns. While several basic science studies exist showing the superiority of bony fixation at time zero in cadaveric models, no clinical studies have been published comparing suture to bony fixation. In our own series, the only significant improvements in outcomes between bony and suture fixation regarding isolated lateral meniscal transplantation was with range of motion, with all other parameters showing no differences (Sekiya JK, Groff YJ, Irrgang JJ, et al., unpublished data, 2004). While we still recommend bony fixation for the horns of our meniscal allograft, the clinical significance may be minimal. One of the authors (JKS) uses bony fixation for both medial and lateral transplants while the senior author (CDH) has abandoned the use of bone plugs for medial transplants.

Recently, one of the authors (JKS) has begun utilizing a femoral distractor to aid in opening of the medial or lateral compartment for debridement of the native meniscus and assistance with graft passage (Sekiya JK, Bonner KF, Kurtz CA, unpublished data, 2004). The femoral distractor can be placed in a fashion as to allow positioning of the knee in a flexed position with varus or valgus stress and to open the medial or lateral compartments, respectively. This significantly improves visualization for allograft fixation, as well as assists with graft passage, particularly with the often difficult posterior bone plug for the medial meniscus.

■ REHABILITATION

Postoperatively the patients are started on a continuous passive motion (CPM) machine 24 hours after surgery and continued until 90 degrees of flexion is obtained. The postoperative range of motion goal is to achieve full extension equivalent to the contralateral knee within 1 week and flexion to 90 degrees by 4 to 6 weeks. A range of motion brace is worn and patients are restricted to partial weight bearing with crutches immediately after surgery. Patients do follow-up with a physical therapist and are started immediately on quadriceps sets, straight leg raises, heel slides, and calf pumps. Crutches are discontinued after approximately 4 to 6 weeks provided the patient has full knee extension without quadriceps lag, minimal swelling, flexion to 90 degrees, and is able to walk without a bent-knee gait. Closed chain exercises are started 6 weeks postoperatively from 0 degrees to 45 degrees of flexion and slowly increased to 75 degrees. Postoperative physical therapy is continued for 2 to 3 months with emphasis on restoration of full range of motion and strength. After 8 weeks low impact aerobic exercises are allowed to include stationary bike. Patients are allowed to resume running at approximately 6 months but return to strenuous sports is not recommended.

■ OUTCOMES AND FUTURE DIRECTIONS

Our results in the recent literature for both isolated meniscal transplantation and for those performed in conjunction with ACL reconstruction have been promising. Yoldas et al.[23] published a 2-year follow-up on 31 meniscal transplants of which 20 were combined with ACL reconstructions. Thirty of the 31 patients had a normal or nearly normal rating according to International Knee Documentation (IKDC)

knee function and activity level and 19 of 20 combined procedures were normal or nearly normal according to IKDC stability testing. Average single leg hop and vertical jump was 85% of the contralateral limb and no progressive joint space narrowing was seen with radiographic examination.

Sekiya et al. evaluated 25 patients that had undergone isolated lateral meniscal transplantation at an average follow-up of 3.3 years (Sekiya JK, Groff YJ, Irrgang JJ, et al., unpublished data, 2004). Seventeen patients had bony fixation and 8 patients had suture fixation of the anterior and posterior horns of the meniscal allograft. Ninety-six percent of patients felt that their overall function and activity level were improved following surgery. The SF-36 physical and mental component summary scores were higher for these subjects than age- and gender-matched scores from the general population. No significant joint space narrowing of the transplanted lateral compartments was seen when compared with the joint space narrowing of the lateral compartment of the contralateral knee. Interestingly, preoperative and postoperative radiographic joint space measurements of the involved lateral compartment were significantly correlated with subjective assessment, symptoms, sports activity score, Lysholm score, and final IKDC rating at latest follow-up. In addition, patients fixed using the bony technique had significantly better range of motion according to IKDC criteria at latest follow-up compared to the suture fixation group.

Sekiya et al.[18] also evaluated 28 combined meniscal transplantations with ACL reconstructions at an average follow-up of 2.8 years. Eighty-six percent to 90% of the patients had normal or nearly normal scores according to IKDC overall subjective and symptoms assessment, while the average SF-26 physical and mental component summary scores were at higher levels in the patients compared to their age and sex-matched population. Lachman and pivot shift testing were normal or nearly normal in 90%, and KT-1000 testing at both 20 pounds and maximal manual revealed an average of 1.5 mm of increased anterior translation compared with the normal, contralateral knee. As in prior studies, no joint space narrowing was observed over time with radiographic examination.

Graf et al.[17] evaluated 9 patients following combined medial meniscal transplantation and ACL reconstruction with an average follow-up of 10 years. One meniscal allograft was removed postoperatively due to a presumed low-grade infection, although cultures failed to identify an organism. IKDC symptoms were normal or nearly normal in 7 of 8 patients, and 7 of the 8 patients also remained at their preoperative radiographic scores without progression. Six of 8 patients had normal or nearly normal scores according to IKDC functional testing, were extremely pleased with the function of their knees, and were very active in recreational sports. All 8 patients would recommend the procedure to a friend and would undergo the procedure again if under similar circumstances.

Meniscal transplantation continues to evolve as a viable treatment for difficult meniscal injuries requiring partial or total meniscectomy, often performed in conjunction with ACL reconstruction. Surgical techniques stress the importance of indications/contraindications, limb alignment and stability, graft sizing, graft placement, and graft fixation. Studies to evaluate technical aspects of surgery and long-term clinical outcomes remain in progress as this procedure continues to evolve.

■ REFERENCES

1. Allen CR, Wong EK, Livesay GA, et al. Importance of the medial meniscus in the anterior cruciate ligament-deficient knee. J Orthop Res. 2000;18:109–115.
2. Fukubayashi T, Kurosawa H. The contact area and pressure distribution pattern of the knee: a study of normal and osteoarthritic knee joints. Acta Orthop Scand. 1980;51:871–879.
3. Hsieh HH, Walker PS. Stabilizing mechanisms of the loaded and unloaded knee joint. J Bone Joint Surg. 1976;58A:87–93.
4. Levy IM, Torzilli PA, Warren RF. The effect of medial meniscectomy on anterior posterior motion of the knee. J Bone Joint Surg. 1982;64A:883–887.
5. Markolf KL, Mensch JS, Amstutz HC. Stiffness and laxity of the knee—the contributions of supporting structures. J Bone Joint Surg. 1976;58A:583–594.
6. Walker PS, Erkman MJ. The role of the meniscus in force transmission across the knee. Clin Orthop. 1975;109:184–192.
7. Fairbank TJ. Knee joint changes after meniscectomy. J Bone Joint Surg. 1948;30B:664–670.
8. Allen PR, Denham RA, Swan AV. Late degenerative changes after meniscectomy: factors affecting the knee after the operation. J Bone Joint Surg. 1984;66B:666–671.
9. Appel H. Late results after meniscectomy in the knee joint: a clinical and roentgenologic follow-up investigation. Acta Orthop Scand Suppl. 1970;133.
10. Johnson RJ, Kettlekemp DB, Clark W, et al. Factors affecting late results after meniscectomy. J Bone Joint Surg. 1974;56A:719–729.
11. Tapper EM, Hoover NW. Late results after meniscectomy. J Bone Joint Surg. 1969;69A:517–526.
12. Milachowski KA, Weismeier K, Wirth CJ. Homologous meniscus transplantation: experimental and clinical results. Int Orthop. 1989;13:1–11.
13. Garrett JC. Meniscal transplantation: a review of 43 cases with 2- to 7-year follow-up. Sports Med Arthrosc Rev. 1993;2:164–167.
14. Jackson DW, Windler GE, Simon TM. Cell survival after transplantation of fresh meniscal allografts: DNA probe analysis in a goat model. Am J Sports Med. 1993;21:540–549.
15. Pollard ME, Kang Q, Berg EE. Radiographic sizing for meniscal transplantation. Arthroscopy. 1995;11:684–687.
16. Shaffer B, Kennedy S, Klimkiewicz J, et al. Preoperative sizing of meniscal allografts in meniscal transplantation. Am J Sports Med. 2000;28:524–533.
17. Graf KW, Sekiya JK, Wojtys EM. Long-term results following meniscal allograft transplantation: minimum eight and one half-year follow-up. Arthroscopy. 2004;20:129–140.
18. Sekiya JK, Giffin RJ, Irrgang JJ, et al. Clinical outcomes after combined meniscal allograft transplantation and anterior cruciate ligament reconstruction. Am J Sports Med. 2003;31(6):896–906.
19. Shelbourne KD, Gray T. Results of anterior cruciate ligament reconstruction based on meniscus and articular cartilage status at the time of surgery: five- to fifteen-year evaluations. Am J Sports Med. 2000;28:446–452.
20. Shelbourne KD, Stube KC. Anterior cruciate ligament (ACL)-deficient knee with degenerative arthrosis: treatment with isolated autogenous patellar tendon ACL reconstruction. Knee Surg Sports Traumatol Arthrosc. 1997;5:150–156.
21. Johnson DL, Swenson TM, Livesay GA, et al. Insertion-site anatomy of the human menisci: gross, arthroscopic, and topographical anatomy as a basis for meniscal transplantation. Arthroscopy. 1995;11:386–394.
22. Sekiya JK, Elkousy HA, Harner CD. Meniscal transplant combined with anterior cruciate ligament reconstruction. Op Tech Sports Med. 2002;10:157–164.
23. Yoldas EA, Sekiya JK, Irrgang JJ, et al. Arthroscopically assisted meniscal allograft transplantation with and without combined anterior cruciate ligament reconstruction. Knee Surg Sports Traumatol Arthrosc. 2003;11:173–182.

52

HIGH TIBIAL OSTEOTOMY

STEPHEN J. FRENCH, MD, J. ROBERT GIFFIN, MD, PETER J. FOWLER, MD

■ HISTORY OF THE TECHNIQUE

High tibial osteotomy (HTO) for knee pain or disability related to arthrosis is a time-tested procedure. It is generally agreed that in the lower limb, arthrosis is frequently associated with malalignment, that the load across the knee joint is a function of alignment, and that changes in the axial alignment of the femur or tibia in either the coronal or sagittal plane will influence the distribution of this load, resulting in abnormal stresses on articular cartilage.[1] It follows that the assessment and correction of alignment, if indicated, must be at the forefront in the treatment algorithm when considering the management of knee arthrosis.

A primary goal of osteotomy, regardless of anatomical site or technique, is to reposition the weight-bearing line so that the load distribution through the knee is normal or as close to normal as possible, minimizing stresses on the affected compartment.[2,3] While "appropriate" postoperative alignment has been studied extensively, there is no clear consensus as to the correction angle when performing an osteotomy in the younger patient with a cartilage defect.[4-6]

It has been recently suggested by some that in valgus producing high tibial osteotomy, the weight-bearing line should be relocated from the middle to outer third of the lateral compartment.[7] We would argue that this amount of correction is excessive, and based on the work of Dugdale et al.,[8] in the patient with arthrosis, we prefer a weight-bearing line that intersects at a point 62% of the tibial width from the edge of the medial plateau to produce a mechanical axis of 3 degrees to 5 degrees. One should be cautioned against the recommendations of Coventry,[9] Cass and Bryan,[10] and Rudan and Simurda[11] to accept an anatomic valgus of greater than 10 degrees. In the younger patient with

malalignment and articular cartilage lesions, an excessively large correction angle may not be required, and repositioning the weight-bearing line to neutral or just beyond, medially or laterally, is sufficient.

■ INDICATIONS AND CONTRAINDICATIONS

With respect to realignment osteotomy about the knee, Morrey[12] reported that valgus osteotomy can be offered with confidence in those with secondary degenerative arthritis, a varus knee, and localized medial joint pain. The indications for knee osteotomy **(Table 52-1)**, however, are not confined to a deviation in mechanical axis (malalignment) with arthrosis. When knee instability is associated with malalignment, a realignment osteotomy may help restore stability, improve symptoms, and possibly delay the progression of arthrosis.[13] Sagittal imbalance can be of particular interest in instability, and in these situations the role of the tibial slope must be taken into consideration and addressed when a corrective osteotomy is planned. Malalignment in the setting of any articular cartilage restoration procedure is a clear indication for an osteotomy prior to or in combination with the cartilage restoration or "protection" procedure such as meniscal allograft or anterior cruciate ligament reconstruction.

The treatment options for younger patients with isolated cartilage lesions are unfortunately limited. Consequently, the list of contraindications to knee osteotomy in this group is relatively short. Although a realignment osteotomy through the knee to transfer the load bearing axis away from the lesion may be a viable treatment, severe degeneration in the opposite tibiofemoral compartment and a gross loss of

TABLE 52-1	Indications for Knee Osteotomy

Malalignment *and* Arthrosis	Malalignment *and* Instability	Malalignment *and* Arthrosis *and/or* Instability	Malalignment *and* Articular Cartilage Procedure *and/or* Instability

range of motion will certainly affect the outcome and are relative contraindications. A valgus osteotomy should be avoided in those who have previously undergone a lateral meniscectomy.[14] However, in the very young patient this should be considered only a relative contraindication, and in the case of severe varus alignment, a high tibial osteotomy to correct to a neutral alignment will preserve favorable joint mechanics **(Table 52-1 and Table 52-2)**.

■ SURGICAL TECHNIQUES

Alignment is determined by the line extending from the center of the hip to the center of the ankle (i.e., the mechanical axis of the limb).[15] This line typically passes immediately medial to the center of the knee, and by definition, malalignment occurs when this line does not lie close to the center of the knee.[16,17] Sagittal plane alignment should also be evaluated by measuring the posterior tibial slope angle (i.e., the angle between a line perpendicular to the mid-diaphysis of the tibia and the posterior inclination of the tibial plateau on a lateral radiograph). The average tibial slope angle has been shown to be 10 ± 3 degrees.[18]

■ VARUS KNEE

Techniques to realign the varus knee include the classic lateral closing wedge osteotomy, medial opening wedge

osteotomy (preferred in most situations by the senior authors), and osteotomy with external fixation.

Lateral Closing Wedge High Tibial Osteotomy

Currently, our only indication for this procedure is a previous lateral closing wedge osteotomy of the contralateral limb. When required, our preferred method for a lateral closing wedge as described by Coventry,[3] is performed through an incision made along a line from the lateral epicondyle over the Gerdy tubercle extending distally just lateral to the tibial tubercle. This incision is slightly curved if the knee is flexed at 90 degrees, and straight when the knee is in the extended position **(Fig. 52-1A,B)**. The iliotibial band is identified distally and partially elevated by sharp dissection off the Gerdy tubercle. The common peroneal nerve is identified by palpation posterior to the fibular head. It is not routinely dissected free, however, careful attention to its protection throughout the procedure is required. The fibular head is not routinely osteotomized, but if this is required to close the osteotomy, the proximal tibiofibular joint is released. Soft tissues from the posterior aspect of the tibia are also released. A retractor is placed subperiosteally and posteriorly to protect the neurovascular structures and to facilitate carrying out the osteotomy under direct vision. The upper limb of the osteotomy is made 2 cm below and parallel to the joint line. The appropriate-sized wedge is then marked, cut, and removed, and any remaining posterior cortical bone and medial cancellous bone are removed using bone rongeurs, small curettes, and up-cutting Kerrison rongeurs.

Appropriate wedge size is calculated using a modification of the Noyes method, wherein the wedge removed is measured as the height of the angle subtended by the axes of the femur and tibia from the point of the desired position of the weight-bearing axis in the knee following the corrective osteotomy.[19] The measured length of the proposed osteotomy is transposed to a measure along the axis of the femur, and the distance between the femoral and tibial axis at this point is the width of the wedge to be removed.

TABLE 52-2	Specific Indications for Individual Osteotomy Techniques					
	Varus <25°	Varus >25°	Valgus <15°	Valgus >15°	Increased tibial slope	Decreased tibial slope
Medial opening HTO	X					
Lateral closing HTO	X					
Medial closing HTO			X			
Lateral opening HTO			X			
Ex-fix HTO		X			X	X
Anterior closing HTO					X	
Anterior opening HTO						X

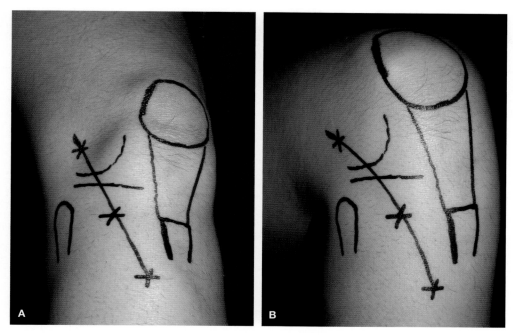

Fig. 52-1. Surface anatomy and approach for lateral tibial closing wedge osteotomy. **A:** Incision made along a line from the lateral epicondyle over the Gerdy tubercle extending distally just lateral to the tibial tubercle. **B:** This incision is slightly curved if the knee is flexed at 90 degrees and straight when the knee is in the extended position.

The osteotomy is closed with the knee in extension and fixed with one or two stepped staples **(Fig. 52-2A,B)**. Care is taken to ensure that the posterior tibial slope has not been decreased due to failure to complete the osteotomy posteriorly, to remove cortical bone from the osteotomy site, or to adequately release the proximal tibiofibular joint, when required.

Technical Alternatives and Pitfalls

Technical points to be appreciated include: adequate visualization anteriorly beneath the patellar tendon to confirm osteotomy of the anterior cortex; complete exposure of the posterior tibia; protection of the neurovascular structures

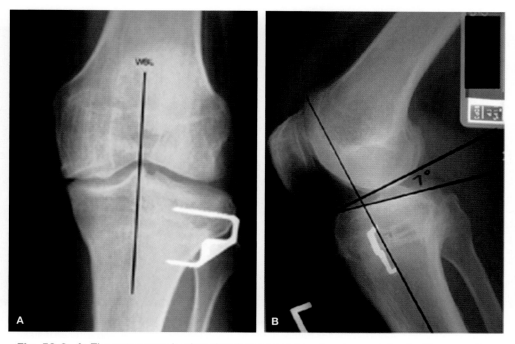

Fig. 52-2. A: The osteotomy is closed with the knee in extension and fixed with one or two stepped staples. **B:** Care is taken to ensure that the posterior tibial slope has not been decreased.

TABLE 52-3	Perils and Pitfalls Corrective Osteotomy	
	Perils	**Pitfalls**
All osteotomies	Adequate exposure Use of intra-op fluoroscopy and guide pins Accurate pre-op planning and radiographic evaluation	Violation of opposite cortex Making asymmetrical bone cuts in sagittal plane Opening the osteotomy before the anterior and posterior cortices are osteotomized
High tibial lateral closing	Make osteotomy 2 cm distal to lateral joint line Complete posterior cortical resection in piecemeal fashion with Kerrison rongeurs	Decreasing tibial slope inadvertently
High tibial medial opening	Use oscillating saw to breach cortex only Make osteotomy below the guide pin Pay particular attention when securing osteotomy plate	Suboptimal guide pin positioning Neglecting the posterior tibial slope when making the osteotomy

with a curved, blunt retractor placed directly on the bone and for large corrections, adequate exposure, and mobilization of the proximal tibiofibular joint **(Table 52-3)**. The osteotomy is made 2 cm distal to the lateral joint line to ensure that the proximal fragment is sufficiently large to avoid the risk of avascularity and violation of the tibial tubercle.

As with all osteotomies of the proximal tibia, there is a tendency to alter the tibial slope if careful attention is not paid to maintain the tibial slope when creating the osteotomy. Fluoroscopy to confirm that the osteotomy has been completed along the anterior and posterior tibial margins and that the medial tibial cortex has been left intact will help avoid an unstable construct. If the medial cortex is breeched, the osteotomy must be considered to be "unstable" and to have a greatly increased risk of nonunion, and plate and screw, rather than staple fixation, is then recommended. As mentioned, completion of the posterior cortical bone

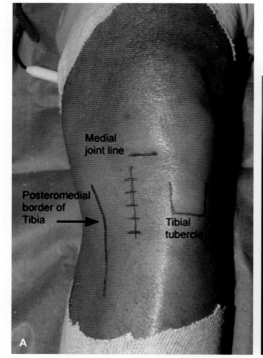
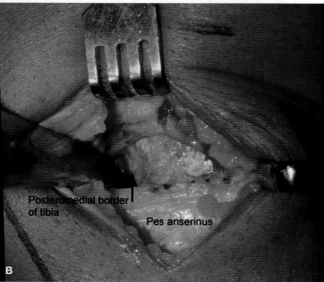

Fig. 52-3. The surgical approach to medial opening wedge HTO is shown. **A:** The skin incision is centered between the posteromedial border of the tibia and the tibial tubercle and extends distally from the medial joint line. **B:** The posteromedial border of the tibia is exposed with a blunt retractor placed deep to the superficial MCL. The pes anserinus is left intact.

resection with pituitary and Kerrison rongeurs or small bone curettes will minimize risk of damage to the posterior neurovascular structures.

Medial Opening Wedge High Tibial Osteotomy

Our preferred technique of medial opening wedge high tibial osteotomy is a modification of the technique described by Puddu et al.[20] This method allows correction of deformity in all planes and in particular allows planned alterations to tibial slope in the sagittal direction.

The procedure is carried out through a vertical skin incision, which extends 5 cm distally from the medial joint line and is centered between the anterior tubercle and the posteromedial border of the tibia **(Fig. 52-3A)**. The gracilis and semitendinosus tendons and the superficial medial collateral ligament are preserved and retracted medially to expose the posteromedial border of the proximal tibia (Fig. 52-3B). A guide pin is inserted obliquely along a line proximal to the tibial tubercle from approximately 4 cm below the medial joint line in the region of the transition between metaphyseal and diaphyseal cortical bone on radiographs extending to a point 1 cm distal to the lateral joint line.

Figure 52-4 illustrates the opening wedge technique, which is monitored throughout with a mobile, low-dose ionizing radiation fluoroscopy unit. The osteotomy is made below the guide pin using a small oscillating saw to breech the medial, anteromedial, and posteromedial cortices. This is followed by narrow, sharp, thin, flexible osteotomes to a point just 1 cm short of the lateral cortex. Frequent imaging helps prevent violation of the lateral cortex or misdirection of the osteotome. The osteotomy is

opened gradually to the desired correction angle first with distracting osteotomes to confirm the mobility of the osteotomy and then a calibrated wedge to the appropriate measured distraction. The distracted osteotomy is then fixed with a 4-hole Puddu plate secured with two 6.5-mm cancellous screws proximally and two 4.5-mm cortical screws distally. Bone grafting is recommended in all opening wedge osteotomies greater than 7.5 mm. Allograft cancellous bone chips or tricortical blocks may be used unless there is an expressed desire by the patient for autograft bone. In our practice osteotomies less than 7.5 mm are rarely grafted.

Technical Alternatives and Pitfalls

Dissection of the most superior fibers of the patellar tendon insertion on the tibial tubercle improves exposure and protects the patella tendon when completing the anterior extent of the corticotomy, which must be distal to the patella tendon insertion. The use of a low-dose ionizing radiation fluoroscope throughout the procedure is critical to ensure all of the following: proper guide-pin placement; prevention of lateral cortex violation; avoidance of osteotome misdirection; avoidance of intra-articular screw placement, and adequate sealing of the bone graft and filling of the defect (Table 52-3).

The tip of the fibular head is a helpful reference when aiming the guide pin. The correct obliquity of the osteotomy relies on proper placement of the guide pin. For larger corrections, placement should be more horizontal. Greater obliquity increases the risk of fixation failure but, on the other hand, provides increased depth, which may be appropriate for smaller corrections.

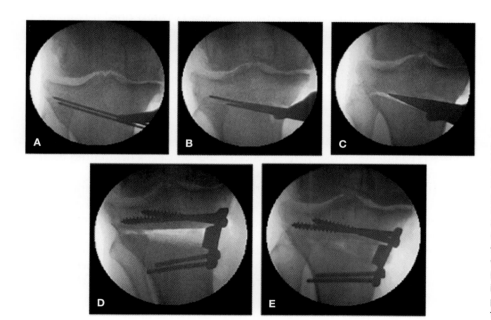

Fig. 52-4. The use of intraoperative fluoroscopy during medial opening wedge HTO is shown. **A:** The guide pin is directed toward the tip of the fibular head and from a point 4 cm distal to the medial joint line. Placement should be optimal before proceeding. **B:** The osteotomy is made *below* the guide pin. **C:** The osteotomy is gradually opened to the desired width using a calibrated wedge. **D:** Fixation is achieved with a 4-hole Puddu plate. Care is taken to avoid intra-articular or intraosteotomy screw placement. **E:** Here the defect has been filled with tricortical bone graft.

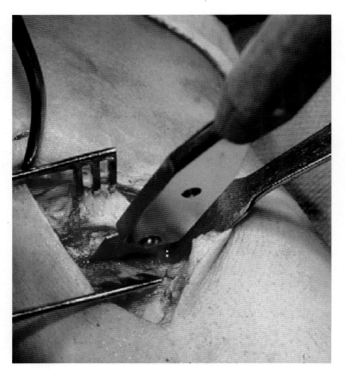

Fig. 52-5. Thin flexible osteotomes used to complete the osteotomy. The osteotomy can then subsequently be opened with distracting osteotomes to the desired correction. This applies less distraction on the initial bone cut and thus decreases the chance of intra-articular fracture.

The osteotomy should always be carried out parallel to the joint line in the sagittal plane and below the guide pin to help prevent intra-articular fracture. The use of thick, traditional type osteotomes can apply a greater distraction moment when completing the osteotomy and carries an inherent risk of creating an extra or intra-articular fracture. This is considerably minimized with thin, flexible osteotomies **(Fig. 52-5)**. However, these should be advanced with frequent fluoroscopy checks to avoid misdirection.

To avoid altering the posterior tibial slope, the distraction of the osteotomy anteriorly (at the tibial tubercle), should be approximately one half its distraction posteromedially. This is facilitated by using trapezoidal distraction block Puddu plates rather then the traditional rectangular version. The plate should be positioned as far posterior as possible along the medial cortex to ensure that the distraction is maximized posteromedially and minimized anteriorly. Careful attention to this detail will help decrease the risk of increasing tibial slope upon distraction of the osteotomy.

Tension of the medial collateral ligament (MCL) should be assessed during distraction, and lengthening by fenestration (of the MCL) may assist in achieving larger corrections.

Finally, strict attention to detail is necessary to avoid intra-articular or intraosteotomy screw penetration during fixation of the plate and to ensure that the defect is completely obliterated with bone graft or a substitute. Frequent rechecks with fluoroscopy are beneficial.

Osteotomy with External Fixation Systems

Various external fixation devices may be employed to address large or multiplanar deformities. As described by Catagni et al.,[21] the Ilizarov frame in the treatment of genu varum addresses both the bony and soft tissue components of the deformity. According to these authors, osteotomy distal to the tibial tuberosity allows slight lateral translation of the tibia, which decreases the amount of angular correction required and allows for correction of the tension on the ligamentous and capsular structures. While medial compartment arthritis and posttraumatic deformity are most amenable to acute correction, skeletally mature patients with residual Blount disease deformity and the younger population with idiopathic genu varum may be best treated with gradual correction.

External frames are recommended for deformities greater than 20 degrees to 25 degrees of mechanical varus requiring gradual correction. For the adult population with unicompartmental arthrosis or joint line obliquity and ligament deficiency we do not routinely employ external fixators for correction.

■ VALGUS KNEE

Realignment of the valgus knee may be approached from the femoral or tibial side. Each of these approaches, according to some authors, may have a negative mechanical consequence.[18] All techniques, femoral or tibial, opening or closing, have a place in the treatment of the valgus deformity. Varus-producing proximal tibial osteotomy in patients with lateral compartment arthrosis has been regarded as controversial due to the tendency to result in joint line obliquity.[9,22]

Coventry,[9] taking both the anatomical axis and the tilt of the plateau into consideration, recommended a supracondylar femoral varus osteotomy if the valgus deformity is more than 12 degrees or if the postoperative tilt of the tibiofemoral joint surface exceeds 10 degrees. Chambat et al.,[23] on the other hand, advocates that all valgus deformities be corrected from the tibial side.

Here, too, although opinions are more uniform than in proximal tibial valgus osteotomy, the degree of correction suggested varies. Several authors recommend correcting the valgus knee to a 0 degree tibiofemoral angle.[22,24] According to Morrey and Edgerton,[25] in the valgus knee the mechanical axis should be repositioned medial to the medial spine. Phillips and Krakow[26] recommend a mechanical axis of 4 degrees varus.

Proximal Tibial Varus Osteotomy

A proximal tibial varus osteotomy is recommended for smaller valgus deformities or those localized to the tibia (which can occur after trauma or lateral meniscectomy).[27] One can perform a lateral opening wedge rather than the medial closing wedge of Coventry,[9] Shoji and Insall,[28] or Chambat et al.[23] The senior authors prefer an opening wedge treatment with the benefits of restoration of the anatomy in the circumstance of primarily a tibial deformity. The incidence of delayed or nonunion of the osteotomy site has not been an issue.

Lateral Opening Wedge Osteotomy

The lateral opening wedge osteotomy is carried out through an oblique skin incision similar to that for the lateral closing wedge made with the knee extended. The osteotomy is oblique, starting 4 cm distal to the lateral joint line just distal to the proximal tibiofibular joint and above the insertion of the patellar tendon and ending 1 to 2 cm distal to the medial articular surface. The fibula is not osteotomized. Residual medial laxity secondary to lengthening of the MCL ligament is less commonly encountered with this technique. This procedure is valuable for corrections of less then 10 mm. The medial structures are not weakened as they are with a medial closing wedge procedure, and dissection around the pes anserinus is avoided.

Medial Closing Wedge Osteotomy

The approach for the medial closing wedge osteotomy is similar to medial opening wedge with posterior retraction of the pes anserinus tendons and the superficial MCL. The osteotomy is made 2 to 3 cm distal to the joint line and then a wedge of predetermined size is removed. The superficial MCL is not violated and reefing or plication of the ligament is not required. Fixation is achieved with one or two osteotomy staples. With respect to alignment, Coventry[9] states that overcorrection is undesirable, and that one should aim for a postoperative weight-bearing line that passes through the center of the knee. This approach may be appropriate for small corrections such as an osteotomy for joint leveling combined with an anterior cruciate ligament (ACL) reconstruction.

■ ALTERED TIBIAL SLOPE

While less clinically prevalent, altered tibial slope in the sagittal plane can add to knee instability and create an altered wear pattern and arthrosis. It may be encountered in the primary ligament deficient knee or in the case of a revision of a failed reconstruction and must be corrected to create a stable joint for ligament reconstruction.

Excessive tibial slope, greater then 13 degrees, results in translation of the tibia and creates an increased chondral wear pattern and alters the joint mechanics and meniscal load sharing. Similarly, decreased tibial slope of less then 7 degrees as a unilateral deformity is considered pathologic.[29] These cases of abnormal alignment will stress the cruciate ligaments and could contribute to graft failure in the setting of an ACL or posterior cruciate ligament (PCL) reconstruction.

Joint realignment procedures for altered tibial slope are approached anteriorly, with either an anterior closing wedge osteotomy for increased tibial slope or an opening wedge osteotomy for decreased tibial slope.

Closing Wedge Osteotomy

Utilizing a similar incision as that used for the medial opening wedge osteotomy, drawn slightly more anterior, the pes tendons are retracted and exposure is carried back to the posteromedial border of the tibia. Adequate visualization across the anterior tibia must be attained to guide the osteotomy. The osteotomy is completed immediately proximal to the tibial tubercle, and the appropriate-sized wedge of bone is removed (1 mm anterior wedge for 1.5 degrees to 2 degrees correction), with the posterior cortex maintained intact initially. The posterior cortex is then fenestrated with a 3.2-mm drill (with careful attention to the adjacent neurovascular structures) to allow a controlled fracture of the posterior cortex while closing the osteotomy to avoid destabilization. The osteotomy is then fixed with one or two staples. Decreasing tibial slope would shift the tibia posteriorly and improve ACL instability.

Opening Wedge

The skin incision is carried down along the medial border of the patellar tendon. The osteotomy is done at the proximal pole of the tibial tubercle. A tibial tubercle osteotomy can be very beneficial for exposure and the reattachment can be done at a length which will not change the position of the patella relative to the femur. The principal tibial osteotomy is oblique, based on the guide pin position. It runs anterior to posterior from distal to proximal, starting roughly 40 mm distal to the joint line and ending 7 to 10 mm from the joint line posteriorly. This avoids the posterior fibers of the PCL and negates any disruption of the proximal tibiofibular joint.

The osteotomy is opened to the desired correction with careful maintenance of the posterior cortex, which is fenestrated with a 3.2-mm drill to increase the flexibility of the hinge while avoiding destabilization of the osteotomy. The osteotomy is packed with bone graft when required and fixed with an anterior Puddu plate and screws. Increasing tibial slope would shift the tibia anteriorly and improve PCL instability.

■ TECHNICAL ALTERNATIVES AND PITFALLS

Complications and Management

The list of possible intraoperative, early postoperative, and late postoperative complications following any realignment procedure around the knee is exhaustive. Some common surgical complications have been outlined that may occur and require supervised or active intervention. We would agree with Coventry[30] that the early complications of upper tibial osteotomy are those of any other surgical operation on the lower extremity. These, as well as some complications that require specific mention, should be included in any list of complications of osteotomy around the knee, namely: infection, neurovascular injury, delayed or nonunion, deep vein thrombosis, and pulmonary embolus.

Also, the possible intraoperative complications of any osteotomy are especially prevalent with osteotomy around the knee. These include intra-articular fracture, intra-articular screw placement, and violation of the opposite cortex with resultant instability of the osteotomy. Prevention of these complications by continuous fluoroscopy use is the best form of management. Otherwise, early recognition and immediate management would be suggested.

Uncontrolled Fracture

Intra-articular fracture should be assessed intraoperatively with fluoroscopy and a decision made whether interfragmentary screw stabilization is required.

A fracture detected postoperatively may require internal fixation with or without revision of the osteotomy or a simple modification of the postoperative rehabilitation protocol with immobilization and nonweight bearing for a period with radiographic monitoring of the fracture.

Violation of the opposite cortex in an opening wedge osteotomy of the tibia usually does not require any additional treatment. In a closing wedge osteotomy of the tibia, the opposite cortex, if violated and unstable, may require additional fixation or modification of the postoperative protocol to prevent loss of correction. If during a distal femoral osteotomy stability is lost due to a violation of the opposite cortex, this opposite cortex should be secured with internal fixation through a separate approach.

Complications of distal femoral osteotomy are essentially the same as in proximal tibial osteotomy: delayed or nonunion, infection, and under- or overcorrection are the main concerns.[26]

Under- or Overcorrection

Numerous authors have discussed overcorrection into valgus.[4,23,28,31,32] Because, cosmetically, producing a valgus deformity is less well tolerated than producing varus alignment, it is best to err on the side of "avoiding excessive valgus."

Critical assessment of the alignment both intraoperatively and in the early postoperative period should take place, and if "overcorrection" or "excessive" varus or valgus correction has occurred, the osteotomy should be revised, as the primary surgical goals have not been attained.

Thromboembolic Event

The frequency of thromboembolic disease is lower following osteotomy than total knee arthroplasty, and the proper method of prophylaxis is controversial.[7] We currently do not use chemical prophylaxis in patients undergoing knee osteotomy. Mobilization is encouraged on postoperative day 1. Patients with specific risk factors for deep venous thromboembolism (DVT) or pulmonary embolism (PE) are anticoagulated with low molecular weight heparin given subcutaneously for the perioperative period and undergo lower limb venous studies prior to discharge from hospital. Patients with a past history of DVT or PE are anticoagulated for 6 weeks with warfarin sodium.

■ REHABILITATION

Early postoperative knee range of motion (ROM) exercises benefit joint healing and articular cartilage nourishment, as well as lower limb neuromuscular function. In addition, the return to normal weight bearing is essential for healthy bone turnover and healing. Postoperative physical therapy programs should focus on these components while respecting the desired outcomes of the realignment procedure, which include union and restoring and maintaining alignment **(Table 52-4)**.

Range of Motion

The restoration of full ROM is an important factor in the long-term success of the surgical procedure and we encourage ROM exercises to begin as soon as possible. Full extension should be achieved by postoperative week 6. If progress is behind schedule, active exercises with slight volitional overpressure are recommended.

Weight Bearing

The weight-bearing progression will depend on the type of osteotomy and any other cartilage restoration procedure performed. Following opening wedge osteotomy patients are restricted to touch weight bearing equivalent to 25 to 40 lb for the first 6 weeks. If any osteocartilaginous procedure has been performed in combination, the opening wedge protocol takes preference. Following closing wedge osteotomy, we allow protected weight bearing for the first 6 weeks. If a cartilage restoration procedure has also been performed, a partial weight-bearing protocol should take preference.

TABLE 52-4	Postoperative Rehabilitation Guidelines

Timeline	Exercise
0–3 wk	• Passive range of motion using slider board • Pedal rocking on bicycle • Isometric quadriceps setting
3–6 wk	• Full circle pedaling on bicycle—very light resistance • Active range of motion • Side lying gluteus medius strengthening • Hip ab/adduction, flexion and extension with resistance fixed above knee, i.e., pulley or resistance tubing • Pool exercises—hip ab/adduction, flexion and extension, knee flexion and extension • Gait pattern training with crutches focusing on proper heel strike/toe off • Pool—deep water running or cycling • Leg press or squat with weight off-loaded to 24–40 lb (watch ROM restriction associated with any cartilage/meniscus restoration/repair)
6–9 wk	• Pool—shallow water walking as weight-bearing restrictions allow • As a general guideline when 60% of body is submerged, 60% of body weight is off-loaded • Standing/seated calf raise • Bilateral wobble board balancing as weight-bearing status allows • Knee flexion/extension with very light resistance
Upon full weight bearing	• Gait training to restore normal gait • Step up and step down to work on alignment and eccentric control • Elliptical trainer and bicycle for cardiovascular conditioning

From the 6-week mark, the progression of weight bearing is dependant on the appearance of the radiograph of the osteotomy. It would be anticipated that any closing wedge osteotomy could progress to weight bearing as tolerated with the use of a cane or a single crutch, if consolidation and progression to union are occurring. An opening-wedge osteotomy should progress to partial weight bearing for 3 weeks and then to protected weight bearing for 3 weeks if consolidation is evident on the radiograph and there is no evidence of hardware loosening or change in position (Table 52-4).

Neuromuscular Rehabilitation

Neuromuscular programs aimed at maintaining surrounding joint strength and muscle function, as well as pain management modalities, should be employed during the initial postoperative 6 weeks.

During weeks 6 to 12, a more functional program can be instituted and methods to improve muscular endurance can be instituted after postoperative week 12. Gait retraining and returning to a fully functional state should be additional goals throughout the rehabilitation process. More directed therapy to correct other functional impairments in addition to the above should also take place after week 12.

■ RESULTS

Successful long-term results following realignment osteotomy are linked to careful patient selection, accurate surgical technique, appropriate surgical correction, and dedicated postoperative rehabilitation (Table 52-5).[7] The current literature reports on the results of series of patients treated with osteotomy for unicompartmental arthrosis; however, few have looked at the results of osteotomy around the knee in combination with a cartilage restoration procedure.

Many clinical series for osteomies about the knee have been presented, however, the influence of a nonhomogenous patient population, nonstandardized operative procedures and rehab protocols, the variety of indications for osteotomy, patient selection, and technical challenges make long-term outcomes difficult to interpret. The objective results of an osteotomy must be examined in respect to the surgical goals of the procedure. When reviewing the data surrounding osteotomies, we have found it very useful to interpret presented series in respect to the stated goals of the series rather then as results of a procedure in general.

Valgus High Tibial Osteotomy

Hernigou et al.[4] reported their results in a group of 93 knees that had been treated by proximal tibial opening wedge osteotomy for varus deformity and medial compartment osteoarthritis. After a mean follow up of 11.5 years, symptomatic relief had deteriorated with time, at an average of 7 years after the osteotomy. Alignment, however, was also found to be a determinant of long-term results. After 5 years 90% of the knees had good or excellent results, while after 10 years, only 45% (42 knees) were good or excellent. In the 20 knees with a postoperative hip-knee-ankle angle of 183 degrees to 186 degrees, there was no pain and no progression of

TABLE 52-5 | **Results**

Author	Date	Type	Number of knees	Avg. F/U (yr)	Avg. Age (yr)	Type of study	Results (%)	Comments
Hernigou et al.[4]	1987	MO	93	11.5	60.3	R	Good or excellent rating: 90% at 5 yr 45% at 10 yr 73% satisfactory 26% failures at 4.5 yr (avg.)	Time and alignment major determinants to long-term results Significant early complications
Morrey[12]	1989	LC	34	7.5	31.3			
Yasuda et al.[32]	1992	LC ex. fix	56	11.25	59.8	R	Survival: 63% at 6 yr 18% at 10+ yr	11 knees evaluated by telephone interview at 10+ years and included only in the clinical analysis of knee function Knee joint function remained favorable for approx. 5–10 yr but deteriorated gradually after 10 yr
Coventry et al.[5]	1993	LC	87	10		R	Survival: 87% at 5 yr 66% at 10 yr	Relative weight (less than 1.7) and angular correction (>5 degree valgus) only risk factors associated with improved duration of survival
Billings et al.[33]	2000	LC*	64	8.5	49	R	33% failures at 5.5 yr (avg.) Survival: 87% at 5 yr 53% at 10 yr	
Shoji and Insall[28]	1973	MC HTO	49	2.6	60.2	R	61% persistent instability 47% persistent pain 6% lacking desired mobility	Results compared to previously published series of HTO for varus deformity and found to be "far inferior"
Coventry[9]	1987	MC HTO	31	9.4	59	R	77% mild/no pain 20% failure (TKA) at 9.8 yr (avg.)	Tibiofemoral angle of >12 degrees or post-op obliquity of joint line of >10 degrees may be indications for DFVO Correction to 0 degrees anatomical tibiofemoral alignment is recommended
Cass et al.[10]	1988		86	Min. 5		R	Satisfactory: 94% at 2 yr 87% at 5 yr 69% at 10 yr 36% failed (TKA)	
Rudan and Simurda[11]	1991	LC	128	7.5	58.5	R	HSS Scores 78% G/E/ at 6–9 yr 70% G/E at 10+ yr 10.9% revision rate	Equal prognosis for men and women in uncontrolled groups No significant difference in results in patients older than 60 yr compared to younger than 60 yr

MO medial opening; G/E good/excellent; HSS Hospital for Special Surgeries; LC lateral closing; LC* calibrated guide + rigid internal fixation; MC medial closing; HTO high tibial osteotomy; DFVO distal femoral varus osteotomy; R retrospective; TKA total knee arthroplasty arthrosis. In those that were undercorrected (an angle of less than 183 degrees), the results were less satisfactory and there was a tendency to a slow deterioration. In the 5 knees that were overcorrected (angle more than 186 degrees), all had progressive degenerative changes in the lateral compartment.

Morrey[12] reported on 34 consecutive lateral closing wedge osteotomies in 33 patients with an average age of 31.3 years with secondary arthritis. At an average follow up of 7.5 years, 24 (73%) were satisfactory with improved pain and mean activity level, while 9 were failures with 5 requiring total knee arthroplasty at a mean of 4.5 years after osteotomy (range 2 to 8 years).

Yasuda et al.[32] showed that overcorrection (femorotibial angle of 164 degrees to 168 degrees) was, in their patients, associated not only with better long-term clinical results but also with a marked decrease in the loss of valgus correction between 1 and 10 years. They evaluated 56 of 86 knees, but only 45 knees clinically and radiographically, with an average follow up of 11 years 3 months, and found an 88% survival at 6 years and a 63% survival at 10 years.

Coventry et al.[5] reported their results on lateral closing wedge proximal tibial osteotomy, a follow up on 87 knees at a median of 10 years. Using moderate or severe pain, or conversion to arthroplasty as a definition of failure, they found an 87% survival free of failure at 5 years, and a 66% survival at 10 years. They found relative patient weight and angular correction to be the only risk factors associated with the duration of survival. If valgus angulation at 1 year was less than 8 degrees in a patient whose weight was more than 1.32 times the ideal weight, the rate of survival decreased to 38% at 5 years and to 19% at 10 years thereafter. While these results indicate that patient body mass and angulation correction factor into the survival of the osteotomy, the number of patients in each subgroup, however, was not reported.

Billings et al.[33] reported the long-term results of 64 knees after valgus osteotomy using a calibrated osteotomy guide and rigid internal fixation at an average of 8.5 years. They found 21 knees (33%) had undergone a total knee arthroplasty at an average of 65 months, and the survivorship analysis showed an expected rate of survival, with conversion to a total knee arthroplasty as the end point, of 85% at 5 years and 53% at 10 years.

Varus High Tibial Osteotomy

Results of proximal tibial varus osteotomy have previously not equaled those of proximal tibial valgus osteotomy.

Shoji and Insall[28] reported "far inferior" results with regards to retention of mobility, relief of pain, and achievement of stability in a group of 49 varus osteotomies that were compared to a previously published series of 63 valgus osteotomies.

Coventry[9] reported 24 (77%) of 31 knees to have no pain or only occasional mild pain at an average of 9.4 years after a closing wedge varus osteotomy for valgus knees with painful osteoarthritis of the lateral compartment. The remaining 7 still had moderate or severe pain at follow up.

Recently, Marti et al.[27] reported 88% good or excellent results at a mean follow up of 11 years using a lateral opening wedge varus osteotomy. These late results are better than those previously described by Harding,[34] and certainly seem to reflect more favorably on the lateral opening wedge osteotomy for correction of valgus deformity less than 15 degrees.

Anterior Opening Wedge High Tibial Osteotomy

Moroni et al.[35] reported on 25 patients, average age 23 years, at an average of 14.5 years after 27 opening wedge osteotomies of the proximal part of the tibia for genu recurvatum. They found that when the osteotomy was performed proximal to the tibial tuberosity with detachment of the tuberosity (18 knees) 78% had good or excellent results, while of the 5 that were performed distal to the tuberosity only 1 had a good result. They also found that in the 21 knees with an entirely or predominantly osseous deformity, 86% achieved a good or excellent result, while those in which the deformity was predominantly in the soft tissues had only fair or poor results because of an increased obliquity of the tibial plateau (overcorrection).

Our experience is similar and we would recommend an osteotomy proximal to the tibial tuberosity for correction of pathologic genu recurvatum.

■ SUMMARY AND FUTURE DIRECTIONS

The natural history of the focal chondral defect in the meniscectomized knee has not been precisely determined.[36] Our knowledge of the postmeniscectomized knee, however, would lead us to look at these knees with additional pathology in the same light. The prognosis, if left untreated, is guarded.

The approach of the orthopaedic surgeon in the treatment of articular cartilage lesions, therefore, should be comprehensive. Not only should it include realignment to "off-load" the diseased compartment, as discussed here, but also procedures to allow regeneration or replacement of articular cartilage.

Our future direction looks at establishing normal alignment and joint stability as the foundation for successful treatment of articular cartilage lesions. It is to be hoped that the combination of joint realignment procedures, in combination with cartilage repair therapies in development, will enable improved results for the treatment of articular cartilage lesions in the knee.

Case 52-1

Thirty-one-year-old male with isolated medial compartment articular cartilage disease, varus malalignment, and intact ACL and PCL. **A:** The AP view shows the weight bearing line (WBL) through the center of the medial compartment and the predicted correction angle. **B:** Postoperatively, the mechanical axis of the limb is normalized.

Case 52-2

Thirty-seven-year-old elite athlete with lateral compartment arthrosis and a PCL deficient right knee. **A:** Preoperative bilateral standing AP views reveal WBL passing directly through the center of the right knee, but more laterally than in the normal contralateral knee. **B:** A varus producing lateral opening wedge HTO was carried out to off-load the diseased lateral compartment. **C:** Pre- and **(D)** postoperative lateral views demonstrate that the proximal tibial slope angle (PTSA) was not altered, despite the patient's PCL deficiency. Posterolateral tibial degeneration was observed on arthroscopic examination and to avoid a flexion deformity.

Case 52-3

Seventeen-year-old female with symptomatic varus hyperextension thrust of the right knee shown in the clinical photo **(A)**. **B:** Preoperative AP radiographs demonstrate varus alignment with opening of the lateral joint space. **C:** The axial alignment has been improved. **D:** The preoperative PTSA of 0 degrees has been increased to 8 degrees **(E)**.

Case 52-4

Thirty-one-year-old male with a recurvatum deformity of the knee as a result of a tibial diaphyseal malunion. **A:** Preoperative radiograph demonstrates a decreased PTSA which exacerbated his symptoms. **B:** Following anterior opening wedge osteotomy performed through the bed of a tibial tubercle osteotomy, the PTSA is increased.

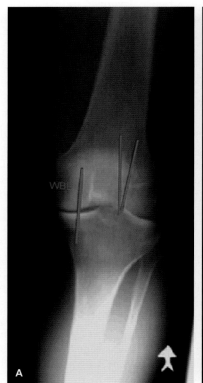
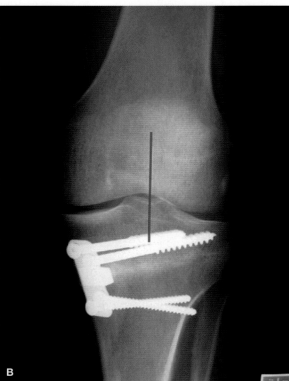

Case 52-1

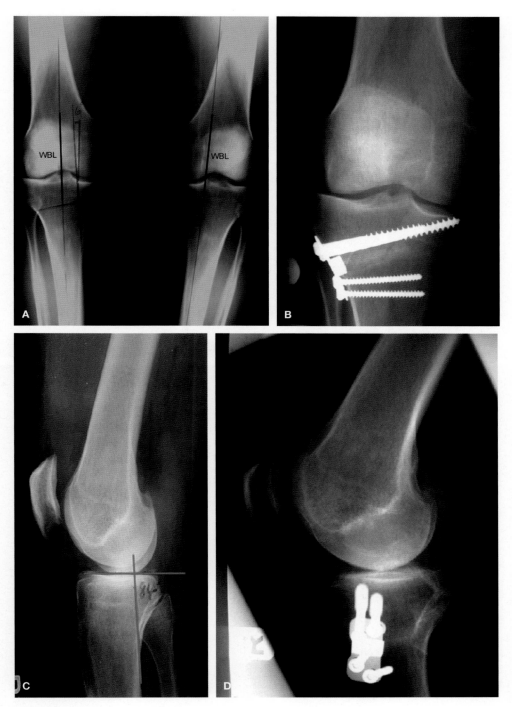

Case 52-2

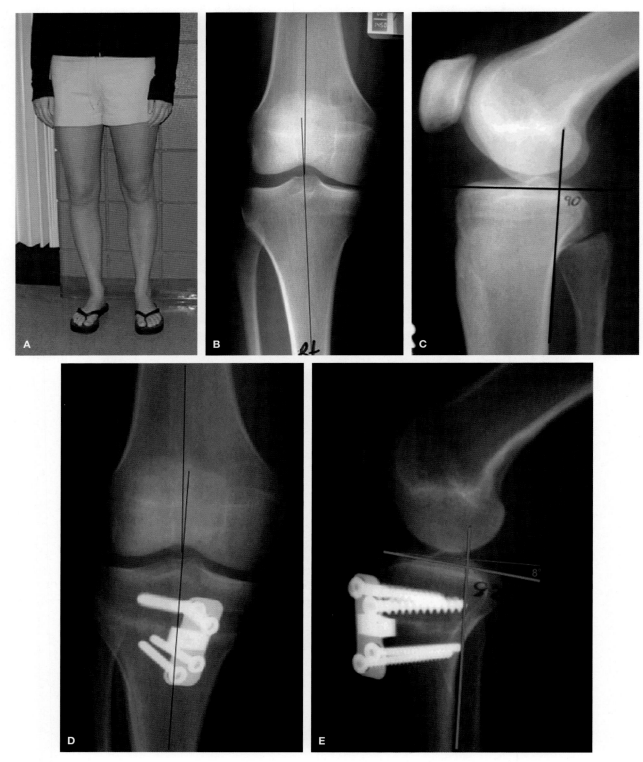

Case 52-3

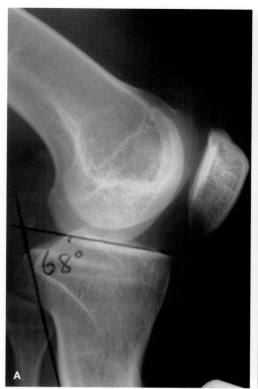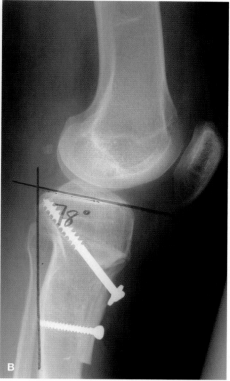

Case 52-4

■ REFERENCES

1. Cooke TDV, Pichora DS. Knee dysplasia: an unusual but important problem associated with progressive arthritis. J Bone Joint Surg Br. 1985;67:332.
2. Maquet P. The biomechanics of the knee and surgical possibilities of healing osteoarthritic knee joints. Clin Orthop Rel Res. 1980;146:102–110.
3. Coventry MB. Upper tibial osteotomy for gonarthrosis. The evolution of the operation in the last 18 years and long term results. Orthop Clin North Am. 1979;10:191–210.
4. Hernigou P, Medevill D, Debeyre J, et al. Proximal tibial osteotomy with varus deformity: a ten to thirteen year follow-up study. J Bone Joint Surg Am. 1987;69:332.
5. Coventry MB, Ilstrup DM, Wallrich SL. Proximal tibial osteotomy: a critical long-term study of 87 cases. J Bone Joint Surg Am. 1993;75:196.
6. Dugdale TW, Noyes FR, Styer D. Pre-operative planning for high tibial osteotomy. Clin Orthop. 1992;274:248–264.
7. Hanssen AD, Stuart MJ, Scott RD, et al. Surgical options for the middle-aged patient with osteoarthritis of the knee joint. AAOS Instr Course Lect. 2001;50:499–511.
8. Dugdale TW, Noyes FR, Styer D. Pre-operative planning for high tibial osteotomy. Clin Orthop. 1992; 274: 248–264.
9. Coventry MB. Proximal tibial varus osteotomy for osteoarthritis of the lateral compartment of the knee. J Bone Joint Surg Am. 1987;69:32–38.
10. Cass JR, Bryan RS. High tibial osteotomy. Clin Orthop Rel Res. 1988;230:196–199.
11. Rudan JF, Simurda MA. Valgus high tibial osteotomy: a long-term follow-up study. Clin Orthop. 1991;268:157–160.
12. Morrey BF. Upper tibial osteotomy for secondary osteoarthritis of the knee. J Bone Joint Surg Br. 1989;71:554–559.
13. Badhe NP, Forster IW. High tibial osteotomy in knee instability: the rationale of treatment and early results. Knee Surg Sports Traumatol Arthrosc. 2002;10:38–43.
14. Morrey BF. Upper tibial osteotomy for secondary osteoarthritis of the knee. J Bone Joint Surg Br. 1989;71:554–559.
15. Paley D, Herzenberg JE, Tetsworth K, et al. Deformity planning for frontal and sagittal plane corrective osteotomies. Orthop Clin North Am. 1994;25:465.
16. Moreland JR, Bassett LW, Hanker GJ. Radiographic analysis of the axial alignment of the lower extremity. J Bone Joint Surg Am. 1987;69:749.
17. Hsu RWW, Himeno S, Coventry MB, et al. Normal axial alignment of the lower extremity and load-bearing distribution of the knee. Clin Orthop Rel Res. 1990;255:215–217.
18. Giffin RJ, Vogrin TM, Zantop T, et al. Effects of increasing tibial slope on the biomechanics of the knee. Am J Sports Med. March 2004;32(2):376–382.
19. Dugdale TW, Noyes FR, Styer D. Preoperative planning for high tibial osteotomy. Clin Orthop. 1992;274:248–264.
20. Puddu G, Franco V. Femoral antivalgus opening wedge osteotomy. Oper Tech Orthop. 2000;8:56–60.
21. Catagni MA, Guerreschi F, Ahmas TS, et al. Treatment of genu varum in medial compartment osteoarthritis of the knee using the Ilizarov method. Orthop Clin North Am. 1994;25:509–514.
22. McDermott GP, Finkelstein JA, Farine I, et al. Distal femoral varus osteotomy for valgus deformity of the knee. J Bone Joint Surg Am. 1988;70:110–116.
23. Chambat P, Selmi TAS, Dejour D, et al. Varus tibial osteotomy. Oper Tech Orthop. 2000;8:44–47.

24. Learmouth ID. A simple technique for varus supracondylar osteotomy in genu valgum. J Bone Joint Surg Br. 1990;72:235–237.

25. Morrey BF, Edgerton BC. Distal femoral osteotomy for lateral gonarthrosis. Instr Course Lect. 1992;41:77–85.

26. Phillips MJ, Krakow KA. Distal varus osteotomy: Indications and surgical technique. AAOS Instr Course Lect. 1999;48:129.

27. Marti RK, Verhagen RAW, Kerkhoffs GMMJ, et al. Proximal tibial varus osteotomy: Indications, technique and five to twenty-one-year results. J Bone Joint Surg Am. 2001;83:164–170.

28. Shoji H, Insall J. High tibial osteotomy for osteoarthritis of the knee with valgus deformity. J Bone Joint Surg Am. 1973;55:963–973.

29. Dejour D, Bonin N, Locatelli E. Tibial antirecurvatum osteotomies. Oper Tech Sports Med. 2000;8(1):67–70.

30. Coventry MB. Upper tibial osteotomy for osteoarthritis. J Bone Joint Surg Am. 1985;67:1140.

31. Insall JN, Joseph DM, Msika C. High tibial osteotomy for varus gonarthrosis: a long-term follow-up study. J Bone Joint Surg Am. 1984;66:1040–1048.

32. Yasuda K, Majima T, Tsuchida T, et al. A 10- to 15-year follow-up observation of high tibial osteotomy in medial compartment osteoarthrosis. Clin Orthop. 1992;282:186–195.

33. Billings A, Scott DF, Camargo MP, et al. High tibial osteotomy with a calibrated osteotomy guide, rigid internal fixation, and early motion. Long-term follow-up. J Bone Joint Surg Am. 2000;82:70–79.

34. Harding ML. A fresh appraisal of tibial osteotomy for osteoarthritis of the knee. Clin Orthop. 1976;114:234.

35. Moroni A, Pezzuto V, Pompili M, et al. Proximal osteotomy of the tibia for the treatment of genu recurvatum in adults. J Bone Joint Surg Am. 1992;74:577–586.

36. Cole BJ, Harner CD. Degenerative arthritis of the knee in active patients: evaluation and management. J Am Acad Orthop Surg. 1999;7:389–402.

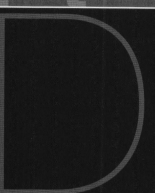

Part

D

PATELLOFEMORAL AND EXTENSOR MECHANISM PROBLEMS

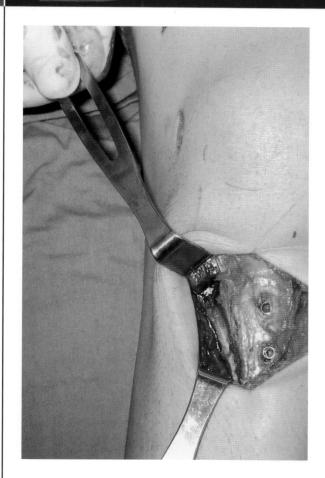

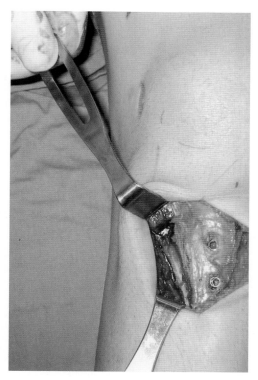

Fig. 53-5. Fixation following the tubercle transfer. Note the tubercle was transferred about 1 cm medially.

amount of distalization is determined by the preoperative 30-degree flexion lateral view.

Once the angle of the cut has been determined, a small oscillating saw is used to perform the osteotomy. The retractors are used to adequately visualize the blade exiting the anterolateral cortex. The distal portion of the cut is not completed, just tapered to a hinge. The proximal portion of the osteotomy, just superior to the patellar tendon insertion, is completed using a quarter-inch curved osteotome. This proximal cut connects the medial and lateral edges of the osteotomy and prevents the osteotomy from extending into the tibial plateau.

Once the osteotomy is complete, a half-inch straight osteotome is used to pivot the tubercle. The bone pedicle is hinged distally and pushed up the inclined plane. Once the tubercle is hinged, it is transferred about 1 cm medially. Again, the amount of translation is determined by the degree of instability and chondrosis.

The tubercle is then temporarily held in place with a 2/32 Steinmann pin. The position is then confirmed by clinical exam, including range of motion, patellar tracking, glide, and tilt. Two parallel 4.5-mm bicortical screws are then used to fix the osteotomy (Fig. 53-5). These screws are placed using the AO technique for compression. The mini C-arm is then used to confirm the position of the osteotomy and the two screws. Patellar height can also be checked with the C-arm.

The patellar glide is rechecked. If excessive lateral patellar glide persists (greater than 2 quadrants), a medial imbrication is performed. The incision for the imbrication is placed just off the medial border of the patella. The incision is carried through the skin and subcutaneous tissue. The bursa is then incised to expose the medial retinaculum/medial patellofemoral ligament (Fig. 53-6). This retinaculum is then incised, taking care to preserve the underlying synovial layer. A pants-over-vest imbrication, using 2-0 Surgidac suture in a horizontal mattress, is performed (Fig. 53-7). The knots are tied in extension. However, range of motion of the knee is checked to confirm that the sutures do not limit flexion.

After thorough irrigation, the fascia of the anterior compartment is then closed with no. 0 absorbable suture. The subcutaneous tissue is then closed with 2-0 absorbable sutures. A running 4-0 absorbable stitch is placed in a subcuticular fashion. Steri-strips are then applied, followed by a sterile dressing and Cryocuff. An ELS brace, locked in full extension, is then applied (Fig. 53-8).

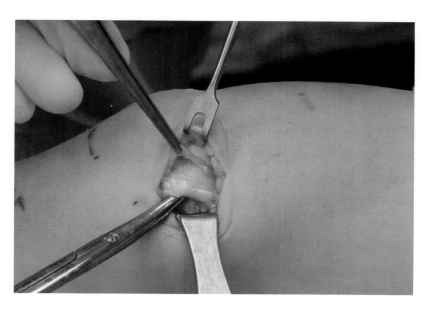

Fig. 53-6. Medial imbrication, showing the bursa superiorly and the medial patellofemoral ligament inferiorly.

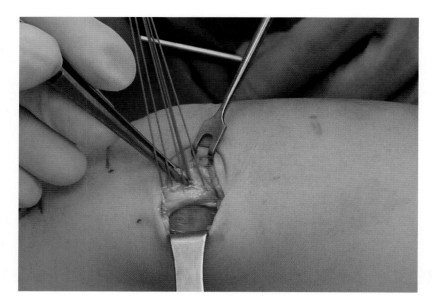

Fig. 53-7. Medial imbrication, following the suture placement.

■ TECHNICAL ALTERNATIVES AND PITFALLS

Arthroscopic lateral release can be performed instead of an open release. The same structures are addressed during both procedures. The superficial and deep layers of the retinaculum need to be sectioned. Care should be taken to limit the release of the most distal fibers of the vastus lateralis (vastus lateralis obliquus). Overrelease of this tendon can result in a prolonged rehabilitation, medial patellar subluxation, and quadriceps weakness.

Common pitfalls exist through every phase of the treatment of patellar instability, including patient selection, operative technique, and postoperative rehabilitation. A few major pitfalls will be reviewed.

It is important to determine the amount of patellar instability and chondrosis from history, clinical examination, and arthroscopic evaluation. Ignoring significant chondrosis and

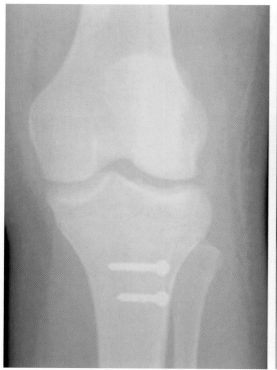
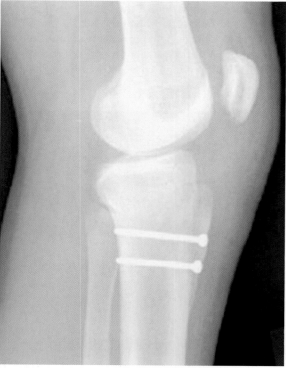

Fig. 53-8. Postoperative AP (A) and Lateral (B) radiographs.

only addressing the instability with a medialization of the tubercle (flat osteotomy) can worsen the patellofemoral chondrosis symptoms. The patellofemoral joint reaction forces are altered with a tibial tubercle transfer. The forces on the lateral patellar facet and distal patellar pole are decreased, while the proximal forces are increased. Therefore, diffuse or proximal patellar chondrosis should not be treated with anteromedialization. The increased joint reaction forces can exacerbate the symptoms and progression of the arthritis.

Another pitfall is the failure to recognize medial patellar instability, which is usually an iatrogenic condition. Medial instability usually results from an extensive lateral release, with injury to the VLO or the vastus lateralis. Treating a patient with medial patellar subluxation with anteromedialization of the tubercle can result in devastating symptoms.

Pitfalls of the lateral release include excessive release, incomplete release, inadequate hemostasis, and releasing a patella to track onto deficient articular cartilage. During the release, whether arthroscopic or open, excellent visualization and hemostasis is mandatory. Postrelease, patellar tilt should be 70 degrees to 90 degrees. Care should be taken to preserve the VLO insertion.

Pitfalls during the osteotomy include too shallow of a cut, which results in little cancellous bone and mostly cortical bone to transfer. This pitfall can lead to a delayed union or nonunion. Another pitfall that can occur during the osteotomy includes not making the proximal cut behind the patellar tendon with the osteotome. This proximal cut connects the medial and lateral edges of the osteotomy and prevents the cut from extending proximally into the metaphysis or tibial plateau.

Postoperative complications, including neurovascular injury, infection, compartment syndrome, deep venous thrombosis, and pulmonary embolism are rare but should be discussed with every patient preoperatively. Pitfalls during rehabilitation include increasing range of motion too quickly, allowing unprotected ambulation without a brace or assistive device, and too early return to play. These pitfalls can lead to a proximal tibia fracture, fixation failure of the osteotomy, delayed union, malunion, or nonunion.

■ REHABILITATION/RETURN TO PLAY RECOMMENDATIONS

The postoperative rehabilitation actually begins before the elective procedure with a thorough discussion between the patient, surgeon, and a physical therapist to outline realistic expectations and anticipated progression to return to play. The therapist and patient are given brochures detailing guidelines for rehabilitation after a proximal-distal realignment. Progression through each phase takes into consideration the patient's individual status as well as the surgeon's advisement. The postoperative rehabilitation is divided into four phases, each with emphasis on regaining quadriceps strength, range of motion, and attainment of goals prior to advancement. The same rehabilitation protocol is followed for proximal and distal realignments with the exception of range-of-motion limitations. For the first 6 weeks, proximal and combined proximal-distal realignments are limited to a range of motion from 0 degrees to 60 degrees, while distal realignments can progress to 90 degrees of flexion.

In phase I (0 to 6 weeks), initial goals are to control pain and the inflammatory process, protect the fixation and soft tissues, and regain quadriceps and VMO control. Rehabilitation begins with the patient being allowed to weight bear as tolerated with the ELS brace locked in extension for all activities except for sleeping. A continuous passive motion (CPM) is used for 2 hours two times a day with range of motion limitations as above. Heel slides in conjunction with CPM limit the adverse effects of immobilization. Other exercises include quadriceps sets and isometric adduction with biofeedback for VMO, straight leg raises in four planes with the brace locked in extension, nonweight-bearing gastrocnemius-soleus and hamstring stretches, and resisted ankle range of motion with Therabands. Patellar mobilization is begun when tolerated with performance of superior, inferior, and lateral tilt of the patella. Inferior mobility is required for knee flexion, and superior patellar mobility is necessary for normalized knee extension. Aquatic therapy is begun at 3 to 4 weeks with emphasis on normalization of gait.

Phase II (6 to 8 weeks after surgery) begins as scheduled if the patient has no signs of active inflammation, a good quadriceps set, and the appropriate amount of allowed flexion. Goals are to increase the range of flexion, avoid overstressing fixation, and increase quadriceps and VMO control for restoration of proper patellar tracking. The brace is removed for sleeping and unlocked for ambulation. CPM is discontinued when flexion is at least 90 degrees, and heel slides are continued with progression to full flexion. In addition to the phase I exercises, the patient begins balance and proprioception exercises, straight leg raises without the brace, and weight-bearing gastrocnemius-soleus stretching. Workouts on a stationary bike can be performed with low resistance and a high seat position to decrease the patellofemoral joint compression forces. Progression also includes short arc quadriceps exercises in pain-free ranges (0 degrees to 20 degrees and 60 degrees to 90 degrees of flexion) and wall slides progressing to mini-squats at 0 degrees to 45 degrees.

Phase III (8 weeks to 4 months after surgery) begins if the patient has good quadriceps tone, no extension lag with straight leg raise, a nonantalgic gait pattern, and good dynamic patellar control. Crutches may be discontinued at this point, and the brace is removed after evidence of radiographic healing and good, active control of the knee are demonstrated. Exercises progress to include step-ups, closed kinetic chain terminal knee extension with resistive tubing or weight machine, hamstring curls, toe raises, and leg press from 0 degrees to 45 degrees of flexion. Flexibility and proprioception exercises are continued. Patients may progress to moderate resistance on the stationary bike with the addition of swimming and a stair climber for endurance.

Phase IV (4 months to 6 months after surgery) encompasses the final supervised rehabilitation phase. At this point, the patient should have good-to-normal quadriceps strength, no evidence of patellar instability, no soft tissue complaints, and a normal gait pattern. The surgeon clears the patient to advance if goals have been met to begin more concentrated closed kinetic chain exercises and resume full or partial activity. The patient advances through functional progression with emphasis on sports-specific rehabilitation with the ultimate goals of return to sport with patellofemoral stability, normal strength, full range of motion, and no complaints of pain.

OUTCOMES AND FUTURE DIRECTIONS

Outcomes after surgical management for patellar instability and LPCS are optimized with appropriate diagnosis, recognition and treatment of associated disorders, and postoperative rehabilitation with emphasis on early motion and attainment of quadriceps strength. Most patients are able to return to sport at or near their previous level of performance. For most patients, patellofemoral stability is restored to the painless knee with the return of normal range of motion and full strength.

Future directions in the treatment of patellar instability include continued advances in arthroscopy and research and trials directed at the MPFL. With arthroscopy, the thorough inspection of the joint for associated lesions with concurrent treatment is performed with less morbidity than the previously advocated open arthrotomy. Newer techniques of arthroscopic all-inside medial reefing and lateral release show promising results in the treatment of patellar instability.[20] Much focus has been given recently to the MPFL as the essential lesion in lateral patellar dislocation. Biomechanical studies have demonstrated its significant contribution as a restraining force against lateral patellar motion.[2] Procedures designed to restore the normal restraints against abnormal lateral motion should repair or reconstruct the MPFL.[21] Studies of repair of the MPFL and other medial patellar stabilizers for acute patella dislocations have produced good short-term results.[3,22] More investigation is needed into the long-term results of these procedures, and further study is needed regarding the MPFL in chronic instability.

REFERENCES

1. Hughston JC. Subluxation of the patella. J Bone Joint Surg. 1968;50A(5):1003–1026.
2. Conlan T, Garth WP Jr, Lemons JE. Evaluation of the medial soft-tissue restraints of the extensor mechanism of the knee. J Bone Joint Surg. 1993;75A:682–693.
3. Sallay PI, Poggi J, Speer KP, et al. Acute dislocation of the patella: a correlative pathoanatomic study. Am J Sports Med. 1996;24(1):52–60.
4. Roux C. Recurrent dislocation of the patella: operative treatment. Rev Chir. 1888;8:682–689.
5. Goldthwait JE. Slipping or recurrent dislocation of the patella: with the report of eleven cases. Boston Med Surg J. 1904;150:169–174.
6. Hauser EDW. Total tendon transplant for slipping patella: a new operation for recurrent dislocation of the patella. Surg Gynecol Obstet. 1938;66:199–214.
7. Cox JS. Evaluation of the Roux-Elmslie-Trillat procedure for knee extensor realignment. Am J Sports Med. 1982;10(5):303–310.
8. Fulkerson JP, Becker GJ, Meaney JA, et al. Anteromedial tibial tubercle transfer without bone graft. Am J Sports Med. 1990;18(5):490–497.
9. Merchant AC, Mercer RL. Lateral release of the patella: A preliminary report. Clin Orthop. 1974;103:40–45.
10. Kolowich PA, Paulos LE, Rosenberg TD, et al. Lateral release of the patella: indications and contraindications. Am J Sports Med. 1990;18(4):359–365.
11. McGinty JB, McCarthy JC. Endoscopic lateral retinacular release: a preliminary report. Clin Orthop. 1981;158:120–125.
12. Metcalf RW. An arthroscopic method for lateral release of the subluxating or dislocating patella. Clin Orthop. 1982;167:9–18.
13. Fu FH, Maday MG. Arthroscopic lateral release and the lateral patellar compression syndrome. Orthop Clin North Am. 1992;23:601–612.
14. Hughston JC, Walsh WM, Puddu G. Patellar Subluxation and Dislocation. Philadelphia: WB Saunders Co; 1984.
15. Cox JS, Cooper PS. Patellofemoral instability. In: Fu FH, Harner CD, Vince KG, eds. Knee Surgery. Vol 1. Baltimore: Williams and Wilkins; 1994:953–999.
16. Dejour H, Walch G, Nove-Josserand L, et al. Factors of patellar instability: an anatomic radiographic study. Knee Surg Sports Traumatol Arthrosc. 1994;(2)1:19–26.
17. Insall J, Salvati E. Patellar position in the normal knee. Radiology. 1971;101:101–104.
18. Merchant AC, Mercer RL, Jacobsen RH, et al. Roentgenographic analysis of patellofemoral congruence. J Bone Joint Surg. 1974;56A(7):1391–1396.
19. Laurin CA, Dussault R, Levesque HP. The tangential x-ray investigation of the patellofemoral joint: x-ray technique, diagnostic criteria and their interpretation. Clin Orthop. 1979;144:16–26.
20. Halbrecht, JL. Arthroscopic patella realignment: an all-inside technique. Arthroscopy. 2001;17(9):940–945.
21. Arendt, EA, Fithian, DC, Cohen E. Current concepts of lateral patella dislocation. Clin Sports Med. 2002;21:499–519.
22. Ahmad, CS, Shubin Stein, BE, Matuz, D, et al. Immediate surgical repair of the medial patellar stabilizers for acute patellar dislocation. Am J Sports Med. 2000;28:804–810.

54

PATELLOFEMORAL REALIGNMENT FOR ARTHRITIS

FRANK V. THOMAS, MD, JOHN P. FULKERSON, MD

■ HISTORY OF THE TECHNIQUE

Patellar arthritis is all too common in the general population. However, rarely does a primary degenerative process affect only the patella. The chondral abnormalities are usually seen in the face of instability or are secondary to a blunt trauma to the front of the knee causing a breakdown of the cartilage. Instability may be posttraumatic or is seen in a number of anatomic or biologic predispositions. A recent case series review by Nomura and Inoue[1] documented cartilage damage in 67 of 70 patients surgically treated for recurrent patellar instability. Because of the strong association, instability will get considerable mention throughout this chapter. In addition, many of the procedures that have been designed to treat one entity have been found to be effective in the treatment of the other.

Understanding patellofemoral anatomy and kinematics is essential to discerning the physical findings, and when warranted, selecting the correct surgical procedure. There is a complex relationship between the bone and soft tissue structures about the extensor mechanism, but only the osseous morphology and soft tissue stabilizers will be reviewed as they are the areas that can be surgically addressed. This will help in understanding the rationale for surgical decision making.

The facets of the patella consist of the lateral, medial, and odd; while there are only two facets of the trochlea—the medial and lateral. On the axial view of the patellofemoral articulation, the wider lateral aspect of the joint can be appreciated. This is where a majority of the pathology is found. There are two retinacula; a medial one and a thicker lateral one. Their major attachment sites are on the femur, but more distally, they become confluent with the capsule and its meniscal attachments. The medial patellofemoral ligament is part of the medial retinaculum and acts as a vital stabilizer against lateral patellar subluxation. The two retinacula not only function to tether the patella from contralateral displacement, but also act to buttress the patella on their respective sides as indicated by the observation that the lateral retinaculum actually helps to prevent lateral translation.[2]

Goodfellow et al.[3] made great contributions to our understanding of the patellofemoral articulation pattern. In full extension the patella articulates with the supratrochlear fat pad. At 10 degrees, the trochlea is first contacted. The lateral facet aligns at 20 degrees, but the central ridge does not articulate until 35 degrees of flexion is reached. These first 20 degrees are when the patella is most at risk for lateral subluxation.[4] From an axial standpoint, the initial contact area on the patella is distal. The patellar articulation is through the central third at 45 degrees and ends up proximally at 90 degrees. Up to this point, the contact area involves the central ridge in addition to the medial and lateral facets of the patella, but only at a flexion arc of 135 degrees does the odd facet become involved. This approximate sequence was arthroscopically supported by Sojbjerg et al.[5]

Pathogenesis of Patellar Instability

The focus of this chapter is the treatment of patellar arthritis. As mentioned, this more often than not is seen in patients with instability or malalignment. Patellar instability can present in several ways. For some, it is a traumatic event that can initiate the condition of recurrent instability. The management of acute dislocations is beyond the scope of this chapter, but it should be noted that as many as one half of these patients will have continued instability or chronic pain.[6] Generalized laxity may be the underlying cause of the instability.[7,8] It is frequently uncovered in patients whose trauma is apparently trivial in nature, and the individuals will often present with bilateral complaints. A genetic predisposition for this has been suggested.[9] Fulkerson[10] originally described a pattern of nerve injury in the peri-patellar retinaculum of some patients with anterior knee pain. Later, Sanchis-Alfonso[11] has done considerable work to identify and quantify the neural innervation of the lateral retinaculum, which may account for much of the pain seen in association with patellar instability.

Patellar tilt is a type of malalignment that can usually be detected on physical examination. It is revealed by a relatively tight lateral retinaculum. A computed tomography (CT) study by Dejour et al.[12] demonstrated tilt in 83% of patients with patellar instability.

There is a frequent association between patella alta and patellar instability. This was found to be present in more than a third of patients with anterior knee pain according to a radiographic review by Davies et al.[13] and was seen in more than half of the patients evaluated by Greenen et al.[14] Trochlear dysplasia, as indicated by a high sulcus angle and a shallow trochlea, was found to be present in a majority of patients in both series. One study suggested that the dysplastic joint may be characterized by a small medial patellar facet and was frequently noted in their series of patients with instability.[15] Dysplasia may have even more of a profound effect on patellar stability than patella alta. We feel that the surgical procedures designed to address these problems (i.e., trochleoplasty, patellar tendon shortening, or tubercle distalization) are not reproducible and carry significant risk of complication.

Ficat[16] first described excessive lateral pressure syndrome (ELPS) in 1978. Insufficient medial or excessively tight lateral restraints leading to lateral instability allow for an increased load to the lateral aspect of the patellofemoral joint throughout the arc of flexion. The result of this process is severe degenerative changes in this region.

Muscle weakness secondary to a pathologic abnormality may also contribute to symptoms in some patients with an unstable patella.[17] This certainly requires further investigation, but probably is one of the inciting factors to a lesser extent.

■ INDICATIONS AND CONTRAINDICATIONS

History

Taking a careful history is crucial to identifying the problem. Patellofemoral abnormalities can give patients a sense of overall knee instability identical to that seen in anterior cruciate ligament (ACL) deficiency. Without a high index of suspicion, it is possible to overlook the patella as a source of instability and focus on evaluating the ligamentous components of the knee. The same pivoting activities can injure either structure. However, most patients with an actual dislocation will provide an accurate history even when spontaneous reduction occurs.

Sometimes pain is the only presenting complaint. Patients who do not have a history of trauma are occasionally unaware that it is their patella causing their sensation of instability. It is important to ascertain whether the knee is

clicking, popping, swelling, or "giving way" without ignoring the patellofemoral joint as a source of these symptoms. At the same time, a snapping chondral lesion may be mistaken for patella subluxation. Identifying exacerbating and alleviating factors will aid in understanding how the problem affects the individual on a daily basis.

Sudden episodes of knee buckling without any forewarning are more indicative of medial than lateral instability. This is critical to note: medial patella subluxation is a complication of previous surgery and may actually be misconstrued as persistent lateral instability.

Physical Examination

Observation should be the initial part of the physical examination. It gives an accurate idea of the severity of the abnormality. Along with monitoring gait, the examiner should also pay attention to the patient's ability to rise from a chair. A meticulous integumentary examination is vital, particularly looking for evidence of reflex sympathetic dystrophy or subcutaneous neuromas in patients with prior surgeries. Many patients with patellofemoral abnormalities have had previous operations. The size, number, appearance, and location of the incisions should be noted. Close observation may yield muscle atrophy. A large percentage of patients with weakness can be successfully cared for with nonoperative means that include physical therapy, reassurance, and bracing.

A quick examination of the hips will sometimes indicate a degenerative process, which may be the true cause of the knee pain. The internal and external range of motion of each hip and any inequality should be noted. This information, in addition to the lower limb alignment both on standing and during gait observation, can help to identify underlying anatomic abnormalities. Either rotational or angular deformities may account for patellar malalignment and instability. Have the patient stand and perform a single-leg knee bend to discern if there is weakness of hip external rotators, which should be addressed during physical therapy.

Asking the patients to simply squat into a catcher's position is helpful in evaluating the overall function of the knee. This is an easy and sensitive test that can quickly determine the condition of the patellofemoral joint. An inability to do this, however, can be caused by a variety conditions such as meniscal, articular cartilage, or cruciate pathology. The presence or absence of a "J sign" can also be determined during this maneuver.

Strength evaluation should be part of any lower extremity exam. In addition to the quadriceps muscles, the hip rotators should be looked at since weakness with external rotation can predispose the patella to lateral tracking.

During palpation of the patellofemoral joint, the examiner should try to identify the area of tenderness and at what degree of motion pain is elicited. Crepitus should be looked for. Ascertaining the degree or degrees of flexion where the crepitus is found will give an idea of the location of the chondral lesions. The soft tissues should not be forgotten since retinacular tenderness may indicate this structure as the primary cause of the knee pain. Patellar tilt may be appreciated by a tight lateral retinaculum. At the same time, insufficient medial restraints may be detected in severe lateral instability. Palpation will define this in a thin individual.

Evaluating patellar tracking is the most difficult part of the exam. First, note whether the patella is starting medially or laterally and then displacing to articulate with the sulcus in flexion or whether the perceived displacement with flexion is actually subluxation out of the sulcus. With the exception of severe instability, every patella will find the groove at some point in flexion. Active extension is also important to observe. The subluxation of the patella may better manifest itself as the knee nears full extension. However, this may be difficult for some very symptomatic patients to achieve.

It is always important to check apprehension in full extension, but, similar to a shoulder evaluation, it should be left for last as it may make the remainder of the examination difficult. Overall ligamentous stability should be determined with particular attention paid to the posterior cruciate ligament (PCL). Chronic PCL laxity frequently presents as anterior knee pain.

Be cognizant of generalized ligamentous laxity as a cause of patellar instability. It is a good idea to quickly evaluate every patient for this condition, which ultimately makes treatment of patellar instability more difficult. Knee, elbow, and metacarpophalangeal hyperextension as well as the ability to touch the forearm with an abducted thumb are quick and easy to perform. Most patients are aware of whether or not they have excessive laxity.

Radiographic Evaluation

Standard x-rays should consist of weight bearing PA and lateral radiographs of the knee as well as a 45-degree axial view. The lateral should not be overlooked as a source of information regarding the patella and its articulation. Patellar height can be determined by looking at several relationships. As a quick matter of reference, an extension of Blumensaat's[18] line should be at or just below the distal pole of the patella with the knee flexed 30 degrees. However, after using it in a handful of cases, it will become easily understood how inconsistent this reference is. The Insall/Salvati[19] index can be measured by dividing the patellar tendon length by the height of the patella. A measurement >1.2 is abnormal. Because this measurement does not take into account the morphology of the distal femur and the tibial tubercle shape and height can be variable, we prefer the Bernageau[20] index. It is a relationship between the distal patellar articular edge and the proximal central trochlea. However, a lateral x-ray in full extension is required for this, which is not a routine part of most knee series. The Blackburne and Peel[21] method of measuring patellar height is probably the most reproducible. It references the tibial plateau height and the

articular portion of the patella, which are more readily identifiable radiographic landmarks. An index >1.06 is considered abnormal. Another advantage is that the degree of flexion can be anywhere from 0 degrees to 60 degrees to obtain this value.

The lateral view can also provide information about the congruence of the joint. With a true lateral x-ray, as indicated by posterior femoral condyle overlap, the medial patellar edge can be viewed in relationship to the median ridge and lateral edge. One study demonstrated a high specificity and sensitivity for determining subluxation and tilt when radiographs were obtained in both flexion and extension.[22] Trochlear depth can also be accurately determined if you have a true lateral.[23]

The axial view may be obtained at 30 degrees or 45 degrees. Both knees should be included on the same cassette. This should be performed in all patients with patella-related complaints. In the case of an acute dislocation, osteochondral fragments may be seen in the gutters, which may warrant early surgical intervention. The presence and location of any joint space narrowing should be noted. Trochlear and patellar morphology may be evaluated as well as tilt and subluxation, which are quantified by measuring patellar congruence as described by Merchant et al.[24] and the sulcus angle. The sulcus angle should be 130 degrees to 137 degrees.[25] A sulcus angle greater than 150 degrees is a sign of trochlear dysplasia and has been reported to be present in conjunction with most other radiographic abnormalities.[13] A congruence angle greater than 16 degrees is felt to be indicative of malalignment. All of these findings will have a definite impact on any planned surgical intervention. One report supported these radiographic indices but was unable to reproduce them when isolated chondromalacia was encountered in the absence of instability.[26]

Our use of CT scan has decreased over the past decade. Nonetheless, if physical exam and radiographs provide inconclusive results, a CT scan can help to define the anatomy of the patellofemoral joint and may also be useful in documenting rotational abnormalities of the lower extremity.[27,28] Midtransverse patellar axial images at 15, 30, and 45 degrees will demonstrate the articular contact pattern of the patella with regard to its angle of engagement and progression during flexion.[29] CT is also excellent for determination of the relationship between the tibial tubercle (TT) and trochlea groove (TG) on the TT–TG relationship.

Patients often present with a magnetic resonance imaging (MRI) report in hand if they have been referred for the evaluation of patellofemoral instability. These are useful in evaluating the condition of the medial patellofemoral ligament (MPFL) or determining the location of a MPFL injury in the case of an acute dislocation.[30] The only time we routinely order an MRI in patients with isolated patellofemoral pathology is if we want to evaluate the chondral surfaces or if primary MPFL injury is suspected.

Nonoperative Treatment of Patellofemoral Arthritis

Cowan et al.[31,32] have done considerable electromyographic work to support the use of physical therapy as a first line of treatment in patellar instability. Rehabilitation should start at the hip. The focus should not only be on vastus medialis obliquus (VMO) strengthening, but also hip external rotator strengthening. The hip musculature acts as a vital core stabilizer that plays a crucial role in the kinetic chain. Hanten and Schulthies[33] have suggested that strengthening the hip adductors will even assist in selective VMO strengthening. A study of 45 high school skiers found that 73% reported complaints of anterior knee pain that decreased to 35% a year later following a formal physical therapy program.[34]

There is a growing understanding of the pathologic significance of proprioceptive loss following injury. The patellar taping technique described by McConnell[35] may assist in regaining this. As with any other joint, working to correct proprioception should be part of the rehabilitative process.

If instability is present, a trial of bracing should be employed in conjunction with other nonoperative modalities. Some literature does exist to support its use.[36,37] We initiate the use of orthotics early in the treatment course, usually at the first visit. Our preferred brace is the Tru-Pull brace (DonJoy, Vista, Calif.), which has several appealing characteristics. The circumferential neoprene sleeve has a soft rubber lining from top to bottom that provides excellent maintenance of the brace's position. Patellar control is accomplished by an adjustable C-shaped, sturdy foam pad that comes in two widths to apply focused pressure to the unstable side of the patella. Once the brace is applied, the tension on the parapatellar pad is adjusted using two hook and loop fasteners.

Overall, the nonoperative treatment of patellar arthritis is more likely to be successful in the absence of anatomic abnormalities.[38]

■ SURGICAL TECHNIQUE

Arthroscopic Evaluation and Chondroplasty

The physical examination will accurately classify the instability pattern in most cases, but the location and extent of degenerative changes is quite difficult to predict, even with diagnostic studies.[39] Since this information greatly influences the treatment and prognosis,[40] we have a systematic method by which we arthroscopically evaluate the patellofemoral joint prior to performing any realignment procedure.

An exam under anesthesia should be obtained, but mainly adds information in patients who are apprehensive. Passive patella tracking can be determined without the interference of patients' quadriceps activity.

With the patient in the supine position, we apply a tourniquet, but rarely need to inflate it. A circumferential leg holding clamp hinders a suprapatellar approach arthroscopically and is not used if an open procedure or an isolated lateral release is being considered as it can make extreme flexion difficult and interferes with patella tracking. A post for valgus stressing is preferable and figure-four positioning is used for any needed varus moment. In general, varus and valgus stressing as well as rotation should be avoided while observing tracking as these maneuvers can affect the patellofemoral congruity.

The concept of the arthroscopic exam is simple; view the tracking from as many portals as possible and do it several times with the knee both infused and drained of irrigation fluid. An outflow cannula is not used because it is felt to be unnecessary with our equipment, and it may affect the patellofemoral tracking by either tethering the soft tissues or applying direct compression to the patella during flexion. We start with a lateral parapatellar portal. At 60 mm Hg pressure, the distention will cause the patella to make initial contact with the trochlea later in the flexion arc, usually not until 30 degrees to 40 degrees of knee flexion. We strive to observe flexion and extension through both the medial and lateral portals with the knee in neutral rotation while the joint is distended and then again without fluid distention. Observing tracking through a superior accessory portal, either medially or laterally, may be helpful when the findings of the tracking through the standard portals are inconclusive. Viewing through multiple portals will also help to define the size and location of cartilage defects. On occasion some infrapatellar fat pad resection will be necessary to completely visualize the articulation.

To treat chondral damage on the patella we use a shaver to debride loose fragments and may perform a microfracture technique if there is exposed bone. The same philosophy is employed on the trochlear side. Two reports have indicated that the success of articular debridement is greater in cases of posttraumatic chondral lesions,[41,42] but we do not limit the use of chondroplasty to these instances.

Experience with osteochondral resurfacing on the patella and trochea has been favorable in selected cases. Often in combination with anteromedial tibial tubercle transfer, articular resurfacing is important in patellofemoral joint preservation surgery.

Lateral Release

Lateral retinacular release is the most commonly performed and written about method of altering patellar tracking. It can also be harmful. The use of an isolated lateral release, either arthroscopic or open, should be limited to cases of mild instability caused by rotational patella malalignment (tilt). The beneficial effects have been supported by several reports.[43–45] Patellar tilt is a sign of mild patellar instability and is commonly found in patients who present with anterior knee pain. As mentioned, physical examination is usually accurate and radiographic examination is ultimately diagnostic. On exam, tilt is characterized by a tight lateral retinaculum that prevents anterior displacement of the lateral facet with the knee in full extension. Furthermore, the lateral retinaculum has been postulated to be a primary source of pain as evidenced by the presence of small nerve injuries and secondary neural growth factors in this region.[10] This may account for some of the improvement following lateral release, which has been documented in a series published by Krompinger and Fulkerson.[46]

The procedure, nonetheless, is overused, resulting in significant morbidity in some situations. Primary medial instability is an absolute contraindication to lateral release. Be aware that trochlear dysplasia may predispose to medial instability postoperatively. A lateral release should also be used judiciously in cases where medial patellofemoral arthrosis predominates as this side of the joint will experience an increase in loading forces following the procedure. Lastly, the results are less predictable when a lateral release has been performed in patients with patella subluxation or, on the other extreme, when there is no evidence of malalignment at all.[47,48]

Technique

In most instances, a circumferential leg holder is not used to allow for ease of knee flexion. A tourniquet is applied but rarely inflated as we prefer to address bleeding immediately and as completely as possible. After a complete arthroscopic evaluation of tilt **(Fig. 54-1)**, tracking, and any areas of chondromalacia, a moment should be taken to define the anatomy of the lateral retinaculum. Debridement of synovial tissue or an enlarged fat pad is sometimes necessary to visualize the distal extent of the retinaculum, which is usually at the level of the lateral parapatellar portal. The vastus lateralis should also be identified to determine the proximal end of the release and should not be violated. Transillumination and palpation will ensure that the quadriceps tendon is avoided centrally.

An arthroscopic thermal ablation device can be used to perform the release. The release should be performed 1 cm from the lateral edge of the patella and the tip of the probe

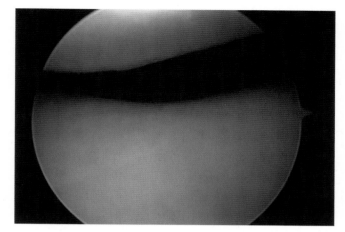

Fig. 54-2. Lateral release: Arthroscopic appearance of tilt.

should be visualized at all times **(Fig. 54-2)**. We prefer to perform the release in layers so that the depth of the release can be monitored during the entire procedure. The capsule is first released, followed by the thick retinaculum **(Fig. 54-3)**. Once adipose tissue is encountered and the edges of the retinaculum have separated, the depth of the release has been determined. If difficulty is encountered in accessing the proximal retinaculum, one may begin the release with the probe in the medial parapatellar portal while viewing through the lateral portal, then switching portals to complete the release.

After the release is completed, the tracking and any concurrent articular lesion contact should be reevaluated **(Fig. 54-4)**. The surgeon must deflate the tourniquet, if used, and look for bleeding, which may come from a lateral geniculate artery. Inflow pressure will tamponade bleeding, even from arteries. Therefore, draining the knee while visualizing the retinacular edges is necessary to ensure hemostasis. It is our routine not to close arthroscopic portals. We apply xeroform gauze (Kendall, Indianapolis, Ind.), sterile gauze, sterile cast padding, and a bias-cut stockinette.

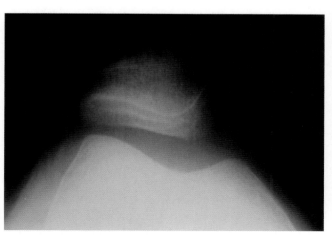

Fig. 54-1. Radiographic evidence of tilt.

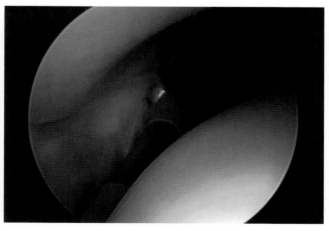

Fig. 54-3. Lateral release: The release is performed 1 cm from the articular edge.

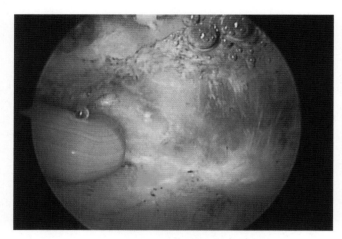

Fig. 54-4. Lateral release: The retinaculum is being released. The exposed fascial fibers are next.

Post-op Management

Early motion is encouraged to combat the effects of prolonged pain and swelling that may accompany this procedure. No brace is used and immediate weight bearing is permitted.

Complications

Despite having relatively low intraoperative and immediate postoperative morbidity, complications can arise. Paying careful attention to hemostasis is crucial as an acute expanding hemarthrosis can be extremely painful and may warrant operative intervention. Being aware of the location of the probe at all times will ensure that the extensor mechanism is not violated, and if the depth of the release is not observed, it is possible to burn the skin from inside. As was mentioned earlier, medial instability is not only a contraindication to undergoing a lateral release, but is a well-described complication.[49,50] The presentation is usually an acute worsening in symptomatology. This complication requires surgical correction.

Arthroscopic Medial Imbrication

The proximal patellar realignment procedure described by Insall et al.[51] is an effective, reproducible procedure for treating lateral patellofemoral articular lesions. Its successful use in the treatment of lateral patellar instability has subsequently been described by Abraham et al.[52] However, their report did bring into question its long-term efficacy. Nevertheless, a large incision and a significant amount of dissection are required.

In 1986, Yamamoto[53] published an arthroscopic technique to address the medial retinaculum in acute lateral dislocations. Small et al.[54] later published promising reports on its efficacy. Henry and Pflum[55] and Ahmad and Lee[56] have presented all-arthroscopic techniques in the literature. Halbrecht[57] described an all-arthroscopic technique in 2001 that is most similar to what we currently use (dis-

cussed below). In the reports by Halbrecht as well as Haspl et al.,[58] no recurrent dislocations or subluxation episodes were encountered at the latest follow-up.

The indication for this procedure is primarily instability, but we have found it to be useful even when significant chondral abnormalities accompany it. One study questioned the use of medial imbrication as an isolated procedure to treat patellar instability in the face of patellofemoral arthritis, certainly when it is advanced.[59] In our series currently being investigated, we have found that the procedure is effective when treating patients with chondral lesions as long as there is no radiographic evidence of degenerative changes. The procedure has not been proven in patients with severe patellar instability, but our greatest rate of success was in patients in whom instability was the primary complaint. Some of the patients had severe instability that manifested as recurrent dislocations. Furthermore, any medial imbrication procedure carries the risk of medial patella overload, as the medial retinaculum is a posteriorly oriented structure.

In addition to radiographic evidence of patellofemoral degeneration, trochlear dysplasia is a relative contraindication. When the sulcus angle nears 180 degrees, medial retinacular imbrication may create a condition of medial instability. Generalized laxity should also be a cause for concern as medial instability may be the end result here as well. A more complex soft tissue balancing in these patients is sometimes necessary. Such problems, as well as a lateral patellar tendon insertion (high TT–TG relationship) increase the need for accurate tibial tubercle transfer.

Technique

With the patient in the supine position, a tourniquet is applied to the proximal thigh. Once again, we do not use a circumferential leg holder. It is easier to rotate the extremity when it is flat on the table.

Diagnostic arthroscopy is very important **(Fig. 54-5)**. A lateral release is usually performed as described above. The tracking should then be reassessed since the release may have corrected the abnormality. If persistent subluxation is seen, we proceed with the medial imbrication. An arthroscopic shaver should be used to clear any tissue that is obscuring the view of the medial retinaculum. Two 1-cm transverse incisions approximately 2 cm apart are needed to place the instruments, and they should be positioned such that the entire retinaculum can be accessed proximally and distally. Starting proximally, an 18 G needle is used to place a 0 PDS monofilament suture (Ethicon Inc., Somerville, N.J.) from outside-in just medial to the edge of the patella **(Fig. 54-6)**. A BirdBeak (Arthrex, Naples, Fla.) grasper is used to retrieve the suture 1.0 to 1.5 cm posteriorly **(Fig. 54-7)**. The PDS is used to shuttle a no. 2 FiberWire suture (Arthrex, Naples, Fla.), which is immediately tied leaving the knot in an extra-articular position. An arthroscopic knot pusher can be helpful in securing the knots blindly in an obese individual. The tissue can be seen

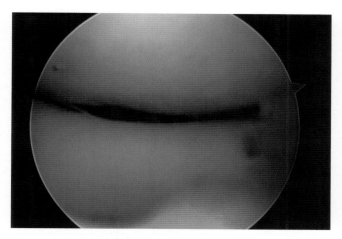

Fig. 54-5. Lateral release: Arthroscopic appearance following a successful release.

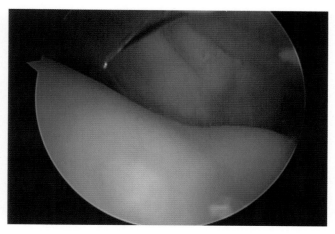

Fig. 54-7. Medial imbrication: The 18 G needle should pass just along the edge of the patella.

arthroscopically to ensure that they are tight. By tying each suture as it is placed **(Fig. 54-8)**, the tracking can be repeatedly evaluated to determine how much more imbrication is required. Typically four or five sutures will be needed to obtain the desired medialization. Through the two incisions, the procedure is repeated retrieving each subsequent PDS suture more or less posteriorly to imbricate more or less tissue. Since the sutures are placed in line with the retinacular fibers, they may cut through the tissue as they are tied. If this occurs, they can be shuttled using a second PDS to create a mattress or figure-eight configuration. Once the desired tracking pattern has been achieved **(Fig. 54-9)**, the tourniquet is deflated and the knee is observed for bleeding, especially at the lateral retinacular edges.

Increasingly now, we prefer a mini-open technique through a 3–4 cm incision over the proximal medial patella. By elevating the VMD, the medial patellofemoral ligament (MPFL) may be palpated to assure continuity. This, then, may be simply advanced on the patella side,

along with VMD. This produces a very secure repair. We have been impressed how often the MPFL is intact, although elongated.

We close the medial incisions with a subcuticular pull-out nylon suture, but not the two parapatellar portals. All incisions are covered with xeroform gauze (Kendall, Indianapolis, Ind.) and sterile gauze, which is secured with sterile cast padding. A bias-cut stockinette is applied followed by a cold therapy device and a knee immobilizer.

Post-op Management

Strict immobilization is prescribed for 2 weeks with no limitation in weight bearing. After this time, we encourage one 90-degree passive flexion arc daily with no active extension for 4 more weeks. An x-ray is obtained at the 6-week post-op visit at which point strengthening exercises are begun. Usually another 4 to 6 weeks are required to regain the strength necessary to resume daily activity, and 4 to 6 months total are needed to return to vigorous activity.

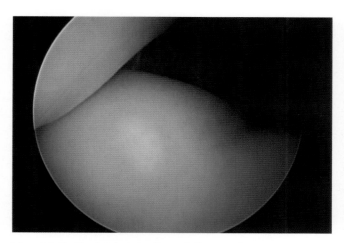

Fig. 54-6. Medial imbrication: Arthroscopic appearance of subluxation.

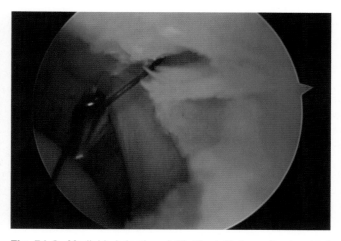

Fig. 54-8. Medial imbrication: A BirdBeak (Arthrex, Naples, Fla.) grasper is used to retrieve the suture 1 to 1.5 cm posteriorly.

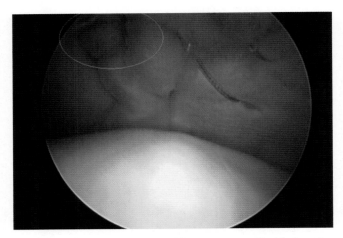

Fig. 54-9. Medial imbrication: The sutures are tied before the next is passed. In the circle, the imbricated tissue is seen. A figure-eight configuration is demonstrated here as well.

Complications

The complications from an arthroscopic patellar realignment procedure are the same as those encountered from a lateral release, but may also include stiffness or articular overload related to the imbrication.

Oblique Tibial Tubercle Osteotomy

Tibial tubercle anteromedialization (AMZ) is a versatile patellar realignment osteotomy that was originally described by the senior author in 1983.[60] There are several attractive aspects to this osteotomy. First, the flat cut incorporates a large surface area to facilitate healing and allow for multiple points of fixation. Second, the oblique angle of the cut can be adjusted toward either the sagittal or coronal plane to allow for more anteriorization or more medialization, respectively. By obtaining a combination of these, not only can lateral instability be corrected, but distal lesions can be unloaded (Figs. 54-20 and 54-21). Lastly, the distal taper minimizes the

metaphyseal insult thereby decreasing the risk of iatrogenic fracture. In 1990, Fulkerson et al.[34] reported on 30 patients who were more than 2 years post-op and found that more than 90% of patients had good to excellent results. Encouragingly, even 75% of the patients with significant degenerative changes obtained good to excellent results.

The indication for an AMZ is a combination of distal or lateral patellar arthritis and lateral subluxation.[61] Also, some physicians will routinely add this procedure when performing an autologous cartilage implantation in the patella or femoral trochlea to gain exposure and decrease contact stresses. In the case of severe instability, a proximal realignment may be needed in addition to the AMZ.

Advanced proximal or medial patellofemoral arthrosis is a contraindication to an AMZ as is medial instability. Smoking and diabetes may present difficulty with bone and wound healing in this area, which is often deficient of subcutaneous adipose tissue. Obese patients are at an increased risk of tibia fractures and should be encouraged to lose weight preoperatively.

Technique

With the patient in the supine position a tourniquet is applied to the thigh. After prepping and free-draping, the tourniquet is inflated. An arthroscopic evaluation is routinely performed to evaluate the patellofemoral joint. Occasionally, advanced proximal or medial patellar arthrosis is discovered and the procedure is aborted.

Once the indication is supported by direct visualization, an 8- to 10-cm longitudinal midline or slightly lateral incision is made (Fig. 54-10). The proximal end of the incision is positioned at the distal pole of the patella. The incision is taken sharply down to the extensor mechanism. The paratenon is maintained. A lateral retinacular release is then created, preferably with the Bovie, up to the level of the proximal pole of the patella. With an Army-Navy retractor, the release can be performed without extending the skin incision proximally.

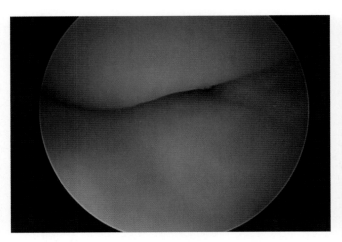

Fig. 54-10. Medial imbrication: The subluxation has been corrected.

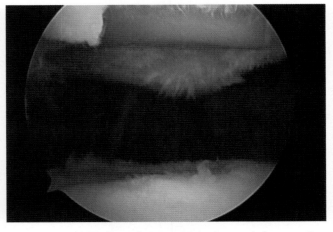

Fig. 54-11. AMZ: Opposing areas of advanced degeneration laterally.

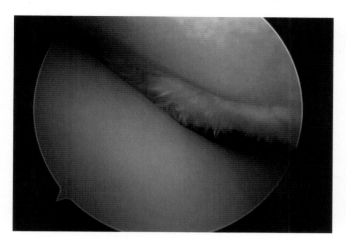

Fig. 54-12. AMZ: Following the AMZ, the small area of intact cartilage on the proximal patella can now be seen articulating with the trochlea.

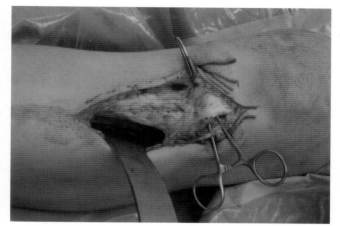

Fig. 54-14. AMZ: Tracker (Mitek, Norwood, Mass.) retractor in place with the tendon isolated.

The patellar tendon is skeletonized to protect it. Metzenbaum scissors are used to dissect the fat pad off of its posterior surface. The Bovie is then used to incise the anterior compartment fascia at the edge of the tibial crest. This should be extended 5 to 6 cm distal to the tibial tubercle, which will be the size of the fragment. Using a Cobb elevator, the anterior tibialis muscle is elevated subperiosteally off the proximal aspect of the tibia. The Tracker (Mitek, Norwood, Mass.) retractor is placed around the posterolateral corner of the tibia **(Fig. 54-11)** to protect the muscle and anterior tibial artery. The Bovie is used to outline the medial edge of the osteotomy starting at the medial border of the distal patellar tendon edge. The osteotomy is tapered toward the anterior tibial crest in both the sagittal and coronal planes to a point 5 to 6 cm distal to the tibial tubercle. The Tracker osteotomy guide is used to obtain a plane for the osteotomy that must be strictly adhered to **(Fig. 54-12)**. The guide is placed in line with the medial Bovie mark, and the anterior-posterior tilt is adjusted depending on whether the tubercle needs to be more anteriorized or medialized.

Distal patella articular lesions require anteriorization of the tibial tubercle.

The guide is secured with two pins. If desired, the posterolateral exit point can be predetermined with the outrigger **(Fig 54-13)**. An oscillating saw with a 1-in. blade is used to begin the osteotomy **(Fig. 54-14)**. If the plane is more sagittally oriented, threatening the posterior tibial cortex, the osteotomy is stopped at the cortex and an osteotome is used to back-cut the cortex laterally. Once the plane of the osteotomy has been established, the guide is removed and the saw is used to extend the cut proximally to just above the level of the tubercle **(Fig. 54-15)**. Distally, the cut is carried to a point where the taper results in a thin bridge of bone that is only 2 to 3 mm thick. Osteotomes are used to connect the cuts. A half-inch osteotome is used to cut the cortex transversely behind the tendon with the retractor in place **(Fig. 54-16)**. This osteotome is tilted so that the cut is angled from anterior-proximal to posterior-distal. Otherwise the fragment may not be mobile. A 1-in. osteotome is then used to connect the proximal edge of the posterolateral cut to the

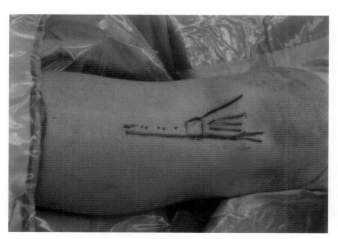

Fig. 54-13. AMZ: Marked-out skin incision.

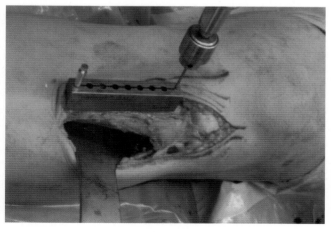

Fig. 54-15. AMZ: Tracker osteotomy guide in place.

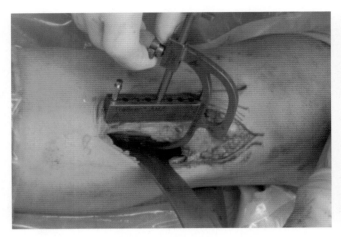

Fig. 54-16. AMZ: The osteotomy guide outrigger can be used to determine the location of the osteotomy posterolaterally.

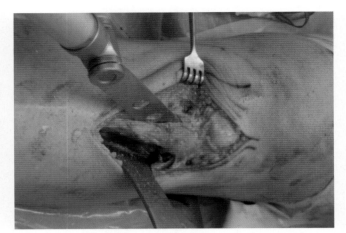

Fig. 54-18. AMZ: Once the osteotomy plane has been established, the guide is removed to complete the cut proximally and distally.

transverse cut **(Fig. 54-17)**. It is important to cut posteriorly through the transverse cut in order to prevent fracture of the metaphyseal portion of the tuberosity. Finally, an osteotome is placed through the medial cut to lever the fragment loose, again maintaining the distal periosteal hinge.

The loose fragment is anteriorized around 1 cm on average **(Fig. 54-18)**. The medialization is not adjustable at this point since the displacement must be along the line of the osteotomy. If needed and planned for, over 1 cm of medial translation can be routinely achieved by cutting more in the coronal plane. Fixation is performed using two AO 4.5-mm fully threaded cortical screws that are placed using the lag technique. A countersink is employed to decrease the amount of irritation experienced **(Fig. 54-19)**. The first screw is placed in the midportion of the tubercle, not in the metaphyseal region. This is done for two reasons; the bone quality is better distally, and in the event of a tuberosity fracture, the more proximal region remains for salvage fixation. Following placement of the first screw, the tracking is

arthroscopically re-evaluated. If the alignment is acceptable, the second screw is placed distal to the first.

The tourniquet is deflated prior to closure, and the knee is inspected for bleeding. The retinacular edges and the parapatellar fat pad are the usual locations. A drain is not routinely used, unless bleeding is excessive. The anterior compartment fasciotomy is left open, and only the subcutaneous adipose tissue is approximated with a 0 or 2-0 Vicryl (Ethicon Inc, Somerville, N.J.). We prefer to close the skin with a running subcuticular suture using a 3-0 monofilament suture to be removed in a week. Full-length Steri-strips (3M, St. Paul, Minn.) are applied, and the arthroscopic portals are covered with xeroform gauze. Sterile gauze is secured with sterile Webril or cast padding, and the leg is wrapped from the toes to the thigh with an elastic bandage.

Post-op Management
A majority of the time, patients are discharged the same day. Only toe-touch weight bearing is allowed for 6 weeks. On

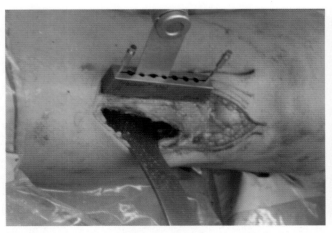

Fig. 54-17. AMZ: An oscillating saw with a 1-in. blade is used for the osteotomy.

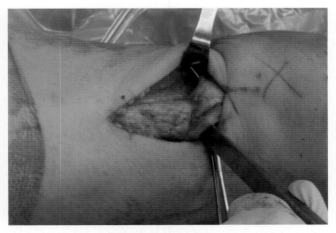

Fig. 54-19. AMZ: A half-inch osteotome is used to cut the cortex behind the patellar tendon.

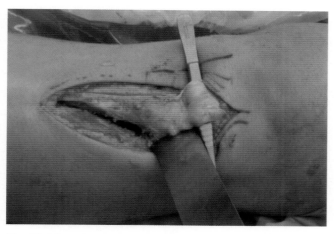

Fig. 54-20. AMZ: A 1-in. osteotome is used to connect the transverse and posterolateral cuts.

post-op day 1, the patient is encouraged to perform a passive flexion arc of 90 degrees once a day. Otherwise, a long-leg knee immobilizer is used for 6 weeks, and no active extension is permitted during this time.

An x-ray is obtained at the first postoperative visit, but serial radiographs are not routinely taken to evaluate the osteotomy. Because of the secure fixation of the sizable opposed cancellous surfaces, very little or no callous will be appreciated. In our experience the screws will need to be removed in 75% of the cases due to discomfort despite countersinking. We like to wait until 1 year postoperatively to do this.

Complications

There are many significant complications that can arise following this procedure. For one, anterior compartment syndrome is a risk. Fortunately, we have not experienced this, but the violation of the anterior compartment makes this possible. This is the rationale behind not closing the muscular fascia and meticulously inspecting the wound for bleeding.

Second, fracture of the fragment or nonunion of the osteotomy can occur. For this reason we are strict about prohibiting active extension for the first 6 weeks. A tibial metaphyseal fracture has been encountered as far as 6 months postoperatively. The senior author ( ) has performed over 500 anteromedialization procedures and has encountered metaphyseal fractures in slightly more than 2% of the cases. Of note, obesity has been consistently a factor in our experience. Stetson et al.[62] reported six fractures in their series of 234 cases. Thrombophlebitis, infection, and neurovascular injury can occur. We are aware of one case of injury to the deep peroneal nerve, but we have not seen this in our large series.

Trillat Tibial Tubercle Osteotomy

The primary indication for the osteotomy that Trillat et al.[63] described in 1964 is pure lateral instability with no chondromalacia or minimal cartilage damage confined to the proximal, lateral aspect of the patella **(Fig. 54-23)**. If isolated distal arthrosis or advanced lateral arthrosis is present, an AMZ is better indicated to shift the patellar loading proximally. However, even when diffuse lateral disease is seen in the face of severe instability, a Trillat osteotomy may be the only viable option, despite inconsistent results published on it usage in patients with painful instability.[64] A variation of the technique we use was shown to improve not only recurrent instability, but was also shown to have a radiographically profound affect on the congruence angle.[65–67]

A cadaveric study demonstrated increased contact pressures following isolated medialization.[68] Therefore, the procedure should be avoided in patients with medial chondral abnormalities. We have seen medial instability after a Trillat osteotomy and recommend caution when considering it in patients with trochlear dysplasia or global laxity.

Technique

Supine positioning and a tourniquet are once again used. With the leg prepped and the extremity free-draped, the

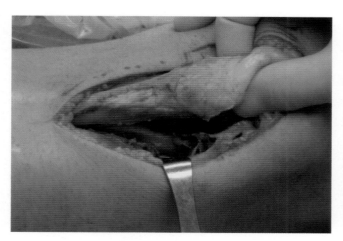

Fig. 54-21. AMZ: The fragment is displaced roughly 1 cm along the plane of the osteotomy.

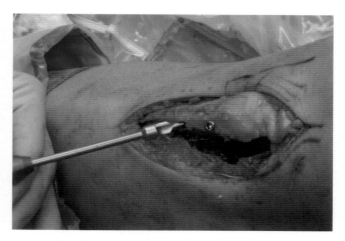

Fig. 54-22. AMZ: The countersink is used to minimize screw prominence.

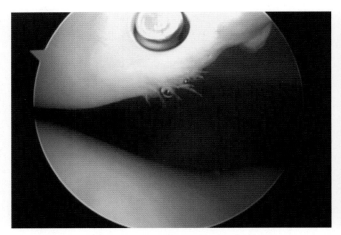

Fig. 54-23. Trillat: Arthroscopic appearance of subluxation in a patient with recurrent dislocations.

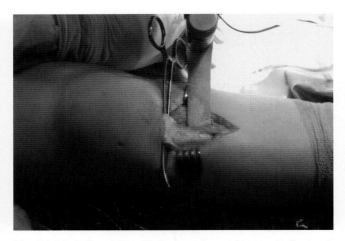

Fig. 54-25. Trillat: An oscillating saw is used to create the coronal osteotomy.

tourniquet is inflated. Following arthroscopic examination, a 6- to 7-cm midline incision is created. A lateral release can first be performed arthroscopically or subcutaneously through the incision. The patellar tendon is isolated for protection, as it is in the AMZ **(Fig. 54-22)**. In the Trillat, the plane of the osteotomy is near coronal. If anything, a tendency toward a slight anterior progression should be the only deviation, because the tubercle may otherwise deviate posteriorly as it is medially displaced. If allowed, this will result in an increase in contact pressures.

An oscillating saw is used to create the osteotomy **(Fig. 54-24)**. The dimensions of the tubercle fragment should be 1.5 cm thick and 5 cm in length with a taper to 1 cm in width distally. The overall width will be determined by the morphology of the tubercle. This sizing will allow ample room for fixation using two 4.5-mm fully threaded cortical AO screws that are placed using the lag technique to obtain posterior cortical fixation **(Fig. 54-25)**. One centimeter of medialization can be routinely obtained without sacrificing cancellous bone opposition. By rotating the fragment at its

proximal end, the tapered end of the fragment can remain in place to minimize the postoperative bony prominence. As with the AMZ, a countersink should be utilized and arthroscopic evaluation should be performed prior to placement of the second screw **(Fig. 54-26)**. Closure is no different from that used following an AMZ, with the adipose tissue being the deepest layer addressed. A knee immobilizer is applied in the operating room.

Postoperative Management

Toe-touch weight bearing is recommended, and crutches for 6 weeks. Active extension is prohibited during this time, but a daily 90-degree arc of passive motion is encouraged starting the day after surgery. The screws, like the AMZ, frequently need to be removed.

Complications

Since the anterior compartment of the lower leg is not violated, the risk of iatrogenic compartment syndrome is minimal. Wound healing may once again be an issue due to

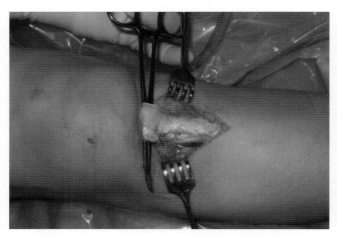

Fig. 54-24. Trillat: The tibial tubercle is exposed and the tendon is isolated.

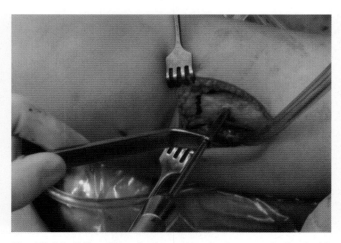

Fig. 54-26. Trillat: After displacement, the fragment is fixed with two AO cortical screws using the lag technique.

the bony prominence and usual lack of subcutaneous tissue. Tubercle fractures and osteotomy nonunions are possible issues that are rare when a strict postoperative course is adhered to. As mentioned, medial instability may result in a small number of cases.

Medial Patellofemoral Ligament Reconstruction

A MPFL reconstruction is used for severe lateral patellar instability, which, as mentioned earlier, is usually accompanied by degenerative changes. Under most circumstances, proximal soft tissue or tibial tuberosity realignment will suffice. However, when instability persists or the medial restraints are found to be inadequate, reconstructing the medial patellofemoral ligament may be warranted, particularly when there is trochlear dysplasia. A small series reported by Muneta et al.[69] demonstrated its success as a corrective procedure when instability was refractory to tibial tubercle transfer. We have used it in combination with tubercle transfers to help in the surgical management of complex patellofemoral instability when dysplasia coexists. Arendt, Fithian, and Cohen have reviewed MPFL reconstruction and its proper use.[70]

There is one instance, in particular, in which painful instability could be worsened by a MPFL reconstruction. Medial facet chondromalacia is most common in severe recurrent patellar instability. Therefore, considering that the medial facet will experience increased contact pressures postoperatively, this procedure should be avoided in this situation. MPFL reconstruction does not give the option of unloading symptomatic medial facet articular lesions and requires more clinical studies to support its regular use.

Technique

With the patient in the supine position, a tourniquet is applied to the proximal thigh. The knee is prepped with the extremity free-draped, after which the tourniquet is inflated. A small longitudinal incision is made over the pes anserinus to harvest the semitendinosus. The quadriceps tendon can also be used, but the length needed is easier to obtain from the semitendinosus. The tendon is prepared by first scraping the muscle off with a Cobb elevator. If necessary, it can be tubularized with a small Vicryl suture. The length is determined intraoperatively to account for the length of the MPFL plus 2 cm for each tunnel. The graft length will be 80 to 100 mm on average. The graft is doubled and the free ends are whipstitched with no. 2 FiberWire. The other end is sutured with a no. 2 FiberWire and a no. 2 Ethibond (Ethicon, Somerville, N.J.) in a locking Krackow fashion over 1.5 cm. These are tied over an EndoButton (Smith-Nephew, Andover, Mass.) with the goal of acquiring 2 cm of graft in the patellar tunnel after it is drilled and measured (see below).

Two parallel 4-cm longitudinal skin incisions are made over the medial retinaculum; one at the patellar edge and one over the medial epicondyle **(Figs. 54-27** and **54-28)**. If the skin is mobile, the procedure can be performed through one incision (illustrated in the accompanying photos).

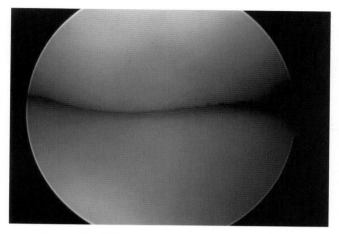

Fig. 54-27. Trillat: The tracking has been corrected.

Blunt subcutaneous dissection should be used to protect the saphenous neurovascular structures. The anatomic regions to be identified for tunnel placement are the junction of the proximal and middle third of the patella on its medial border, and the medial condyle midway between the epicondyle and adductor tubercle. There is a distinct ridge delineating the MPFL origin **(Fig. 54-29)**. To expose the site for the graft placement, the retinaculum is transversely incised in line with its fibers while the capsule is maintained **(Fig. 54-30)**.

The graft is sized and the appropriate width femoral tunnel is reamed to a depth of 30 mm. A guide wire is used on the patellar side where the hole is reamed at the above-mentioned landmark where the soft tissues attach **(Fig. 54-31)**. The 5-mm EndoButton reamer is passed over the guide wire and the tunnel is measured before the graft can finally be secured to the EndoButton.

Two lead sutures are placed in the EndoButton to pass it through the tunnel using a Beath pin or a suture passer **(Fig. 54-32)**. The knee is placed through a range of motion to evaluate isometry and tension. The femoral side is ultimately

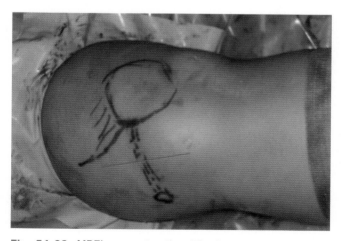

Fig. 54-28. MPFL reconstruction: The line indicates the skin incision when a single incision technique is used.

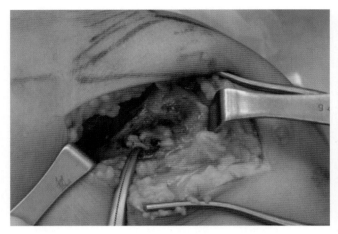

Fig. 54-29. MPFL reconstruction: The femoral origin of the MPFL is located at the tip of the clamp.

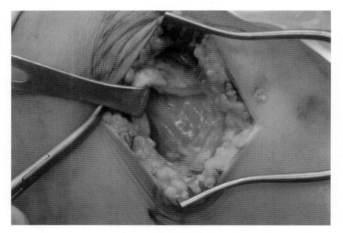

Fig. 54-30. MPFL reconstruction: The retinaculum is transversely incised to expose but maintain the capsule.

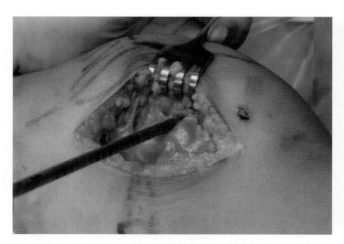

Fig. 54-31. MPFL reconstruction: The patellar tunnel is reamed over the Beath pin at the junction of the proximal and middle third to a depth of 20 or 25 mm. Do not violate the lateral cortex.

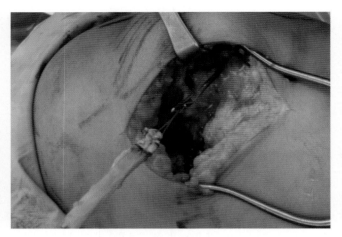

Fig. 54-32. MPFL reconstruction: The lead/toggle sutures are passed through the patellar tunnel with the Beath pin.

secured with a Biotenodesis screw (Arthrex, Naples, Fla.) **(Figs. 54-33** and **54-34).**

The tourniquet is deflated prior to closure to ensure that bleeding is controlled. The dermis is closed with a 2-0 Vicryl suture and the skin is closed with a running subcuticular suture. Steri-strips and sterile gauze are applied followed by sterile cast pad, an elastic bandage, and a knee immobilizer.

Postoperative Management

The postoperative course we pursue is the same as that employed following an arthroscopic realignment. Two weeks of strict immobilization is followed by a once daily 90-degree arc of passive flexion. Weight bearing is not limited. At 6 weeks, active extension is allowed. Typically 6 months will be needed before strenuous activity can be resumed. Radiographs are obtained at the 6-week follow-up visit.

Complications

The two most common complications following a MPFL reconstruction are that it does not decrease the lateral

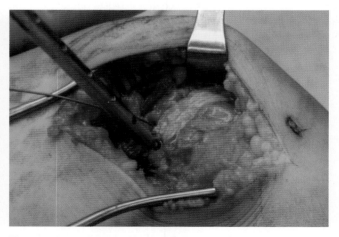

Fig. 54-33. MPFL reconstruction: After the knee has been ranged to verify isometry and determine tension, the femoral side is fixed with a Biotenodesis screw (Arthrex, Naples, Fla.).

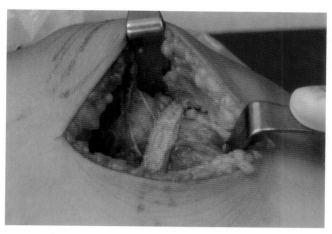

Fig. 54-34. MPFL reconstruction: The quadriceps tendon graft appearance following fixation.

instability or it worsens the pain from overloading a worn medial facet. We have concerns about the risk of a nonisometric reconstruction or excessive posteriorly directed forces created by this tenodesis procedure.

Patellofemoral Arthroplasty

Patellofemoral arthroplasty is a viable option when there are diffuse patellofemoral degenerative changes that cannot be adequately treated by tibial tubercle transfer and/or articular resurfacing and joint preservation. Isolated, diffuse arthritis of a properly aligned patellofemoral joint is the best indication for articular resurfacing, but this scenario is quite uncommon. If concomitant malalignment is encountered, we recommend addressing it first. These concepts were illustrated in a follow-up study by Arciero and Toomey[71] evaluating 25 arthroplasties. They appreciated the detrimental effects of malalignment and multicompartmental disease on long-term results.

■ SUMMARY

Degenerative patellofemoral disorders are difficult to treat. However, with careful evaluation and planning, consistently good results can be obtained when surgical intervention is warranted. Differentiating instability from arthrosis and identifying the cases where they coexist are essential steps in the treatment process. Anteromedial tibial tubercle transfer is particularly helpful, as it both realigns and unloads the patellofemoral joint. Supplementation with selective articular cartilage resurfacing expands the possibilities for patellofemoral joint preservation.

■ REFERENCES

1. Nomura E, Inoue M. Cartilage lesions of the patella in recurrent patellar dislocation. Am J Sports Med. 2004;32(2):498–502.

2. Desio SM, Burks RT, Bachus KN. Soft tissue restraints to lateral patellar translation in the human knee. Am J Sports Med. 1998; 26(1):59–65.

3. Goodfellow JW, Hungerford DS, Zindel M. Patello-femoral mechanics and pathology: I. functional anatomy of the patellofemoral joint. J Bone Joint Surg. 1976;58B:287.

4. Senavongse W, Farahmand F, Jones J, et al. Quantitative measurement of patellofemoral joint stability: force-displacement of the human patella in vitro. J Orthop Res. 2003;21(5):780–786.

5. Sojbjerg JO, Lauritzen J, Hvid I, et al. Arthroscopic determination of patellofemoral malalignment. Clin Orthop. 1987 Feb;(215): 243–247.

6. Hawkins RJ, Bell RH, Anisette G. Acute patellar dislocations. The natural history. Am J Sports Med. 1986;14(2):117–120.

7. Zimbler S, Smith J, Scheller A, et al. Recurrent subluxation and dislocation of the patella in association with athletic injuries. Orthop Clin North Am. 1980;11(4):755–770.

8. Runow A. The dislocating patella. Etiology and prognosis in relation to generalized joint laxity and anatomy of the patellar articulation. Acta Orthop Scand Suppl. 1983;201:1–53.

9. Borochowitz Z, Soudry M, Mendes DG. Familial recurrent dislocation of patella with autosomal dominant mode of inheritance. Clin Genet. 1988;33(1):1–4.

10. Fulkerson J, Tennant R, Jaivin J, et al. Histologic evidence of retinacular nerve injury associated with patellofemoral malalignment. Clin Orthop. 1985;187:196–205.

11. Sanchis-Alfonso V, Rosello-Sastre E, Monteagudo-Castro C, et al. Quantitative analysis of nerve changes in the lateral retinaculum in patients with isolated symptomatic patellofemoral malalignment. a preliminary study. Am J Sports Med. 1998;26(5):703–709.

12. Dejour H, Walch G, Nove-Josserand L, et al. Factors of patellar instability: an anatomic radiographic study. Knee Surg Sports Traumatol Arthrosc. 1994;2(1):19–26.

13. Davies AP, Costa ML, Shepstone L, et al. The sulcus angle and malalignment of the extensor mechanism of the knee. J Bone Joint Surg Br. 2000;82(8):1162–1166.

14. Greenen E, Molenaers G, Martens M. Patella alta in patellofemoral instability. Acta Orthop Belg. 1989;55(3):387–393.

15. Cross MJ, Waldrop J. The patella index as a guide to the understanding and diagnosis of patellofemoral instability. Clin Orthop. 1975;110:174–176.

16. Ficat, P. [The syndrome of lateral hyperpressure of the patella] Acta Orthop Belg. 1978;44(1):65–76.

17. Floyd A, Phillips P, Khan MR, et al. Recurrent dislocation of the patella: histochemical and electromyographic evidence of primary muscle pathology. J Bone Joint Surg Br. 1987;69(5): 790–793.

18. Blumensaat C. Die lageabweichungen und verrenkungen der kniescheibe. Ergeb Chir Orthop. 1938;31:149.

19. Insall JN, Salvati E. Patella position in the normal knee joint. Radiology. 1971;101:101.

20. Bernageau J, Goutallier D. *Affections Femoro-Patellaires.* Encyclopedic Med. Chir, Radiodiagnostic II. 1977;31:312.

21. Blackburne JS, Peel TE. A new method of measuring patellar height. J Bone Joint Surg Br. 1977;59(2):241–242.

22. Murray TF, Dupont JY, Fulkerson JP. Axial and lateral radiographs in evaluating patellofemoral malalignment. Am J Sports Med. 1999;27(5):580–584.

23. Malghem J, Maldague B. Depth insufficiency of the proximal trochlear groove on lateral radiographs of the knee: relation to patellar dislocation. Radiology. 1989;170(2):507–510.

24. Merchant AC, Mercer RL, Jacobsen RH, et al. Roentgenographic analysis of patellofemoral congruence. J Bone Joint Surg Am. 1974;56(7):1391–1396.

25. Galland O, Walch G, Dejour H, et al. An anatomical and radiological study of the femoropatellar articulation. Surg Radiol Anat. 1990;12:119.

26. Dowd GS, Bentley G. Radiographic assessment in patellar instability and chondromalacia patellae. J Bone Joint Surg Br. 1986;68(2):297–300.

27. Tsujimoto K, Kurosaka M, Yoshiya S, et al. Radiographic and computed tomographic analysis of the position of the tibial tubercle in recurrent dislocation and subluxation of the patella. Am J Knee Surg. 2000;13(2):83–88.

28. Davids JR, Marshall AD, Blocker ER, et al. Femoral anteversion in children with cerebral palsy: assessment with two and three-dimensional computed tomography scans. J Bone Joint Surg Am. 2003;85–A(3):481–488.

29. Pinar H, Akseki D, Karaoglan O, et al. Kinematic and dynamic axial computed tomography of the patello-femoral joint in patients with anterior knee pain. Knee Surg Sports Traumatol Arthrosc. 1994;2(3):170–173.

30. Hinton RY, Sharma KM. Acute and recurrent patellar instability in the young athlete. Orthop Clin North Am. 2003;34(3):385–396.

31. Cowan SM, Bennell KL, Crossley KM, et al. Physical therapy alters recruitment of the vasti in patellofemoral pain syndrome. Med Sci Sports Exerc. 2002;34(12):1879–1885.

32. Cowan SM, Bennell KL, Hodges PW, et al. Simultaneous feedforward recruitment of the vasti in untrained postural tasks can be restored by physical therapy. J Orthop Res. 2003;21(3):553–538.

33. Hanten WP, Schulthies SS. Exercise effect on electromyographic activity of the vastus medialis oblique and vastus lateralis muscles. Phys Ther. 1990;70(9):561–565.

34. Bergstrom KA, Brandseth K, Fretheim S, et al. Activity-related knee injuries and pain in athletic adolescents. Knee Surg Sports Traumatol Arthrosc. 2001;9(3):146–150.

35. McConnell, J. The management of chondromalacia patellae. J Physiother. 1986;32:215–223.

36. Shellock FG, Mink JH, Deutsch AL, et al. Effect of a newly designed patellar realignment brace on patellofemoral relationships. Med Sci Sports Exerc. 1995;27(4):469–472.

37. Cherf J, Paulos LE. Bracing for patellar instability. Clin Sports Med. 1990;9(4):813–821.

38. Hvid I, Andersen LI, Schmidt H. Chondromalacia patellae: the relation to abnormal patellofemoral joint mechanics. Acta Orthop Scand. 1981;52(6):661–666.

39. Pidoriano AJ, Fulkerson JP. Arthroscopy of the patellofemoral joint. Clin Sports Med. 1997;16(1):17–28.

40. Grana WA, Hinkley B, Hollingsworth, S. Arthroscopic evaluation and treatment of patellar malalignment. Clin Orthop. 1984;186:122–128.

41. Ogilvie-Harris DJ, Jackson RW. The arthroscopic treatment of chondromalacia patellae. J Bone Joint Surg Br. 1984;66(5):660–665.

42. Federico DJ, Reider B. Results of isolated patellar debridement for patellofemoral pain in patients with normal patellar alignment. Am J Sports Med. 1997;25(5):663–669.

43. Sherman OH, Fox JM, Sperling H, et al. Patellar instability: treatment by arthroscopic electrosurgical lateral release. Arthroscopy. 1987;3(3):152–160.

44. Aglietti P, Pisaneshci A, Buzzi R, et al. Arthroscopic lateral release for patellar pain or instability. Arthroscopy. 1989;5(3):176–183.

45. Schonholtz GJ, Zahn MG, Magee CM. Lateral retinacular release of the patella. Arthroscopy. 1987;3(4):269–272.

46. Krompinger WJ, Fulkerson JP. Lateral retinacular release for intractable lateral retinacular pain. Clin Orthop. 1983 Oct;(179):191–193.

47. Strand T, Alho A, Raugstad TS, et al. Patellofemoral disorders treated by operations. Acta Orthop Scand. 1983;54(6):914–916.

48. Shea KP, Fulkerson JP. Preoperative computed tomography scanning and arthroscopy in predicting outcome after lateral retinacular release. Arthroscopy. 1992;8(3):327–334.

49. Nonweiler DE, DeLee JC. The diagnosis and treatment of medial subluxation of the patella after lateral retinacular release. Am J Sports Med. 1994;22(5):680–686.

50. Shellock FG, Mink JH, Deutsch A, et al. Evaluation of patients with persistent symptoms after lateral retinacular release by kinematic magnetic resonance imaging of the patellofemoral joint. Arthroscopy. 1990;6(3):226–234.

51. Insall J, Bullough PG, Burstein AH. Proximal "tube" realignment of the patella for chondromalacia patellae. Clin Orthop. 1979;144:63–69.

52. Abraham E, Washington E, Huang TL. Insall proximal realignment for disorders of the patella. Clin Orthop. 1989;248:61–65.

53. Yamamoto, RK. Arthroscopic repair of the medial retinaculum and capsule in acute patellar dislocations. Arthroscopy. 1986;2(2):125–131.

54. Small NC, Glogau AI, Berezin MA. Arthroscopically assisted proximal extensor mechanism realignment of the knee. Arthroscopy. 1993;9(1):63–67.

55. Henry JE, Pflum FA. Arthroscopic proximal patella realignment and stabilization. Arthroscopy. 1995;11(4):424–425.

56. Ahmad CS, Lee FY. An all-arthroscopic soft-tissue balancing technique for lateral patellar instability. Arthroscopy. 2001;17(5):555–557.

57. Halbrecht JL. Arthroscopic patella realignment: an all-inside technique. Arthroscopy. 2001;17(9):940–945.

58. Haspl M, Cicak N, Klobucar H, et al. Fully arthroscopic stabilization of the patella. Arthroscopy. 2002;18(1):E2.

59. Albuquerque RF, Pacheco A, Hernandez AJ, et al. Appraisal of surgical treatment of 47 cases of patellofemoral instability. Rev Hosp Clin Fac Med Sao Paulo. 2002;57(3):103–107.

60. Fulkerson, JP. Anteromedialization of the tibial tuberosity for patellofemoral malalignment. Clin Orthop. 1983;177:176–181.

61. Pidoriano AJ, Weinstein RN, Buuck DA, et al. Correlation of patellar articular lesions with results from anteromedial tibial tubercle transfer. Am J Sports Med. 1997;25(4):533–537.

62. Stetson WB, Friedman MJ, Fulkerson JP, et al. Fracture of the proximal tibia with immediate weightbearing after a Fulkerson osteotomy. Am J Sports Med. 1997;25(4):570–574.

63. Trillat A, Dejour H, Couette A. [Diagnosis and treatment of recurrent dislocations of the patella]. Rev Chir Orthop Reparatrice Appar Mot. 1964;50:813–824.

64. Kumar A, Jones S, Bickerstaff DR, et al. Functional evaluation of the modified Elmslie-Trillat procedure for patello-femoral dysfunction. Knee. 2001;8(4):287–292.

65. Rillmann P, Dutly A, Kieser C, et al. Modified Elmslie-Trillat procedure for instability of the patella. Knee Surg Sports Traumatol Arthrosc. 1998;6(1):31–35.

66. Shelbourne KD, Porter DA, Rozzi W. Use of a modified Elmslie-Trillat procedure to improve abnormal patellar congruence angle. Am J Sports Med. 1994;22(3):318–323.

67. Wootton JR, Cross MG, Wood DG. Patellofemoral malalignment: a report of 68 cases treated by proximal and distal patellofemoral reconstruction. Injury. 1990;21(3):169–173.

68. Kuroda R, Kambic H, Valdevit A, et al. Articular cartilage contact pressure after tibial tuberosity transfer: a cadaveric study. Am J Sports Med. 2001;29(4):403–409.

69. Muneta T, Sekiya I, Tsuchiya M, et al. A technique for reconstruction of the medial patellofemoral ligament. Clin Orthop. 1999;Feb;(359):151–155.

70. Arendt E, Fithian D, Cohen E. Current concepts of lateral patella dislocation. Clin Sports Med. 2002;21:499–519.

71. Arciero RA, Toomey HE. Patellofemoral arthroplasty: a three- to nine-year follow-up study. Clin Orthop. 1988 Nov;(236):60–71.

Part

E

ARTICULAR CARTILAGE INJURIES

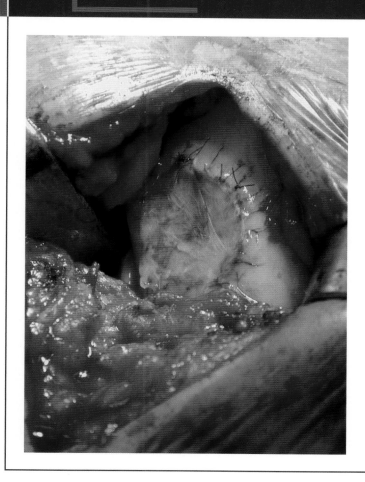

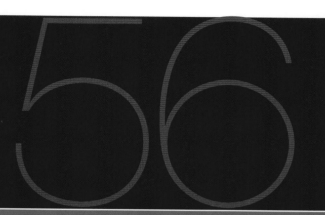

56

SURGICAL TREATMENT OF OSTEOCHONDRITIS DISSECANS OF THE KNEE

■ CHRISTINA R. ALLEN, MD, MARC R. SAFRAN, MD

■ HISTORY OF THE TREATMENT OF OSTEOCHONDRITIS DISSECANS

Osteochondritis dissecans (OCD) of the knee is a condition that causes separation or fragmentation of a segment of sub-chondral bone and overlying cartilage from the remaining underlying subchondral bone. With progression of the con-dition, this pathology may result in signs or symptoms cor-relating with the disease stage as it impacts on the integrity of the overlying articular cartilage.

Early signs or symptoms associated with intact cartilage over an OCD lesion may be related to cartilage softening or an alteration in the mechanical properties of the cartilage. At this early stage, the patient may complain of vague ante-rior knee pain and a variable amount of swelling that is typ-ically intermittent and often related to activity level. In later stages, due to lack of underlying support of the cartilage, the patient may present with signs or symptoms of articular car-tilage separation (cartilage flaps or "loose bodies" causing locking or catching symptoms), inflammatory synovitis, or a persistent or intermittent effusion. Because lesions may become symptomatic, surgical intervention may often be required. In 1840, Paré was the first to describe the removal of joint loose bodies, which were presumably osteochondral fragments.[1] Operative treatment for unstable lesions has been traditionally attributed to Smillie,[2] who developed a nail for open reduction and internal fixation of displaced and unstable lesions.

The incidence of OCD has been estimated at between 0.02% to 0.03% (based on a survey of knee radiographs) and 1.2% (based on knee arthroscopies).[3,4] The highest rates appear among patients between 10 and 15 years of age, with rare instances in children under 4 or patients over 50 years of age. Higher rates among males are historically reported, with an approximate 2:1 ratio compared with

females, though recent data suggest that this difference is lessening.[5] Bilateral lesions, typically in different phases of development, are reported in 15% to 30% of cases and mandate assessment of both knees in all those presenting with this diagnosis.[6] OCD lesions of the knee most com-monly involve the lateral aspect of the medial femoral condyle (Fig. 56-1A,B). The lateral femoral condyle is less frequently involved, and patellar OCD lesions are even more rare.[6,7]

The etiology of osteochondritis dissecans remains unclear. König[8] originally described the condition in 1888 and gave it a name indicative of his initial belief that OCD was due to an inflammatory reaction of both the bone and the cartilage. Current consensus regarding etiology is debatable, although an inflammatory etiology is unlikely, as recognized by König a decade later. Repetitive microtrauma, ischemia, epiphyseal abnormalities, osteochondral fracture, genetic predisposition, and endocrine abnormalities have all been postulated as potential contributors to development of OCD.

Clinically, Cahill[5] and Mubarak and Carrol[9] emphasized a distinction between two types of OCD as recognized by the osseous age of the patient at the time of symptom onset. Those with open physes are considered to have juvenile onset OCD, while those who are skeletally mature at the time of symptom onset have the adult form. Paradoxically, adult onset OCD may simply be a delayed onset of previ-ously asymptomatic juvenile OCD that failed to heal and manifests later with loosening and joint degeneration. Skeletal age at onset of symptoms appears to be the most important determinant of prognosis and remains an essen-tial factor directing the timing and nature of treatment deci-sions. Paletta et al.[10] found that all patients with open phy-seal plates and increased activity on bone scan were more likely to heal their OCD lesion, while those without increased activity did not heal. In contrast, among patients

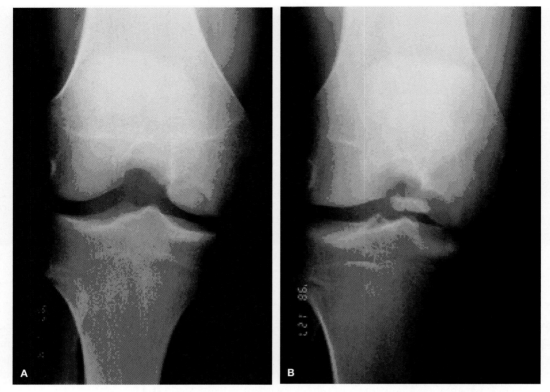

Fig. 56-1. The classic location for osteochondritis dissecans. AP radiographs demonstrates a lateral aspect of the medial femoral condyle OCD lesion before **(A)** and after **(B)** displacement.

with closed growth plates only 33% healed despite having a similar increase in activity within the lesion.

Both radiographic and surgical classification systems for OCD lesions have been described, with few having clear prognostic significance. Using plain radiographs of the talus, Berndt and Harty[11] classified OCD in four stages that describe the condition and position of the osteochondral fragment, ranging from compression of the subchondral bone to complete detachment of the fragment (loose body). Cahill and Berg[12] describe a method of dividing the AP and lateral radiographs into 15 distinct zones. This alphanumeric system provides standardization for research and descriptive purposes, but has found limited clinical application to date with regard to treatment or prognosis.[5]

DiPaola et al.[13] classified lesions according to appearance on magnetic resonance imaging (MRI) and correlated specific findings with the potential for fragment detachment. They described lesions containing fluid (high T2 signal) behind the subchondral fragment as potentially unstable, as this suggested a breach of the cartilage surface. The presence of a low T2 signal behind the fragment suggests that there is no fluid behind the fragment, indicating a stable fibrous attachment and potentially intact cartilage surface. Other reports suggest a similarly high level of confidence for predicting lesion stability using intra-articular gadolinium contrast.[14]

DiPaola's classification system has proven to be reasonably accurate and predictive of the stability of lesions on arthroscopic examination. O'Connor et al.[15] found an 85% correlation between preoperative MRI findings using DiPaola's criteria and arthroscopic findings graded with Guhl's arthroscopic classification system for OCDs. In Guhl's[16] system, OCD stages are defined by cartilage integrity and fragment stability. Type I lesions have softening of cartilage but no breach of the cartilage surface; type II lesions have breached cartilage but are stable. Type III osteochondral defects have a definable fragment that remains partially attached (flap lesion), type IV lesions constitute an osteochondral defect at the donor site with a resultant loose body in the knee joint.

■ INDICATIONS AND CONTRAINDICATIONS

No randomized, controlled clinical trials exist for either operative or nonoperative interventions for OCD of the knee. In general, physis maturity, dissection of the lesion from the adjacent subchondral bone or stability, size, and location of lesions and cartilage surface integrity have been used as predictive criterion for necessity of operative intervention.

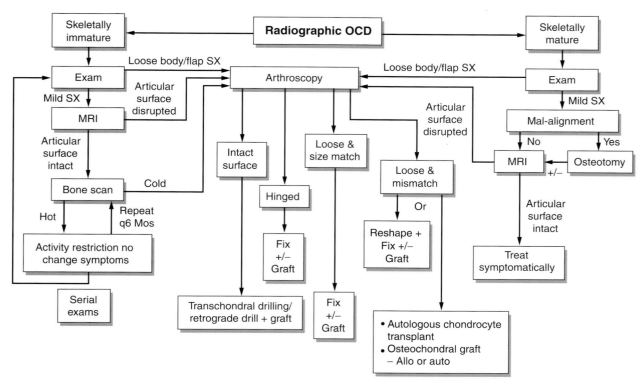

Fig. 56-2. Treatment algorithm for knee OCD.

Recently, a large multicenter review of the European Pediatric Orthopedic Society's experience with treatment of OCD lesions was performed.[6] Lessons from this study are derived from the knees of 318 juvenile patients and 191 adults. The authors of the study made several important distinctions and conclusions. They determined that if there are no signs of dissection (loosening), the prognosis is significantly better and that pain and swelling are not good indicators of fragment dissection. Additionally, plain radiographs and computed tomography (CT) scan are not useful in predicting dissection. Sclerosis on plain radiographs predicts a poor response to drilling. Further analysis demonstrated that lesions greater than 2 cm in diameter had a worse prognosis, and when there is evidence of dissection, surgical treatment results are better than nonsurgical. Lesions in the classical location of the lateral aspect of the medial femoral condyle had a better prognosis. Finally, although patients with adult onset symptoms had a higher proportion of abnormal findings on radiographs after the treatment period (42%), more than one in five of those with open epiphyseal plates (22%) had abnormal knee radiographs at an average of 3 years after starting treatment.

An algorithm for treatment decisions is outlined in **Fig. 56-2**, with the primary goal being to promote healing of lesions in situ and preventing displacement.

Nonoperative treatment through activity modification may include a wide spectrum of approaches that have his-torically included crutches for limited weight bearing, braces, or even casts for non-compliant patients. In patients without significant sports participation, prescribing a non–weight-bearing status and range of knee motion exercises may be beneficial to cartilage and help avoid the potential disaster of "cast disease" and arthrofibrosis. Our approach is to limit sports activities without immobilization, casting, or crutches, except for the noncompliant patient.

Choosing surgical intervention for managing OCD of the knee and selecting a strategy for repair, reconstruction, or removal of osteochondral lesions depends upon the stability of the osteochondral lesion and the integrity of the overlying cartilage. Essentially, the indications for operative treatment in skeletally immature patients are a symptomatic osteochondral fragment that is attached but not healing, a partially or completely detached fragment with a disrupted articular surface, and loose bodies. In skeletally mature individuals, lesions are less likely to heal with conservative treatment once fluid is dissecting under the fragment; therefore, symptomatic lesions and loose bodies are generally treated surgically.

■ PREOPERATIVE IMAGING STUDIES

Three standard roentgenograms of the knee, bilateral posterior-anterior (PA) 30-degree bent knee (Rosenberg or notch view), axial (Merchant) view, and lateral weight-bearing exams are routine in the initial evaluation for OCD.[17] Lesions of the weight-bearing surface of the femur are best seen with a flexed knee PA view and may help identify the lesions in the posterior condyles (Fig. 56-1A,B). Lateral radiographs allow recognition of the relative anterior-posterior location and identification of normal benign accessory ossification centers in the skeletally immature patient as described by Caffey et al.[18] An axial view of the patella should be added, as it may uncover the unusual patella lesion. Plain radiographs also allow a baseline assessment of the lesion size, presence or absence of sclerosis, presence or absence or lesions in the contralateral knee, potential dissection, and assignment to one of several classification systems that are based on radiographic criteria.

MRI studies are also useful in quantifying the size of the lesion. Again, the studies of DiPaola et al.[13] have shown that lesions containing fluid (high T2 signal) behind the subchondral fragment tend to be unstable and may require surgical treatment **(Fig. 56-3)**, whereas lesions that demonstrate a low T2 signal behind the fragment indicate a stable fibrous attachment.

The use of bone scans may be beneficial in monitoring the healing progress of a stable lesion and may also be useful in predicting the healing potential of a lesion. As previously noted, Paletta et al.[10] found that all patients with open physeal plates and increased activity on bone scan went on to

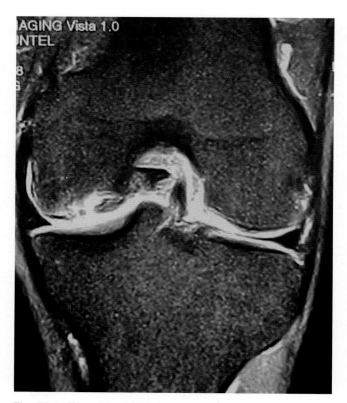

Fig. 56-3. T2-weighted MRI of the knee demonstrating high signal behind osteochondral fragment, indicating an unstable fragment.

heal their OCD lesions, while those without increased activity did not heal without surgical intervention. In contrast, among patients with closed growth plates only 33% healed despite having a similar increase in activity within the lesion.

■ SURGICAL TECHNIQUES

Surgical treatment of osteochondral defects is usually performed under general anesthesia, possibly supplemented with a femoral nerve block for postoperative pain relief. Arthroscopic treatment is preferable because of decreased morbidity, although it may be necessary to perform a mini-arthrotomy or full arthrotomy in order to gain adequate access to the osteochondral defect for repair. Posterior condyle lesions and the less common patella and tibial plateau lesions are particularly difficult to fix arthroscopically and an arthrotomy should be used in order to ensure precise access, exposure, reduction, and fixation of the lesion. A 30-degree arthroscope is generally utilized and standard inferomedial and inferolateral arthroscopic portals are established. It may be beneficial to establish the arthroscopic viewing portal first (viewing from the portal opposite the OCD lesion) and then use a spinal needle to localize direct access to the OCD lesion before establishing the working portal on the same side of the knee as the defect. Anterior synovitis and hypertrophic fat pads should be excised with a shaver in order to allow adequate visualization of and access to the OCD lesion. The OCD lesion is then probed for stability, which will dictate the method of treatment. The meniscus of the affected compartment should be carefully examined for injury and stability. Likewise the surrounding cartilage on the tibial and femoral sides should be examined and probed for defects, flaps, and evidence of softening. If loose bodies are encountered, every attempt should be made to remove them intact, as they could possibly be salvaged and utilized to repair the osteochondral defect.

■ TREATMENT OF STABLE LESIONS

Operative treatment for stable or intact lesions with normal articular cartilage involves drilling of the subchondral bone with the intention of stimulating vascular ingrowth and subchondral bone healing. Retrograde techniques (defined as methods that avoid articular cartilage disruption using a transosseous approach) have given way to arthroscopically assisted antegrade (transchondral) methods that have proven to be highly efficacious in skeletally immature patients. In general, drilling is more effective in promoting healing in skeletally immature patients than in older patients, but is still worth attempting in all patients with a persistently symptomatic lesion with intact articular cartilage.

Arthroscopically assisted antegrade drilling may be performed with a 0.062-in. Kirschner wire to a minimum

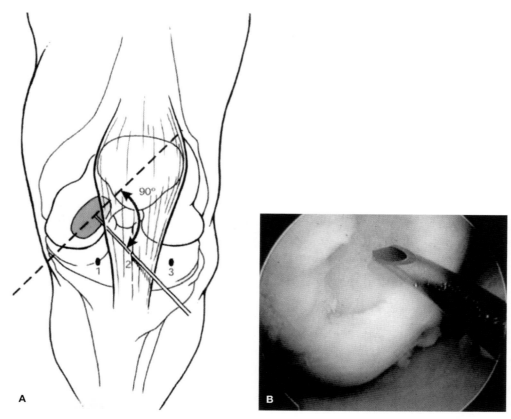

Fig. 57-8. A: Illustration of planned transpatellar tendon portal using a spinal needle to confirm perpendicular access to lesion bed. (Reprinted from Hangody L, Rathonyi G, Duska Z, et al. Autologous osteochondral mosaicplasty. J Bone Joint Surg Am. March 2004;(suppl 1):86, with permission.) **B:** Arthroscopic view of spinal needle to determine portal placement for perpendicular access to chondral defect. (Reprinted from Hangody L, Rathonyi G, Duska Z, et al. Autologous osteochondral mosaicplasty. J Bone Joint Surg Am. March 2004;(suppl 1):86, with permission.)

analyzing ten recommended sites for osteochondral harvest using pressure-sensitive film through a functional range of knee motion. They found the sites with least contact pressure were the superior lateral aspect of the lateral femoral condyle followed by the superior medial aspect of the intercondylar notch. Importantly they also reported that none of the donor sites harvested were free from significant contact pressure. They did not evaluate the superior and medial edges of the femur. All of the above mentioned sites are acceptable for donor grafts **(Fig. 57-7)**, however, it must be remembered that long-term follow-up on donor site morbidity is limited.

Planning before graft harvest is vital and includes determining the number of grafts, graft diameter, and the convexity or concavity of donor and recipient surfaces. It must be remembered that the periphery of the femur gives convex cores and the notch area produces grafts with concave articular surfaces. A key goal in resurfacing is matching the surface ultrastructure of the transplanted grafts with the normal surface topography of the joint in the area of the lesion. This allows accurate re-creation of the joint surface anatomy to restore contact pressures and joint mechanics to normal.

Donor Graft Harvest

When performing core harvest arthroscopically, portal selection is crucial. It is essential that the tube harvester be oriented perpendicular to the donor articular cartilage. This may be accomplished by using a spinal needle to ensure perpendicular access prior to making the portal **(Fig. 57-8A,B)**. Portals may be made safely over much of the knee region as long as care is taken not to damage healthy underlying articular cartilage or meniscus. Hangody et al.[68,80] prefer to use the medial border of the medial femoral condyle in arthroscopic harvesting as it is easier to access since the patella generally is displaced laterally with knee distension. The periphery of the lateral femoral condyle and the intercondylar notch also may be accessed arthroscopically with the use of accessory portals.

When performing an arthrotomy or mini-arthrotomy, access to the desired donor site area must be kept in mind when planning the amount of exposure available with the planned skin incision. A contralateral portal is used for viewing the portal site and ensuring a perpendicular alignment. The knee is extended to access more superior donor

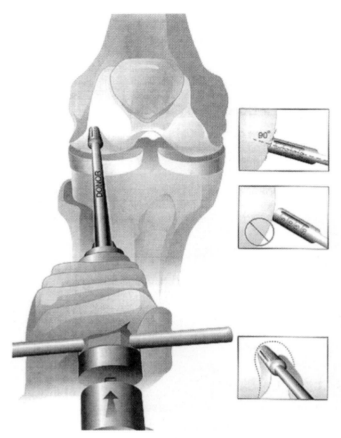

Fig. 57-9. Harvest technique using Arthrex OATS system. (Reprinted from Bobic V, Morgan C, Carter T. Osteochondral autologous graft transfer. Oper Tech Sports Med., 2000;8(2), Elsevier Inc, with permission.)

the portal and placed over the selected donor cartilage. Once position is confirmed a mallet is used to seat the harvester to a depth of 15 mm for chondral defects and 25 mm for osteochondral defects. The additional 10 mm provides adequate cancellous bone to replace subchondral bone loss in osteochondral lesions.

While seating the harvester one must clearly see the depth markings on the barrel to procure accurately sized grafts **(Fig. 57-9)**. During impaction the angle and rotation of the harvester tube must remain constant and perpendicular. This ensures that the graft will have a symmetric cartilage cap that will fit congruently in the lesion being filled. Depending on the system being used, the harvester is then toggled 5 degrees with no rotation (Acufex MOSAICplasty), rotated 90 degrees clockwise and counterclockwise (Arthrex OATS), or rotated 720 degrees (Inovasive COR) to fracture the cancellous bone at the base of the graft. The harvester is then removed and the osteochondral graft is ready to be transplanted. The Acufex system requires removal of the graft from the harvester, which must be pushed out from the osseous end to avoid cartilage injury **(Fig. 57-10A,B)**. The Arthrex and Inovasive sets do not require free handling of the grafts as they remain in the harvester tube for transplantation. Six to 8 mm grafts seem to be optimal for creating a congruent articular surface while limiting the total amount of fill tissue between grafts in the lesion.

Recipient Socket Preparation

The principle of recipient bed preparation is to prepare a socket in the subchondral bone that enables a secure press-fit osteochondral graft to be placed. No additional fixation is used, thus graft size and socket size are created to achieve a secure press-fit fixation upon seating of each core. Duchow et al.[83] evaluated the stability of press-fit grafts in porcine femoral condyles with the Arthrex OATS system. They controlled for graft size in diameter and length. They

sites and flexed progressively to reach the more inferior areas. The sulcus terminalis identifies the inferior limit for graft harvest on both the lateral and medial femoral condyles. The correctly sized tubular graft harvester is introduced through

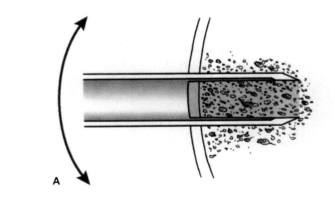

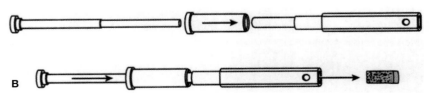

Fig. 57-10. Illustration of harvest technique using Acufex MOSAICplasty system. **A:** Chisel in donor site with graft being harvested. **B:** Harvesting chisel instrumentation with graft removed after harvest. (Reprinted from Hangody L, Rathonyi G, Duska Z, et al. Autologous osteochondral mosaicplasty. J Bone Joint Surg Am. March 2004(suppl 1):86, with permission.)

also looked at harvesting technique and the effect of repeated graft insertion after pullout to see if stability changed. They found that 15- and 20-mm grafts were significantly more stable than those 10 mm in length. They demonstrated that larger diameter grafts were more stable than smaller ones and that reinsertion after pullout significantly reduced primary fixation strength. When the harvest was performed and levering was used, as opposed to the recommended rotation with this system, stability was also compromised. When multiple grafts are to be transplanted it is vital that each one is completed before the creation of additional recipient sockets to avoid fracture of the recipient tunnel walls. The recipient tube harvester is placed on the prepared subchondral bed of the lesion in perpendicular position and driven into bone to a depth of 13 mm (Arthrex OATS). The harvester is next rotated, not levered, and then pulled out removing cancellous bone from the base of the tunnel **(Fig. 57-11A,B)**.

The donor harvester tubes are 1 mm larger than the recipient harvester tubes, allowing for press-fit insertion of grafts. Additionally, creating recipient sockets slightly more shallow than donor grafts allows better accuracy when seating grafts flush with surrounding cartilage. When utilizing the Acufex and Inovasive systems, a universal guide is positioned in the bed of the lesion and an appropriate-sized drill bit is used to drill the initial recipient tunnel. This is followed by a dilator that leaves the tunnel slightly undersized compared to the core graft being inserted **(Fig. 57-12)**. At this point one recipient socket is prepared and ready to accommodate one core graft.

Perpendicular alignment of the harvester or universal guide is crucial to create a graft transfer that is going to be flush with the intact cartilage around the defect. The harvester and universal guide are designed with atraumatic cutting edges so as not to damage peripheral cartilage while creating recipient sockets. Some authors believe drilling is not ideal due to thermal damage and subsequent necrosis. Miniaci et al.[84] showed that manual punch techniques of graft harvest and socket creation improved chondrocyte survival over power techniques.

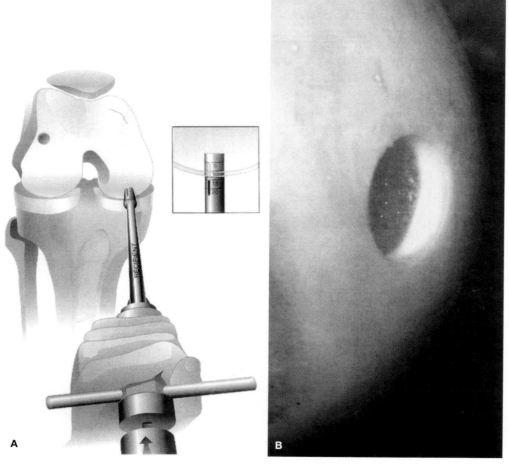

Fig. 57-11. A: Recipient socket preparation with Arthrex OATS system. (Reprinted from Bobic V, Morgan C, Carter T. Osteochondral autologous graft transfer. Oper Tech Sports Med. 2000;8(2), Elsevier Inc, with permission.) **B:** Recipient socket created within lesion with the Arthrex OATS system. (Reprinted from Bobic V, Morgan C, Carter T. Osteochondral autologous graft transfer. Oper Tech Sports Med. 2000;8(2), Elsevier Inc, with permission.)

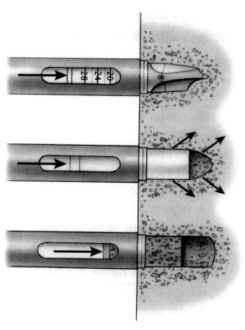

Fig. 57-12. Recipient socket preparation using universal guide from Acufex MOSAICplasty instrumentation. (Reprinted from Hangody L, Rathonyi G, Duska Z, et al. Autologous osteochondral mosaicplasty. J Bone Joint Surg Am. March 2004;(suppl 1):86, with permission.)

Osteochondral Graft Insertion

As mentioned the transfer of grafts must be done sequentially with graft harvest followed by recipient socket creation and graft insertion. It must be remembered not to harvest multiple grafts or create multiple recipient sockets at the same time as problems may be encountered. The goal is optimal fill of the defect, and this is best achieved with sequential graft transfer to enable accurate graft sizing and avoid recipient tunnel fracture. The OATS system has alignment rods that may be used to measure the depth of the socket and confirm alignment for graft insertion. The donor harvester with the core graft is reinserted in the driver assembly. The impaction cap is unscrewed and a collared pin is exposed, which advances the graft into the socket. The harvester has a beveled leading edge that is easily inserted into the recipient socket. This seats the harvester and serves to stabilize it for final graft seating. A mallet is used to gently tap the collared pin for seating of the graft **(Fig. 57-13)**. It is recommended

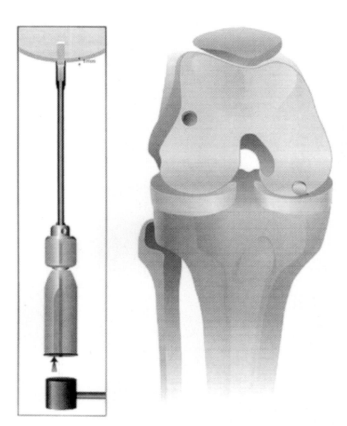

Fig. 57-13. Graft insertion with Arthrex OATS system. (Reprinted from Bobic V, Morgan C, Carter T. Osteochondral autologous graft transfer. Oper Tech Sports Med. 2000;8(2), Elsevier Inc, with permission.)

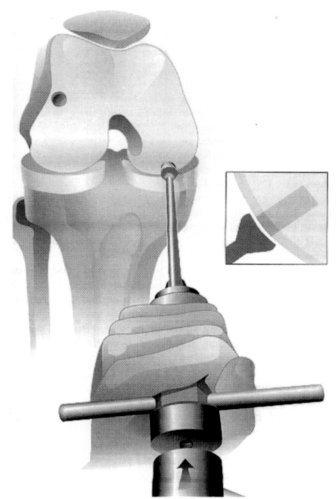

Fig. 57-14. Final graft seating performed with over-sized tamp from Arthrex OATS set. (Reprinted from Bobic V, Morgan C, Carter T. Osteochondral autologous graft transfer. Oper Tech Sports Med. 2000;8(2), Elsevier Inc, with permission.)

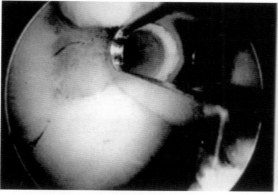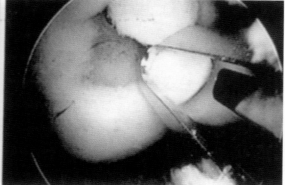

Fig. 57-15. Acufex MOSAICplasty universal guide used for graft insertion. (Reprinted from Hangody L, Rathonyi G, Duska Z, et al. Autologous osteochondral mosaicplasty. J Bone Joint Sur Am. March 2004;(suppl 1):86, with permission.)

that the graft be left 1 mm exposed and final seating be performed with an oversized tamp **(Fig. 57-14)**.

Once a flush, congruent position is achieved, this graft transfer is complete. It is extremely important not to over-seat the graft in a recessed position or leave the graft proud as either of these will adversely affect contact pressures. If a graft is seated too deeply one should prepare the adjacent recipient socket and use a probe to elevate the prior graft until it is flush.[80] When the graft is slightly raised it should be further seated until exactly flush with the surrounding surface. Alternatively, with the Acufex and Inovasive systems a universal guide is used for socket creation, and this guide remains in place. The core graft is then inserted into the guide with the cartilage surface on

the outside, and an adjustable plunger is used for final graft seating **(Fig. 57-15)**.

Graft transfers are continued until the defect is filled adequately and congruency is achieved with the surrounding articular surface. Multiple grafts of varying sizes allow the surgeon to achieve the most complete filling of defects and shape the grafts such that they are congruent with all edges of the lesion **(Fig. 57-16)**. Recessed areas and grafts that are slightly raised are problematic as they do not restore articular contact pressures adequately.[85] Raised grafts are also of concern as micromotion and remodeling may occur and interfere with graft incorporation.[86]

Donor Site Care

Donor harvest sites have routinely been left open, although some describe filling them with cancellous plugs obtained from socket preparation.[87] Kim and Shin[87] described the formation of loose bodies requiring arthroscopy after filling donor sites with osseous plugs. Donor sites left open have been shown to reliably fill in with cancellous bone and fibrocartilage and are found level with surrounding cartilage at repeat arthroscopy[68,71] **(Fig. 57-17)**. Leaving donor sites open is recommended to avoid increasing technical difficulty and creating potential complications associated with filling of these lesions.

Arthrotomy/Closure/Immediate Postoperative Care

When difficulty is encountered or lesion size precludes a completely arthroscopic approach a mini-arthrotomy or arthrotomy should be used without hesitation. Mini-arthrotomy incisions may be placed either medially or laterally, and a medial parapatellar approach is recommended for formal arthrotomy **(Fig. 57-18A,B)**. The technique of lesion preparation, graft harvest, recipient socket preparation, and graft insertion are all identical, regardless of which approach is

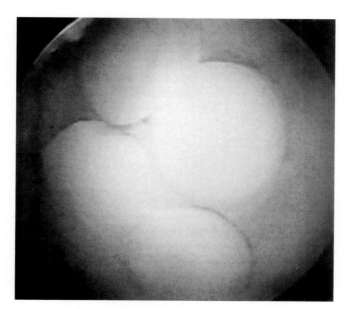

Fig. 57-16. Multiple osteochondral core grafts after final seating within lesion. (Reprinted from Bobic V, Morgan C, Carter T. Osteochondral autologous graft transfer. Oper Tech Sports Med, 2000;8(2), Elsevier Inc, with permission.)

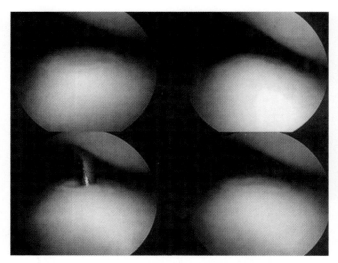

Fig. 57-17. Repeat arthroscopy 1 year after mosaicplasty procedure. Donor evaluation reveals fibrocartilage repair tissue level with remainder of joint surface with stability upon probing. (Reprinted from Bobic V, Morgan C, Carter T. Osteochondral autologous graft transfer. Oper Tech Sports Med. 2000;8(2), Elsevier Inc, with permission.)

chosen. Portal closure is standard for any arthroscopy, and arthrotomy incisions are closed in layers ensuring tight closure of the retinaculum. Drains are routinely placed and left for 24 hours or until output is minimal. Cold therapy is used in all patients for up to 7 to 10 days for control of swelling and pain relief. Pain control with narcotics and anti-inflammatory agents is standard, and prophylaxis against thromboembolism is recommended. Immediate continuous passive motion is started in the hospital and continued upon discharge. Hospital stay is planned for 23-hour observation and modified as appropriate for each individual patient. Weight bearing is prevented over the first couple of weeks, and

crutches are used for ambulation. After 2 to 3 weeks partial weight bearing is allowed.

■ OATS OUTSIDE THE KNEE JOINT

Osteochondral autologous grafts were initially designed for use in the knee joint to replace defects in the articular cartilage of the weight-bearing portion of the femoral condyles. This was quickly extended to the patellofemoral joint after initial good results. Over time this procedure was applied to lesions of the tibia and the talus. More recently attempts have been made to use this technology for lesions involving the femoral head, humeral head, and humeral capitellum.[68]

The technique of mosaicplasty outside the knee is identical to that already described, although the approach to the lesion is joint specific. The ipsilateral knee is used for donor grafts. This creates some concern about potential morbidity to an otherwise healthy knee joint. This concept is not dissimilar from techniques described using contralateral patellar-tendon autografts for ACL reconstruction, which have reportedly low morbidity in the knee where the graft was harvested.[88]

When proximal tibial or patellofemoral mosaicplasty is performed an open arthrotomy is sometimes necessary to acquire good access to the lesion and donor sites. For treatment of lesions in the tibia, talus, and other joints, arthroscopic graft harvest is performed in the knee and an open approach to the joint being treated is performed. This provides the best exposure for graft transplantation in the articular surface of the proximal and distal tibia, talus, humeral and femoral heads, and humeral capitellum. It is possible to access lesions in the tibia without a formal arthrotomy. This may decrease some of the morbidity associated with open surgery. An ACL guide is positioned in the center of the

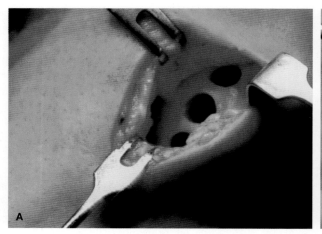
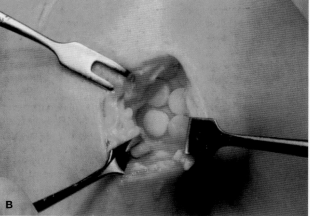

Fig. 57-18. A: Mini-arthrotomy approach demonstrating donor sites after harvest. (Reprinted from Hangody L, Rathonyi G, Duska Z, et al. Autologous osteochondral mosaicplasty. J Bone Joint Surg Am. March 2004;(suppl 1):86, with permission.) **B:** Mini-arthrotomy approach showing lesion after graft transplantation. (Reprinted from Hangody L, Rathonyi G, Duska Z, et al. Autologous osteochondral mosaicplasty. J Bone Joint Surg Am. March 2004;(suppl 1):86, with permission.)

defect during arthroscopy, and a guide pin is drilled through the tibia into the center of the lesion after abrasion arthroplasty is complete. A cannulated reamer matching the size of the defect is used to ream the defect in a retrograde manner.

Graft harvest is performed from the periphery of the femoral trochlea at the angle corresponding to the angle set on the ACL guide. Subsequently, the core graft is inserted retrograde from the cortical window on the tibia and seated flush to the articular surface with press fit technique. The tunnel defect under the graft is then supported with a cancellous bony cylinder graft, which may be fixed with a bioabsorbable screw. Ueblacker et al.[89] reported this technique in five patients for lesions in the proximal and distal tibia without complications and Matsusue et al.[90] performed this successfully in one patient with a tibial plateau lesion. The retrograde approach should be used with caution as the technical difficulty is significant and fixation of the core grafts must be supported by further grafting due to retrograde entry. This approach has been used with good results for arthroscopic drilling of talar lesions, but it remains to be seen if congruent stable grafts may be reliably implanted in this manner without significant complications.

■ ALLOGRAFT TRANSPLANTATION WITH MOSAICPLASTY TECHNIQUE

Allograft osteochondral transplantation also provides a hyaline cartilage plug to restore surface congruity in chondral and osteochondral lesions. Many authors have used allograft for reconstruction of large lesions and reported good results. Czitrom et al.[91] found chondrocyte viability in allografts, although survival decreased over time. He found living chondrocytes in 60% of grafts after 2 years and in 37% after 6 years. Other authors have reported good clinical results ranging from 63% to 77% after large allograft reconstruction for osteoarticular defects.[58,59,92] Allograft avoids the problem of donor site morbidity and circumvents the limitations on tissue availability. Larger lesions may be treated with allograft as more tissue is available for graft harvest. The size and depth of the lesion still must be considered when evaluating the indications for the OATS procedure, but lesions from 40 to 80 mm^2 may be amenable to OATS with allograft. Bulk allograft is better suited than mosaicplasty for defects encompassing the majority of the weight-bearing surface of the joint.

The operative technique is no different with allograft and is easier than harvesting autograft. Lesion preparation is performed followed by sequential allograft core harvest. Recipient socket creation is done to match the core and transplantation is completed. Sequential transplantation is carried out to fill the defect maximally and progressively contour the new surface created by the grafts. Allograft tissue adds expense to the surgery, and there is a limited availability of age-appropriate donor tissue. Other concerns include risk of disease transmission, immune reaction, and infection.

■ TECHNICAL PEARLS FOR MOSAICPLASTY

As with any surgical procedure, and especially those requiring arthroscopy, there is a learning curve when performing OATS. It is suggested that one familiarize him- or herself with the commercially available systems prior to using them in the operating room and decide which one works best in your hands. As with any procedure, strict attention to indications and contraindications will improve outcome.

There are some technical points that warrant specific mention to optimize success with this method of treatment. Graft harvest and implantation require perpendicular alignment for flush congruent surfaces to be obtained. Failure to maintain perpendicularity will produce asymmetric cores resulting in step-offs in the new articular surface. Success with this depends on portal placement when performing harvest arthroscopically. A spinal needle must be used along with varying viewing angles from the contralateral portal to ensure optimal portal placement. The use of either 30- or 70-degree arthroscopes is recommended to obtain the best view of the lesion.

The manufacturers' instructions are also vital as different systems call for different techniques of graft harvest to obtain ideal cores. When difficulty is encountered with arthroscopic harvest do not hesitate to make a mini-arthrotomy or arthrotomy if required. Graft implantation is also vital for success, and meticulous attention should be paid to seating of the grafts. Recessing grafts and leaving grafts proud are both problematic as neither adequately restores surface contact pressures to normal. Grafts should be seated flush with the surrounding cartilage surface. It has been suggested in the past that leaving grafts slightly raised may be acceptable as they may be driven flush upon initiation of range of motion and weight bearing. Recent evidence has demonstrated that contact pressures are significantly abnormal with raised grafts, and this technique cannot be recommended.[85]

Close packing of grafts is ideal to increase the percentage of hyaline fill in the defect, with a goal being greater than 80% with the mosaicplasty technique **(Fig. 57-19)**. Lesion preparation is equally important. Vertical walls of intact hyaline cartilage should be sharply created around the periphery of the defect with a curette or knife followed by abrasion in the lesion to viable subchondral bone. A normal shoulder surrounding the lesion is important to define the periphery of the defect and provide a site for integration of hyaline graft tissue with intact cartilage. Drilling should be avoided when possible to avoid thermal necrosis in the recipient socket and surrounding cartilage. Manual harvesting and recipient socket creation with current systems avoids the need for power instrumentation and prevents potential thermal damage.

It must be recognized that the larger the lesion being treated the more potential for donor site morbidity and the more difficult to create a new articular surface without step-offs. Recognizing when a lesion is suitable for this technique

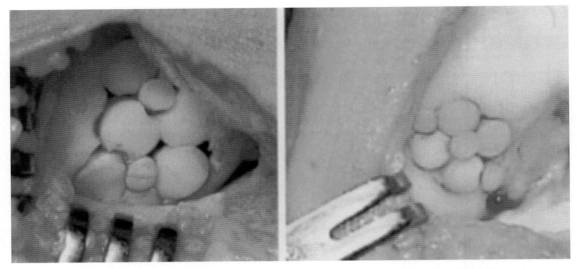

Fig. 57-19. Arthrotomy utilized for mosaicplasty. Lesion fill is over 80%. (Reprinted from Hangody L, Rathonyi G, Duska Z, et al. Autologous osteochondral mosaicplasty. J Bone Joint Surg Am. March 2004;(suppl 1):86, with permission.)

is important and guidelines should be followed; lesions less than 20 mm^2 are ideal, defects between 20 and 40 mm^2 are appropriate, and lesions larger than 40 mm^2 should be approached with caution and other approaches considered.

■ TECHNICAL ALTERNATIVES AND PITFALLS

The armamentarium available for treating injury to articular cartilage includes a vast array of procedures. Authors disagree as to which approach offers the best clinical outcome, though most concur on the ultimate goal of treatment: to repair the damaged cartilage and underlying subchondral bone with new hyaline cartilage capable of restoring normal contact pressures and reproducing the biomechanical properties of native joint cartilage. The limited ability of hyaline cartilage to regenerate after injury mandates surgical attempts to restore the joint surface to normal.

The simplest approach to chondral lesions is arthroscopic lavage and debridement chondroplasty. Chondroplasty is most appropriate for small grade II and III lesions by the Outerbridge classification.[73] It improves the surface congruity in these partial lesions and prevents unstable pieces of cartilage from detaching and becoming loose bodies. Surface delamination in these lesions can be halted and surface debris eliminated. Mechanical chondroplasty is the recommended technique as radiofrequency thermal techniques have been shown to lead to chondrocyte death even when used at recommended "cartilage" settings.[93]

Mechanical debridement is quick, easy, and cost-effective. It burns no bridges in regard to future treatment options for patients with progression of disease. It may be more effective in lower demand patients with normal alignment.[94]

Marrow-stimulating techniques take advantage of cartilage's natural response to injury by enhancing mesenchymal cell recruitment into the defect.

Various techniques exist to create access channels to the subchondral vasculature, including drilling, abrasion arthroplasty, and microfracture. These techniques are generally indicated for grade IV lesions and some grade III lesions with limited remaining cartilage cover. They are all technically easy and cost-effective and can be done arthroscopically in a single stage. Drilling has the disadvantage of difficult access to some lesions and the potential for thermal injury. All three of these techniques depend heavily on a postoperative non–weight-bearing protocol for best results, and many patients find this aspect of care to be overconstraining. The repair tissue generated is of limited quality as it consists predominantly of fibrocartilage, which lacks the durability and strength of normal hyaline cartilage.[18]

Perichondrium and periosteum have been used to fill defects in articular cartilage. An autogenous graft of tissue is taken and sewn to the defect. Initially Homminga et al.[37] reported good results at 1 to 2 years with perichondrium, although they found late calcification of the grafts with significant deterioration in clinical results over time. O'Driscoll et al.[36] have reported on periosteal grafting and continuous passive motion with some formation of hyaline like tissue. Periosteum provides an autogenous source of mesenchymal cells for cartilage repair. There is uncertainty about the durability of this repair tissue and overgrowth may be a problem. This is a technically demanding procedure without long-term results, which many consider to still be experimental.

Autologous chondrocyte implantation (ACI) has been used more extensively over the past decade. It has the benefit of being applied to both small and large defects from 20 mm to 100 mm^2. It can be used alone or in combination with bone grafting if subchondral damage is extensive. It requires cartilage biopsy and in vitro growth of chondrocytes, which are placed into the lesion at a second surgery. A watertight periosteal patch is sewn over the defect followed by chondrocyte injection beneath the patch. It is attractive as a source of hyalinelike tissue,[38] although some have reported follow-up biopsy that demonstrated predominantly fibrocartilage in the lesions.[55] This technique provides autologous chondrocytes for restoration of variable-sized chondral lesions with no donor site morbidity. It is, however, technically demanding, requires two-staged procedures including an arthrotomy, and is extremely expensive. Another concern is the risk of infection introduced into a joint after in vitro culture of chondrocytes. A reoperation rate of up to 20% has been reported for graft hypertrophy, delamination, and joint arthrofibrosis.

Osteochondral grafting has long been used for defects in weight-bearing joints to restore the articular surface.[48–51] The guiding principle is that a loss of articular cartilage is being replaced with identical hyaline cartilage tissue that has the same biomechanical characteristics. The OATS technique provides an arthroscopic approach to treat focal chondral and osteochondral lesions and maintain hyaline viability. An ideal lesion for OATS may be the limited osteochondritis dissecans (OCD) lesion where replacing subchondral bone will provide the most complete healing. It can be done in one sitting and is much more cost-effective than chondrocyte implantation.

It is technically demanding and sometimes difficult to precisely contour the articular surface. A major limitation is the availability of autogenous tissue for OATS and the concern over donor site morbidity. It has been shown that all recommended donor sites do experience significant contact stresses.[82] Clinical studies have not shown significant donor morbidity, and second-look arthroscopy has found fibrocartilage tissue repair in all donor sites.[68,71,72]

Challenges continue regarding the ideal donor site to exactly match surface topography, contour, and articular cartilage thickness in the lesion. OATS is not indicated for lesions larger than 40 mm^2, and integration of the grafts to one another and surrounding hyaline cartilage is not always complete.

Allografts may be used for small and large chondral and osteochondral lesions with no donor site morbidity. These grafts may be incorporated with the OATS technique or transferred in bulk for very large defects. Cadaveric tissue adds expense to the procedure and raises issues of disease transmission, infection, and immunologic reaction. Furthermore chondrocyte viability and graft integration are areas of concern in the use of allograft tissue.

■ REHABILITATION

Rehabilitation after OATS varies depending upon the surgeon. Postoperative care should always be tailored to the individual lesion and patient. Some feel that there should be no restrictions on range of motion or weight bearing if the grafting was done correctly with a good press-fit technique.[71] A more conservative approach is adopted by others who permit immediate range of motion but keep a non–weight-bearing protocol for the first 3 weeks.[55,68] Partial weight bearing is progressed over the next 2 to 3 weeks, followed by full weight bearing. Brace use is not recommended as part of the routine postoperative protocol with mosaicplasty. When mosaicplasty is combined with ligament reconstruction or osteotomy, brace use is required and the protocol includes immediate motion with restricted weight bearing. Straight leg raises and isometrics may begin early, and quadriceps and hamstring strengthening constitute the final phases of therapy. Return to athletics should be delayed in order for adequate graft integration and healing to occur. Once quadriceps strength has been regained and symptoms are absent, return to play is allowed around 6 to 9 months.

■ OUTCOMES AND FUTURE DIRECTIONS

Much attention has been given to chondral and osteochondral injuries in the knee and other joints. Although the natural history is still somewhat controversial, MRI and arthroscopy have brought these injuries and their optimal treatment into question.[20–22,78] It has been shown that even small chondral lesions can lead to significant pain, swelling, and mechanical symptoms that do respond well to treatment.[19] Many methods of treatment exist, and each lesion and patient must be approached individually.

Patient age and activity demands are important as are the size and location of the chondral injury when determining the most appropriate treatment. Arthroscopy has improved our ability to treat these lesions while limiting the morbidity of open surgery. Outcome studies with longer follow-up are now becoming available and must be utilized to support our rationale for each procedure.

Marrow stimulating techniques are the simplest and most cost-effective measures for full-thickness chondral lesions. Rodkey and Steadman[95] reported on 203 patients with at least 3 years follow-up. This group was 75% improved, 19% unchanged, and 6% worse after microfracture 3 years earlier. They correlated poorer prognosis with preoperative loss of joint space, increasing age, chronic lesions, and failure to use continuous passive motion after surgery. This is a case series and among other limitations lacked a control group.

Autologous chondrocyte implantation has been performed now for almost 10 years and more studies are starting to emerge on its results. Brittberg et al.[38] initially reviewed 23 patients 66 months after ACI and found 16 of 23 maintained good or excellent results. Biopsy was performed in half of these patients, which showed hyalinelike cartilage. The patellar defects performed worse in this group. Peterson[96] reported 90% good to excellent results in

219 patients treated with ACI at an average of 4 years from surgery. Knutsen et al.[97] recently reported a randomized clinical trial comparing microfracture with ACI with 2-year follow-up. There were 40 patients in each group evaluated with clinical scoring systems and repeat arthroscopy with biopsy and histology. Both groups had significant clinical improvement at 2 years with 76% of patients having less pain. The SF-36 score showed significantly better outcomes in the microfracture group. Patients underwent repeat arthroscopy at 2 years, which revealed no significant differences upon viewing and probing of the repair tissue. Histologic comparison revealed no differences in the repair tissue between groups. There was a hybrid of hyalinelike tissue and fibrocartilage present in both groups with some tendency for the ACI group to have more hyalinelike cartilage. Also of significance was a 25% unplanned reoperation rate in the ACI group. Most of these consisted of arthroscopic debridement for hypertrophy of repair tissue.

Hangody et al.[52–54] developed the concept of mosaicplasty utilizing osteochondral autograft plugs from "less weight-bearing" areas of the knee joint. They have performed 831 mosaicplasty procedures over a 10-year period for chondral lesions in various joints.[68] The distribution of these lesions are as follows: 597 in the femoral condyles, 118 in the patellofemoral joint, 76 of the talar dome, 25 in the tibial condyles, 6 of the humerus at the capitellum, 6 of the femoral head, and 3 of the humeral head. Clinical scores in these patients showed 92% good to excellent results for femoral condylar lesions, 87% for tibial lesions, 79% for patellofemoral defects, and 94% for talar surgery. There was minimal morbidity from donor site harvesting. This was evaluated using cases where the ipsilateral knee was used for

grafts to be implanted elsewhere. This allowed symptoms in the knee to be reliably attributed to donor harvest. Histologic follow-up revealed good survival of hyaline cartilage. Areas between individual grafts and between grafts and surrounding article cartilage were integrated with fibrocartilage fill tissue **(Fig. 57-20)**. Donor sites were repaired with fibrocartilage tissue that was flush with the joint surface. Complications included four deep infections and 36 postoperative hematomas. These outcomes are limited by the lack of prospective design and no control group.

Two studies have been reported recently that were prospectively designed and randomized to compare mosaicplasty with ACI. Horas et al.[55] evaluated 2-year outcomes in 40 patients with lesions of the femoral condyles. Patients underwent either OATS or ACI and were followed with clinical scores and histologic evaluation of repair tissue. The Lysholm score showed slower recovery in the ACI group, although the Meyers and Tegner scores were similar for the two groups. Histology revealed predominantly fibrocartilage in the ACI patients and viable hyaline cartilage at the core grafts in the OATS patients. There was a persistent gap between the core grafts and the surrounding articular surface, demonstrating a lack of complete integration with the OATS technique. In contrast to Horas's report, Bentley et al.[98] performed a similar comparison between these techniques and showed better improvement at 1 year for the ACI group. One hundred patients were evaluated clinically with the Cincinnati and Stanmore scoring systems, and 60 patients underwent a second arthroscopy to grade the repair tissue according to the International Cartilage Research Society grading system. They reported 88% clinical and 82% arthroscopic improvement for ACI patients versus 69% and 35% respectively for OATS patients. Both of these reports have only short-term follow-up and caution must be used in interpreting the data.

Long-term outcomes on cartilage repair techniques are lacking. Most reports are case series that lack prospective design and fail to include suitable controls. Best outcomes will be achieved when proper indications are used when deciding upon optimal treatment for each individual patient. Mosaicplasty is a useful technique that has shown good clinical results over the past 10 years and should be considered for patients with focal, unipolar lesions smaller than 40 mm^2.

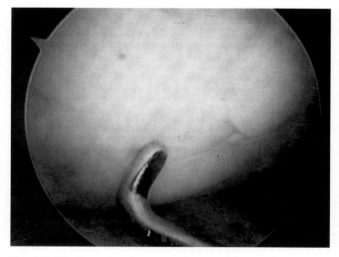

Fig. 57-20. Repeat arthroscopy 1 year after mosaicplasty for lesion in medial femoral condyle. Probing demonstrates a new chondral surface with good osteochondral graft survival and fibrocartilage repair around grafts. (Reprinted from Hangody L, Fules P. Autologous osteochondral mosaicplasty for the treatment of full-thickness defects of weight-bearing joints. J Bone Joint Surg Am. March 2003;(suppl 2):85, with permission.)

■ SUGGESTED READINGS

Bentley G, Biant LC, Carrington RWJ, et al. A prospective, randomized comparison of autologous chondrocyte implantation versus mosaicplasty for osteochondral defects in the knee. J Bone Joint Surg Br. 2003;85:223–230.

Bobic V, Morgan C, Carter T. Osteochondral autologous graft transfer. Oper Tech Sports Med. 2000;8(2):168–178.

Brittberg M, Lindahl A, Nilsson A, et al. Treatment of deep cartilage defects in the knee with autologous chondrocyte transplantation. New Eng J Med. 1994;331:889–895.

Brittberg M, Peterson L, Sjouml E, et al. Articular cartilage engineering with autologous chondrocyte transplantation. J Bone Joint Surg Am. 2003;85:109–115.

Buckwalter JA, Mankin HJ. Articular cartilage. J Bone Joint Surg Am. 1997;79:600–632.

Essentials of alignment and cartilage repair of the knee. Drez D, DeLee J, eds. Oper Tech Sports Med. 2000;8(2).

Hangody L, Feczko P, Bartha L, et al. Mosaicplasty for the treatment of articular defects of the knee and ankle. Clin Orthop. 2001;391 (suppl):328–336.

Hangody L, Fules P. Autologous osteochondral mosaicplasty for the treatment of full-thickness defects of weight-bearing joints. J Bone Joint Surg Am. 2003;85(suppl 2):25–32.

Hangody L, Kish G, Karpati Z, et al. Arthroscopic autogenous osteochondral mosaicplasty for the treatment of femoral condylar articular defects: a preliminary report. Knee Surg Sports Traum Arthrosc. 1997;5:262–267.

Hangody L, Kish G, Karpati Z, et al. Mosaicplasty for the treatment of articular cartilage defects of the knee. Orthopedics. 1998;22:751–756.

Hangody L, Rathonyi GK, Duska Z, et al. Autologous osteochondral mosaicplasty: surgical technique. J Bone Joint Surg Am. 2004;86: 65–72.

Horas U, Pelinkovic D, Herr G, et al. Autologous chondrocyte implantation and osteochondral cylinder transplantation in cartilage repair of the knee joint: a prospective, comparative trial. J Bone Joint Surg Am. 2003;85:185–192.

Knutsen G, Engebretsen L, Ludvigsen TC, et al. Autologous chondrocyte implantation compared with microfracture in the knee: a randomized trial. J Bone Joint Surg Am. 2004;86:455–464.

Minas T, Nehrer S. Current concepts in the treatment of articular cartilage defects. Orthopedics. 1997;20:525–538.

Potter HG, Linklater JM, Allen AA, et al. Magnetic resonance imaging of articular cartilage in the knee. J Bone Joint Surg Am. 1998;80:1276–1284.

■ REFERENCES

1. Buckwalter JA, Mankin HJ. Articular cartilage. J Bone Joint Surg Am. 1997;79:600–632.

2. Buckwalter JA, Rosenberg LC, Hunziker EB. Articular cartilage: composition, structure, response to injury, and methods of facilitating repair. In: Ewing JW, ed. *Articular Cartilage and Knee Joint Function. Basic Science and Arthroscopy.* Bristol-Myers/Zimmer Orthopaedic Symposium. New York: Raven Press; 1990:19–56.

3. Buckwalter JA, Hunziker EB, Rosenberg LC, et al. Articular cartilage: composition and structure. In: Woo SLY, Buckwalter JA, eds. *Injury and Repair of the Musculoskeletal Soft Tissues.* Park Ridge, Ill.: American Academy of Orthopaedic Surgeons; 1988:405–425.

4. Jeffery AK, Blunn GW, Archer CW, et al. Three-dimensional collagen architecture in bovine articular cartilage. J Bone Joint Surg Br. 1991;73:795–801.

5. Kuettner KE, Schleyerbach R, Peyron JG, et al. *Articular Cartilage and Osteoarthritis.* New York: Raven Press; 1992.

6. Hunter W. Of the structure and disease of articulating cartilages. Philos Trans R Soc Lond. 1743;42:514–521.

7. Mankin HJ. The response of articular cartilage to mechanical injury. J Bone Joint Surg Am. 1982;64:460–466.

8. Buckwalter JA, Mow VC. Cartilage repair in osteoarthritis. In: Moskowitz RW, Howell DS, Goldberg MV, et al, eds. *Osteoarthritis, Diagnosis and Medical/Surgical Management.* Vol. 2. Philadelphia: W.B. Saunders; 1992:71–107.

9. Bennett GA, Bauer W, Maddock SJ. A Study of the repair of articular cartilage and the reaction of normal joints of adult dogs to surgically created defects of articular cartilage. Am J Pathol. 1932;8:499–524.

10. Calandruccio RA, Gilmer WS. Proliferation, regeneration, and repair of articular cartilage of immature animals. J Bone Joint Surg Am. 1962;44:431–455.

11. Campbell CJ. The healing of cartilage defects. Clin Orthop. 1969;64:45–63.

12. DePalma AF, McKeever CD, Subin SK. Process of repair of articular cartilage demonstrated by histology and autoradiography with tritiated thymidine. Clin Orthop. 1966;48:229–242.

13. Mankin HJ. The reaction of articular cartilage to injury and osteoarthritis. Parts 1 and 2. N Engl J Med. 1974;291:1285–1292, 1335–1340.

14. Buckwalter JA, Lohmander S. Current concepts review. Operative treatment of osteoarthrosis: current practice and future development. J Bone Joint Surg Am. 1994;76:1405–1418.

15. Buckwalter JA, Einhorn TA, Bolander ME, et al. Healing of musculoskeletal tissues. In: Rockwood CA Jr., Green D, eds. *Fractures.* Philadelphia: J.B. Lippincott; 1996:261–304.

16. Shapiro F, Koide S, Glimcher MJ. Cell origin and differentiation in the repair of full thickness defects of articular cartilage. J Bone Joint Surg Am. 1993;75:532–553.

17. Wakitani S, Goto T, Pineda SJ, et al. Mesenchymal cell-based repair of large, full-thickness defects of articular cartilage. J Bone Joint Surg Am. 1994;76:579–592.

18. Minas T, Nehrer S. Current concepts in the treatment of articular cartilage defects. Orthopedics. 1997;20:525–538.

19. Levy AS, Lohnes J, Sculley S, et al. Chondral delamination of the knee in soccer players. Am J Sports Med. 1996;24:634–639.

20. Curl WW, Krome J, Gordon ES. Cartilage injuries: a review of 31,516 knee arthroscopies. Arthroscopy. 1997;13:456–460.

21. Potter HG, Linklater JM, Allen AA, et al. Magnetic resonance imaging of articular cartilage in the knee. J Bone Joint Surg Am. 1998;80:1276–1284.

22. Fowler PJ. Bone injuries associated with anterior cruciate ligament disruption. Arthroscopy. 1994;10:453–460.

23. Johnson DL, Urban WP Jr., Caborn DNM, et al. Articular cartilage changes seen with magnetic resonance imaging-detected bone bruises associated with acute anterior cruciate ligament rupture. Am J Sports Med. 1998;26:409–414.

24. Bobic V. Arthroscopic osteochondral autograft transplantation in anterior cruciate ligament reconstruction: a preliminary clinical study. Knee Surg Sports Traumat Arthrosc. 1996;3:262–264.

25. Terry GC, Flandry F, Manen JWV, et al. Isolated chondral fractures of the knee. Clin Orthop. 1988;234:170–177.

26. Lippiello L, Hall D, Mankin HJ. Collagen synthesis in normal and osteoarthritic human cartilage. J Clin Invest. 1977;59:593–600.

27. Buckwalter JA, Mow VC, Ratliff A. Restoration of injured or degenerated articular surfaces. J Am Acad Orthop Surg. 1994;2:192–201.

28. Woo SLY, Buckwalter JA, eds. *Injury and Repair of the Musculoskeletal Soft Tissues.* Park Ridge, Ill.: American Academy of Orthopaedic Surgeons; 1988.

29. Pridie K. A method of resurfacing osteoarthritic knee joints. J Bone Joint Surg Br. 1959;41:618–619.

30. Magnuson PB. Joint debridement surgical treatment of degenerative arthritis. Surg Gynecol Obstet. 1941;73:1–9.

31. Steadman JR, Briggs KK, Rodrigo JJ, et al. Outcomes of microfracture for traumatic chondral defects of the knee: average 11-year follow-up. Arthroscopy. 2003;19:477–484.

32. Friedman MJ, Berasi CC, Fox TM, et al. Abrasion arthroplasty in osteoarthritic knee. Clin Orthop Relat Res. 1984;182:200–205.

33. Bert J, Maschka K. The arthroscopic treatment of unicompartmental gonarthrosis: a five-year follow-up study of abrasion arthroplasty plus debridement and arthroscopic debridement along. Arthroscopy. 1989;5:25–32.

34. Steadman J, Sterett W. The surgical treatment of knee injuries. Med Sci Sports Exerc. 1995;27:328–333.

35. O'Driscoll SW, Salter RB. The repair of major osteochondral defects in joint surfaces by neochondrogenesis with autogenous

osteoperiosteal grafts stimulated by continuous passive motion: an experimental investigation in the rabbit. Clin Orthop. 1986;208: 131–140.

36. O'Driscoll SW, Keeley FW, Salter RB. Durability of regenerated articular cartilage produced by free autogenous periosteal grafts in major full-thickness defects in joint surfaces under the influence of continuous passive motion: a follow up report at one year. J Bone Joint Surg Am. 1988;70:595–606.

37. Homminga GN, Bulstra SK, Bouwmeester PM, et al. Perichondral grafting for cartilage lesions of the knee. J Bone Joint Surg Br. 1990;72:1003–1007.

38. Brittberg M, Lindahl A, Nilsson A, et al. Treatment of deep cartilage defects in the knee with autologous chondrocyte transplantation. New Eng J Med. 1994;331:889–895.

39. Peterson L, Menche D, Grande D, et al. Chondrocyte transplantation-an experimental model in the rabbit. Trans Orthop Res Soc. 1984;9:218.

40. Brittberg M, Peterson L, Sjouml E, et al. Articular cartilage engineering with autologous chondrocyte transplantation. J Bone Joint Surg Am. 2003;85:109–115.

41. Gross AE. Fresh osteochondral allografts for post-traumatic knee defects: surgical technique. Oper Tech Orthop. 1997;7:334.

42. Bugbee WD. Fresh osteochondral allografting. Oper Tech Sports Med. 2000;8:158–162.

43. Ghazavi MT, Pritzker KP, Davis AM, et al. Fresh osteochondral allografts for post-traumatic osteochondral defects of the knee. J Bone Joint Surg Br. 1997;79:1008–1013.

44. Beaver RJ, Mahomed M, Backstein D, et al. Fresh osteochondral allografts for post-traumatic defects in the knee: a survivorship analysis. J Bone Joint Surg Br. 1992;74:105–110.

45. Mahomed M. The long term success of fresh, small fragment osteochondral allografts used for intraarticular post-traumatic defects in the knee joint. Orthopedics. 1992;15:1191–1199.

46. McDermott AG, Langer F, Pritzker KP, et al. Fresh small-fragment osteochondral allografts: long-term follow-up study on first 100 cases. Clin Orthop. 1985;197:96–102.

47. Garrett JC. Fresh osteochondral allografts for treatment of articular defects in osteochondritis dissecans of the lateral femoral condyle in adults. Clin Orthop. 1994;303:33–37.

48. Campanacci M, Cervellati C, Donati U. Autogenous patella as replacement for a resected femoral of tibial condyle: a report of 19 cases. J Bone Joint Surg Br. 1985;67:557–563.

49. Fabbricciani C, Schiavone PA, Delcogliano A, et al. Osteochondral autograft in the treatment of osteochondritis dissecans of the knee. In: American Orthopaedic Society for Sports Medicine Annual Meeting, Orlando, Fla.: AOSSM; 1994:78–79.

50. Outerbridge HK, Outerbridge AR, Outerbridge RE. The use of a lateral patellar autologous graft for the repair of a large osteochondral defect in the knee. J Bone Joint Surg Am. 1995;77:65–72.

51. Yamashita F, Sakakida K, Suzu F, et al. The transplantation of an auto-geneic osteochondral fragment for osteochondritis dissecans of the knee. Clin Orthop. 1985;201:43–50.

52. Hangody L, Karpati Z. New possibilities in the management of severe circumscribed cartilage damage in the knee. Hungarian. Magy Traumatol Ortop Kezseb Plasztikai. 1994;37:237–243.

53. Hangody L, Kish G, Karpati Z, et al. Autogenous osteochondral graft technique for replacing knee cartilage defects in dogs. Orthopedics. 1997;5:175–181.

54. Bodo G, Kaposi AD, Hangody L, et al. The surgical technique and the age of the horse both influence the outcome of mosaicplasty in a cadaver equine stifle model. Acta Vet Hung. 2001;49:111–116.

55. Horas U, Pelinkovic D, Herr G, et al. Autologous chondrocyte implantation and osteochondral cylinder transplantation in cartilage repair of the knee joint: a prospective, comparative trial. J Bone Joint Surg Am. 2003;85:185–192.

56. Goldberg VM, Caplan AI. Cellular repair of articular cartilage. In: Kuettner KE, Goldberg VM, eds. Osteoarthritic Disorders:

Workshop, April 1994. Monterey, Calif.: Rosemont, Ill.: American Academy of Orthopaedic Surgeons; 1995:357–364.

57. Brittberg M, Nilsson A, Lindahl A, et al. Rabbit articular cartilage defects treated with autologous cultured chondrocytes. Clin Orthop. 1996;326:270–283.

58. Beaver RJ, Gross AE. Fresh small-fragment osteochondral allografts in the knee joint. In: Aichroth PM, Cannon WD Jr., eds. Knee Surgery. Current Practice. Deutscher: Arzte-Verlag Koln; 1992:464–471.

59. Meyers MH, Akeson W, Convery FR. Resurfacing of the knee with fresh osteochondral allograft. J Bone Joint Surg Am. 1989;71: 704–713.

60. Czitrom AA, Langer F, VcKee N, et al. Bone and cartilage allotransplantation: a review of 14 years of research and clinical studies. Clin Orthop. 1986;208:141–145.

61. Lexer E. Substitution of whole or half joints from freshly amputated extremities by free plastic operation. Surg Gynecol Obstet. 1908;6:601–609.

62. DePalma AF, Sawyer B, Hoffmann JD. Fate of osteochondral grafts. Clin Orthop. 1962;22:217–221.

63. Wilson WJ, Jacobs JE. Patellar graft for severely depressed comminuted fractures of the lateral tibial condyle. J Bone Joint Surg Am. 1952;34:436–442.

64. Aichroth PM, Ellis H. Transplantation of joint surfaces by cartilage grafts. Br J Surg. 1970;57:855.

65. Muller W. Osteochondrosis dissecans. In: Hastings DE, ed. Progress in Orthopaedic Surgery, Vol. 3, New York: Springer; 1978:135.

66. Hangody L, Feczko P, Bartha L, et al. Mosaicplasty for the treatment of articular defects of the knee and ankle. Clin Orthop. 2001;391(suppl):328–336.

67. Bodo G, Hangody L, Szabo Z, et al. Arthroscopic autologous osteochondral mosaicplasty for the treatment of subchondral cystic lesion in the medial femoral condyle in a horse. Acta Vet Hung. 2000;48:343–354.

68. Hangody L, Fules P. Autologous osteochondral mosaicplasty for the treatment of full-thickness defects of weight-bearing joints. J Bone Joint Surg Am. 2003;85(suppl 2):25–32.

69. Bobic V. Osteochondral autologous graft transplantation in the treatment of focal articular cartilage lesions. Sem Arthroplasty. 1999;10(1):21–29.

70. Hangody L, Kish G, Karpati Z, et al. Arthroscopic autogenous osteochondral mosaicplasty for the treatment of femoral condylar articular defects: a preliminary report. Knee Surg Sports Traum Arthrosc. 1997;5:262–267.

71. Bobic V, Morgan C, Carter T. Osteochondral autologous graft transfer. Oper Tech Sports Med. 2000;8(2):168–178.

72. Hangody L, Kish G, Karpati Z, et al. Mosaicplasty for the treatment of articular cartilage defects of the knee. Orthopedics. 1998;22:751–756.

73. Outerbridge R. The etiology of chondromalacia patella. J Bone Joint Surg Br. 1961;43:752–767.

74. Noyes FR, Barber-Westin SD. Anterior cruciate ligament reconstruction with autogenous patellar tendon graft in patients with articular cartilage damage. Am J Sports Med. 1997;25:626–634.

75. Geissler WB, Whipple TL. Intra-articular abnormalities in association with posterior cruciate ligament injuries. Am J Sports Med. 1993;21:846–849.

76. Pareolie JM, Bergfield JA. Long-term results of non-operative treatment of isolated posterior cruciate ligament injuries in the athlete. Am J Sports Med. 1986;14:35–38.

77. Tetsworth K, Paley D. Malalignment and degenerative arthropathy. Orthop Clin North Am. 1994;25:367–377.

78. Disler DG, McCauley TR, Wirth CR, et al. Detection of knee hyaline cartilage defects using fat-suppressed three-dimensional spoiled gradient-echo MR imaging: comparison with standard MR imaging and correlation with arthroscopy. Am J Roentgenol. 1995;165:377–382.

79. Disler DG, McCauley TR, Kelman CG, et al. Fat-suppressed three-dimensional spoiled gradient-echo MR imaging of hyaline cartilage defects in the knee: comparison with standard MR imaging and arthroscopy. Am J Roentgenol. 1996;167:127–132.

80. Hangody L, Rathonyi GK, Duska Z, et al. Autologous osteochondral mosaicplasty: surgical technique. J Bone Joint Surg Am. 2004;86:65–72.

81. Hangody L, Sukosd L, Szigeti I, et al. Arthroscopic autogenous osteochondral mosaicplasty. Hung J Orthop Trauma. 1996;39:49–54.

82. Simonian PT, Sussmann PS, Wickiewicz TL, et al. Contact pressures at osteochondral donor sites in the knee. Am J Sports Med. 1998;26:491–494.

83. Duchow J, Hess T, Kohn D. Primary stability of press-fit-implanted osteochondral grafts. Influence of graft size, repeated insertion, and harvesting technique. Am J Sports Med. 2000;28:24–27.

84. Miniaci A, Evans P, Hurtig M. Proceedings of the 17th AANA Annual Meeting, Orlando, Fla., 1998.

85. Koh JL, Wirsing K, Lautenschlager E, et al. The effect of graft height mismatch on contact pressure following osteochondral grafting: a biomechanical study. Am J Sports Med. 2004;32:317–320.

86. Pearce SG, Hurtig MB, Kalra MS, et al. A comparison of two techniques for optimizing graft congruency in mosaic arthroplasty. Proceedings of the 18th AANA Annual Meeting, Vancouver, BC, Canada, 1999.

87. Kim S-J, Shin S-J. Loose bodies after arthroscopic osteochondral autograft in osteochondritis dissecans of the knee. Arthroscopy. 2000;16(7):online short reports, E16.

88. Rubinstein RA Jr., Shelbourne KD, VanMeter CD, et al. Isolated autogenous bone patellar tendon bone graft site morbidity. Am J Sports Med. 1994;22:324–327.

89. Ueblacker P, Burkart A, Imhoff AB. Retrograde cartilage transplantation on the proximal and distal tibia. Arthroscopy. 2004;20:73–79.

90. Matsusue Y, Kotake T, Nakagawa Y, et al. Case report: arthroscopic osteochondral autograft transplantation for chondral lesion of the tibial plateau of the knee. Arthroscopy. 2001;17:653–659.

91. Czitrom AA, Keating S, Gross AE. The viability of articular cartilage in fresh osteochondral allografts after clinical transplantation. J Bone Joint Surg Am. 1990;72:574–579.

92. Gross AE, McKee N, Pritzker KPH, et al. Reconstruction of skeletal defects at the knee: a comprehensive osteochondral transplant program. Clin Orthop. 1983;174:96–106.

93. Lu Y, Edwards RB III, Cole BJ, et al. Thermal chondroplasty with radiofrequency energy: an in vitro comparison of bipolar and monopolar radiofrequency devices. Am J Sports Med. 2001;29:42–49.

94. Hubbard M. Articular debridement versus washout for degeneration of the medial femoral condyle. J Bone Joint Surg Br. 1996;78:217–219.

95. Rodkey W, Steadman J. The microfracture technique to treat full-thickness articular cartilage defects: biological basis and long term clinical results. Presented at 18th Annual AANA meeting, Vancouver, BC, Canada, April 16, 1999.

96. Peterson L. Autologous chondrocyte transplantation articular cartilage regeneration and transplantation. Presented at the AAOS Annual Meeting, New Orleans, La., 1998.

97. Knutsen G, Engebretsen L, Ludvigsen TC, et al. Autologous chondrocyte implantation compared with microfracture in the knee: a randomized trial. J Bone Joint Surg Am. 2004;86:455–464.

98. Bentley G, Biant LC, Carrington RWJ, et al. A prospective, randomized comparison of autologous chondrocyte implantation versus mosaicplasty for osteochondral defects in the knee. J Bone Joint Surg Br. 2003;85:223–230.

58

MICROFRACTURE FOR CHONDRAL LESIONS

MICHAEL A. TERRY, MD, J. RICHARD STEADMAN, MD,
WILLIAM G. RODKEY, DVM, KAREN K. BRIGGS, MBA, MPH

■ HISTORY OF THE TECHNIQUE

The microfracture technique was initially developed by the senior author (JRS) in the mid-1980s to treat full thickness cartilage defects in the knee. These defects are common and have been shown rarely to heal spontaneously.[1,2] The microfracture technique has been modified to its current format over the past 20 years and has been used to treat cartilage lesions in the hip, talus, elbow, and shoulder.[3–7] The procedure began with puncture holes created in exposed bone with a simple awl. The most dramatic modification in technique came after animal studies revealed the importance of removal of the calcified cartilage layer.[8] The other significant modifications also involve bed preparation, as discussed below. The rehabilitation protocol has remained essentially the same aside from minor modifications and is also described below.

■ INDICATIONS AND CONTRAINDICATIONS

Indications for microfracture chondroplasty include full thickness articular cartilage defects in the weight-bearing area between the tibia and femur or in the contact area between the patella and femoral condyles.[9,10] Unstable cartilage flaps in these regions that extend to the subchondral bone are also lesions that are suitable for the microfracture technique. Microfracture can be performed on any size lesion, but Steadman et al.[10] reported trends of better results with lesions smaller than 400 mm^2 without statistical significance. It is preferable, but not required, to have articular cartilage surrounding the lesion that forms an appropriate border for the lesion rather than a lesion that gradually transitions to a full thickness defect. These borders provide some degree of protection and containment for the marrow elements and clot that provide the repair tissue.

Patients with acute injuries to the knee that result in full thickness cartilage loss are treated as soon as appropriate and practical. Patients with chronic lesions or degenerative lesions in the knee are treated conservatively initially for a period of at least 12 weeks. Conservative management for these types of lesions includes: activity modification, physical therapy, nonsteroidal anti-inflammatory medications, and joint injections, as appropriate. Patients who have failed conservative treatment for chronic or degenerative lesions then become candidates for microfracture.

Microfracture should only be performed in patients who are able and willing to undergo the specified postoperative rehabilitation described below. Patients who are unreliable or are unable to complete the rehabilitation required are less likely to benefit from the procedure. Another relative contraindication is malalignment, which could leave the regenerating region under inappropriately high stress during the early phase of repair when the tissue is less durable.[11] Advanced age can be a relative contraindication if completion of the rehabilitation protocol is not possible, and it has been demonstrated that age is significant in outcome after microfracture.[9,12] Generalized degenerative changes, inflammatory arthritis, and unstable knees are also relative contraindications. None of these are absolute contraindications because of the low morbidity associated with the procedure, but appropriate patient expectations must be created before the procedure is undertaken.[9,10,12–14]

■ SURGICAL TECHNIQUES

Microfracture can be performed on patients with either regional or general anesthesia. Microfracture under local anesthesia with sedation has not been studied and should be used with care because of the potentially adverse environment created by the local analgesia.

We place our patients in a supine position on a standard operating room table for knee arthroscopy. We apply a tourniquet but generally do not inflate it for microfracture procedures.

Standard arthroscopic portals can be used for microfracture. We make three portals: a superior and medially placed inflow portal and medial and lateral parapatellar portals. Accessory portals are occasionally made as needed for lesions in difficult locations. We perform a standard and thorough diagnostic arthroscopy of the knee prior to microfracture. If other pathology is present in the knee that requires treatment, we complete such treatment prior to microfracture, with the exception of ligament reconstruction. This technique decreases the amount of time that the microfractured bone is exposed to the elevated intra-articular pressures and fluid flow that can decrease the formation of the clot, which is critical to success.

Once a lesion is identified for microfracture **(Fig. 58-1)**, it is probed thoroughly to ensure that all bordering cartilage is stable **(Fig. 58-2)**. It is then debrided of all loose flaps of cartilage using a shaver **(Fig. 58-3)**. Creation of stable full-thickness borders of cartilage surrounding a central lesion is optimal for microfracture as it provides some degree of protection to the regenerating tissue that is forming in the treated lesion. All loose cartilage and cartilage flaps should be removed regardless of border conditions.

The removal of the calcified cartilage layer is important and is usually performed carefully using a hand held curette **(Fig. 58-4)**.[8] Care must be taken at this stage. Subchondral bone destabilization or loss of the articular morphology results from overly aggressive debridement. Debridement and bed preparation that are inadequate will leave cartilage on the underlying bone, potentially inhibiting the regeneration process.[8]

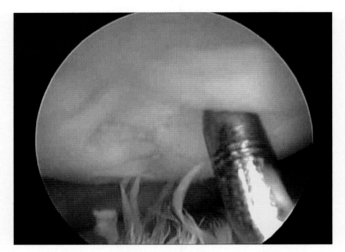

Fig. 58-2. The edges of each defect selected for microfracture must be thoroughly probed to ensure that the cartilage along the border is stable.

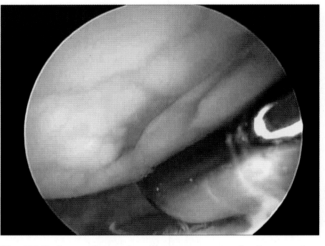

Fig. 58-3. Loose flaps of cartilage are removed using a motorized shaver.

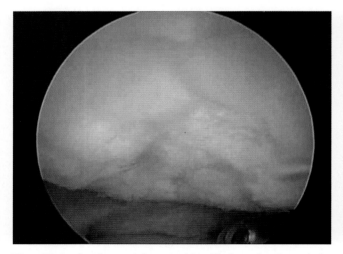

Fig. 58-1. Cartilage defect is identified and selected for microfracture.

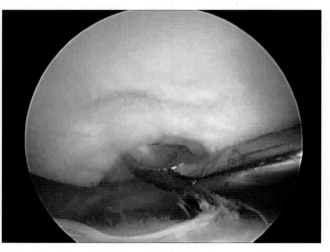

Fig. 58-4. The remaining cartilage, including the calcified cartilage layer, is removed using a hand-held curette.

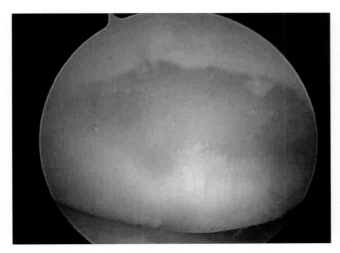

Fig. 58-5. The microfracture bed after preparation.

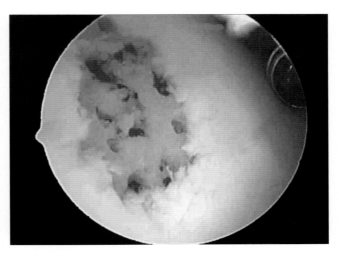

Fig. 58-7. The microfracture grid is completed with central holes after the peripheral holes are created. The microfracture holes should be as close together as possible without becoming confluent with each other.

After the bed is prepared **(Fig. 58-5)**, arthroscopic awls are used to complete the microfracture chondroplasty. These specifically designed manual devices are used rather than powered devices to minimize thermal damage to the surrounding tissue and maximize control. A 30- or 45-degree device is most commonly employed, but 90-degree awls are also used (most commonly on the patella). The awls are advanced through the subchondral bone to create multiple small holes or "microfractures" to a depth that allows the return of fat droplets or blood from the cancellous bone. The depth required is typically 2 to 4 mm. The holes in the bone are made as close together as possible without breaking one into the next. A mallet is generally used with the awls to produce these holes, but manual advancement of the awls is sometimes helpful and should be used at all times with the 90-degree awl. The peripheral microfractures are made first at the junction of the surrounding cartilage and the exposed

bone **(Fig. 58-6)**. Finally, the central holes are made to complete the grid **(Fig. 58-7)**.

The microfracture awl produces a roughened surface in the subchondral bone to which the marrow clot can adhere more easily. The integrity of the subchondral plate is also maintained during this process when done correctly. Microfracture chondroplasty using awls virtually eliminates thermal necrosis that could occur with power drills. The various awls with different angles also allow subchondral penetration at all locations within the knee. The awls provide not only perpendicular holes but also improved control of depth penetration compared to drilling.

After all holes are made, the arthroscopic fluid pump pressure should be reduced and the entire microfracture grid should be observed **(Figs. 58-8** and **58-9)** for bleeding and fat

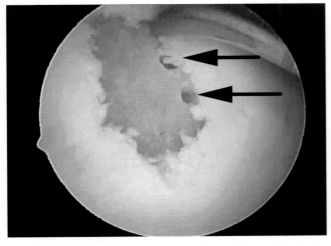

Fig. 58-6. Microfracture begins in the periphery of a lesion *(arrows)*. Holes are created initially at the junction of the lesion and the border cartilage.

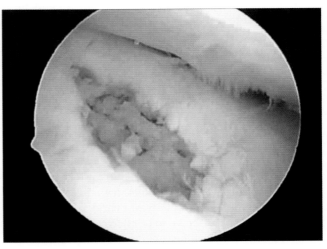

Fig. 58-8. The final microfracture grid after completion and prior to the reduction of the arthroscopic fluid pump pressure.

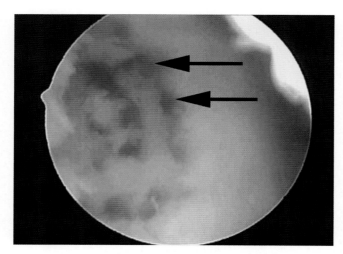

Fig. 58-9. The microfracture grid after the arthroscopic fluid pump pressure is reduced. Blood or marrow elements should be observed to be coming from each of the microfracture holes *(arrows)* with the pump pressure reduced. This observation ensures that the holes are of appropriate depth.

droplet leakage into the joint from each hole. If blood and marrow contents are noted to return to the joint, the holes are sufficiently deep. If there is no return to the joint, the holes can be deepened and rechecked.

Once the microfracture is complete, the arthroscopic equipment is removed from the joint. Intra-articular drains should not be used because the goal of the procedure is to keep the marrow clot in the joint at the site of the lesion. We close all portal sites with an absorbable suture and dress the wounds appropriately. We use a cooling device in nearly all patients as a component of the postoperative therapy.

■ TECHNICAL ALTERNATIVES AND PITFALLS

Alternatives to the microfracture procedure are numerous and include autogenous chondrocyte implantation, osteochondral autograft transplantation, osteochondral allograft transplantation, simple chondroplasty without microfracture, limited or total arthroplasty, or continued conservative treatment. The appropriate procedure to perform will depend on the patient and the defect.[15] Microfracture has many advantages. The results obtained with the microfracture technique have been shown to be reliable and durable.[9,10,14] The procedure is technically relatively simple when compared to autograft placement, autologous chondrocyte implantation (ACI), or allograft placement.[12,16–18] There is no requirement for arthrotomy or multiple procedures with the microfracture technique. Simple chondroplasty or debridement-type procedures have not been shown to be effective.[19]

Pitfalls and complications are rare, usually resolve within a short period of time, and are generally not severe.[9,10,12–14] Patients will occasionally experience transient pain, most commonly after microfracture in the patellofemoral joint.[13] Clicking, catching, or gritty sensations have also occasionally been noticed after microfracture. Usually these symptoms are transient and not associated with pain. Effusions in the knee after microfracture usually resolve within 2 months after surgery, but effusions and swelling may recur when the patient begins weight bearing after the initial period of limited weight bearing. The effusions are also generally self-limiting and usually do not require treatment.

Care must be taken during the operative procedure not to debride stable cartilage and not to destabilize or alter the geometry of the subchondral bone. It is equally important, however, to debride all cartilage including the calcified cartilage layer in lesions to be treated. Care should be exercised with the awls and motorized shaver as well. Awls can skive during the procedure, resulting in injury to surrounding healthy cartilage or fracture of one hole into another. The most common pitfall associated with microfracture is not an operative one, but rather it is incomplete or inappropriate rehabilitation.

■ REHABILITATION/RETURN TO PLAY RECOMMENDATIONS

The rehabilitation program after the microfracture procedure is critical to its success.[9,10,13,14,20] The postoperative protocol is designed to provide the optimal environment for the differentiation of the marrow elements and the production of the extracellular matrix. These two processes are intimately involved in the generation of durable repair tissue.

The rehabilitation protocol is also frequently modified for specific patients. Patients that have concurrent surgical procedures will most often complete some variation of our two main programs, which are detailed below.

Rehabilitation after microfracture of lesions in the weight-bearing regions of the femur or tibia is different from that after microfracture of lesions in the contact area of the patellofemoral articulation.[10,20] After microfracture of lesions on the weight-bearing surfaces of the femoral condyles or tibial plateaus, continuous passive motion (CPM) is started immediately after surgery in the recovery room. The initial range of motion (ROM) typically is 30 degrees to 70 degrees, and then it is increased as tolerated by 10 degrees to 20 degrees until full passive ROM is achieved. The rate of the machine is usually one cycle per minute, but the rate can be varied based on patient preference and comfort. We apply the CPM during the night for those who tolerate its use at night and exclusively during the day for those who do not have night tolerance. The goal is to use the CPM for 6 to 8 hours every 24 hours. If a CPM is unavailable or not appropriate for some other reason, we will instruct the patient to undergo approximately 500 cycles of passive ROM three times daily. Full passive motion is achieved in all cases as soon as possible.

Patients with weight-bearing lesions are also prescribed toe-touch weight bearing with crutches for 6 to 8 weeks. This regimen may be modified for small lesions, but caution must be taken when decreasing this period because of the fragility of the newly formed and immature repair tissue.[11] We generally do not use a brace for these patients during the immediate postoperative period, but we often use braces to unload the treated regions after the initial postoperative period as the patient begins to increase activity levels.

Patients begin stationary biking without resistance and a deep-water exercise program at 1 to 2 weeks after microfracture. The deep-water exercises include use of a kick board and a flotation vest for deep-water running. Patients progress to full weight bearing after 8 weeks and begin a more vigorous program of active motion of the knee and strengthening of the periarticular muscles. They also begin elastic resistance cord exercises at approximately 8 weeks after microfracture. We generally allow patients to begin weight training after they have reached an appropriate level with the above-described protocol, but not before 16 weeks postoperatively. If patients are to consider weight training, we emphasize proper form and an interval type program. Athletes will return to sports involving cutting or pivoting at 4 to 6 months after microfracture.

Rehabilitation after microfracture of lesions in the patellofemoral is significantly different from that after microfracture in a weight-bearing region. Patients who have undergone microfracture in the patellofemoral joint are treated in a locking brace with flexion limited to 20 degrees for at least 8 weeks. We limit the motion of the knee in these patients to 20 degrees in order to eliminate shear forces across the treated lesion that would occur at increased flexion angles with active quadriceps function during walking. We allow removal or unlocking of the brace only for passive range of motion and utilization of the CPM. These patients generally also achieve full range of motion rapidly despite the use of the brace because of the passive range of motion and CPM programs.

Patients are treated initially with crutches, but they rapidly progress to weight bearing as tolerated after treatment of patellofemoral lesions. All weight bearing is to be completed in a brace locked as described above for the first 8 weeks. The brace is then discontinued after full range of motion is gradually achieved over approximately 1 week.

We allow the patients to begin strengthening after the brace is discontinued. In patients with patellofemoral lesions, the contact areas are observed arthroscopically during knee motion and recorded. The ranges of motion of the knee during this contact are avoided during strengthening exercises for 4 months postoperatively.

We use cryotherapy for all microfracture patients in the postoperative period for 1 to 7 days in an effort to decrease inflammation, maximize rehabilitation, and control postoperative pain regardless of the location of the treatment. Anti-inflammatory medications and physical therapy modalities are also prescribed as appropriate.

■ OUTCOMES AND FUTURE DIRECTIONS

Steadman et al.[9] presented results of microfracture in 75 knees. This study presented long-term follow-up (7 to 17 years, average 11.3 years) on patients with traumatic chondral defects in the knee treated with microfracture. Patients were excluded from the study if other pathology existed that required surgical treatment. The patients averaged 30 years of age and had lesions averaging 277 mm^2. The authors report an improvement in pain, swelling, and Lysholm scores. Improvements were also reported in patients' ability to perform activities of daily living, strenuous work, and sports.

A recent prospective randomized study compared autologous chondrocyte implantation and microfracture in 80 patients without generalized osteoarthritis and with stable knees.[12] This study compared the two methods of cartilage defect treatment histologically and using various outcome measures. The authors found no significant difference in improvements in Lysholm scores, visual analog scale pain scores, or histological evaluation. The authors reported that microfracture patients achieved significantly better results based on the short form 36 Physical Component score.

Animal and human studies have demonstrated promising results regarding histological and cellular analysis of microfracture regeneration tissue.[8,11,12] There have been no studies to date, however, that demonstrate regeneration tissue that is identical to normal hyaline cartilage. More research is needed to enhance key matrix component production after microfracture.

■ REFERENCES

1. Hjelle K, Solheim E, Strand T, et al. Articular cartilage defects in 1,000 knee arthroscopies. Arthroscopy. 2002;18:730–734.
2. Buckwalter JA. Articular cartilage: injuries and potential for healing. J Orthop Sports Phys Ther. 1998;28:192–202.
3. Byrd JW, Jones KS. Osteoarthritis caused by an inverted acetabular labrum: radiographic diagnosis and arthroscopic treatment. Arthroscopy. 2002;18:741–747.
4. Navid DO, Myerson MS. Approach alternatives for treatment of osteochondral lesions of the talus. Foot Ankle Clin. 2002;7:635–649.
5. Bradley JP, Petrie RS. Osteochondritis dissecans of the humeral capitellum: diagnosis and treatment. Clin Sports Med. 2001;20: 565–590.
6. Bishop JY, Flatow EL. Management of glenohumeral arthritis: a role for arthroscopy? Orthop Clin North Am. 2003;34:559–566.
7. Siebold R, Lichtenberg S, Habermeyer P. Combination of microfracture and periostal-flap for the treatment of focal full thickness articular cartilage lesions of the shoulder: a prospective study. Knee Surg Sports Traumatol Arthrosc. 2003;11:183–189.
8. Frisbie DD, Trotter GW, Powers BE, et al. Arthroscopic subchondral bone plate microfracture technique augments healing of large chondral defects in the radial carpal bone and medial femoral condyle of horses. Vet Surg. 1999;28:242–255.
9. Steadman JR, Briggs KK, Rodrigo JJ, et al. Outcomes of microfracture for traumatic chondral defects of the knee: average 11-year follow-up. Arthroscopy. 2003;19:477–484.

10. Steadman JR, Rodkey WG, Briggs KK. Microfracture chondroplasty: indications, techniques, and outcomes. Sports Med Arthrosc Rev. 2003;11:236–244.

11. Frisbie DD, Oxford JT, Southwood L, et al. Early events in cartilage repair after subchondral bone microfracture. Clin Orthop Rel Res. 2003;407:215–227.

12. Knutsen G, Engebretsen L, Ludvigsen TC, et al. Autologous chondrocyte implantation compared with microfracture in the knee: a randomized trial. J Bone Joint Surg Am. 2004;86:455–464.

13. Steadman JR, Rodkey WG, Briggs KK. Microfracture to treat full-thickness chondral defects: surgical technique, rehabilitation, and outcomes. J Knee Surg. 2002;15:170–176.

14. Steadman JR, Miller BS, Karas SG, et al. The microfracture technique in the treatment of full-thickness chondral lesions of the knee in National Football League players. J Knee Surg. 2003;16: 83–86.

15. Cole BJ, Lee SJ. Complex knee reconstruction: articular cartilage treatment options. Arthroscopy. 2003;19(suppl 1):1–10.

16. Barber FA, Chow JC. New frontiers in articular cartilage injury. Arthroscopy. 2003;19(suppl 1):142–146.

17. Sgaglione NA, Miniaci A, Gillogly SD, et al. Update on advanced surgical techniques in the treatment of traumatic focal articular cartilage lesions in the knee. Arthroscopy. 2002;18(suppl 1):9–32.

18. Brittberg M, Lindahl A, Nilsson A, et al. Treatment of deep cartilage defects in the knee with autologous chondrocyte transplantation. N Engl J Med. 1994;331:889–895.

19. Moseley JB, O'Malley K, Petersen NJ, et al. A controlled trial of arthroscopic surgery for osteoarthritis of the knee. N Engl J Med. 2002;347:81–88.

20. Steadman JR, Rodkey WG, Rodrigo JJ. Microfracture: surgical technique and rehabilitation to treat chondral defects. Clin Orthop Rel Res. 2001;391S:S362–S369.

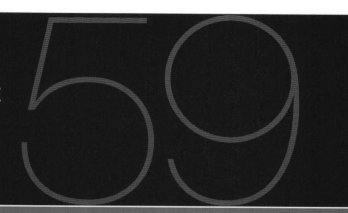

AUTOLOGOUS CHONDROCYTE IMPLANTATION

■ J. WINSLOW ALFORD, MD, BRIAN J. COLE, MD, MBA

■ HISTORY OF THE TECHNIQUE

Historically, the initial treatment of chondral injury included arthroscopic debridement to smooth the surface and remove debris that might promote an inflammatory response. Reparative techniques such as marrow stimulation offer another option that involves penetration of the subchondral bone to stimulate bleeding and recruitment of pluripotent mesenchymal marrow stem cells that differentiate and form fibrocartilage.[1] Restorative options used to replace the damaged cartilage include osteochondral autograft and allograft transplantation. Finally, autologous chondrocyte implantation (ACI), the subject of this chapter, involves the biologic replacement of articular cartilage. First reported clinically by Brittberg et al.[2] in 1994 and subsequently by several other authors,[3-5] ACI has become an acceptable treatment option in appropriately indicated patients with symptomatic chondral defects.

The procedure involves an arthroscopically performed biopsy of articular cartilage followed by implantation of cultured chondrocytes beneath a periosteal patch. At this juncture, ACI is considered a first-generation technology and advances in biologic carriers, cell-seeded scaffolds, and single-stage biological techniques are sure to replace ACI within the next 5 to 10 years depending upon regulatory pathways. Although the vast majority of the clinical experience with these technologies is with the treatment of chondral injuries of the knee, our experience is beginning to include other weight-bearing diarthrodial joints as well.

Preclinical Experience

In the 1980s, several groups reported the results of ACI performed in rabbit articular cartilage defects.[6,7] In shallow defects, an average of 82% of the surface area of the defect was covered by reformed cartilage. More recently, Brittberg et al.[8] placed periosteal patches on rabbit patellar defects with and without implanting chondrocytes. After 1 year, the periosteal grafts with chondrocytes had resulted in an average repair area of 87% of the total area of the defect compared to 31% in the animals treated without chondrocytes. In addition, the tissue produced by the chondrocytes and periosteal flap had a hyalinelike appearance compared to a fibrous appearance in the group without chondrocytes.

In contrast, Breinan et al.[9] found no difference at 12 or 18 months in coverage area or histologic appearance of defects repaired with either empty periosteal patches or chondrocyte-filled patches. In this study, a substantial number of defects involved violation of the subchondral bone, resulting in the creation and evaluation of osteochondral defects. Since this work, the importance of avoiding violation of the subchondral bone and antecedent bleeding has been implicated as a key feature of the ACI procedure. With respect to the longevity of the chondrocytes, studies monitoring the fate of labeled chondrocytes have demonstrated that implanted chondrocytes contribute to the formation of repair tissue and are integrated into surrounding normal articular cartilage up to 18 months following implantation.[10]

■ INDICATIONS AND CONTRAINDICATIONS

Overview

Traumatic focal chondral lesions are rarely found in isolation. A thorough evaluation of the involved extremity is essential. Assessment of associated ligament injuries, meniscal deficiency, and coexisting mechanical axis malalignment or patellofemoral maltracking must be identified with a strategy for correction incorporated into the overall surgical plan and postoperative rehabilitation.

Patient evaluation and identification of candidates for ACI treatment remain challenging. This is in part due to the fact that the natural history of commonly found asymptomatic lesions is unclear. In general, incidentally discovered articular cartilage lesions are well tolerated and rarely become symptomatic.[11] It is generally accepted that a symptomatic cartilage lesion that fails to respond to conservative care or initial arthroscopic measures is likely to persist or worsen without treatment.[12–14] Alternatively, the likelihood of a cartilage lesion detected incidentally on magnetic resonance imaging (MRI) or at arthroscopy becoming symptomatic depends on its location, depth, geographic configuration, the physical demands of the patient, subjective pain tolerances, and the presence of co-morbidities. Added to the unpredictable nature of the incidental lesion, the tendency for articular cartilage to respond to injury with a disordered and often incomplete repair response is likely to be related to the variability of symptoms that patients demonstrate following cartilage injury.[1,2,15]

Obtaining a history of the mechanism of injury, the onset and pattern of symptoms, prior treatments and the response to these treatments, as well as a thorough review of previous operative reports, arthroscopic images, and video is an important part of the initial patient evaluation. For example, Peterson et al.[16] demonstrated that the typical patient indicated for ACI had an average of 2.1 previous treatments. The senior author (BJC) has had a similar experience in more than 120 ACI procedures, and we have learned that direct verbal or written communication with the most recent treating physician is extremely useful.

The etiology of chondral lesions is variable and includes blunt trauma, focal wear, or chronic conditions (i.e., osteochondritis dissecans). Variable etiology and associated biology are further affected by prior treatments rendered, functional expectations of the patient, and unique patient personality characteristics. For these reasons, identifying candidates for ACI remains challenging. For a specific patient at a particular point in time there may be several reasonable treatment options. A central tenant of cartilage restoration is that a selected treatment must not "burn bridges" but rather allow for further treatments should they prove necessary. It is essential to avoid "linear reasoning" when evaluating a particular patient. There are often several potential etiologies that lead to patient complaints of knee pain, and, thus, incidental defects must not be inappropriately labeled as responsible for a patient's symptoms.

In addition to lesion characteristics, an evaluation of the relative severity of commonly occurring co-morbidities such as ligament and meniscal insufficiency and malalignment of the patellofemoral or tibiofemoral joints must also occur. This coexisting pathology must be addressed in conjunction with the articular cartilage pathology or in an appropriately

staged fashion. Left untreated, coexisting pathology remains a contraindication to ACI. Ligament reconstruction, corrective osteotomies, or meniscal transplants are frequently required in addition to an ACI procedure. A comprehensive plan to address all features of the patient's joint pathology must be devised and discussed at length with the patient before proceeding. Treating co-morbidities greatly enhances a patient's possibility of achieving a good outcome by providing a symbiosis of two or more mutually beneficial procedures. The decision to perform multiple procedures concomitantly or in a staged manner requires the judgment of an experienced articular cartilage surgeon.

Imaging

Radiographic evaluation should include standing anterior to posterior, non–weight-bearing 45-degree flexion lateral, patellar skyline (i.e., Merchant), 45-degree flexion posterior-anterior (PA) weight bearing, full-length alignment views. The PA weight bearing 45-degree (tunnel or Rosenberg) view is essential because it brings the posterior femoral condyle into a tangential position relative to the tibial plateau and x-ray beam. A normal appearing joint in a standing AP x-ray may reveal severe articular cartilage loss in the region of the posterior femoral condyle when viewed with the knee in 45 degrees of flexion.

Recent advancements in cartilage-specific MRI technology permit precise diagnosis and measurement of articular cartilage pathology. High-resolution fast spin echo sequencing techniques provide a high level of accuracy in predicting defect location, size, and depth.[17] Techniques using fat saturation in T2 protocols or fat suppression in T1 protocols combined with ionic gadolinium diethylene triamine penta-acetic acid (Gd-DTPA) contrast allow for inferences of biomechanical and biochemical changes involved in matrix degradation and formation.[18,19] Improvements in MRI technology allow for a more accurate preoperative determination of lesion characteristics and also may allow for the postoperative assessment of actual glycosaminoglycan content and an assessment of the overall biochemical quality of the healing tissue.

Animal studies investigating the utility of ultrasound technology in the evaluation of articular surfaces were modeled to evaluate degenerative lesions, and the reliability of ultrasound for the evaluation of focal chondral lesions is unproven at this time.[20] Nuclear medicine studies are of limited value due to the nonspecific nature of the information it provides. However, in the presence of osteochondritis dissecans (OCD), a completely different pathophysiology exists and a bone scan can provide information about biologic activity and healing potential.

Arthroscopy

An examination under anesthesia will allow for an assessment of co-morbidities that may need to be addressed. A thorough arthroscopic evaluation is valuable to determine the location, topical geography, surface area, and depth of a defect in addition to providing a formal assessment of comorbidities such as the condition of the opposing articular surface, ligament and meniscus status, and an evaluation for other unsuspected defects. Grading of articular cartilage lesions depends on direct visual assessment and has inter- and intraobserver variability. In addition to the rating systems of Outerbridge,[21] Insall,[22] Baur,[23] and Noyes and Stabler,[24] which are frequently cited in the literature, the International Cartilage Repair Society (ICRS) has offered a grading system to be used as a universal language when surgeons are communicating about cartilage lesions.[25] Verbal or written grading of articular surfaces should specify which grading system is being used and should be accompanied by a written and diagrammatic description of the lesion.

If the lesion is located in the patellofemoral joint, careful arthroscopic analysis of patellofemoral tracking and mechanical alignment is important because a combined anteromedialization of the tibial tubercle is generally recommended in conjunction with ACI of the patellofemoral joint.

Indications

The overall assumption is that identified defects are at least in part responsible for the patient's signs and symptoms at the time of clinical evaluation. Smaller acute defects (i.e., less than 3 cm²) are typically treated initially with other modalities, whereby ACI is employed when these treatments fail to improve upon the patient's clinical presentation following adequate time for recovery and response. ACI is ideal for symptomatic, unipolar, full thickness, or nearly full thickness chondral or shallow osteochondral defects. Commonly, patients have failed previous treatments. Occasionally, larger symptomatic lesions in high demand patients are indicated for ACI as a first line treatment. ACI is traditionally indicated for treatment of focal defects in the knee, but its off-label use has recently been expanded to include the treatment of chondral defects in the ankle, shoulder, elbow, wrist, and hip.[26-30] In the knee, off-label usage for the patella and tibia has also met with success rates that parallel the femoral condyle and trochlea. Bipolar lesions (greater than grade II changes on the opposing surface) are a relative contraindication to ACI. As already discussed, malalignment, ligament instability, and meniscus deficiency are not considered contraindications to ACI as long as they are addressed concomitantly or in a staged fashion.

Patellofemoral lesions are commonly treated with simultaneously performed anteromedialization of the tibial tubercle. It is important to determine the desired ratio of anteriorization to medialization required from the distal realignment as this will determine the angle of the tubercle osteotomy performed at the time of implantation.

OCD is not a contraindication for ACI provided that bone loss is less than 6 to 8 mm. Greater degrees of bone loss are corrected with bone grafting in a single- or two-stage procedure. A "sandwich technique" where the cells are injected between two opposing layers of periosteum placed over a bone graft to re-establish the subchondral bed has been utilized in a single stage, but the senior author (BJC) prefers to first graft the lesion and biopsy at that time only to return if necessary to perform the ACI procedure no sooner than 6 months following the index treatment.

■ SURGICAL TECHNIQUES

Stage I

Prior to biopsy, we make every effort to obtain insurance approval for both phases of the ACI procedure. We rarely will biopsy a patient without the explicit intention to definitively treat the defect with ACI. The first stage involves an arthroscopic evaluation of the focal chondral lesion to assess containment, depth, and potential bone loss **(Fig. 59-1)**. A biopsy of normal hyaline cartilage is obtained from either the superomedial edge of the trochlea,[31] or our preferred site, the lateral side of the intercondylar notch (i.e., where bone is removed for an ACL notchplasty) using a curved bone-graft harvesting gouge **(Fig. 59-2)**. If the biopsy is obtained from the trochlear ridge, it is recommended that a ring curette be used to allow for visualization of the biopsy process. The total volume of the biopsy should be approximately 200 to 300 mg preferably in three "Tic-Tac-sized" fragments. It is preferable to penetrate to the subchondral bone to ensure that the deep chondrocytes are included in the biopsy. The prepared shipping container has a collection vial that is clearly

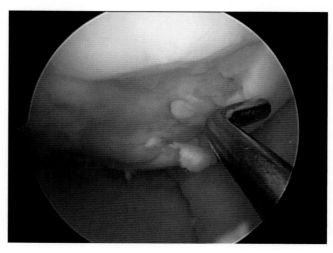

Fig. 59-1. An arthroscopic evaluation of focal chondral lesion provides direct measurement and assessment of lesion containment and potential bone loss.

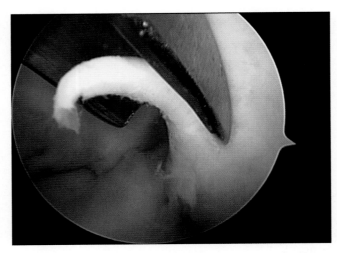

Fig. 59-2. An arthroscopic biopsy of articular cartilage cells is taken from the non–weight-bearing portion of lateral femoral condyle in a left knee.

marked to indicate adequate biopsy volume **(Fig. 59-3)**. As when performing an ACL notchplasty, it is important not to violate the weight-bearing articular cartilage. The biopsy is sent to Genzyme Biosurgery Corp (Cambridge, Mass) for processing and cellular expansion.

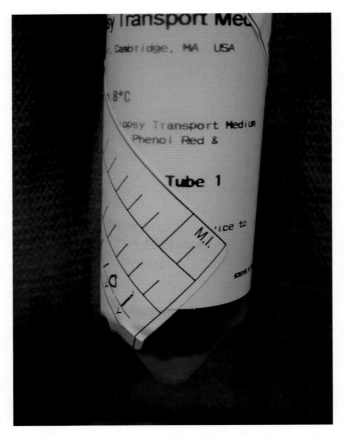

Fig. 59-3. Prepared shipping vial, demonstrating proper collection to assess adequate biopsy volume.

Stage II

The second stage of the procedure is cell implantation, which takes place between 1 and 18 months following the biopsy. A tourniquet is typically used until after the defect is prepared and the periosteal patch is harvested. The surgical exposure depends upon defect location. Patellofemoral (PF) lesions are approached through a midline incision allowing a simultaneously performed tibial tubercle osteotomy. We prefer to access PF lesions through a lateral retinacular release without formally everting the patella 180 degrees. We also avoid disruption of the fat pad and dissection around the patellar tendon to reduce complications related to postoperative stiffness. The tibial tubercle osteotomy does afford some increased patellar mobility facilitating access to the defect, but we intentionally avoid complete elevation and "flipping" of the tibial tubercle to minimize trauma to the fat pad and patellar tendon.

Femoral condyle lesions are addressed through limited ipsilateral parapatellar arthrotomies. For medial defects, we use a limited subvastus medialis approach, which has, in our experience, reduced the magnitude of postoperative pain allowing earlier and more complete return of motion. Lateral defects are approached through a limited lateral retinacular release. We then utilize a separate 3-cm incision beneath the pes anserine tendon insertion to harvest the periosteal patch. These recent modifications have allowed us to perform the majority of our ACI procedures on an outpatient basis.

Defect preparation involves removing the loose cartilage flaps and leaving healthy surrounding hyaline cartilage to form stable vertical walls shouldering the lesion. Circular or oval-shaped prepared defects are biomechanically more stable.[31] A no. 15 scalpel and sharp ring curettes are used to incise the defect border to, but not through, the level of the subchondral bone **(Fig. 59-4A,B)**. Hemostasis is controlled with the use of neuropatties soaked with a dilute 1:1,000 epinephrine solution.

The periosteal patch is harvested through a 3-cm incision on the proximal medial tibia, 2 fingerbreadths distal to the pes anserine tendon attachments. More distal and anteromedial locations tend to provide the best source for the periosteal patch. If a simultaneous tibial tubercle osteotomy is performed, we use a single extensile incision and harvest the periosteum prior to performing the osteotomy. Superficial subcutaneous fat is carefully removed with sharp dissection from the periosteum on the antero-medial tibia to avoid inadvertent penetration. Smokers tend to have poor quality periosteum and obese patients have a larger amount of adherent adipose tissue to separate from the periosteum, which will require extra care. In addition, older patients tend to have very thin periosteum. A patch that is at least 2 mm larger than the defect is harvested to account for slight shrinkage following detachment. The patch edges are scored to bone with a no. 15 scalpel on three sides, leaving it attached proximally, and elevated with a sharp curved periosteal elevator beginning distally and

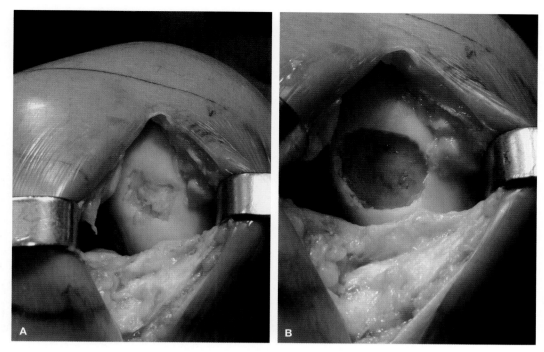

Fig. 59-4. Defect before **(A)** and after **(B)** preparation.

moving toward the inferior edge of the pes and overlying sartorius fascia **(Fig. 59-5)**. The character of the periosteum will change as the sartorius fascia fibers are encountered. It is recommended that the fat and small blood vessels found on the periosteum be dissected off after the periosteum is safely elevated from the bone, but before detaching the final proximal edge. The outer surface is marked to distinguish it from the inner cambium layer. Additional sources for periosteum, if necessary, are the distal femur, which is

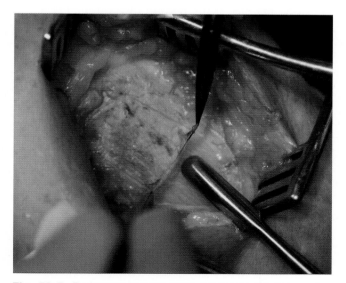

Fig. 59-5. Periosteal harvest from anteriomedial tibia, using curved-tipped elevator to minimize risk of penetrating periosteum during harvest.

thicker and more vascular than the periosteum on the proximal tibia, or the contralateral leg, which carries the disadvantage of a second surgical site. In extreme cases, two periosteal patches may be sewn together, taking care to minimize suture bulk at the seam.

The tourniquet is then deflated and meticulous hemostasis is obtained. The patch is then sewn onto the cartilage with the cambium layer facing the defect. The periosteum is secured with a 6-0 absorbable Vicryl suture on a P-1 cutting needle. The suture should be coated in sterile glycerin or mineral oil to prevent adherence to the surgical gloves, periosteum, and articular cartilage, allowing smooth suture passage without tissue tearing. The suture is passed through the patch edge first and then through the surrounding articular cartilage. The needle should enter the cartilage perpendicular to the inside wall of the defect at a depth of 2 mm below the articular surface and exit the articular surface 3 to 4 mm from the edge of the defect. The goal is to anchor the periosteum flush with the surrounding articular cartilage surface. One strategy is to first secure the four corners of the defect and then fill in the gaps with sutures every 3 mm, leaving one 4- to 6-mm gap to perform water tightness testing and injection of the cells. The location of this "gap" region should be selected to allow for easy syringe and catheter orientation. The patch should be taught over the defect to create a potential space to accept the cell suspension. In the trochlear groove, however, overtightening will cause a loss of concavity and result in a prominence, which can impinge on the patella. If small holes are inadvertently created in the periosteum patch, they may be carefully repaired with a single 6-0 Vicryl suture. If the surrounding cartilage is unable to hold suture, microanchors loaded with absorbable suture may be used or if at the edge of an articular surface, small bone tunnels may be created with a 0.45 K-wire to pass transosseous sutures. Uncontained osteochondritis dissecans is typically on the lateral edge of the medial condyle and extending into the notch. Grafting these lesions may require that patch sutures be placed into the synovium surrounding the posterior cruciate ligament.

Water tightness testing is performed with a nonantibiotic saline-filled tuberculin syringe and 18-guage catheter. The patched cavity must be watertight to ensure cell containment and to prevent cell cavity contamination from postoperative hemarthrosis. After the saline is injected for the water tightness test, it should be removed completely. Additional sutures are placed at leakage locations and, after gently drying the cartilage surrounding the patch, the edges of the patch are sealed with fibrin glue (Tisseel, Baxter Healthcare Corp, Glendale, Calif) and a second water tightness test is performed as previously described. Do not prime the fibrin glue syringe needle prior to injection because the needle bore will clog, requiring tip replacement.

The chondrocytes are delivered and stored in vials that should remain upright at all times. Meticulous attention to sterile technique is paramount during this step as the vial's exterior is not sterile. The vials are held vertical without dis-

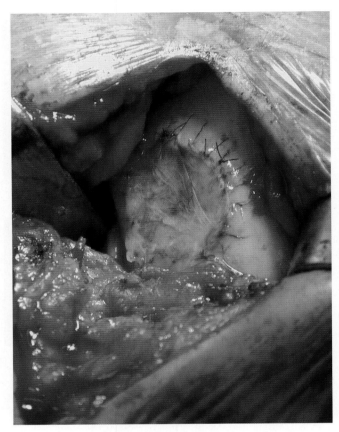

Fig. 59-7. After cell implantation, the sutured periosteal patch is sealed with fibrin glue.

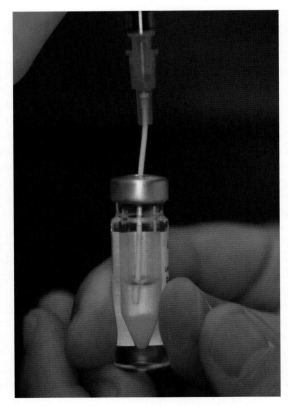

Fig. 59-6. Angio-catheter tip is submerged in fluid while the vial containing chondrocytes is held vertical. Meticulous attention to sterile technique during this step is paramount.

turbing the pellet of cells in the bottom of the vial. The lid is removed, and the top is thoroughly sterilized with ethanol alcohol. An 18-gauge angio-catheter is inserted into the vial and advanced so the tip is submerged in the fluid, but above the pellet of cells in the bottom of the vial. The metal trochar is withdrawn, leaving the plastic catheter in the vial. Next, a 3-cc syringe is attached to the external portion of the catheter and only the fluid is aspirated into the syringe, leaving the pellet of cells behind **(Fig. 59-6)**. This fluid is gently injected back into the vial atraumatically, suspending the cells in the fluid. This process is methodically repeated until a homogeneous suspension is achieved. The entire contents of the vial are then drawn into the syringe. The syringe and catheter are carefully withdrawn from the vial while maintaining negative pressure in the syringe to prevent inadvertent escape of the chondrocyte suspension. The catheter tip is then discarded and replaced with a fresh sterile angio-catheter tip for implantation.

To implant the cells into the prepared defect, the catheter is placed through the opening at the top of the defect and advanced to the distal end. The cells are slowly injected into the bed of the defect with a side-to-side motion for even dispersal while the catheter is slowly withdrawn. The opening is then closed with additional sutures and sealed with fibrin glue **(Fig. 59-7)**.

■ TECHNICAL ALTERNATIVES AND PITFALLS

Most defects are easily accessible on the weight-bearing surface of the femoral condyle through a standard parapatellar arthrotomy. However, far posterior condylar lesions or focal cartilage defects of the tibial plateau may require additional strategies for exposure, including an open submeniscal approach or even en block osteotomy of the collateral ligaments, which are repaired with interference screws at the completion of the procedure.

ACI has traditionally been applied to treat relatively shallow lesions of articular cartilage without involvement of the subchondral bone. For osteochondral defects of more than 8 to 10 mm in depth, bone grafting is recommended. The bone graft may be performed at the time of biopsy, and the implantation may be delayed to allow for bone graft consolidation. Alternatively, the "sandwich technique" has been utilized to replace bone and resurface the defect in a single step. A complete description of the procedure is reported elsewhere.[32] With that technique, the bone defect is filled with bone graft, periosteum is sutured on top of the bone graft at the level of the subchondral bone plate, a second layer of periosteum is placed over the cartilage defect, and the chondrocytes are then placed between the layers of periosteum. The result is a cancellous grafted bone defect covered by two layers of watertight periosteal patches with the cambium layers facing each other and into the cavity filled with autologous chondrocytes.

It is commonly believed that for all of these techniques, realignment osteotomy should be performed as an adjunct procedure if the lesion is in a compartment under more than physiologic compression.[33] Outcome data clearly indicate that poorer results are expected if mechanical axis or patellofemoral joint malalignment is left uncorrected at the time of the cartilage restoration procedure.[33]

Patellofemoral joint realignment with a tibial tubercle osteotomy is a familiar procedure and has been in the mainstream of orthopedics for decades.[34] We recommend that any cartilage restoration procedure performed on the PF joint be combined with a distal realignment procedure that anteriorizes the patella to unload the newly resurfaced PF joint. Any associated PF maltracking or instability must be appreciated preoperatively and corrected at the time of the distal realignment. Whether performing the distal realignment to anteriorize the patella and unload the PF joint or to medialize it to correct lateral instability associated with a pathologic Q angle, the surgeon must be intimately familiar with each patient's PF mechanics to choose the proper osteotomy angle. Flatter angles will medialize more than anteriorize, and steeper angles will provide more anteriorization than medialization. A lateral release should be performed in addition to the distal realignment. There are commercially available surgical instruments to make the procedure technically easier to perform with precision (Tracker AMZ guide, Mitek, Norwood, Mass).

A high tibial osteotomy is required when performing a cartilage restoration procedure in the medial compartment of a varus knee. Many of these patients are relatively young and do not desire or tolerate large cosmetic changes in their lower extremity alignment. Unlike standard high tibial osteotomy for isolated medial compartment osteoarthritis, in which the aim is to correct the mechanical axis laterally to 62% of the width of the tibial plateau in the lateral compartment,[35] high tibial osteotomies combined with cartilage restoration in the medial compartment should correct the mechanical axis to neutral or just beyond. Because of its simplicity and reduced morbidity, we prefer an opening medial osteotomy to create a valgus correction rather than the traditional closing lateral osteotomy. Commercially available instrumentation (Arthrex, Inc, Naples, Fla) allows for a technically simple, rapidly performed osteotomy with precision and rigid fixation. Similarly, laterally based defects in a valgus knee are corrected with a simultaneously performed opening wedge distal femoral osteotomy.

When performing a corrective osteotomy combined with a cartilage restoration procedure, it is critical to establish a preoperative plan that allows for a stepwise incorporation of both procedures. For example, when performing an ACI of the PF joint with a combined distal realignment, the periosteal patch must be harvested from the anteromedial tibia prior to making the osteotomy of the tubercle through that area. Articular cartilage lesion preparation, graft suturing, and cell implantation require subluxation or eversion of the patella and should be performed prior to establishing rigid fixation of the tubercle osteotomy distally.

Uncorrected ligamentous instability is a contraindication to ACI. Methods of ligament reconstruction are well established and will not be reviewed here. When performing an ACL reconstruction in the setting of an ACI, periosteal patch harvest would occur before hamstring harvest or tibial drilling. If treating patellar or trochlear defect with ACI and distal realignment, hamstring autograft or patellar tendon allograft would be required as the osteotomized tibial tubercle insertion would be unavailable as an ACL graft source.

In complex cases, a guideline of two procedures per operation and staging subsequent procedures should be followed. When staging procedures, osteotomies should be performed first with a 4- to 6-month healing interval to allow for complete bone healing and remodeling. Subsequent hardware removal should be incorporated into the overall surgical plan.

■ REHABILITATION

The rehabilitation protocol for ACI in the knee is based on the three phases of the natural maturation process of the graft.[36–38] The proliferative phase occurs soon after the cells are implanted, followed by the matrix production phase during which the tissue becomes incorporated and integrated into the host. To assist cellular orientation and to prevent adhesions, early continuous passive motion is crucial and begins at least 6 hours after the procedure is completed and continues for up to 6 weeks at 6 hours per day. The graft must be protected from mechanical shear, and closed chain strengthening exercises are initiated to allow for a functional gait. Patients are allowed passive motion and touch down weight bearing until 4 to 6 weeks when progression to full weight bearing is allowed. Weigh bearing in extension for PF lesions theoretically could be permitted early in the process, but we remain concerned about the potential for sustaining a tibial fracture through the tibial tubercle osteotomy site. The third phase is the maturation phase, which results in graft stiffness that more closely resembles the surrounding articular cartilage. During this extended phase, various impact-loading activities are phased in with increased strength work. Concomitant procedures do not generally change the rehabilitation protocol.

■ OUTCOMES AND FUTURE DIRECTIONS

It is estimated that ACI has been performed on 10,000 patients worldwide.[33] Micheli et al.[39] reported on 50 patients who were followed for a minimum 36 months and demonstrated a significant improvement of 5 points on the Modified Cincinnati scale measuring overall knee function (10-point scale). Eighty-four percent had an improvement in their condition, 2% were unchanged, and 13% deteriorated. One third of these patients had failed a previous marrow stimulation procedure. Peterson et al.[40] published his results on 94 patients with 2- to 9-year follow-up. The results varied considerably based upon defect location. The results of ACI when treating the patella initially were 62% good to excellent. However, later in the series, simultaneously performed tibial tubercle osteotomy was performed and results improved to 85% good and excellent. Twenty-four out of the 25 isolated femoral condyle lesions were graded as having good to excellent results with a 92% success rate. In the OCD group, 16 of 18 patients were rated good to excellent representing an 89% success rate. The majority of follow-up biopsies revealed hyalinelike tissue that demonstrated type II collagen on immunohistochemical staining. In 10% to 15% of cases, the biopsy site demonstrated an exaggerated healing response in the notch, resulting in discomfort and catching that may occur between 3 and 9 months. This routinely responded well to simple arthroscopic debridement.

To study the long-term durability of ACI, Brittberg et al.[32] followed 61 patients for a mean of 7.4 years after ACI. Good or excellent results were found in 81% at 2 years, and 83% at 5- to 11-year evaluation. The total failure rate was 16%, all of which occurred in the first 2 years. In this series, patients with the longer outcome were early patients who underwent ACI before full maturation of the surgical technique. As all failures occurred before 2 years, this study illustrates the durability of results at 2 years.

To compare microfracture to ACI, Knutsen et al.[41] randomized 80 patients with focal chondral defects in nonarthritic knees to receive either ACI or microfracture. At 2 years, arthroscopic evaluation, biopsy, and clinical evaluation, using Tegner, Lysholm, ICRS, and SF-36, demonstrates significant improvement in both groups, with significant difference between groups, favoring microfracture. In this series, both groups of patients were allowed immediate partial weight bearing (up to 50 lb), which may be disruptive for the fragile ACI patch. In addition, multiple surgeons were included in the study, all of whom included their early ACI patients for comparison. Longer term results will be needed from this study to determine the ability of microfracture to endure, given historical questions of its durability.

Horas et al.[42] compared ACI to osteochondral autograft transplantation at 2 years in 40 patients with a single femoral condyle chondral defect. Both treatments decreased symptoms, but the improvement provided by ACI lagged behind that provided by the osteochondral autograft transplant. Histologically, the ACI tissue was primarily fibrocartilage, whereas the osteochondral transplants retained their hyaline character. There was a persistent gap and lack of integration between the bone plugs and the surrounding articular cartilage. This study had a small number of patients in each group, a relatively short follow-up, and no control group.

To compare mosaicplasty to ACI, Bently et al.[43] randomized 100 patients with an average age of 31.3 with isolated traumatic focal chondral defects to receive ACI or mosaicplasty. Modified Cincinnati scores and clinical assessment measures rated good to excellent results in 88% of ACI patients and only 69% of the mosaicplasty patients. Arthroscopy at 1 year demonstrated 82% healing among ACI patients, but only 34% healing among mosaicplasty patients. This is the only prospective, randomized controlled comparison of ACI and mosaicplasty, and it appears to demonstrate the superiority of ACI over small-plug autologous mosaicplasty.

In the future, techniques utilizing minimally invasive implantation will spare the patient the morbidity of an open arthrotomy. All arthroscopic techniques have been reported, but are not currently implemented in the United States.[44] The technique is based on implanting a 2-mm thick polymer fleece, preloaded with autologous chondrocytes in a fibrin gel, that is anchored to the condyle arthroscopically. Lee has implemented in vitro culturing of a chondrocyte-laden scaffold prior to implantation. In a canine model, he evaluated full thickness focal chondral defects without bone involvement 15 weeks after implantation of an autologous articular chondrocyte-laden type-II collagen scaffold that had been cultured in vitro prior to implantation.[45] In these cultured scaffolds, the reparative tissue formed from the scaffolds filled 88% ± 6% of the cross-sectional area of the original defect, with hyaline cartilage accounting for 42% ± 10% (range, 7% to 67%) of the defect area. Further work is necessary to identify the specific culture and cell density parameters needed to maximize this advantage of in vitro scaffold culture prior to final implantation compared to the results of noncultured implantation.[46,47] In the future, allogeneic sources of cells or single-stage biologic techniques may offer the added advantage of eliminating the need for biopsy prior to implantation. As ACI technology becomes more mainstream and techniques improve, it will likely be used more routinely to treat other joint surfaces as well as the knee.

■ SUGGESTED READINGS

Bentley G, Biant LC, Carrington RW, et al. A prospective, randomised comparison of autologous chondrocyte implantation versus mosaicplasty for osteochondral defects in the knee. J Bone Joint Surg Br. 2003;85:223–230.

Brittberg M. ICRS Clinical Cartilage Injury Evaluation System—2000. Paper presented at Third International Cartilage Repair Society Meeting, April 28, 2000.

Brittberg M, Lindahl A, Nilsson A, et al. Treatment of deep cartilage defects in the knee with autologous chondrocyte transplantation. N Engl J Med. 1994;331(14):889–895.

Brittberg M, Peterson L, Sjogren-Jansson E, et al. Articular cartilage engineering with autologous chondrocyte transplantation: a review of recent developments. J Bone Joint Surg Am. 2003;85-A(suppl 3):109–115.

D'Amato M, Cole BJ. Autologous chondrocyte implantation. Orthop Techn. 2001;11:115–131.

Erggelet C, Sittinger M, Lahm A. The arthroscopic implantation of autologous chondrocytes for the treatment of full-thickness cartilage defects of the knee joint. Arthroscopy. 2003;19(1):108–110.

Fulkerson JP. Anteromedialization of the tibial tuberosity for patellofemoral malalignment. Clin Orthop. July–August 1983;177:176–178.

Knutsen G, Engebretsen L, Ludvigsen TC, et al. Autologous chondrocyte implantation compared with microfracture in the knee: a randomized trial. J Bone Joint Surg Am. March 2004;86-A(3):455–464.

Lee CR, Grodzinsky AJ, Hsu HP, et al. Effects of a cultured autologous chondrocyte-seeded type II collagen scaffold on the healing of a chondral defect in a canine model. J Orthop Res. 2003;21:272–281.

Messner K, Maletius W. The long-term prognosis for severe damage to weight-bearing cartilage in the knee: a 14-year clinical and radiographic follow-up in 28 young athletes. Acta Orthop Scand. 1996;67(2):165–168.

Peterson L, Minas T, Brittberg M, et al. Treatment of osteochondritis dissecans of the knee with autologous chondrocyte transplantation: results at two to ten years. J Bone Joint Surg Am. 2003;85(suppl 2):17–24.

Peterson L, Minas T, Brittberg M, et al. Two- to 9-year outcome after autologous chondrocyte transplantation of the knee. Clin Ortho Rel Res. 2000;374:212–234.

Romeo AA, Cole BJ, Mazzocca AD, et al. Autologous chondrocyte repair of an articular defect in the humeral head. Arthroscopy. October 2002;18(8):925–929.

Shelbourne KD, Jari S, Gray T. Outcome of untreated traumatic articular cartilage defects of the knee: a natural history study. J Bone Joint Surg Am. 2003;85-A(suppl 2):8–16.

■ REFERENCES

1. Buckwalter JA. Were the Hunter brothers wrong? Can surgical treatment repair articular cartilage? Iowa Orthop J. 1997;17:1–13.

2. Brittberg M, Lindahl A, Nilsson A, et al. Treatment of deep cartilage defects in the knee with autologous chondrocyte transplantation. N Engl J Med. 1994;331(14):889–895.

3. Gillogly SD. Autologous chondrocyte implantation: current state-of-the-art. In: Imhoff AB, Burkart A, eds. *Knieinstabilität-knorpelschaden.* Darmstadt, Germany: Steinkopff; 1998:60–66.

4. Minas T. Chondrocyte implantation in the repair of chondral lesions of the knee: economics and quality of life. Am J Orthop. 1998;27:739–744.

5. Mandelbaum BR, Browne JE, Fu F, et al. Articular cartilage lesions of the knee. Am J Sports Med. 1998;26:853–861.

6. Peterson L, Menche D, Grande D, et al. Chondrocyte transplantation—an experimental model in the rabbit. Trans Orthop Res Soc. 1984;9:218.

7. Grande DA, Pitman MI, Peterson L, et al. The repair of experimentally produced defects in rabbit articular cartilage by autologous chondrocyte transplantation. J Orthop Res. 1989;7(2):208–218.

8. Brittberg M, Nilsson A, Lindahl A, et al. Rabbit articular cartilage defects treated with autologous cultured chondrocytes. Clin Orthop. 1996;326:270–283.

9. Breinan HA, Minas T, Hsu HP, et al. Effect of cultured autologous chondrocytes on repair of chondral defects in a canine model. J Bone Joint Surg Am. 1997;79:1439–1451.

10. Dell'Accio F, Vanlauwe J, Bellemans J, et al. Expanded phenotypically stable chondrocytes persist in the repair tissue and contribute to cartilage matrix formation and structural integration in a goat model of autologous chondrocyte implantation. J Orthop Res. 2003;21:123–131.

11. Shelbourne KD, Jari S, Gray T. Outcome of untreated traumatic articular cartilage defects of the knee: a natural history study. J Bone Joint Surg Am. 2003;85-A(suppl 2):8–16.

12. Linden B. Osteochondritis dissecans of the femoral condyles: a long-term follow-up study. J Bone Joint Surg Am. 1977;59(6):769–776.

13. Messner K, Maletius W. The long-term prognosis for severe damage to weight-bearing cartilage in the knee: a 14-year clinical and radiographic follow-up in 28 young athletes. Acta Orthop Scand. 1996;67(2):165–168.

14. Shelbourne KD, Jari S, Gray T. Outcome of untreated traumatic articular cartilage defects of the knee: a natural history study. J Bone Joint Surg Am. 2003;85(suppl 2):8–16.

15. Sahlstrom A. The natural course of arthrosis of the knee. Clin Orthop. 1997;340:152–157.

16. Peterson L, Minas T, Brittberg M, et al. Treatment of osteochondritis dissecans of the knee with autologous chondrocyte transplantation: results at two to ten years. J Bone Joint Surg Am. 2003;85(suppl 2):17–24.

17. Potter H, Linklater J, Answorth A. Magnetic resonance imaging of articular cartilage in the knee: an evaluation with use of fast-spin-echo imaging. J Bone Joint Surg Am. 1998;80:1276–1284.

18. McCauley T, Disler D. Magnetic resonance imaging of articular cartilage of the knee. J Am Acad Orth Surg. 2001;9:2–8.

19. Burstein D, Bashir A, Gray ML. MRI techniques in early stages of cartilage disease. Invest Radiol. 2000;35:622–638.

20. Laasanen MS, Töyräs J, Vasara AI, et al. Mechano-acoustic diagnosis of cartilage degeneration and repair. J Bone Joint Surg Am. 2003;85(suppl 2):78–84.

21. Outerbridge RE. The etiology of chondromalacia patellae. J Bone Joint Surg Br. 1961;43:752–759.

22. Insall J. Patellar pain. J Bone and Joint Surg. 1982;64A(1):147–152.

23. Baur M. Chondral lesions of the femoral condyles: a system of arthroscopic classification. Arthroscopy. 1988;(4):97–102.

24. Noyes F, Stabler C. A system for grading articular cartilage lesions at arthroscopy. Am J Sports Med. 1989;17(4):505–513.

25. Brittberg M. ICRS Clinical Cartilage Injury Evaluation System—2000. Paper presented at Third International Cartilage Repair Society Meeting, April 28, 2000.

26. Koulalis D, Schultz W. Massive intraosseous ganglion of the talus: reconstruction of the articular surface of the ankle joint. Arthroscopy. 2000;16:E14.

27. Giannini S, Buda R, Grigolo B, et al. Autologous chondrocyte transplantation in osteochondral lesions of the ankle joint. Foot Ankle Int. 2001;22:513–517.

28. Romeo AA, Cole BJ, Mazzocca AD, et al. Autologous chondrocyte repair of an articular defect in the humeral head. Arthroscopy. October 2002;18(8):925–929.

29. Nilsson A, Lindahl A, Peterson L, et al. Autologous chondrocyte transplantation of the human wrist. In: Hunziker E, Mainil-Varlet, eds. *Updates in Cartilage Repair: A Multimedia Production on Cartilage Repair on 6 CD-roms.* Philadelphia: Lippincott Williams and Wilkins; 2000.

30. Johansen O, Lindahl A, Peterson L, et al. Hip osteochondritis treated by debridement, suture of a periosteal flap and chondrocyte implantation: a case report. In: Hunziker E, Mainil-Varlet, eds. *Updates in Cartilage Repair: A Multimedia Production on Cartilage Repair on 6 CD-roms.* Philadelphia: Lippincott Williams and Wilkins; 2000.

31. D'Amato M, Cole BJ. Autologous chondrocyte implantation. Orthop Techn. 2001;11:115–131.

32. Brittberg M, Peterson L, Sjogren-Jansson E, et al. Articular cartilage engineering with autologous chondrocyte transplantation: a review of recent developments. J Bone Joint Surg Am. 2003;85-A(suppl 3):109–115.

33. Gross AE. Repair of cartilage defects in the knee. J Knee Surg. 2002;15(3):167–169.

34. Fulkerson JP. Anteromedialization of the tibial tuberosity for patellofemoral malalignment. Clin Orthop. July–August 1983;177: 176–178.

35. Lobenhoffer P, Agneskirchner JD. Improvements in surgical technique of valgus high tibial osteotomy. Knee Surg Sports Traumatol Arthrosc. May 2003;11(3):132–138.

36. Gillogly SD, Voight M, Blackburn T. Treatment of articular cartilage defects of the knee with autologous chondrocyte implantation. J Orthop Sports Phys Ther. 1998;28(4):241–251.

37. Minas T, Chiu R. Autologous chondrocyte implantation. Am J Knee Surg. 2000;13(1):41–50.

38. Minas T, Peterson L. Advanced techniques in autologous chondrocyte transplantation. Clin Sports Med. 1999;18(1):13–44.

39. Micheli LJ, Browne JE, Erggelet C, et al. Autologous chondrocyte implantation of the knee: multicenter experience and minimum 3-year follow-up. Clin J Sport Med. October 2001;11(4): 223–238.

40. Peterson L, Minas T, Brittberg M, et al. Two- to 9-year outcome after autologous chondrocyte transplantation of the knee. Clin Ortho Rel Res. 2000,374:212–234.

41. Knutsen G, Engebretsen L, Ludvigsen TC, et al. Autologous chondrocyte implantation compared with microfracture in the knee: a randomized trial. J Bone Joint Surg Am. March 2004;86-A(3):455–464.

42. Horas U, Pelinkovic D, Herr G, et al. Autologous chondrocyte implantation and osteochondral cylinder transplantation in cartilage repair of the knee joint: a prospective, comparative trial. J Bone Joint Surg Am. 2003;85:185–192.

43. Bentley G, Biant LC, Carrington RW, et al. A prospective, randomised comparison of autologous chondrocyte implantation versus mosaicplasty for osteochondral defects in the knee. J Bone Joint Surg Br. 2003;85:223–230.

44. Erggelet C, Sittinger M, Lahm A. The arthroscopic implantation of autologous chondrocytes for the treatment of full-thickness cartilage defects of the knee joint. Arthroscopy. 2003;19(1):108–110.

45. Lee CR, Grodzinsky AJ, Hsu HP, et al. Effects of a cultured autologous chondrocyte-seeded type II collagen scaffold on the healing of a chondral defect in a canine model. J Orthop Res. 2003;21: 272–281.

46. Peterson L, Menche D, Grande D, et al. Chondrocyte transplantation—an experimental model in the rabbit. Trans Orthop Res Soc. 1984;9:218.

47. Brittberg M, Nilsson A, Lindahl A, et al. Rabbit articular cartilage defects treated with autologous cultured chondrocytes. Clin Orthop. 1996;326:270–283.

4

HIP AND GROIN

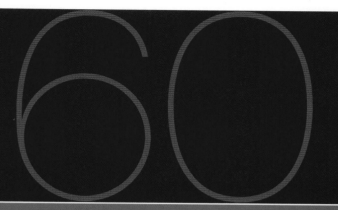

HIP ARTHROSCOPY AND THE MANAGEMENT OF NONARTHRITIC HIP PAIN

BRYAN T. KELLY, MD, PETE DRAOVITCH, PT, AT, KEELAN R. ENSEKI, MS, PT, ROBROY L. MARTIN, PhD, PT, RICHARD ERHARDT, PhD, MARC J. PHILIPPON, MD

■ HISTORY OF THE TECHNIQUE

Within the discipline of sports medicine, the hip has received considerably less attention than other joints, largely due to the difficulty that practitioners have traditionally had in assessing intra-articular pathology around the hip. Traditionally, young people with hip pain were given a diagnosis of "early arthritis," with very little consideration for soft tissue anatomy and injury in and around the joint. Arthroscopic examination of the hip is significantly more challenging than similar surgery around the shoulder and knee, primarily due to the anatomical constraints **(Fig. 60-1)**. The femoral head is deeply recessed in the bony acetabulum and is convex in shape. The thick fibrocapsular and muscular envelopes around the hip joint increase the amount of force required for distention of the hip during arthroscopy; the relative proximity of the sciatic nerve, lateral femoral cutaneous nerve, and femoral neurovascular structures make portal placement more challenging.[1,2]

Nonetheless, over the past several years hip arthroscopy has begun to gain considerable interest within the orthopedic community. The advent of better diagnostic tools, especially magnetic resonance imaging (MRI), has helped in the detection of intra-articular hip pathology in a more predictable fashion. Technical advances in appropriate portal placement, needle positioning, distraction techniques, and patient set up have all improved the accessibility of the hip joint. New techniques and instrumentation have facilitated the visualization and treatment of these intra-articular lesions by hip arthroscopy. Most notably, the recent adaptation of arthroscopy equipment to create flexible scopes and instruments specifically designed for the hip has led to improved safety, visualization, and accessibility of this joint[3] **(Fig. 60-2A,B)**. These improvements in technology have led

to a more detailed understanding of the specific intra-articular soft tissue lesions that lead to nonarthritic hip pain. This chapter discusses the current clinical and radiographic methods to detect early hip joint disease and the current indications and surgical techniques of hip arthroscopy.

■ INDICATIONS AND CONTRAINDICATIONS

Athletes subject their bodies to extreme forces; their lower extremity joint may experience joint reactive forces in excess of five times body weight during activities such as running and jumping.[4] The mechanisms of injuries can be from repetitive motion or direct trauma. Subtle radiographic evidence of hip dysplasia or decreased head-neck junction offset may place the athlete at underlying risk for intra-articular injury.[5–9] A source of intra-articular pathology should be investigated in patients with unremitting hip pain lasting greater than 4 weeks. The senior author (MJP) has performed over 2,500 hip arthroscopies and has had significant experience with the arthroscopic treatment of elite and amateur athletes from a wide variety of sporting endeavors including: golf, football, ice hockey, baseball, basketball, tennis, skateboarding, gymnastics, weightlifting, ballet, soccer, tae kwon do, Olympic yachting, and figure skating.[4,10–12]

Hip arthroscopy offers a less invasive alternative for hip procedures that would otherwise require surgical dislocation of the hip. In addition, this procedure allows surgeons to address intra-articular derangements that were previously undiagnosed and untreated. In our experience, hip arthroscopy has been very effective for the treatment of numerous athletic injuries including labral tears, capsular laxity with iliofemoral ligament deficiency, femoral-acetabular

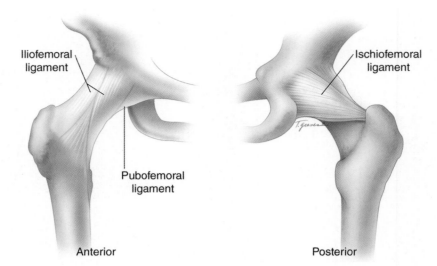

Fig. 60-1. Anatomical constraints of the hip. The anterior ligamentous constraints of the hip are seen in the anterior view and include the iliofemoral and pubofemoral ligaments. The ischiofemoral ligament is the primary posterior restraint. (Reprinted with permission from Kelly BT, Williams RJ III, Philippon MJ. Hip arthroscopy: current indications, treatment options, and management issues. Am J Sports Med. November–December 2003;31(6):1020–1037.)

impingement and decreased femoral head neck junction offset, lateral impact injury and chondral injuries, injuries to the ligamentum teres, extra-articular conditions (internal and external snapping hip), and loose bodies. Other less common indications for hip arthroscopy include management of osteonecrosis of the femoral head (Avascular Necrosis [AVN]), synovial chondromatosis and other synovial abnormalities, crystalline hip arthropathy (gout and pseudogout), infection, management of posttraumatic intra-articular debris, and in extremely rare cases, management of mild to moderate hip osteoarthritis. In addition, patients with long-standing, unresolved hip joint pain and positive physical findings may benefit from arthroscopic evaluation.[3,5,7–9,13–24] Hip arthroscopy is contraindicated in patients with hip fusions, advanced arthritis, open wounds or cellulitis, obesity, stress fractures in the femoral neck, severe dysplasia, and stable AVN.

Appropriate patient selection is of paramount importance to a successful outcome after hip arthroscopy. Injuries to the hip in athletes are often categorized as muscle strains or soft tissue contusions. However, hip pain, particularly in the young adult, may arise from a number of soft-tissue

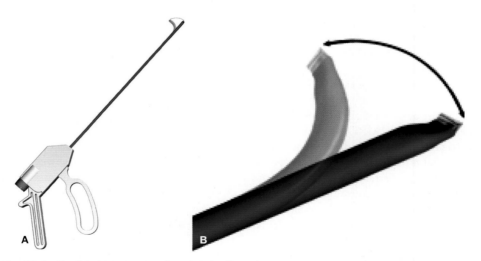

Fig. 60-2. Flexible instruments allow for significantly improved access to most structures within the hip joint during routine arthroscopy. (Reprinted with permission from Kelly BT, Williams RJ III, Philippon MJ. Hip arthroscopy: current indications, treatment options, and management issues. Am J Sports Med. November–December 2003;31(6):1020–1037.)

Hip Pain with Preservation of Joint Space

 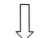

Primary Labrum	**Primary Chondral**	**Primary Capsule**	**Extra-articular**	**Systemic**
Trauma	Lateral impact	Laxity	Snapping Hip	Hormonal
Laxity	Subluxation / Dislocation	Adhesive Capsulitis	Internal	Rheumatoid
Bony Impingement	AVN	Synovitis / Inflammation	External	Polyarticular
Dysplasia	Loose bodies		Trochanteric Bursitis	Autoimmune
Degenerative	Synovial Chondromatosis		Ischial Bursitis	RSD
	Chondrocalcinosis		Psoas Bursitis	Regional Pain
	Degeneration		Osteitis Pubis	Syndrome
			Sports Hernia	
			Piriformis Syndrome	
			SI Joint	
			Pelvic Obliquity	
			Leg Length Inequality	
			Chronic Tendonitis	
			Hip Flexor	
			Adductor	
			Abductor	
			Gluteus Medius Tear	
			Referred Pain	
			Back	
			Genitourinary	
			Endometriosis	

Fig. 60-3. Diagnostic algorithm for categorizing and treating nonarthritic hip pain.

structures in and around the hip joint. It is important to be able to differentiate extra-articular from intra-articular pathology. Based upon our clinical experience and review of patient outcomes we have come up with a detailed algorithm for categorizing nonarthritic hip pain **(Fig. 60-3)**. Injuries to the hip are classified based upon the primary soft-tissue problem: labrum, chondral, capsule, extra-articular, or systemic. Within each primary problem, underlying causes or abnormalities are identified. This comprehensive assessment algorithm provides a rational approach to patient evaluation and improves clinical decision making and treatment plans.

Labral Injury

In our experience, injuries to the labrum are the most common source of hip pain identified at the time of arthroscopy. In the review of 300 recent cases, labral tears were present in 90% of them **(Fig. 60-4)**. Dynamic forces acting across the injured hip will result in hip pain, decreased athletic performance, and limitations in activities of daily living. The diagnosis of a labral tear remains largely clinical and is analogous to those patients who present with meniscal pathology. These patients often present with mechanical symptoms (catching and painful clicking) as well as restricted range of motion. Sometimes their presentation is more subtle, with symptoms of dull, activity-induced, positional pain that fails to improve with rest.[20,25] Classic symptoms of hip clicking

may be misdiagnosed as a labral tear when the etiology is in fact from a different source (snapping iliotibial band tendon or a hypermobile psoas tendon). Patients who have persistent hip pain for greater than 4 weeks, clinical signs, and radiographic findings consistent with a labral tear are candidates for hip arthroscopy. No radiographic study, however, including high-contrast gadolinium-enhanced arthrography MRI scanning, is entirely sensitive or specific in the detection

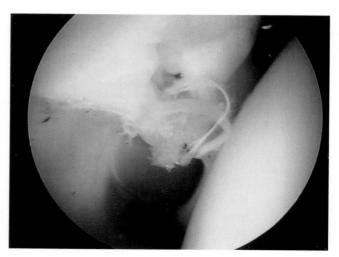

Fig. 60-4. Typical appearance of a labral tear in the anterior superior weightbearing zone.

of labral tears.[26] Thus, a high clinical suspicion of positive physical findings is essential for proper treatment.

In order to effectively treat patients with labral tears, the underlying cause of the labral injury must be identified. Based upon our clinical experience and comprehensive review of 300 recent cases, we have identified at least five causes of labral tears: (a) trauma, (b) laxity/hypermobility, (c) bony impingement, (d) dysplasia, (e) degeneration. Capsular laxity or hypermobility of the hip is the most common underlying cause for labral injury in our experience, resulting in 34% of the cases.[3,27] Femoral-acetabular impingement is the second most common cause for labral injury and was the underlying cause in 33% of the reviewed cases. Bony impingement can result from decreased femoral head neck junction offset (CAM effect), overhang of the anterior superior acetabular rim (pincer lesion), a retroverted acetabulum, or a combination of these bony deformities.[5,7–9,28] Specific traumatic events such as twisting, falling, or other lower extremity loads may precede the onset of symptoms. However, isolated traumatic labral tears were less common overall (14%), although they were the most common type of tears seen in high level athletes.

It has been shown that labral tears are associated with acetabular dysplasia.[29,30] In our practice, this subgroup of patients represented 5% of the labral tears seen at the time of arthroscopy. Although Byrd and Jones[29] report that the results of hip arthroscopy in the presence of dysplasia compare favorably with the results reported for the general population, we believe that extreme dysplasia (center edge angle <17 degrees) is a contraindication to the procedure. The final factor commonly associated with the presence of a labral tear is global hip joint degeneration. Degenerative labral tears were present in 11% of the patients in our series. Isolated treatment of labral tears without addressing the underlying causative factor will likely result in poor outcomes. These associated causative factors must be identified preoperatively and treated appropriately at the time of surgery.

Chondral Injury

Although chondral injury is an appropriate indication for hip arthroscopy, these lesions can be an elusive source of hip pain.[31,32] Traditionally, chondral damage around the hip has been associated with either progressive joint deterioration (osteoarthritis or rheumatoid arthritis) or trauma. However, acute isolated traumatic articular surface injuries can occur from impact loading across the hip joint. There appears to be a particular propensity for this injury pattern in young physically fit adult males who suffer impact loading over the greater trochanter in association with sport or activity. The so-called lateral impact injury occurs following a blow to the greater trochanter, which, due to its subcutaneous location, has minimal ability to absorb large forces. The high bone density of this region allows impact on this area to transfer energy and load to the joint surface, resulting in

chondral lesions of the femoral head or acetabulum without associated osseous injury. Arthroscopic findings in this clinical scenario will commonly support this lateral impact mechanism.[32]

In most cases of chondral injuries in the hip joint, symptom onset is immediate; however, in some cases the injury will appear innocuous with variable associated dysfunction. Persistent symptoms such as intermittent catching or pain elicited by provocative maneuvers should prompt a more extensive diagnostic workup. Although gadolinium-enhanced MR arthrography is currently the most promising imaging modality, it still has some limitations in reliably demonstrating chondral injuries perhaps due to the static nature of the imaging study and the lack of hip joint distraction during the test. Potter et al.[33] have demonstrated the utility of cartilage sensitive MRI for the detection of these lesions, which can be performed successfully without the use of gadolinium.

Primary chondral sources of intra-articular hip pain may also be due to loose bodies or synovial chondromatosis. Removal of these cartilaginous loose bodies can be successfully performed arthroscopically with very satisfying results. Focal AVN may be treated effectively with hip arthroscopy if the lesion is identified prior to collapse. In these cases, arthroscopically assisted core drilling and bone grafting can be performed to revascularize the necrotic region. Arthroscopic evaluation of the core tract allows for a direct assessment of the presence of bleeding bone.

Capsule Pathology

Hip instability can be a difficult disorder to diagnose and can be of traumatic or atraumatic origin. Professional athletes may develop overuse injuries of the hip from abnormal stresses on normal anatomy resulting in hip pain with associated subtle rotational hip instability.[3,4,12] Injuries or soft-tissue abnormalities such as labral tears or iliofemoral ligament insufficiency can disturb the complex buffer mechanism in the hip and result in increased tension in the joint capsule and its ligament and decreased ability to absorb stress or overstress.

Instability of the hip joint is much less common than in the shoulder, but can be a source of great disability. The hip joint relies much less on its adjacent soft tissue for stability because of the intrinsic osseous stability. It is apparent that any deviation from "normal" bony anatomy will lead to more dependence on the capsular tissue and labrum for stability. The labrum helps to contain the femoral head in extremes of range of motion, especially flexion. The labrum and capsule also act as load-bearing structures during flexion, causing a hip with a deficient labrum to be subject to instability if capsular laxity is present.[3,27] Takechi et al.[34] have demonstrated that the labrum may enhance stability by providing negative intra-articular pressure in the hip joint. Ferguson et al.[35,36] have further identified a stabilizing role of the labrum using a poroelastic finite element model to demonstrate that the

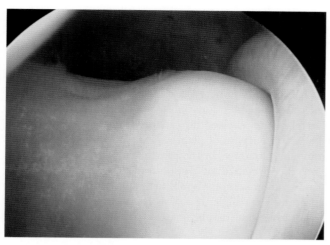

Fig. 60-5. View of the normal suction seal of the labrum on the femoral head with the traction released.

labrum provides some structural resistance to lateral and vertical motion of the femoral head within the acetabulum and helps to form a suction seal around the femoral head **(Fig. 60-5)**. Since the labrum appears to enhance joint stability and preserve joint congruity, there is a significant concern about the potential for rotational instability or hypermobility of a hip associated with a deficiency of labral tissue. This instability may result in redundant capsular tissue and create a potential abnormal load distribution due to a transient incongruous joint resulting from subtle subluxation.[3]

Even less common than hypermobility of the hip is global capsular tightness. These patients present with a capsular pattern of decreased motion and closely resemble the clinical findings associated with adhesive capsulitis of the shoulder. They typically have significant synovitis associated with their decreased motion. Nonoperative management should be the mainstay of treatment for these patients, focusing on physical therapy to regain motion and anti-inflammatory medications to decrease the inflammation. Fluoroscopically guided corticosteroid injections directly into the hip joint may help decrease the local inflammation. If patients are unresponsive to nonoperative treatment, they may be considered for arthroscopic capsular release; however, we have mixed results in these cases.

Extra-articular Sources of Pain

Extra-articular sources of hip pain are perhaps more common than intra-articular sources. A thorough evaluation is necessary to identify any associated extra-articular problems prior to the time of arthroscopy. Sources of extra-articular hip pain include: internal snapping hip (iliopsoas over the iliopectineal eminence); external snapping hip (iliotibial band over the greater trochanter); trochanteric and ischial bursitis; chronic tendonitis involving the hip flexors, adductors, and abductors; gluteus medius tears; osteitis pubis and sports hernia; piriformis syndrome; SI joint dysfunction;

pelvic obliquity; leg length inequality; and referred pain from sources including the back, genitourinary, and endometriosis.

Systemic Sources of Pain

Systemic sources of hip pain include complex regional pain syndrome or reflex sympathetic dystrophy, rheumatoid arthritis, polyarticular arthritides, diabetes, and hormonal factors. Identifying a systemic cause of the hip pain should lead the treating surgeon away from surgical intervention, unless a discreet mechanical factor is identified.

Clinical Exam

Prior to a formal history and physical examination, all patients complete pre-evaluation subjective questionnaires to report the location and nature of the symptoms, as well as the intensity of the symptoms over the prior 24 hours (Appendices 1, 2, and 3). A comprehensive patient history should be performed to assess the qualitative nature of the discomfort (pain, clicking, catching, instability, stiffness, weakness, or decreased performance), the specific location of the discomfort, the timing of the onset of symptoms, the precipitating cause of the symptoms, and assessment of any referred or systemic causes of hip pain (Appendix 4).[37–39] An intra-articular etiology causing intractable hip pain in the adult can present in a variety of ways. Patients may have pain in the anterior groin, anterior thigh, buttock, greater trochanter, or medial knee. Other symptoms include persistent clicking, catching, locking, giving way, or restricted range of motion. Symptoms may be preceded by a traumatic event, either a fall or twisting injury; however, insidious onset of hip pain may also be reported. Symptoms are typically exacerbated with activity and improved with rest.

A comprehensive physical examination form may be used to record all findings (Appendix 4). The initial portion of the exam should asses the patient's gait and posture and is best performed when the patient is unaware that they are being watched. Antalgic gait patterns result in shortening of the stance phase, as well as shortening of the length of the step on the affected side secondary to pain. During a Trendelenburg gait, functionally or physiologically weakened gluteus medius forces shift the upper body to the involved side so as to move the center of gravity over the painful hip and decrease the moment the arm forces across the hip joint.[40] Evaluation of posture and limb position should look for pelvic obliquity, limb length inequality, muscle contractures, and scoliosis and includes both static and dynamic evaluations.[39] Iliac crest heights are determined in both the standing and sitting positions for the purpose of differentiating pelvic obliquity from leg length inequality. Several lumbar movements are performed after a base line of symptoms is established to determine if the lumbar motions elicit any of the symptoms. If suspicion is present for lumbar involvement, lower extremity deep tendon reflexes and manual muscle testing should be performed in the seated and supine position. Straight leg testing and femoral nerve stretch testing should be performed to rule out a radicular source of pain.

Examination of the hip joint itself begins with palpation of specific regions of the hip to localize sites of tenderness, to delineate the integrity of the muscular structures about the hip, and to identify any areas of gross atrophy. If the source of the pain is truly intra-articular, palpable pain can rarely be elicited. Active and passive range of motion of both hips should be evaluated in the seated and supine positions. Any asymmetry in adduction, abduction, flexion, extension, external rotation, and internal rotation should be noted as well as any reproduction of symptoms in these positions.

Several tests can be exercised to identify specific hip pathology. The Thomas test will help to identify the presence of a hip flexion contracture by eliminating the effects of excessive lumbar lordosis on the perceived extension of the hip.[40] Typically, passive range of motion should match or exceed active range of motion; however, provocative maneuvers performed during passive range of motion evaluation may result in limited motion secondary to pain and are highly suggestive of intra-articular pathology. Painful hip flexion, adduction, and internal rotation can indicate acetabular rim problems or labral tears, especially if clicking or groin pain is present. The Faber test involves flexion, abduction, and external rotation of the hip and suggests sacroiliac pathology or iliopsoas spasm. The Ober test is used to evaluate tightness in the iliotibial band and may elicit symptoms in the presence of trochanteric bursitis. The test is positive when the leg remains in the abducted position after the hip is passively extended and abducted with the knee extended. The piriformis test is performed by flexing the hip to 60 degrees, stabilizing the hip, and exerting a downward pressure on the knee. If the piriformis is tight, pain is elicited; and if the sciatic nerve is compressed (piriformis syndrome), the patient experiences radicularlike symptoms.[39,40] Mechanical symptoms attributable to intra-articular pathology can also be elicited by loading the hip joint with both a resisted leg raise in the supine position as well as forced internal rotation while applying an axial load. Both of these maneuvers can load the hip joint anterolaterally, which is the most common location for labral tears.

The complete physical examination should include motor strength testing of both hips in order to detect subtle differences from side to side. Finally, a neurovascular examination should be performed to rule out referred pain secondary to radicular symptoms or vascular etiology. In most patients, hip pain goes away over time if the patient complies with conservative treatment. If a patient's hip pain persists, is reproducible on physical examination, and does not respond to appropriate conservative measures (including rest, ambulatory support, nonsteroidal anti-inflammatory drugs, and physical therapy), hip arthroscopy may be of substantial value.[41,42] A subset of patients may have persistent symptoms despite negative or uncertain radiographic studies. Arthroscopy can lead to definitive diagnoses such as focal degenerative arthritis, chondromalacia, chondral flap tears, nonossified loose bodies, synovitis, labral lesions, and synovial chondromatosis in as many as 40% of these cases.[21,43]

All patients undergo a standard series of plain x-rays including standing anteroposterior (AP) pelvis, cross-table lateral of the involved hip, and a 90-degree flexion lateral. The main purpose of plain x-rays is to rule out significant joint space narrowing, the presence of acetabular dysplasia, and the presence of femoral-acetabular impingement. Radiographic indices should include the center-edge angle and the Sharp angle. If acetabular dysplasia is suspected, a false-profile view may be obtained to look for loss of anterior coverage.[44]

MRI has become the examination of choice for the evaluation of unexplained hip pain. Its unique ability to provide detailed images of soft tissue and marrow-based abnormalities in multiple planes of view makes it superior to other modalities employed in intra-articular hip imaging. Gadolinium-enhanced MR arthrography of the hip may be performed when evaluation of the capsulolabral structures or articular surfaces is most important. Intra-articular injection of 10 to 15 cc of gadolinium solution, followed by routine MRI may increase the sensitivity and specificity of detecting intra-articular hip pathology.[38,44] Czerny et al.[45] compared conventional MRI with MR arthrography in the diagnosis of labral tears. They reported a sensitivity and accuracy of 80% and 65% for conventional MRI compared to 95% and 88% with MR arthrography. Results such as these suggest that MR arthrography may have a significant advantage over conventional MRI for the evaluation of capsulolabral structures in the hip. More recent cartilage imaging methods, described by Potter et al.,[33] may obviate the need for intra-articular gadolinium in the MRI detection of chondral lesions of the hip.

■ SURGICAL TECHNIQUES

Hip arthroscopy may be performed in either the supine or lateral position depending upon surgeon preference. In either case, distraction of the femoral head from the acetabulum must be performed to fully visualize the articular surfaces. Either general or spinal anesthesia may be used; however, it is necessary to maintain complete skeletal muscle relaxation at all times to minimize the amount of traction force required for distraction. A thorough understanding of the anatomic relationships around the hip joint with special attention to neurovascular structures and tissue planes is of paramount importance. Specialized instruments including flexible probes, extra long cannulas, and extra long specialized instruments such as shavers, burs, drills, and loose body retrievers; all have improved accessibility of the joint and increase the versatility of procedures available to the surgeon (Fig. 60-2A,B). Initial insertion of long spinal needles

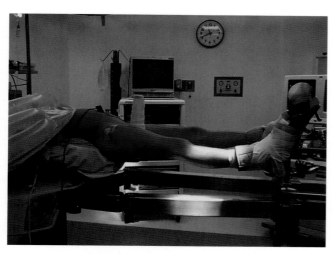

Fig. 60-6. The modified supine position: the hip is in 10 degrees flexion, 15 degrees internal rotation, 10 degrees lateral tilt, and neutral abduction.

(6-inch 16 gauge) allows release of the negative pressure vacuum phenomenon created with joint distraction and also allows for injection of sterile saline for joint distention.

We perform hip arthroscopy in the modified supine position in which the hip is placed in a position of 10 degrees flexion, 15 degrees internal rotation, 10 degrees lateral tilt, and neutral abduction **(Fig. 60-6)**. A minimum of 8 to 10 mm of distraction is recommended to avoid any iatrogenic injury to the chondral surfaces or labrum. Adequate traction typically requires between 25 and 50 lb of force **(Fig. 60-7)**.[31] Gentle countertraction is also applied

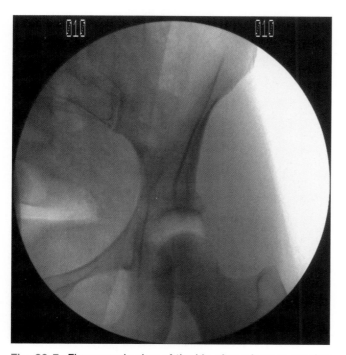

Fig. 60-7. Fluoroscopic view of the hip after adequate traction has been applied. A minimum of 8 to 10 mm is necessary to avoid iatrogenic injury to the cartilage surfaces or the labrum.

to the contralateral limb. All of the intra-articular structures in the hip joint can be seen through the combined use of 70- and 30-degree arthroscopes as well as by the interchange of portals.[20]

Portal Placement

Accurate portal placement is essential for optimal visualization of all intra-articular structures and safe access to the hip joint. Typically, three basic portals are used: anterolateral, anterior, and posterolateral **(Fig. 60-8A,B)**. The vast majority of procedures performed within the joint can be accomplished with just two portals: the anterolateral and the anterior. Two accessory portals (proximal lateral and distal lateral) are useful for releases of the iliotibial band (ITB) and osteochondroplasty for decreased head-neck junction offset respectively.

Anterolateral Portal

The anterolateral portal has also been described as the anterior paratrochanteric portal as it is referenced off the greater trochanter. This portal is traditionally described as being approximately 1 to 2 cm superior and 1 to 2 cm anterior to the anterosuperior "corner" of the greater trochanter depending upon the patient's weight and size. In our experience, we have found the portal to be more useful if placed directly off the anterosuperior portion of the greater trochanter. This portal allows for optimal visualization of the iliofemoral ligament, femoral head, anterior superior labrum, ligamentum teres, transverse ligament, and most of the acetabulum. Typically a 70-degree scope is used through this portal for greatest visualization.

Anterior Portal

The anterior portal is typically the second portal to be established and allows for visualization of the posterior-superior capsule, posterior superior labrum, the posterior recess, the femoral head, and the ligamentum teres. This portal is also the optimal location for viewing the head-neck junction, the anterior femoral neck, the zona orbicularis, and the distal insertion of the capsular ligaments on the intertrochanteric line. Again, use of the 70-degree arthroscope will allow for optimal visualization. The portal is established by identifying the intersection of the vertical line drawn from the anterior superior iliac spine distally and the horizontal line drawn from the superior surface of the femoral greater trochanter medially. This portal presents the greatest risk to the lateral femoral cutaneous nerve, which lies within several millimeters of the cannula. In addition, the lateral femoral circumflex artery and femoral neurovascular bundles must be protected.[1] Care must be taken not to place this portal too anterior or deep, as this places the femoral neurovascular bundle at risk.[46] The localization of the femoral pulse distal to the inguinal ligament helps prevent inadvertent injury to these structures.

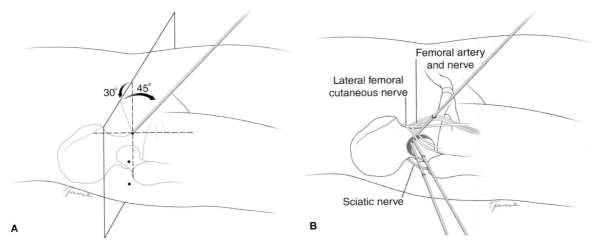

A   **B**

Fig. 60-8. Three portals are traditionally used (anterolateral, posterolateral, and anterior). The anterior portal coincides with the intersection of a sagittal line drawn distally from the anterior superior iliac spine and a transverse line across the superior margin of the greater trochanter. **A:** The anterolateral and posterolateral portals lie anterior and posterior to the superior tip of the greater trochanter. **B:** Careful attention to proper portal placement is essential for avoidance of nearby neurovascular structures. (Reproduced with permission from Kelly BT, Williams RJ III, Philippon MJ. Hip arthroscopy: current indications, treatment options, and management issues. Am J Sports Med. November–December 2003;31(6):1020–1037.)

Posterolateral Portal

The posterolateral portal is also described as the posterior paratrochanteric portal as it is also referenced off the greater trochanter. The entry site is 2 to 3 cm posterior to the tip of the greater trochanter at the same level as the anterolateral portal. Direct visualization of entry into the joint is possible with the scope in the anterolateral portal. The anterolateral and posterolateral portals should be established parallel to one another. The greatest risk with this portal is injury to the sciatic nerve, which lies within approximately 3 cm.[46,47] Advancing the trocar with the femur in a neutral or slightly internally rotated position can protect the nerve, as this maneuver rotates the nerve away from the posterior margin of the greater trochanter. This portal is used for visualization of the posterior aspect of the femoral head, the posterior labrum, posterior capsule, and the inferior edge of the ischiofemoral ligament.[1]

Proximal Lateral Accessory

The proximal lateral accessory portal is used for ITB releases. It is placed approximately 2 cm distal and in line with the anterolateral portal. The 30-degree arthroscope is placed in the anterolateral portal, and the accessory portal is established as a working portal for additional instruments required for the release. The ITB can be clearly visualized through the anterolateral portal, and the release can be performed under direct visualization through the accessory portal.

Distal Lateral Accessory

The distal lateral accessory portal is used for an osteochondroplasty performed in patients with decreased femoral head-neck junction offset. It is placed at the midpoint between the anterior and anterolateral portals and approximately 4 cm distal. The portal typically enters the capsule at around the level of the zona orbicularis and allows for direct access to the anterior neck. This portal can be established under direct visualization with the 70-degree arthroscope placed in the anterior portal **(Fig. 60-9)**.

Once traction is applied, the anterolateral portal is established under fluoroscopic guidance using the landmarks described above. Immediate visualization of the anterior

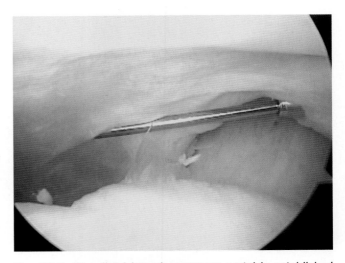

Fig. 60-9. The distal lateral accessory portal is established under direct visualization. The entry point is at the level of the zona orbicularis and allows for direct access of the anterior femoral head neck junction.

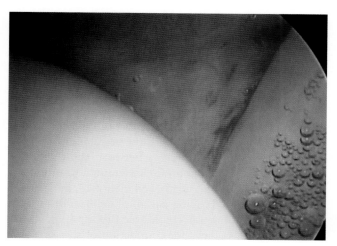

Fig. 60-10. Visualization of the anterior triangle is achieved upon entry into the joint through the anterolateral portal.

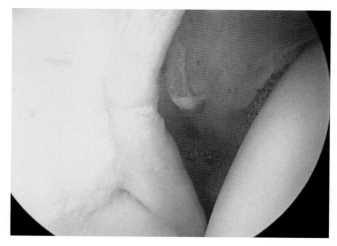

Fig. 60-12. The location of the psoas tendon can be appreciated at the level of the "psoas U" and is found behind a thin veil of capsular tissue.

triangle is established through this portal **(Fig. 60-10)**. The anterior triangle represents the intra-articular portion of the lateral limb of the iliofemoral ligament. The anterior portal is established under direct visualization, as the spinal needle is directed between the lateral and medial limbs of the Y-ligament **(Fig. 60-11)**.

Systematic Arthroscopic Examination

A systematic evaluation of the anterior structures of the joint can be performed with the arthroscope in the anterolateral portal. Starting anteromedially the entire circumference of the labrum can be visualized including the recess between the labrum and the capsule. The anterior portion of the femoral head is completely inspected and should include a complete evaluation of the fovea capitis, the ligamentum

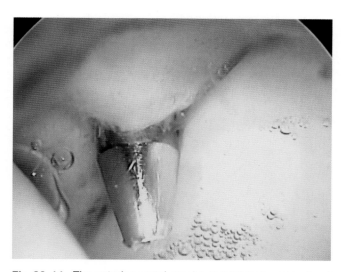

Fig 60-11. The anterior portal can be established under direct visualization from the anterolateral portal. The placement of the portal should be between the lateral and medial limbs of the Y-ligament.

teres, the transverse acetabular ligament, the fat pad, and the central aspect of the acetabulum. The psoas tendon or bursae may be intra-articular in approximately 20% of people **(Fig. 60-12)**; if it is extra-articular, the psoas tendon lies immediately medial to a thin veil of capsular tissue and can be easily palpated with a probe.

Once the inspection is complete from the anterolateral portal, the arthroscope is switched to the anterior portal for a more complete view of the posterior aspect of the joint. From this portal a more complete evaluation of the posterior labrum, the normal posterior sulcus, and the posterior superior capsule can be performed. The posterior recess can be inspected for loose bodies, which is a common resting ground for any intra-articular debris, and the posterior aspect of the femoral head can be more clearly evaluated with the arthroscope in this position.

Once the intra-articular examination is complete, the scope is left in the anterior portal and the traction is slowly released so that the head-neck junction can be evaluated. The anterior aspect of the hip may be adequately visualized with minimal traction. With hip flexion to 45 degrees and external rotation to 30 degrees, the anterior capsule becomes relatively patulous and can be distended with saline, making visualization of the head and neck relatively easy. As the traction is slowly released, an upward pressure must be maintained on the arthroscope to avoid articular cartilage injury. Once the traction is completely released, the arthroscope can be slid into the head-neck junction recess **(Fig. 60-13)**. From this position, a clear view of the anterior femoral neck and the associated vincula and the normal labrum suction seal (Fig. 60-5) can be established. If any work needs to be performed in the head neck junction recess, it is best accomplished through the distal lateral accessory portal described above (Fig. 60-9).

If there is concern regarding pathology associated with the ITB, gluteus medius, or piriformis, a proximal lateral

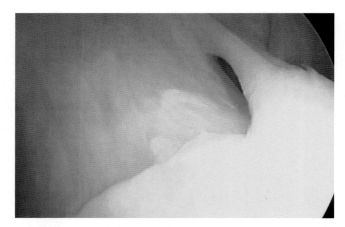

Fig. 60-13. The head neck junction recess is best visualized from the anterior portal with the traction released, and the hip flexed to 45 degrees and externally rotated.

portal is established approximately 2 cm distal and in line with the anterolateral portal. A 30-degree arthroscope is placed in the anterolateral portal, which allows for adequate visualization of the ITB. If the ITB is released, the arthroscope can be driven into the trochanteric bursae for evaluation and inspection of the gluteus medius and piriformis.

Arthroscopic Management of Labral Tears

The goal of arthroscopic debridement of a torn labrum is to relieve pain by eliminating the unstable flap tear that causes the observed hip discomfort. As such, the surgeon seeks to debride all torn tissue and leave as much healthy labrum intact as possible **(Fig. 60-14A,B)**. The majority of the vascular supply to the labrum comes from the capsular contribution,[48] while the articular surface of the labrum has decreased vascularity and has limited synovial covering. The labrum is thinner in the anterior inferior section and thicker and slightly rounded in appearance posteriorly. In the posterior superior portion of the acetabulum, an inferior recess is present. A recess between the acetabular labrum and the hip extends circumferentially around the labrum. Once the labral tear is well identified, the margins need to be defined. Probing and focal delineation by heat treatment with a monopolar flexible probe will complete this process. This allows for contraction of the torn portion of the labrum. A flexible ligament chisel is then used to cut the torn part of the labrum, leaving only a small portion attached. A motorized shaver is then used to complete the debridement and remove the torn portion of the labrum.[12]

We now have significant experience with over 250 labral repairs **(Fig. 60-15A,B)**. Two techniques are utilized. If the labrum is detached from the bone, a bioabsorbable suture anchor is placed on the rim of the acetabulum. Typically, placement of the anchor needs to be extracapsular in order to achieve an appropriate angle that will not result in penetration of the anchor into the joint. Fluoroscopy may be used during this portion of the procedure to ensure appropriate placement. Once the anchor is placed, the suture material is passed through the split in

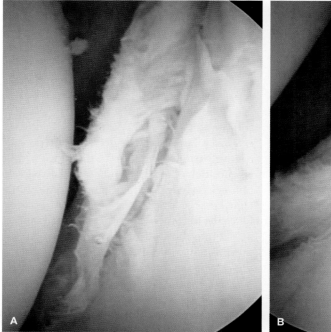
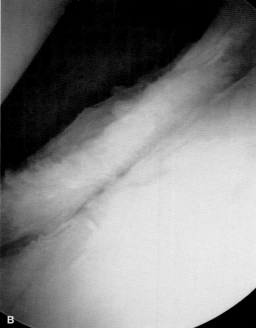

Fig. 60-14. Debridement of labral tears **(A)** should remove all degenerative tissue and leave as much viable tissue as possible **(B)**.

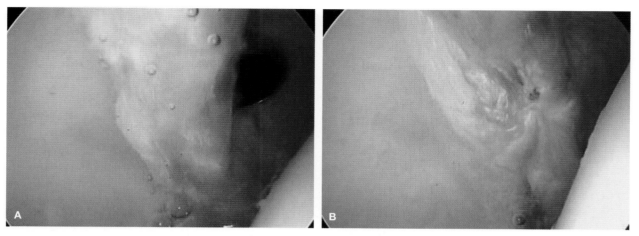

Fig. 60-15. Arthroscopic labral repair. The labrum is seen detached off of the bony acetabulum **(A)** and is repaired back using a suture anchor and mattress suture around the labral tissue **(B)**.

the labrum, and then the suture is retrieved and passed through the labrum a second time, thus resulting in a vertical mattress suture. The suture is tied down using standard arthroscopic knot-tying techniques. The second technique is performed if there is an intrasubstance split in the labrum. In this case, a bioabsorbable suture is passed around the split using a suture lasso or similar suture passing instrument. The suture is tied, thus reapproximating the split labral tissue.

Arthroscopic Management of Femoral-Acetabular Impingement

Femoral-acetabular impingement is a significant cause of labral tears. It is related to decreased offset at the femoral head-neck junction. This results in impingement of the head-neck junction against the rim of the acetabulum in the position of flexion and internal rotation, leading to injury to the labrum as well as the adjacent cartilage on the rim of the acetabulum. The deformity may be secondary to previously undiagnosed "silent slips" of the femoral epiphysis or from other congenital reasons.[5,7–9,28] Ganz et al.[28] has popularized the open surgical dislocation technique for removal of the impinging osteophyte. The procedure can be effectively performed arthroscopically using the anterior arthroscopic portal and the distal lateral accessory portal as previously described. Once the head-neck recess is clearly visualized, the location of the decreased offset can be clearly identified **(Fig. 60-16)**. Sequential removal of the impinging osteophyte can be performed with precision **(Fig. 60-17A,B)**. Oftentimes the location of the labral tear can act as a marker for the precise location of the bony impingement. As the osteochondroplasty proceeds laterally, caution must be exercised to avoid injury to the lateral retinacular vessels. At the completion of the procedure, dynamic fluoroscopy is performed to ensure that all impinging bony lesions have been removed.

Arthroscopic Management of Capsular Laxity

Arthroscopic thermal modification of collagen in the hip capsular tissue appears to be a treatment option for patients with hip instability. We have significant experience with its use in athletes with rotational instability associated with labral tears.[10,11,27] It also may be of benefit in patients with posttraumatic instability from hip dislocation or subluxation, as well as in patients with atraumatic instability associated with generalized ligament laxity. In addition to focal thermal treatment, we now perform arthroscopic capsular plication of the iliofemoral ligament in patients with significant capsule redundancy and laxity.[3] This procedure is performed by placing a no. 2 Vicryl suture through both limbs of the iliofemoral ligament (medial and lateral bands of the Y-ligament of Bigelow) using a suture lasso technique. Once the suture is appropriately placed, the traction is released, the hip is placed into full internal rotation, and the suture is tensioned. Tightening of the anterior capsule typically

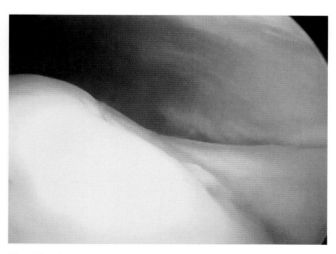

Fig. 60-16. Head-neck junction osteophyte.

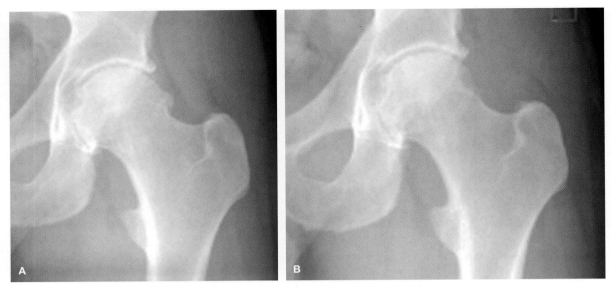

Fig. 60-17. Preop **(A)** and postop **(B)** radiograph of a hip with femoral-acetabular impingement. Removal of the osteophyte can be very effectively accomplished arthroscopically.

results in decreased external rotation of the involved foot at the completion of the procedure. Short-term results appear promising; however, more studies are required to determine the long-term efficacy and potential shortcomings of this treatment approach.[3]

Arthroscopic Management of Chondral Lesions

As in other joints, the long-term consequences of chondral lesions are concerning. The difficulty in diagnosing these lesions as well as the inability to improve symptoms with conservative management provide a reasonable rationale for the use of arthroscopic hip surgery in the treatment of chondral injuries. In the presence of persistent symptoms, hip arthroscopy has been useful for the evaluation and staging of chondral injury as well as the debridement of loose flaps and removal of free cartilage fragments. Larger cartilage defects may be amenable to cartilage resurfacing procedures that have been applied in the knee. We have limited experience with autologous chondral transplantation from the lateral femoral condyle. These surgeries have been technically successful, and early follow-up has been encouraging. Microfracture of medium-sized defects has been performed in many patients with full-thickness lesions **(Fig. 60-18A,B)**. Although symptomatic improvement from arthroscopic debridement of unstable cartilage flaps is encouraging, future advancement in surgical techniques will focus on more predictable cartilage resurfacing procedures to not only alleviate mechanical symptoms, but also promote the long-term overall health of the hip joint.[32]

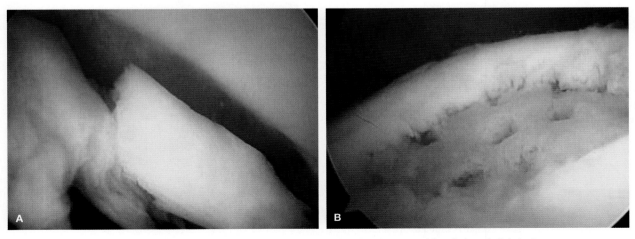

Fig. 60-18. A: Chondral lesion of the femoral head. **B:** Microfracture of focal chondral defect.

Arthroscopic Management of Snapping Hip

Snapping hip is characterized by an audible snap or pop that usually occurs when the hip is brought through a range of motion. It is often accompanied by pain and generally occurs during physical activity. Three sources of snapping have been described including: external (lateral), internal (medial), and intra-articular, with the external type being the most common.[49,50] The external type is caused by snapping of either the posterior border of the iliotibial band or the anterior border of the gluteus maximus over the greater trochanter when the hip is flexed from an extended position.[49,51,52] The internal type is most commonly associated with painful displacement of the iliopsoas tendon over the iliopectineal eminence[53] or over the femoral head.[52,53] The intra-articular type is commonly a clicking sensation caused by a loose body in the joint, such as a fracture fragment, a torn piece of labrum, a chondral flap, or synovial chondromatosis.

The history and physical examination are usually diagnostic of the source of the snapping hip. Internal snapping is generally localized over the anterior part of the groin; external snapping is localized over the greater trochanter; and intra-articular clicking can be elicited with hip rotation. Nonoperative management, including physical therapy and anti-inflammatory medications, is often adequate to relieve symptoms; however, refractory cases may require surgical intervention.[50] Surgical treatment of these conditions has historically required open procedures to lengthen either the iliopsoas tendon or iliotibial band,[50,53–55] or remove the offending intra-articular pathology.[50] Current arthroscopic techniques allow for both transarticular iliopsoas and extra-articular iliotibial band releases.

The iliopsoas tendon can be clearly identified at the level of the "psoas U," as previously described (Fig. 60-12). Patients with symptomatic internal snapping typically have significant inflammation of the capsule around the psoas and may demonstrate true impingement of the tendinous portion of the psoas at the labral-femoral interface. The tendinous portion of the psoas can be carefully transected through a 1-cm medial capsular window adjacent to the anterior portal entry point using an Orthopedic Beaver Mini Blade (Becton Dickinson, Franklin Lakes, NJ). The muscle fibers of the psoas are left intact with this technique (Fig. 60-19A,B). ITB releases are typically performed using the proximal lateral accessory portal as described previously. Use of a 30-degree arthroscope allows for clear visualization of the ITB. The posterior third of the band is released at the location of the symptomatic snapping over the greater trochanter.

Additional Procedures

Additional arthroscopic procedures include: debridement of partial or complete ligamentum teres injuries; removal of loose bodies and synovial chondromatosis; removal of focal pigmented villonodular synovitis lesions; and repair of gluteus medius tears. Management of patients with mild to moderate arthritic changes should be performed with caution, as the results of this procedure are less predictable unless a clear mechanical factor is identified. Loss of greater than 50% of the joint space should be considered a contraindication to an arthroscopic procedure.

■ POSTOPERATIVE CARE

Patients are allowed to leave the hospital the same day of surgery. Weightbearing status is predicated upon the extent of the procedure and will be described in detail in the rehabilitation section. Soft tissue surgery generally requires only

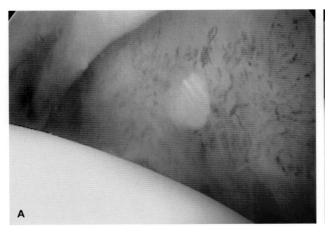 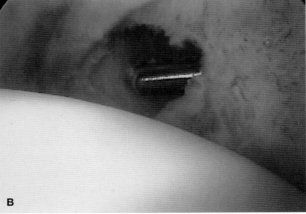

Fig. 60-19. Iliopsoas tendon releases can be performed arthroscopically for symptomatic internal snapping hip. The intra-articular portion of the iliopsoas tendon can be seen in **(A)**. After localization of the tendon the intra-articular portion can be released using a beaver blade through a small capsular window **(B)**.

10 days of restricted weightbearing (20 lb, foot flat). If an extensive bony resection (osteochondroplasty) or microfracture procedure is performed, then 4 to 6 weeks of restricted weightbearing is prescribed. The patient is placed in a continuous passive motion (CPM) machine for 4 hours per day for 4 weeks. This is used to maintain motion and eliminate postoperative stiffness. Early range of motion on a stationary bike is initiated in the recovery room prior to discharge. The patient is placed in a hip brace to avoid hyperextension during the first 10 days after surgery, and immobilization night boots are placed on patients who underwent capsular tightening procedures to help prevent excessive external rotation of the feet during the nighttime. Postoperative medications include: a narcotic, an anti-inflammatory, and a blood thinner (dalteparin sodium or enteric-coated aspirin) to prevent postoperative deep venous thrombosis. Sutures are removed on postoperative day 10, and follow-up visits are scheduled for 6 weeks, 12 weeks, 6 months, and 1 year.

■ TECHNICAL ALTERNATIVES AND PITFALLS

There are very few open procedure alternatives to the currently indicated arthroscopic hip procedures. The one notable exception is the open surgical dislocation for femoral-acetabular impingement. All of the other procedures discussed in this chapter do not have an "equivalent" open procedure. Thus, the only technical alternatives, in the majority of cases, are nonoperative management protocols. We reserve hip arthroscopy for patients who have recalcitrant symptoms resistant to nonoperative treatment, and clearly identifiable pathology based upon their clinical exam and radiographic studies. In the appropriately indicated patient, and with careful attention to surgical details, hip arthroscopy is a very safe procedure. Although many vital neurologic and vascular structures are at risk during hip arthroscopy, the majority of the complications associated with this surgical procedure are related to traction and fluid management.[56] Nonetheless, a thorough understanding of the anatomic vicinity of these neurovascular structures is necessary to avoid injury due to inadvertent portal placement. Catastrophic complications, such as femoral vascular injury and permanent femoral or sciatic nerve damage should be easily avoided with appropriate surgical planning and preparation.

Clarke et al.[57] performed a prospective review of 1,054 consecutive hip arthroscopies and reported an overall complication rate of 1.4%. Complications included neurapraxia, portal wound bleeding, portal hematoma, trochanteric bursitis, and instrument breakage. The only major complication was one case of septic arthritis.

Samson[56] reviewed complications in 530 cases of hip arthroscopy and found a total complication rate of 5.5% (34). Of these, 0.5% (3) were considered permanent and 5%

(27) were transient. The most common complications were transient neuropraxia of the peroneal, femoral, sciatic, lateral femoral cutaneous, and pudendal nerves secondary to traction. These typically resolved in 2 to 3 days.

Rodeo et al.[58] reviewed the complications from arthroscopy and also reported that most complications were neuropraxias resulting from excessive or prolonged traction. Direct trauma to cutaneous nerves, such as the lateral femoral cutaneous nerve, was also identified as a potential source of nerve injury that typically occurs during portal placement. Additional complications related to the application of traction include pressure necrosis of the foot, scrotum, or perineum. These problems can be avoided with close attention to the force and duration of traction, as well as the intermittent release of traction throughout a prolonged procedure. Careful placement and padding of the perineal post as well as adequate padding on the foot will help avoid intraoperative injury to these regions.

Bartlett et al.[59] reported one case of cardiac arrest as a result of intra-abdominal extravasation of fluid during arthroscopic removal of a loose body from the hip joint of a patient with an acetabular fracture. This case required emergent laparotomy to relieve excessive intra-abdominal pressure. Careful attention to both the arthroscopy pump and fluid outflow will reduce the incidence of this complication. Infection is a potential complication of any surgical procedure; however, it has not been reported and is likely to be as rare during hip arthroscopy as it is with arthroscopic procedures of other joints due to the copious amounts of fluid used throughout the procedure. Several authors have suggested that there is a risk of accelerating avascular necrosis of the femoral head during hip arthroscopy, and some have even stated that hip arthroscopy is a relative contraindication in patients with an established diagnosis of avascular necrosis.[41,60]

■ REHABILITATION/RETURN TO SPORTS RECOMMENDATIONS

General

As a general guideline, we recommend 3 months of supervised therapy after arthroscopic hip procedures. During month 1 we prescribe 1 day of therapy each week, during month 2 patients receive therapy 2 days per week, and during the final month, where return of strength, coordination, and endurance are emphasized, patients have therapy 3 times per week. Month 1 is the tissue healing phase and focuses on decreasing inflammation, allowing the tissue to heal properly, and regaining full range of passive motion. Month 2 is the early strengthening phase, and month 3 focuses on return of full strength, endurance, and coordination.

Due to the complex nature of the hip joint (27 muscles crossing the hip) and the significant weakness that can occur after these procedures, we feel that supervised therapy is essential for full return of function. In comparing the outcomes of our patients who receive the full rehabilitation protocol versus those who have shortened or less intense programs, we have found significantly faster and more complete return to full function with the comprehensive program. The duration of therapy may be lengthened or shortened based upon the successful achievement of therapeutic goals. In high-level athletes we are often able to have a return to full activity between 3 and 4 months (depending upon the procedure and the nature of the sport); however, in more sedentary individuals, full function may not return until 6 to 8 months. Appropriate patient education regarding expectations is critical for complete patient satisfaction.

Labral Injury

Rehabilitation following arthroscopic surgery to address labral injuries should take into consideration all of the tissues involved during the procedure. The rehabilitation principles discussed here will assume an individual is undergoing an isolated debridement or repair of the labrum. Rehabilitation considerations for other procedures, including those that may be combined with labral procedures, will be discussed in following sections. When procedures are performed in combination, utilization of the most conservative approach for each aspect of rehabilitation (range of motion, strength, weightbearing) is recommended and is chosen based on tissue healing properties.

The goals of immediate postoperative care are to control inflammation, maintain range of motion, and avoid muscle atrophy of the lower extremities. A combination of modalities and nonsteroidal anti-inflammatory drugs are often used to control inflammation. Early range of motion may be obtained and preserved through a number of approaches. A continuous motion apparatus is often utilized. The use of a stationary bike immediately after surgery can help obtain range of motion without excessive compressive or shear forces at the joint. Excessive range of motion may be avoided through the use of a brace and a night immobilization system. The use of gentle isometrics can help to prevent excessive atrophy of lower extremity musculature.

In patients who have had an isolated labral resection procedure performed, the main factors that affect regaining range of motion and strength are soft tissue damage created by the surgical instrumentation when entering the joint and the effects of immobility. After the soft tissue healing process has begun, a progression from passive range of motion to stretching can be initiated. A major concern during this phase of rehabilitation is to avoid initiating an inflammatory response in the joint. Avoidance of excessive flexion or abduction is a concern. These motions are limited in order to avoid impingement of capsular and soft tissue that has not yet healed. Excessive motion in these planes results in an uncomfortable pinching sensation. We generally recommend beginning stretching as tolerated around 3 to 4 week after surgery. In cases where other procedures

were performed in combination with a labral resection procedure, additional limitations may exist.

The weightbearing progression during rehabilitation is dependent on several issues. The area of the tear and subsequent debridement or repair must be taken into consideration. Most tears in the North American population occur in the anterior-superior weightbearing region of the labrum. A short period of limited weightbearing is usually recommended. We usually recommend a range from 10 to 28 days of foot flat (approximately 20 lb) weightbearing. Complete nonweightbearing precautions in patients undergoing isolated labral procedures are usually not suggested. Gentle compression aids in providing an environment of optimal loading to promote healing. Weight-shifting activities early in rehabilitation help to create this compression without the risks of damage that may occur with the shear forces that are created with ambulation.

Aquatic activities have proven to be an effective component of the rehabilitation process. Early ambulation in the pool allows patients to focus on gait symmetry in a deweighted environment. Active range of motion within pain-free limits can also be initiated in the water. For those individuals concerned with preservation of their cardiovascular fitness, such as distance runners, jogging in an aquatic vest can be initiated as tolerated. Aquatic activities have proven to be an excellent tool to aid in the transition from limited weightbearing to functional activities on dry land.

Active range of motion and open chain resistive exercises can be utilized after the appropriate range of motion and control of baseline symptoms has been established. We recommend an early emphasis on gluteus medius strengthening activities. Open chain knee extension and flexion activities should be progressed as tolerated. Those patients undergoing additional soft tissue release procedures may have precautions regarding specific motions.

After full weightbearing status has been achieved, functional progression is primarily dictated by symptoms. Gait training is often required to ensure symmetrical weightbearing and terminal extension of the affected hip. Careful attention should be given to ensure that a Trendelenburg gait does not exist. Weightbearing exercises should be progressed to closed chain progressive resistance exercises as tolerated. Movement in all planes of motion should be addressed with special attention to rotary stability. We often utilize weightbearing hip rotation activities, and will apply resistance through elastic tubing to increase difficulty. Open and closed chain proprioception should be addressed. The superficial layers of the labrum are innervated, and compromise of this tissue could be implicated in proprioceptive deficits.[61] In patients undergoing isolated labral resection, we will initiate single leg stance activities approximately 10 days to 3 weeks after surgery. Perturbation and functional activities are added as tolerated.

The progression to running varies significantly among individuals. Factors such as preoperative condition, extent of injury, and body composition can affect return to running.

Using devices such as the elliptical trainer or stepper may be useful in providing a transitional period to running. We typically initiate these activities 4 to 6 weeks after surgery as tolerated. In our experience running may be initiated as early as 8 weeks, but more often is initiated closer to 12 weeks after surgery. During the running progression, an individual may develop those conditions of the hip joint region common to runners such as tendonitis and bursitis. If conditions such as these develop, they should be addressed promptly to optimize the running progression. The concept of relative rest should be emphasized to the patient.

Particular attention should be given to patient symptoms during any phase of transition. Such phases include the transition from crutches to full ambulation and from normal activity to higher level activity or return to training in athletes. We have observed that individuals who have made attempts to push excessively through discomfort often develop tendonitis (iliopsoas, rectus femoris, iliotibial band), bursitis, or synovitis. In these cases, activity must be significantly decreased until symptoms have subsided to baseline. Avoiding such situations should be a primary concern as a significant amount of rehabilitation time may be lost in the case of their occurrence.

Many patients who have had labral tears may report a history of low-back pain or symptoms consistent with sacroiliac dysfunction. Such problems should be addressed as indicated by physical examination. Stabilization techniques to enhance lumbo-pelvic stability can be utilized as per patient tolerance. Manual techniques as indicated for the lumbar spine and sacroiliac regions are often found to be useful in addressing symptoms of the sacroiliac and low back regions. Leg length discrepancies may also exist. Orthotic intervention should be considered as indicated in these cases.

The rehabilitation process following repair of the labrum does not vary significantly from that following a resection procedure. A limited weightbearing status may be prolonged depending on the extent and location of the repair. Large tears requiring an extensive repair may have a partial weightbearing status for 4 to 6 weeks. This may hold particularly true for individuals who had tears on the anterior-superior (weightbearing) portion of the labrum. After the repair is believed to be stable, functional progression should parallel the process described for labral resection procedures.

Femoral-Acetabular Impingement

Osteochondroplasty for femoral-acetabular impingement can be successfully performed arthroscopically. These injuries are usually associated with labral pathology, and the rehabilitation guidelines discussed above hold true for these patients. However, due to the bone resection along the femoral head-neck junction and the potential for either subcapital or femoral neck fractures, a longer period of protected weightbearing is indicated (4 to 6 weeks of 20 lb, foot flat). We typically obtain plain x-rays prior to advancing the

weightbearing status. In these patients, more aggressive early passive range of motion can be performed with particular attention to flexion and internal rotation.

Chondral Injury

Rehabilitation of patients undergoing debridement of chondral flaps with microfracture procedures carries particular concerns. The primary concern is to allow healing of the affected articular surfaces. An attempt should be made to create an environment that minimizes compressive and particularly shear forces. Articular damage is often on the weightbearing surface of the femur or acetabulum. A non- or partial weightbearing status for 6 to 8 weeks is usually assigned to the patient. This may vary depending on the extent and location of the chondral lesion. Weight-shifting activities may be initiated earlier; however, caution should be exercised with early ambulatory activities. The combination of weightbearing and rotational motion can create potentially damaging shear forces. When transitioning from a limited weightbearing status to ambulating independently, the patient should be monitored for any symptoms indicative of joint inflammation. If allowed to persist without a period of relative rest, this condition can become extremely difficult to control. In cases where such symptoms do occur, it is recommended that the patient temporarily resume a partial weightbearing status and utilize prescribed anti-inflammatories and modalities as indicated. A therapeutic pool can be utilized to begin early gait training and weightbearing activities. Range of motion progression for microfracture procedures is usually similar to those guidelines followed for a labral resection or repair. If performed in conjunction with a capsular modification procedure, additional range of motion restrictions may be recommended.

Capsular Laxity

The most significant issue of rehabilitation for those patients undergoing capsular modification procedures is early limitation of range of motion to allow appropriate healing and re-establishment of capsular tension characteristics. Weightbearing and strength progression is typically similar to the protocol described for labral procedures. Often capsular modification is performed in conjunction with a labral procedure. Depending on the extent of the procedure, a partial weightbearing status may be assigned from 10 days to 4 weeks after surgery. Protected early range of motion is imperative. There are particular concerns with excessive external rotation and extension. Both of these positions can potentially put an inappropriate amount of tension through the anterior portion of the capsule. Excessive flexion or abduction should also be performed cautiously, as these positions may cause impingement of unhealed anterior capsular tissue into the joint, creating discomfort and potentially aggravating tissue inflammation. We typically limit movement from neutral to 90 degrees of flexion in the sagittal plane, with minimal movement in other planes for the first 7 to 14 days of treatment.

Approximately 7 to 14 days after surgery, rotation is gently initiated through active rotation with the affected knee resting on the exam stool or floor in a quadriped position. Internal rotation should be initiated prior to external rotation. The patient is instructed to rotate the hip using the knee as an axis only within a range of motion that is comfortable. A gradual increase of motion in the sagittal plane can be initiated at approximately 7 to 14 days after surgery. The authors have noted most patients can achieve greater flexion without discomfort using a rocking to heel method in quadriped compared to supine flexion-based activities. Stretching may be initiated as tolerated around 21 to 28 days after the surgery. Gentle joint distraction techniques for the purpose of relieving pain can be initiated around 21 days postoperatively. Direction-specific mobilization techniques may be utilized if indicated after approximately 28 days. Caution should be exercised when utilizing these procedures. Full range of motion as tolerated is typically recommended at approximately 4 to 5 weeks after surgery.

After a patient has reached full weightbearing status, the rehabilitation process for an isolated capsular procedure, or combined labral-capsular procedure typically follows the same course as an isolated labral procedure. Functional progression is based heavily on symptomatic reaction to activity.

Extraarticular Procedures

The primary concerns following tissue release and lengthening procedures are controlling the postoperative inflammatory response and allowing appropriate healing time for those tissues being released. When performed with other procedures such as labral resection or repair and capsular modification, the postoperative concerns that occur with such procedures apply. Specific weightbearing and range of motion may apply in these cases. Early pain free range of motion is indicated. In order to allow appropriate healing and to avoid initiating an exaggerated inflammatory response, early stretching is usually avoided. Stretching is typically initiated as tolerated 4 weeks after surgery. An attempt is made to initiate stretching in a manner and time frame that promotes maintenance of the appropriate tendon length while avoiding an inflammatory response. Isometric exercise for those muscle groups not directly affected by the surgical procedure can be initiated immediately. Submaximal isometric exercises for the involved structures are typically initiated 3 weeks after surgery. This includes isometric flexion for an iliopsoas lengthening procedure and abduction for an iliotibial band lengthening procedure. Straight leg raise activities in the plane of action for the involved musculotendinous structures are usually avoided for a minimum of 4 weeks. Our experience has been that early initiation of such activities is associated with an inflammatory type response resembling tendonitis. Once tolerance of gentle isometrics and active range of motion has been

established, a progression of weightbearing, progressive strengthening exercises, and functional activities should be initiated.

■ OUTCOMES AND FUTURE DIRECTIONS

Several reports have demonstrated the efficacy of hip arthroscopy in the treatment of labral tears, capsular laxity, loose bodies, and chondral injuries.[3,20,29,62,63] However, improvements in outcome scoring criteria and more prospective evaluation are necessary to further advance this field. The University of Pittsburgh, in conjunction with Duquesne University, is in the process of establishing a comprehensive outcome scoring system for all the patients with musculoskeletal hip disorders. This scoring system will contain discriminative, predictive, and evaluative self-report instruments. The discriminative component will categorize patients, the predictive component will help determine the patient prognosis, and the evaluative component will measure the changes in the patient's status over time. A process is currently in place at the UPMC Sports Medicine Hip Disorder Center that allows for uniform collection of demographic, general health, past medical history, history of current hip problems, objective information, as well as information from a battery of items in a self-report format.

The items contained on the self-report instruments are grouped together according to the nature of the questions. The first group of items serves to subjectively assess the nature of the patient's symptoms in a uniform manner (Appendix 1). This information will serve as an evaluative instrument, allowing a change in the patient's symptoms to be monitored over time. As a discriminative instrument, information from these items can be clustered together to help categorize patients based on the characteristics of their symptoms. Information about the patient's complaints will also serve in a predictive capacity assessing for indicators that will predict final outcome. One might expect patients who report more severe limitations in multiple categories to have a poorer outcome. Such categorization will allow the surgeon to more effectively educate the patient regarding expected patient outcomes and the probability of success after surgical intervention.

The second group of items assesses self-reported physical performance, and together is a separate instrument called the Hip Outcome Score (HOS). The HOS is comprised of two scales: the Activity of Daily Living (ADL) and Sports scales (Appendix 2). The primary purpose of the HOS is to function as an evaluative instrument assessing the change in the patient's physical performance over time. At the present time there is not a comprehensive self-report evaluative instrument appropriate for all patients with hip disorders. There are a number of instruments for arthritic conditions and one instrument for nonarthritic conditions. The HOS serves as an evaluative outcome instrument appropriate for individuals with a wide range of musculoskeletal hip-related pathologies, both arthritic and nonarthritic. With respect to individuals with labral-related pathology, they generally function at a high level and have very little limitations except for sports-related activities. Therefore, a sports-specific scale was developed in an effort to be more responsive to changes in the physical performance of these individuals. The reliability, validity, and responsiveness of the HOS are currently being investigated.

As an evaluative instrument the HOS needs to have appropriate psychometric properties, including an appropriate factoral structure, the ability to provide information across all ability levels, and the ability to detect change across the spectrum of ability. It has been hypothesized that the Sport scale deals with activities that require a higher level of ability, while the ADL scale deals with activities that require a lower level of ability. These questions have been addressed in preliminary psychometric analysis. The analysis has consisted of evaluating the items for unidimensionality using factor analysis. Item Response Theory is used to evaluate items for their potential responsiveness and information contribution. Data have been collected on 315 patients, consisting of 192 (61%) males and 123 (39%) females with a mean age of 38.1 (SD 12.4 range 15 to 62). The diagnoses of these patients consisted of the following: degenerative hip conditions ($n = 154$), labral tears ($n = 124$), bursitis ($n = 15$), muscle strains ($n = 12$), and avascular necrosis ($n = 10$). Factor analysis found items on the ADL and Sport subscales loaded on one factor. Results of Item Response analysis found the 19 items on the ADL scale and 9 items on the Sport scale contributed to the test information curve and were potentially responsive. The items on the Sport scale collected information at the higher end of ability, while the ADL scale collected information at the lower end of ability. The results of this study support the use of the HOS, ADL, and Sport subscales for individuals with a wide range of hip-related pathologies and varying levels of ability.

A project has also been completed to assess whether it is valid to use the HOS for individuals with labral tears. One hundred and twenty-four patients with the diagnosis of a labral tear completed the HOS and the SF-36. These subjects consisted of 75 (60%) males and 49 (40%) females with a mean age of 34.2 (SD 10.0 range 15 to 49). The Pearson correlation coefficient was used to determine convergent and divergent evidence of validity by examining the relationship of the HOS to the physical function and mental health subscales of the SF-36. Convergent evidence of validity was displayed as the physical function subscale had strong correlations to the HOS ADL ($r = 0.62$) and Sport ($r = 0.73$) scales. Divergent evidence was also displayed as the mental health subscale had weak correlations to the HOS ADL ($r = 0.30$) and Sport ($r = 0.31$) scales. The results of this study offer evidence of validity for the HOS with patients with labral tears of the hip.

The third grouping of questions look to further describe the nature of sports-related hip injuries (Appendix 3). At the current time there is little information regarding the relation of hip injuries to leg dominance, particular sports or positions, time of the sports season, and level of competition.

Demographic information related to the hip classification systems has been collected. It was hypothesized that the five categories of the classification system could be differentiated by age, gender, body mass index (BMI), duration of symptoms, activity level, and mechanism of injury. Data have been collected on 204 patients who underwent arthroscopic hip surgery, and the following were found:

1 7% of the subjects were classified as type I and had the following characteristics: 100% had primary labral involvement and associated capsular laxity, all had good cartilage condition without a bone spur, mean age of 28 years, gender: 30% female, 70% male, a duration of symptoms of 3 years, mean BMI of 24, 85% had a high activity level, 57% had an insidious onset, and 43% traumatic onset.

2 20% of the subjects were classified as type II and had the following characteristics: 100% had primary capsular laxity and associated labral involvement, all had good cartilage condition without the presence of a bone spur, mean age of 21 years, gender: 71% female, 29% male, duration of symptoms 1year, mean BMI of 22, 70% had a high activity level, 87% had an insidious onset.

3 23% of the subjects were classified as type III and had the following characteristics: 100% had labral involvement and capsular laxity, all had good cartilage condition without the presence of a bone spur, mean age of 45 years, gender: 75% female, 25% male, duration of symptoms 2 years, mean BMI of 23, 14% had a high activity level, 70% had an insidious onset.

4 12% of the subjects were classified as type IV and had the following characteristics: 100% had primary bone spur, 100% had labral involvement, 50% capsular laxity, 82% had good cartilage condition, mean age of 37 years, gender: 75% female, 25% male, duration of symptoms 5 years, mean BMI of 26, 25% had a high activity level, 82% had an insidious onset.

5 30% of the subjects were classified as type V and had the following characteristics: 100% had primary articular cartilage involvement, 90% had a labral tear, 25% had capsular laxity, 25% had a bone spur, mean age of 48 years, gender: 27% female, 73% male, duration of symptoms 6 years, mean BMI of 27, 8% had a high activity level, 60% had an insidious, and 40% traumatic onset.

Analysis found that these five categories were significantly different with respect to age, gender, and activity level, while BMI, duration of symptoms, and mechanism of injury were not significantly different. These initial data suggest that age, gender, and activity level can be used to define the categories of the classification system. Further evaluation of specific outcome scores will provide insight into the success rates of hip arthroscopy based upon patient type.

The University of Pittsburgh, in conjunction with Duquesne University, continues to work on establishing a comprehensive scoring system. Once this system is in place patients will be better able to be categorized, their prognosis will be better defined, and the changes that occur within patients will be better defined. Ultimately, this system will allow for more significant advancements in surgical indications and technique, as we can rapidly assess the efficacy of new procedures. Hip arthroscopy truly is the final frontier in sports medicine. We are now able to access the hip joint without difficulty, perform increasingly more advanced arthroscopic procedures, and are continuously discovering new soft tissue sources of intra- and extra-articular hip pathology. Soon we hope to be able to treat soft-tissue injuries in and around the hip as effectively and routinely as we are able to treat similar lesions in and around the shoulder and knee. Accurate assessment of patient outcome, improved education within the orthopedic community, and continued scientific investigation at both the basic science and clinical levels will lead to the achievement of this goal.

■ APPENDIX 1: SUBJECTIVE EVALUATION FORM

Please read and answer the questions that pertain to you and your injury.

Do you have clicking or snapping?
_____ Frequently
_____ Occasionally
_____ Never

Please select *one* that describes your condition best:
_____ 1. I do not have clicking or snapping
_____ 2. I have clicking or snapping but it does not limit my activity
_____ 3. I have clicking or snapping and it limits my activity slightly
_____ 4. I have clicking or snapping and it limits my activity greatly
_____ 5. I have clicking or snapping and it prevents me from participating in any activity

Do you have the sensation that your foot/leg is rolling out?
_____ Frequently
_____ Occasionally
_____ Never

Do you have the feeling of instability or giving way?
_____ Frequently
_____ Occasionally
_____ Never

Please select *one* that describes your condition best:
_____ 1. I do not have instability or giving way
_____ 2. I have instability or giving way but it does not limit my activity
_____ 3. I have instability or giving way and it limits my activity slightly
_____ 4. I have instability or giving way and it limits my activity greatly
_____ 5. I have instability or giving way and it prevents from participating in any activity

Do you have trouble balancing or stabilizing yourself on your involved leg?
_____ Yes
_____ No

Select the most appropriates responses that describe the location of your pain:
_____ Groin
_____ Outside
_____ Front
_____ Back

Do you have pain when you are extending your hip when you walk?
_____ Yes
_____ No

Please select *one* that describes your condition best:
_____ 1. I do not have stiffness
_____ 2. I have stiffness but it does not limit my activity
_____ 3. I have stiffness and it limits my activity slightly
_____ 4. I have stiffness and it limits my activity greatly
_____ 5. I have stiffness and it prevents me from participating in any activity

Please select *one* that describes your condition best:
_____ 1. I do not have weakness
_____ 2. I have weakness but it does not limit my activity
_____ 3. I have weakness and it limits my activity slightly
_____ 4. I have weakness and it limits my activity greatly
_____ 5. I have weakness and it prevents from participating in any activity

Since the onset of treatment, how would you describe your condition?
_____ Much improved
_____ Somewhat improved
_____ Slightly improved
_____ Unchanged
_____ Slightly worse
_____ Somewhat worse
_____ Much worse

Over the past few weeks, how would you describe your condition?
_____ Much improved
_____ Somewhat improved
_____ Slightly improved
_____ Unchanged
_____ Slightly worse
_____ Somewhat worse
_____ Much worse

■ APPENDIX 2: THE HIP OUTCOMES SCORE (HOS)

ADL Subscale

Please answer *every question* with *one response* that most closely describes your condition within the past week. If the activity in question is limited by something other than your hip mark not applicable (N/A).

	No difficulty at all	Slight difficulty	Moderate difficulty	Extreme difficulty	Unable to do	N/A
Standing for 15 minutes	☐	☐	☐	☐	☐	☐
Getting into and out of an average car	☐	☐	☐	☐	☐	☐
Putting on socks and shoes	☐	☐	☐	☐	☐	☐
Walking up steep hills	☐	☐	☐	☐	☐	☐
Walking down steep hills	☐	☐	☐	☐	☐	☐
Going up one flight of stairs	☐	☐	☐	☐	☐	☐
Going down one flight of stairs	☐	☐	☐	☐	☐	☐
Stepping up and down curbs	☐	☐	☐	☐	☐	☐
Deep squatting	☐	☐	☐	☐	☐	☐
Getting into and out of a bathtub	☐	☐	☐	☐	☐	☐
Sitting for 15 minutes	☐	☐	☐	☐	☐	☐
Walking initially	☐	☐	☐	☐	☐	☐
Walking approximately 10 minutes	☐	☐	☐	☐	☐	☐
Walking 15 minutes or greater	☐	☐	☐	☐	☐	☐

Because of your hip how much difficulty do you have with:

	No difficulty at all	Slight difficulty	Moderate difficulty	Extreme difficulty	Unable to do	N/A
Twisting/pivoting on involved leg	☐	☐	☐	☐	☐	☐
Rolling over in bed	☐	☐	☐	☐	☐	☐
Light to moderate work (standing, walking)	☐	☐	☐	☐	☐	☐
Heavy work (push/pulling, climbing, carrying)	☐	☐	☐	☐	☐	☐
Recreational activities	☐	☐	☐	☐	☐	☐

How would you rate your current level of function during your usual activities of daily living from 0 to 100 with 100 being your level of function prior to your hip problem and 0 being the inability to perform any of your usual daily activities?

0————————100

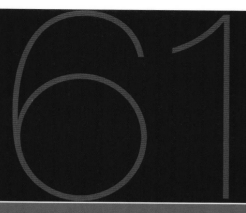

HIP ARTHROSCOPY USING A MINI-OPEN APPROACH

■ RONALD E. DELANOIS, MD, LTCOL, MC, USAF, JON K. SEKIYA, MD

■ HISTORY OF THE TECHNIQUE

Hip arthroscopy has evolved over the past 20 years to address a number of intra-articular abnormalities that result in disabling hip pain. They include symptomatic labral tears, chondral lesions, loose bodies, synovitis, crystalline hip arthropathy, infection, and many more.[1-4] Complications associated with hip arthroscopy have also been well documented.[5] Clarke et al.[1] reported a 1.4% complication rate. They included sciatic neurapraxia, femoral neurapraxia, portal hematoma, infection, failure of adequate access or observation, and arthrotomy. In his series of 1,054 hip arthroscopies, hip access was considered difficult in 18% of the cases. In 2.8% (30 hips) of the cases, the hip joint could not be entered. Two cases, open arthrotomies, had to be preformed for removal of a loose body or for intra-articular debridement. Sekiya et al.[6,7] described hip arthroscopy using the anterior mini-open approach. It was felt that because an open dissection is performed down to the hip capsule, the risk of neurovascular injury is decreased.[6] Also the iatrogenic injury to the articular cartilage or acetabular labrum is potentially reduced. Hawkins[8] described a small anterior exposure to the hip with mini-arthrotomy and subluxation of the femoral head to allow introduction of the arthroscope. Goldman et al.[9] described a limited posterior approach, exposing the posterior hip capsule by releasing the short external rotators to allow the placement of an arthroscope to facilitate the removal of a bullet. In our experience, we have found that hip arthroscopy using the anterior mini-open technique has been an excellent addition to our armamentarium in the management and treatment of hip pathology.

■ INDICATIONS AND CONTRAINDICATION

Hip arthroscopy, using a limited anterior exposure, has similar indications as a standard hip arthroscopy. It is primarily advantageous in the removal of loose bodies or labral tears, patients with synovial chondromatosis, avascular necrosis, infection, and most importantly in patients in which hip access is deemed difficult by standard arthroscopic techniques.[2,4,10–15] In addition, this procedure allows easy conversion to an open technique should it be required. We also feel that patients who are greater than 1.5 times ideal body weight may be best served with this procedure. It allows greater scope mobility and a decreased risk to the neurovascular structures. Sekiya[7] reported no complications in his case series in which a limited anterior exposure was performed. Rehabilitation is extended 2 to 3 weeks to allow for wound healing. Other patients who may be best served with this technique include those with advanced osteoarthritis. These patients have joint capsular contraction, making hip distraction difficult, and thus are at increased risk for articular cartilage damage.

A relative contraindication would include patients in which an altered anterior anatomy exists. These are individuals who have had prior surgery, specifically an osteotomy. Anterior heterotopic bone formation may also be a contraindication for this technique, unless a concomitant open removal is planned.

■ SURGICAL TECHNIQUE

In accordance to the American Academy of Orthopedic Surgeon's recommendation, the operative hip is identified and signed by the surgeon in the holding room. The patient is then brought to the operating room and placed supine on a radiolucent operative table. The patient is than anesthetized as per anesthesia. We prefer a general anesthetic with complete muscle relaxation. A spinal anesthetic can be adequate, but it must provide completed muscle relaxation. Our concern with a spinal anesthetic intraoperatively is that if it begins to wears off, some of the early signs of increased muscle tone can ultimately affect hip exposure. Also, postoperatively the surgeon is unable to perform an immediate neural exam. Once the patient is anesthetized, the sacrum is padded with foam or a gel pad to protect from the development of a sacral decubiti. All the nerves and vessels of the patient's extremities are padded and protected throughout the operation. The arm on the operative side is placed over the patient's chest on top of a pillow. This protects the

extremity and chest and removes the extremity from the operative side. The operative leg is then placed in the traction boot. The leg is abducted between 0 degrees and 20 degrees, depending on the patient's hip anatomy. The foot is maintained in a neutral rotated position. The orientation of the traction must be in line with the perineal post. Otherwise, it may be difficult to generate enough force to adequately distract the hip joint. Also, if the force is not in line with the perineal post, the patient may rotate on the post and again compromise distraction. We prefer to place the nonoperative leg in a traction boot as well to counteract this possible rotation on the perineal post; however, use of a well-leg holder for the nonoperative leg can also be utilized[6,7] **(Fig. 61-1A,B,C,D)**.

Once the patient is appropriately positioned, the extremity is prepped with alcohol then dura-prepped from the knee

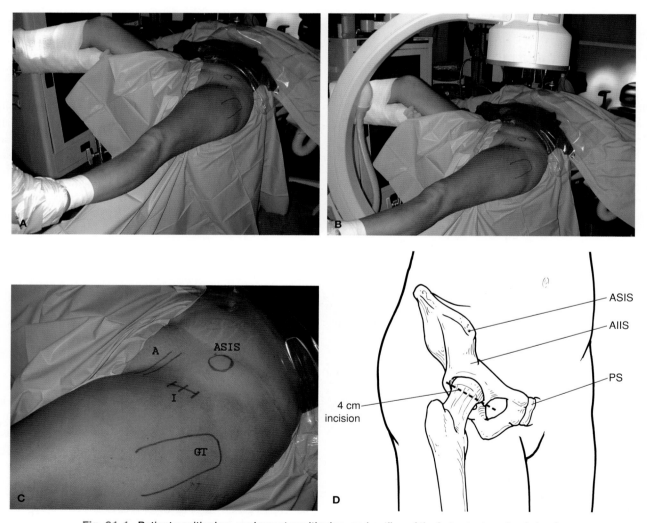

Fig. 61-1. Patient positioning, equipment positioning, and outline of the important anatomic landmarks. **A:** Patient positioned supine on the fracture table with the nonoperative leg in a well-leg holder. **B:** Patient positioned with image intensification in place. **C:** Close-up of landmarks including the greater trochanter *(GT)*, planned incision *(I)*, femoral artery *(A)*, and anterior-superior iliac spine *(ASIS)*. **D:** Drawing depicting planned incision site and landmarks.

to the umbilicus. We use sterile "U" drapes, both proximally and distally, to give exposure to the entire hip, again extending from the umbilicus to the knee. The anterior-superior iliac spine is identified, as well as the pubis. A line is drawn connecting these two anatomic landmarks, which coincide with the inguinal ligament. The femoral pulse is then palpated. Using a marking pen, the femoral artery, vein, and nerve are drawn out. The anterior-inferior iliac spine (AIIS) is also identified and marked using a marking pen. A 4-cm incision is drawn approximately 2 cm below the inguinal ligament, lateral to the neurovascular structures, overlying the femoral head. This incision often falls in line with the hip flexion crease. An image intensifier, fluoroscope, is used to ensure that the incision placement lies directly over the femoral head (Fig. 61-1).

Once we have ensured proper placement of the incision a 10-blade knife is used to incise the skin. The incision is carried down sharply through the dermis and the subcutaneously fat. All bleeders are identified and cauterized. A self-retaining retractor is placed to allow visualization of the sartorius fascia. The fascia can be incised at the junction between the sartorius and the tensor fascia lata muscle **(Fig. 61-2)**. The lateral femoral cutaneous nerve is identified and retracted medially and protected throughout the remainder of the dissection. The inner nervous plane between the tensor fascia lata and the sartorius is then entered using Mayo scissors. The sartorius is taken medially and the tensor fascia lata is taken laterally and held there using two blunt retractors.[16] If an assistant is available, two army-navy retractors work well here. Once these two structures are retracted the next muscle that comes into view should be the direct head of the rectus femoris muscle **(Fig. 61-3)**. Oftentimes you can identify both the direct head and the indirect head. The direct head comes off the AIIS and the indirect head comes off the anterior rim of the acetabulum. These tendons are preserved throughout the operation whenever possible. It is sometimes necessary, though, to detach one

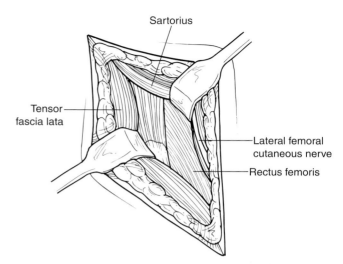

Fig. 61-3. The rectus femoris muscle is identified and retracted. Often, one or both head of the rectus femoris will need to be detached.

or both heads from their origin to gain access to the hip capsule. If the muscles are released from their origin, they need not be repaired since there is minimal retraction and there seems to be no sequelae in the postoperative rehabilitation or in terms of loss of function. One advantage to this approach is that the interval between the sartorius and the iliopsoas muscle can also be explored[17] **(Fig. 61-4)**. This allows exposure to the iliopsoas tendon, which can be lengthened in the case of snapping hip syndrome. A pair of cobra retractors is placed medially and laterally around the femoral head and neck. The hip capsule is freed of all extraneous tissue. Once the hip capsule is under direct visualization, a fluoroscope is used to identify the hip joint. A 60-cc syringe filled with normal saline with an 18-gauge spinal needle is then brought up into the operative field. It is introduced through the hip capsule and

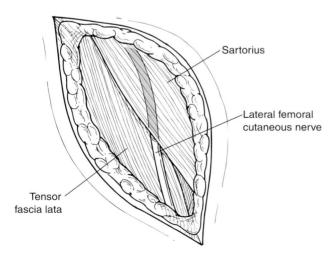

Fig. 61-2. The interval between the tensor fascia lata and sartorius is developed. Care is taken to identify and protect the lateral femoral cutaneous nerve.

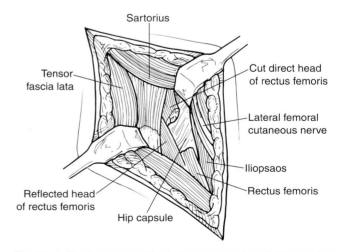

Fig. 61-4. The iliopsoas tendon is then retracted medially exposing the anterior hip capsule. The iliopsoas tendon can be lengthened at this point if it is causing symptomatic snapping or catching.

into the hip joint. This allows insufflation of the hip joint as well as elimination of the negative pressure. Great care is used not to injure the femoral or acetabular cartilage. At this point in time, the nurse in the room or the assistant will apply traction in a longitudinal fashion on the operative extremity. Traction will be applied until there is approximately 1 cm of radiographic clear space between the femoral head and the acetabulum. The amount of force necessary to achieve adequate distraction varies from patient to patient. Eriksson et al.[18] reported a force variation of 300 to 500 N for adequate distraction in the anesthetized patient. Complete muscle relaxation is necessary to minimize this force. Also, elimination of the negative pressure within the hip joint prior to hip distraction can help minimize the force. This is why we prefer to insufflate the hip with saline prior to distraction. Once this has been obtained, the first arthroscopy portal is ready to be made along the anterior capsule. A fluoroscope is used to place an 18-gauge needle into the hip joint. A guide wire from the hip arthroscopy set is passed through the needle. This is checked with the fluoroscope to ensure that no cartilage is injured upon passing the arthroscopy cannula. The arthroscopy cannula is passed into the hip joint followed by the camera. We prefer to have both a 70-degree and a 30-degree scope available to allow visualization of the femoral head and acetabulum. Additional anterior working portals can be utilized along the anterior joint line proximally or distally to our initial portal depending upon the location of the hip pathology. In addition, a percutaneous lateral portal can also be created in a similar fashion to standard all-arthroscopic hip techniques.[19] This is done approximately 1.5 cm anterior and proximal to the greater trochanter at the level of the femoral head. An 11-blade knife is used to make a small stab incision at this location. A Kelly retractor is placed deep within the wound to allow distraction of the soft tissues. Using a similar technique, which was described earlier, a cannula is introduced through this lateral portal and can be used either as a working portal or for camera placement. Oftentimes the cannula can be seen through the anterior incision and is thus more easily passed into the hip joint with injury to the cartilage.

The majority of work can be performed using these portals. The arthroscope is frequently switched back and forth between these portals to improve complete visualization of the hip joint and adequate access to the hip pathology. The posterior portal, which is also described, can be used to facilitate visualization of the posterior hip.[4,20] The risks associated with this portal include injury to the sciatic nerve and the superior gluteal vessels. As a result, it is recommended that this portal be made under direct visualization. We as a routine do not use this portal. With adequate distraction and the use of the other portals, we feel we get excellent visualization of the entire hip joint.

Once the arthroscopy is completed, the arthroscopy equipment is removed from the hip joint and the anterior incision is copiously irrigated with normal saline. If deemed necessary, the rectus tendons can be approximated using a nonabsorbable suture. The remaining tissues are allowed to retract to their normal anatomic position. The subcutaneous tissues are closed using a 2-0 Vicryl suture. The skin incision is then approximated using a 4-0 Monocryl suture. A drain is generally not needed. A sterile dressing is applied, and traction is then removed from the patient's hip joint. The patient is awakened and brought back to the recovery room.

■ TECHNICAL ALTERNATIVES AND PITFALLS

There are several alternatives to this technique. Glick et al.[21] describe hip arthroscopy with the patient in the lateral position. The sited theoretical advantage is that the entire weight-bearing articular surface on the acetabulum and femoral head can be observed via the paratrochanteric portals with a 30-degree scope. Also the lateral femoral cutaneous nerve can be easily avoided because the anterior portal is not used. The three portals described include the proximal trochanteric, the anterior paratrochanteric, and the posterior paratrochanteric. The disadvantage to positioning the patient in this manner is that if the arthroscopy procedure needs to be converted to a mini-open technique, anterior surface anatomy is often difficult to access and orientation is a problem. Hip arthroscopy using a limited anterior exposure is preferably done in the supine position. This allows direct and easy access to the surface anatomy.

The second alternative to this technique is doing the procedure all-open. The sited advantage is that large loose bodies are more accessible. The disadvantage to this technique includes avascular necrosis, nerve damage, muscle damage, heterotopic bone formation, and a prolonged rehabilitation. We reserve this technique for fractures of the femoral head.

Another alternative option is to not use formal traction and to prep the involved leg and hip free. This allows for hip range of motion, which may assist with complete visualization and access of the hip joint. In addition, manual traction can still be applied by an assistant and in our experience, the limited anterior dissection often decreases the need for a formal traction set-up.[7] If joint distraction is found to be inadequate with this method, formal traction can easily be applied.

Pitfalls regarding hip arthroscopy using a limited anterior exposure include inappropriate placement of the starting incision. If placed too medially the femoral nerve and vessels are at increased risk. Also, a medial arthroscopic portal can make it difficult for anterior-superior visualization, the location of most labral tears. If the incision is placed too distal or too proximal, hip entry is again compromised. The surgeon will be either on top of the rim of the acetabulum or on the femoral neck.

■ REHABILITATION

All patients are allowed to weight bear as tolerated postoperatively with a set of crutches. Immediately following surgery, ice is placed onto the anterior incision to reduce swelling. Physical therapy is started on postoperative day 4 with an emphasis on range of motion. Once the patient has established full range of motion and he or she can weight bear without an assistance device, the patient can begin a strengthening program. The patient begins with walking on a treadmill both forward and backward. They then progress to using weights. Quadriceps and hamstring strengthening are encouraged. Most patients return to full activity within 10 to 12 weeks following surgery.

■ OUTCOMES AND FUTURE DIRECTIONS

Sekiya et al.[7] reported their results in five patients using this limited anterior exposure for hip arthroscopy. The procedure either involved the removal of loose bodies or debridement of synovitis, cartilaginous debris, or osteochondral fragments. There were no complications, and all five patients had improvement in their symptoms.

Hip arthroscopy using a mini-open approach combined the advantages of both an open and arthroscopic technique, while minimizing operative risk. This technique allows the occasional hip arthroscopist with an alternative for easier arthroscopic hip access, which is an otherwise very technically difficult procedure to perform.

■ REFERENCES

1. Clarke MT, Arora A, Villar RN. Hip arthroscopy: complications in 1054 cases. Clin Orthop. 2003;1(406):84–88.
2. Kelly BT, Williams RJ III, Philippon MJ. Hip arthroscopy: current indications, treatment options, and management issues. Am J Sports Med. November–December 2003;31(6):1020–1037.
3. Mason JB, McCarthy JC, O'Donnell J, et al. Hip arthroscopy: surgical approach, positioning and distraction. Clin Orthop. 2003; 1(406):29–37.
4. McCarthy JC, Day B, Busconi B. Hip arthroscopy: applications and technique. J Am Acad Orthop Surg. 1995;3(3):115–122.
5. Funke EL, Munzinger U. Complications in hip arthroscopy Arthroscopy. 1996;12:156-159.
6. Sekiya JK, Wojtys EM. Hip arthroscopy using the mini-open approach. Op Tech Sports Med. October 2002;10(4):200–204.
7. Sekiya JK, Wojtys EM, Loder RT, et al. Hip arthroscopy using a limited anterior exposure: an alternative approach for arthroscopic access. Arthroscopy. 2000;16:16–20.
8. Hawkins RB. Arthroscopy of the hip, clinical orthopaedics and related research. 1989;249:44–47.
9. Goldman A, Minkoff J, Price A, et al. A posterior approach to bullet extraction from the hip. J Trauma. 1987;27:1294–1300.
10. Chung WK, Slater GL, Bates EH. Treatment of septic arthritis of the hip by arthroscopic lavage. J Pediatr Orthop. 1993;13(4): 444–446.
11. Ruch DS, Sekiya J, Schaefer WD, et al. The role of hip arthroscopy in the evaluation of avascular necrosis. Orthop Blue J. 2001;24(4): 339–343.
12. Suzuki S, Awaya G, Okada Y, et al. Arthroscopic diagnosis of ruptured acetabular labrum. Acta Orthop Scand. 1986;57:513–515.
13. Keene GS, Villar RN. Arthroscopic loose body retrieval following traumatic hip dislocation. Int J Care Injured. 1994;25(8): 507–551.
14. Byrd JW. Labral lesions: an elusive source of hip pain, case reports and literature review. Arthroscopy. 1996;12:603–612.
15. Sekiya JK, Ruch DS, Hunter DM, et al. Hip arthroscopy in staging avascular necrosis of the femoral head. J South Orthop Assoc. 2000;9(4):254–261.
16. Hoppenfeld S, DeBoer P. *Surgical Exposures I Orthopaedics: The Anatomic Approach*. Philadelphia: JB Lippincott; 1994:325–338.
17. Smith-Petersen MN. Approach to and exposure of the hip joint for mold arthroplasty. J Bone Joint Surg Am. 1949;31:40.
18. Eriksson E, Arvidsson I, Arvidisson H. Diagnostic and operative arthroscopy of the hip. Orthopedics. 1986;9:169–172.
19. Byrd JW, Pappas JN, Pedley MJ. Hip arthroscopy: an anatomic study of portal placement and relationship to the extra'articular structures. Arthroscopy. 1995;11:418–423.
20. Ide T, Akamatsu N, Nakajima I. Arthroscopic surgery of the hip joint. J Arthro Rel Surg. 1991;7(2):204–211.
21. Glick JM, Sampson TG, Gordon RB, et al. Hip arthroscopy by the lateral approach. Arthroscopy. 1987;3(1):4–12.

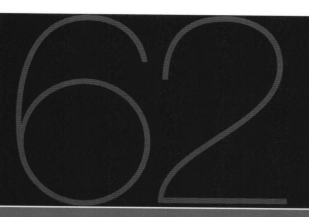

SURGICAL TREATMENT OF OVERUSE INJURIES OF THE LOWER EXTREMITY

ANTHONY A. SCHEPSIS, MD, FREDERICK J. WATSON, MD, WILLIAM R. CREEVY, MD

Overuse injuries of the lower extremity are a commonly seen entity in the sports medicine clinic. Fortunately, only a handful of injured athletes present with a problem that requires surgical intervention to return to the field of play. In this chapter, we will focus on the surgical management of three specific entities—exertional compartment syndrome, anteriorly based "tension" tibial stress fractures, and stress fractures of the fifth metatarsal.

■ EXERTIONAL COMPARTMENT SYNDROME

Historical Perspective

It wasn't until it became clear that the exertional related pain that athletes would experience in the lower extremity could be a result of transient increases in intercompartmental pressure that it became intuitive that fascial release was the only surgical option. As far back as 1956, Mavor[1] successfully treated anterior exertional compartment syndrome by a fascial widening procedure. Subsequently it was recognized that the extensile release necessary in acute compartment syndromes associated with trauma was not necessary and that only the investing fascia contributed to the symptoms in these athletic individuals. There was an evolution from the extensile single incision approach to two incisions with one specific for the anterior and lateral compartments and one specific for the superficial and deep posterior compartments that came into vogue. Many variations in technique have been described, including releasing the affected compartment from one incision, either large or small, or two smaller incisions. Recently endoscopic techniques that minimize morbidity have been introduced, as well as partial fasciectomy, in hopes of minimizing recurrence.

Indications and Contraindications

Exertional lower leg pain may be secondary to many causes; therefore, as in most orthopedic conditions, a careful history, physical examination, imaging studies, and compartment pressure studies are paramount in making the diagnosis before proceeding with operative intervention. Most commonly, the anterior and posterior compartments are involved; however, it is not unusual to have involvement of the lateral and superficial posterior compartments as well, usually in concert with involvement of the adjacent compartment. Most commonly it afflicts young athletes involved in running sports. The patient usually begins to experience a dull ache, crampiness, fullness, or a pressure sensation in the affected compartment that occurs after the individual has been exercising for a period of time. Although this period of time is variable from patient to patient, it usually has a predictable onset for that particular patient. For example, a long-distance runner usually notes that he or she can run at a certain speed and after a predictable period of time will have the onset of the symptoms. The pain usually begins as a dull ache or crampiness with a sensation of fullness. It is usually localized to the entire affected compartment. It usually increases to the point where activity has to be stopped. In some cases, the athlete may report an increase of intensity and duration with training or activity that pushes him or her over the threshold for generation of symptoms.

Sensory or motor disturbances sometimes occur, more commonly when the anterior compartment is affected. Transient "floppiness" of the ankle or a feeling of instability in the ankle and sensory disturbances in the distribution of the superficial peroneal nerve can occur when the anterior compartment is affected. This usually occurs more commonly when the athlete tries to "push through" the pain. In many cases, as symptoms become more chronic, there is a quicker onset of symptoms as the individual meets the maximum tolerability in a shorter period of time. Typically, cessation of exercise will relieve the pain, with more severe pain diminishing over 10 to 15 minutes, but a dull, low-level of symptoms can continue for a significant period of time. Classically, the discomfort will virtually disappear until exercise once again commences. Bilaterality is more common than uncommon. Typically, the pain is felt in the soft tissues and not the bone, and there will be no persistent pain the next day. If the pain is more bony in origin and persists despite the cessation of exercise, stress fracture, or periostitis (medial tibial syndrome), should be considered.[3]

Physical Examination

Unfortunately examination at rest is usually not helpful. Most of these patients are young, healthy athletes who are asymptomatic when they come into the office, making history of paramount importance in the suspicion of the diagnosis. In some cases, the athletes may be overconditioned with hypertrophy of the muscles and a compartment that cannot tolerate the 20% increase in muscle volume that is typically seen with exercise. It is important to look for fascial hernias, more typically seen in patients with anterior or lateral compartment syndrome. It has been reported in anywhere between 15% and 60% of patients. In the author's (AAS) experience, approximately 15% to 20% of patients will have fascial hernias. Oftentimes these are not evident at rest and can only be seen with the patient standing on his or her heel with active dorsiflexion of the foot. This is typically seen at the junction of the mid and distal thirds of the leg, where the superficial peroneal nerve exits through the lateral intermuscular septum to become superficial. It is felt that most likely these fascial hernias represent an enlargement of the foramen through which the superficial peroneal nerve exits. Fascial hernias have a definite association with the development of exertional compartment symptoms.

It is important to examine the whole extremity, including alignment, range of motion, and stability of the knee and ankle, as well as postural foot abnormalities. Manual muscle testing usually reveals no weakness. Careful palpation of the bone is paramount to rule out a stress fracture. In the tibia, the most common location is at the junction of the proximal and mid thirds, with localized tenderness over the posteromedial border of the tibia. Less commonly, a more serious tibial stress fracture in the midshaft, in the anterior cortex, will lead to tenderness and bony fullness on the easily palpable mid and anterior tibial cortices. This more serious stress fracture will be discussed in the next section.

More commonly, patients who present with posterior or posteromedial exertional pain should be carefully examined for medial tibial syndrome.[3] In these cases, there will be dif-fuse tenderness along the distal third of the posteromedial border of the tibia. This is considered to be a periostitis of the muscle attachments. Typically, these patients will also complain of symptoms with activities of daily living with persistent discomfort that gets worse with exercise and does not completely go away with rest. A careful examination of the distal pulses is important, although most of these athletes are young and do not have vascular claudication. The author (AAS) has seen several instances of dynamic popliteal artery entrapment being confused with exertional posterior compartment syndrome. Most commonly, patients will complain of coolness in the foot, but not always. Palpation of the posterior tibial pulse should be performed with the patient at rest and then with the patient actively plantar-flexing the foot with the knee extended. If the pulse diminishes with this maneuver, popliteal artery entrapment syndrome should be suspected and a vascular workup will be necessary. It is the author's (AAS) practice when presented with a patient with exertional calf pain to perform noninvasive Doppler studies as a screening test to look at vascular flow within the posterior tibial artery at rest and then with active plantar flexion of the foot and calculate the ankle brachial indices. In the vast majority of cases, this will be negative; however, if this simple test is done, this entity will not be missed. In this entity, there is a dynamic compression of the popliteal artery as it goes under the soleus, causing transient claudication with exercise.[4]

It is the author's (AAS) routine to examine the patient after reproduction of symptoms. This can be done either at the time of compartment pressure testing or by having the patient leave the office and run up and down stairs until the symptoms are reproduced. This will oftentimes help to substantiate the patient's history and will help the physician to localize the symptoms, particularly if sensory disturbances and motor weakness transiently occurs.

In general, the pain with anterior exertional compartment syndrome tends to be well localized to the anterior compartment. Frequently, however, in a patient with exertional posterior compartment syndrome the pain may be very poorly localized. Therefore, it becomes even more important to rule out bony or vascular etiologies in these cases. Furthermore in patients with profound peroneal nerve weakness with marked weakness of dorsiflexion after exercise, peroneal nerve entrapment at the fibular head should also be suspected.[2] The Tinel sign can usually be elicited in this location in these cases and the diagnosis can be confirmed by nerve conduction velocities of the peroneal nerve across the fibular head at rest and then after exercise.

After physical examination anteroposterior (AP) and lateral radiographs of the leg should be obtained to rule out any bony abnormalities. Chronic stress fractures can often be seen in these radiographs, but not always. It is the author's (AAS) routine to perform a technetium bone scan in all of these patients, particularly if there is any bony tenderness, if they have posterior symptoms, or if they present

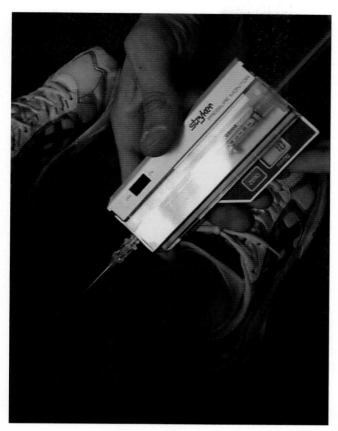

Fig. 62-1. This commercially available testing device is easy to calibrate and use.

measurement system,[5] subsequently we have found that repeated needle insertion via a commercially available slit catheter (Stryker Corp, Kalamazoo, Mich) was more practical than an indwelling catheter that could move or clot off **(Fig. 62-1)**.

Typically, we set up these pressure studies adjacent to a treadmill in the physical therapy department. By previous history and physical examination we have determined which compartments need to be tested. It is crucial that the catheter be inserted into the muscle and not the fascia or tendon. It is crucial to do all pressure measurements with the leg in a consistent position. We perform the pressure testing with the patient supine, with the foot in the neutral position, since it has been well established that foot position can affect the pressure measurements.[6] For the anterior compartment, the catheter should be placed within the muscle belly of the tibialis anterior. The author's (AAS) recommended landmark is the junction of the proximal and mid thirds of the leg, approximately 2 cm lateral to the tibial crest **(Fig. 62-2)**. The skin and subcutaneous tissue are anesthetized with a longer acting anesthetic that will last the duration of the pressure testing. After calibration of the catheter, it is inserted through the fascia, which can be felt with a "pop" into the tibialis anterior muscle. Resting pressure

with a presumed medial tibial syndrome with diffuse tenderness along the posterior third of the distal tibia. In these cases, one would see increased uptake on the delayed images.

Compartment Pressure Testing

The key test in the diagnostic workup is the recording of intracompartmental pressure. Although the etiology can be multifactorial, it is generally agreed that transient ischemia at the capillary level is the responsible culprit for this symptom. During exercise, muscles only get blood flow during the relaxation phase of exercise. With muscle contraction, the pressure is much higher than the capillary perfusion pressure. Theoretically, testing the muscle relaxation pressure would be the most precise method to document muscle ischemia; however, this is not practical to the clinician. There is no role for dynamic measurement of pressures during exercise, since this is affected by the intensity of the muscle contraction as well as the depth of catheter insertion. Therefore, the most clinically useful measurements are to test the pressure before exercise, immediately after exercise, and then at 5 minutes after exercise. The most practical instrument is the slit catheter method. Although in our original clinical studies we used a continuous slit catheter

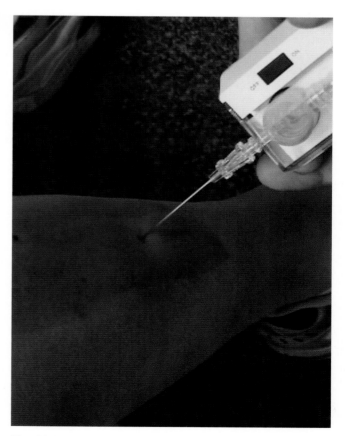

Fig. 62-2. Testing the anterior compartment is best performed by placing the needle in the muscle belly of the tibialis anterior in the proximal portion of the leg.

is recorded. For the lateral compartment, which is tested less commonly, the catheter is inserted at the same level, at the junction of the proximal and mid thirds of the leg, just over the fibular shaft in the muscle belly of the peroneals. For the superficial posterior compartment, placement of the catheter within the fleshy part of the medial head of the gastrocnemius is the easiest.

Compartment pressure testing for the deep posterior compartment is the most difficult, being fraught with error and potential complications. The most volume of muscle is in the proximal portion of the deep posterior compartment; however, placing the catheter blindly in this location can be hazardous because of the adjacent blood vessels. Likewise, there are multiple subcompartments of the deep posterior compartment, particularly the tibialis posterior compartment.[7] If one places a catheter in the distal part of the leg where the deep posterior compartment becomes more superficial, it is unfortunately not uncommon to place the catheter in or adjacent to tendon rather than muscle, making the pressure reading faulty. The author (AAS) usually recommends inserting the catheter carefully just posterior to the tibial shaft at the junction of the mid and distal thirds of the leg, at the location where the soleus bridge ends **(Fig. 62-3)**. The catheter is carefully angled proximally and an initial pass is usually made with a 25-gauge needle to ensure that the vascular structures are not violated. If this trial is passed, the catheter needle is placed in this location, usually in the fleshy portion of the flexor digitorum muscle. Having the patient contract and relax the muscle will assure the examiner that the catheter is in the proper location. Some authors have recommended the use of ultrasound guidance for testing of the deep posterior compartment.[8] Certainly if one would like to test the subcompartments, particularly the tibialis posterior compartment, computed tomography (CT) imaging or ultrasound guidance would be necessary. Davey et al.[7] advocated testing this compartment by inserting the needle anteriorly

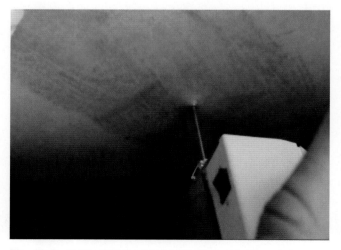

Fig. 62-3. For testing the deep posterior compartment, the needle is inserted into the muscle belly of the FDL, just posterior to the posteromedial border of the tibia.

through the interosseous membrane into the tibialis posterior. We have avoided this because of concerns about the safety of this maneuver. It has not been uncommon in the author's (AAS) experience to have to repeat the deep compartment testing if there is any question as to its validity.

After the resting pressures are obtained, the patient is instructed to run on the treadmill at an increasing cadence until symptoms are maximally reproduced. Usually placing the treadmill at an incline will help to reproduce symptoms faster. It is crucial that symptoms are maximally reproduced and the patient can run no longer before the postexercise pressure measurements are done. An immediate set of measurements after the cessation of exercise (1 minute) and then another set at 5 minutes are performed.

We feel that the pressure criteria set forth by Pedowitz et al.[9] are the most useful. The presence of one or more of the following criteria would be consistent with a diagnosis of exertional compartment syndrome: a resting pressure of ≥ 15 mm Hg, a 1-minute postexercise pressure of ≥ 30 mm Hg, and/or a 5-minute postexercise pressure of ≥ 20 mm Hg.

In summary, the indications for surgical treatment would be a history that is consistent with the diagnosis, compartment pressure testing that is positive in at least one and preferably two out of the three criteria mentioned above, and a patient who is unwilling to modify his or her activity level. Again, it is important to consider all entities in the differential diagnosis, namely nerve entrapment, popliteal artery entrapment, vascular claudication, stress fractures, and medial tibial syndrome. Contraindications would include any vascular insufficiency to the lower extremity, extensive varicosities over the affected compartment, poor skin circulation, and a patient who is unwilling to accept the risks of any potential surgical complications or the potential for an unsuccessful outcome.

Surgical Technique

If the patient truly has exertional compartment syndrome, there really are only two choices: either modify his or her activity to alleviate the symptoms or have a surgical fasciotomy. Obviously the more competitive and avid the athlete, the more likely the patient is to undergo the latter choice. Although different surgical choices have been advocated, it is generally agreed that fasciotomy of the affected compartment is the treatment of choice for this condition. We prefer one incision to release the anterior and/or lateral compartments and one incision to release the deep and superficial posterior compartments of the leg. In those cases in which both the anterior and deep posterior compartments are involved, both incisions are utilized.

Surgical Release of the Anterior and Lateral Compartments

The technique of anterior compartment release involves making one skin incision to release both the anterior and

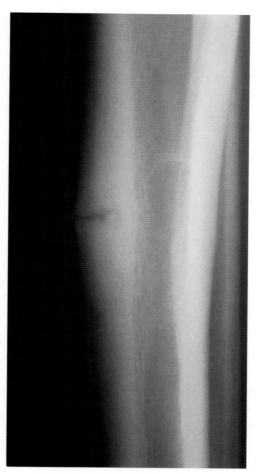

Fig. 62-12. Lateral radiograph of the tibia of a female collegiate basketball player demonstrating the defect of an anterior tibial stress fracture. (Photo courtesy of Robert A. Arciero, MD, Farmington, Conn.)

stress fractures have also been reported. Posteromedial tibial stress fractures usually respond favorably to cessation of the inciting activity. One study suggested that the supplemental use of a pneumatic brace may allow athletes to return to activity sooner than traditional treatment alone.[19]

A less common, but more troublesome location is the anterior cortex (tension side) of the tibia **(Fig. 62-12)**. This site is predisposed to delayed union or nonunion because of the relative hypovascularity of this area and the constant tension applied to it by the posterior musculature. In contrast to compression side (posteromedial) tibial stress fractures, which usually occur in distance runners, tension side (anterior) stress fractures typically occur in athletes involved in sports with repetitive jumping and leaping activities.[17]

Clinical Evaluation

Patients with a tibial stress fracture commonly present with a history of an insidious onset of pain over a period of days to weeks. Pain is usually focal, most commonly in the proximal metaphysis or diaphysis, but diffuse tibial pain is not uncommon. As with all stress fractures, symptoms are typically aggravated by activity and relieved by rest. However, pain at rest and in the evening after stressful activities is also sometimes noted. A careful review of the patient's exercise or training program, especially any recent changes in duration or intensity, as well as an assessment of the patient's general health and nutritional status must be performed. This may help determine whether the injury is the result of overuse (an athlete increasing his or her level of performance) or an overloading injury (a poorly conditioned new athlete with poor muscular development).[20] Also, the menstrual history in female athletes must be assessed, as amenorrhea or oligomenorrhea is associated with stress fractures as part of the "female athletic triad."[17,20]

Localized bone tenderness is commonly found on physical examination. With anterior tibial stress fractures, point tenderness is usually in the central third of the anterior tibia. Stress fractures of both the anterior and posteromedial cortices may exhibit local swelling and palpable periosteal thickening due to their subcutaneous location.[17] A positive "hop-test," in which one-legged hopping reproduces pain at the site of the stress fracture, is frequently seen.[18] An evaluation of limb biomechanics must be performed to identify risk factors such as muscle imbalance, limb-length discrepancy, or excessive foot pronation.[17]

The differential diagnosis of tibial stress fractures includes tibial stress reaction or "medial tibial stress syndrome." Unlike stress fractures, in stress reactions the bone is weakened but not physiologically disrupted. In stress fractures, there is a focal defect in the bone that has the potential to progress to complete fracture.[17,21] Other pathologic processes in the differential include muscle strain, fascial hernia, periostitis, infection, neoplasm, and exertional compartment syndrome.[17,20]

Imaging

As is typical for stress fractures, radiographs can be normal for weeks initially and sometimes may reveal no findings until several months after the onset of symptoms. Periosteal reaction, cortical thickening, cortical lucency, or even a fracture line may be seen on later films. With anterior tibial stress fractures, late films may demonstrate a characteristic "wedge" or V-shaped defect in the anterior cortex (Fig. 62-12, **Fig. 62-13)**. Callus formation is rarely seen on even late radiographs. Once the cortex becomes hypertrophied and the defect widens—the characteristic "dreaded black line"— healing capacity is extremely limited and healing time is markedly prolonged.

Radionucleotide imaging is an extremely useful modality to aid in the diagnosis of tibial stress fractures. The bone scan can be used to differentiate soft tissue from bony

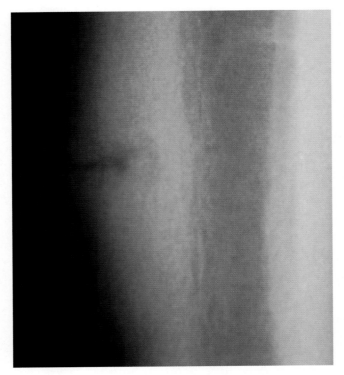

Fig. 62-13. Close-up of the defect. Note the cortical hypertrophy and callus formation. (Photo courtesy of Robert A. Arciero, MD, Farmington, Conn.)

injury with considerable accuracy and may be positive within 6 to 72 hours of the onset of pain. The use of the triple bone scan, with angiogram (phase I), blood pool (phase II), and delayed static images (phase III), allows the differentiation of old stress fractures from acute ones and partial from complete ones. Acute stress fractures are depicted as discrete, localized, sometimes linear areas of increased uptake on all three phases. Soft tissue injuries are characterized by increased uptake on only the first two phases. Minimal activity on the bone scan indicates nonunion of the stress fracture.[17] Medial tibial stress syndrome—"shin splints"—typically demonstrates a more diffuse area of increased activity over the superficial or periosteal layer of the bone on all three phases. Bone scans also provide information on abnormalities that may occur at locations distant from the site of pain in athletes presenting with referred pain. Ultrasound, thermography, computerized tomography (CT), and magnetic resonance imaging (MRI) have all been used in the diagnosis of tibial stress fracture with variable results. These methods are generally not cost-effective. MRI studies, of note, can demonstrate findings that can be falsely suggestive of a tumor. Studies of athletes have shown bone scans to be virtually 100% sensitive in diagnosing stress fractures, although its specificity is slightly lower than the radiograph. Radiographic evaluation, on the other hand, is quite insensitive but very specific. Currently, the diagnostic accuracy of radiography and bone scan used in combination is not improved with the use of the additional diagnostic aids listed above.[18,20]

Treatment

Stress fractures of the anterior cortex of the tibia were first described in ballet dancers by Burrows in 1956.[22] Four of five dancers returned to activity at an average of 15 months following diagnosis. One of the five sustained a complete fracture of the mid tibia 2 weeks after onset of symptoms. Subsequent reports by Friedenberg (1971),[23] Stanitski et al. (1978),[24] and Brahms et al. (1980)[25] described protracted courses and continued symptoms in many high-level collegiate and professional athletes. Brahms et al. reported on a professional football player with an asymptomatic anterior tibial stress fracture who continued to play for three and a half seasons before he sustained a spontaneous complete fracture through the stress fracture area without any trauma. This fracture was treated with closed reduction and casting and the athlete never returned to his sport.

In 1985, Green et al.[21] reported six cases of nonunion of stress fractures of the anterior tibial cortex in athletes. The fractures progressed to complete fractures in five of the six athletes. Five of the six patients had been treated with casting for an average of 6 months. Three patients were treated with bone grafting and healed their fractures within 5 months following surgery. A later study by Rettig et al.[26] described successful treatment of seven of eight competitive basketball players with rest and pulsed electromagnetic field therapy. Only one patient required bone grafting. The average time from initial symptoms to return to competition was 12.5 months.

Initial treatment of anterior tibial stress fractures is generally a period of activity cessation, with or without immobilization. Most agree this period of conservative treatment should continue for a minimum of 4 to 6 months.[17] In 1974, Clement[27] outlined a two-phased rehabilitation program which remains useful today. Phase I includes pain control with local physiotherapy, nonsteroidal anti-inflammatory medication, and ice massage. Modified rest is instituted, which included normal weight bearing for activities of daily living but cessation of the offending activity. Alternative non–weight-bearing activities such as cycling, swimming, and aqua training are recommended to maintain fitness. During this phase, stretching and flexibility training are emphasized, as well as local muscle strengthening and retraining.[18,27]

Phase II begins when the athlete has been free of pain for at least 10 to 14 days and includes the continuation of the modalities of phase I plus a gradual reintroduction of sport.[18,27] Pain has been found to be the most satisfactory guide in assessing progress and increasing the workload in the recovery period. The most important component of phase II treatment is the graded reintroduction of activity. Usually, this means training on an alternate day basis.

Phase II also includes modification of running surfaces, proper footwear, and orthotic control of excessive foot pronation. In the study by Matheson et al.,[18] all 157 tibial stress fractures identified were treated successful with this nonoperative regimen. Three of those cases were treated with electromagnetic radiation for delayed healing. In general, early diagnosis and treatment will allow successful conservative management in the vast majority of patients.

Numerous treatments have been described for treatment of recalcitrant tibial stress fractures. Again, anterior cortical stress fractures are the subset of tibial stress fractures that are most prone to this delay or failure of healing. Lack of healing by 4 to 6 months is an indication to consider more aggressive therapy. As noted earlier, there has been one study that documented successful treatment with pulsed electromagnetic field treatment,[26] while others have shown no benefit.[21] Excision and grafting have been shown to yield successful results.[21] More, recently intramedullary nailing has become a favored approach to recalcitrant anterior tibial stress fractures **(Fig. 62-14)**. Chang and Harris[20] reported good to excellent results in five military personnel treated with reamed unlocked tibial nails. Other studies have also reported success with this technique.[28-31] For the high-level athlete, intramedullary nailing provides an opportunity to return to sport within weeks rather than months and may be worth the inherent risks of the surgery.[32]

Tibial Intramedullary Nailing Operative Technique

Intramedullary nailing is indicated in the athlete with symptomatic tibial stress fracture that has failed nonoperative treatment for a period of at least 3 to 6 months. In the high-level athlete who desires a quicker return to athletic activity or cannot accept prolonged protection, earlier fixation can be considered. The presence of anterior cortical transverse striations—the "dreaded black line"—which signifies a stress fracture that is prone to delayed union, nonunion, and even complete fracture, may be an indication to intervene surgically earlier as well.

The procedure is performed on a radiolucent table. After identification of the correct operative limb and induction of general anesthesia, a padded tourniquet is placed around the upper thigh. The tourniquet is not usually inflated during the procedure. A bump is placed under the ipsilateral buttock to help control against limb external rotation. The operative limb is supported by a bump under the knee (rolled up blankets or any of many commercially available supports) to provide knee flexion during the procedure.

A 4- to 5-cm longitudinal incision is made over the patellar tendon. The approach to the proximal tibia is made medial to the patellar tendon. In this athletic patient population, we advise against a tendon splitting approach favored by many in fracture management. Dissection through the infrapatellar fat pad exposes a flat spot anterior to the tibial plateau and posterior and just proximal to the patellar tendon insertion that is the starting point for nail insertion. Fluoroscopy is used to confirm the correct starting position in the medial-lateral direction. The starting point should lie over the medial tibial spine or its lateral down slope. A curved awl is used to create a starting hole into the proximal tibia. As the awl is inserted, the surgeon should lower his or her hand to ensure anterior position of the hole. If it is angled too posterior, the guide wire may go out the posterior cortex. Fluoroscopy is again used to ensure the correct orientation of the starter hole. It should line up with the medullary canal. The awl is removed and a ball-tipped guide wire is inserted down the medullary canal, stopping at the physeal scar of the distal tibia. Proper position of the guide wire is confirmed on both AP and lateral fluoroscopic images. The medullary canal is then sequentially reamed with flexible reamers over the guide wire. The canal should be reamed up to a diameter in which enough "chatter" is encountered indicating snug fit with the endosteal surface. The nail length is measured with a ruler supplied by the implant manufacturer or by subtracting the exposed length of the guide wire from a second guide wire of the same length. The proximal end of the nail should lie just beneath the cortex at the entry hole. Care must be taken to ensure that the nail does not protrude out of the

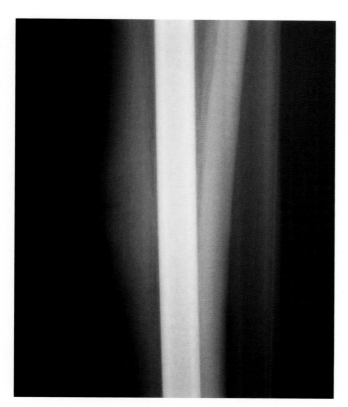

Fig. 62-14. Lateral radiograph 6 months after intramedullary nailing. (Photo courtesy of Robert A. Arciero, MD, Farmington, Conn.)

hole, which could cause abrasion of the patellar tendon. The ball-tipped guide wire is removed and exchanged for a straight-tipped guide wire. Fluoroscopy is again used to confirm position of the new guide wire in the medullary canal. The selected nail is inserted over the guide wire into final position down to the level of the distal tibial physeal scar. Fluoroscopy is utilized to confirm the final position of the nail. We agree with most authors that locking of the nails is unnecessary since there is no rotational instability with these in situ nailings, although, some authors have advocated proximal locking to provide dynamic compression with weight bearing.[30] The guide wire and insertion handle assembly are removed and the wound closed in standard fashion. A compressive dressing is applied.

Patients can generally be allowed to bear weight as tolerated. The athlete can generally be allowed to return to running and jumping activities as early as six weeks after surgery.

Conclusion

Stress fracture of the tibia should always be considered in the differential diagnosis of leg pain in the athlete. Athletes and military recruits involved in running sports seem particularly susceptible to this injury. Posteromedial tibial stress fractures are most common and are generally responsive to activity cessation. Anterior cortex tibial stress fractures, though less common, are more problematic as there is a higher likelihood of prolonged healing or progression to complete fracture. Use of radionucleotide imaging allows early detection and treatment. Conservative management is effective in the vast majority of these injuries, although a few will require surgical intervention. Intramedullary nailing is the preferred method for fixation of recalcitrant anterior tibial stress fractures. The goal in rehabilitation is to return the athlete to sport with a gradual reintroduction of activity at a rate that will allow "remodeling adequate for the osseous system to meet the required physical stresses."[18]

■ FIFTH METATARSAL STRESS FRACTURES

Anatomy and Classification

Fractures of the proximal fifth metatarsal can be divided into three anatomic zones.[33,34] Zone 1 is the cancellous tuberosity and includes the insertion of the peroneus brevis tendon as well as the calcaneometatarsal ligamentous branch of the plantar fascia. These fractures typically extend into the metatarsocuboid joint. Zone 2 is the more distal tuberosity and incorporates the dorsal and plantar intermetatarsal ligaments. Fractures in this area extend into the articulation between the fourth and fifth metatarsals. Zone 3 begins distal to this area and extends distally into the diaphysis.

Variations in the morphology of the proximal fifth metatarsal and its articulations may make it difficult to differentiate the exact border of each zone. However, in general, these anatomic zones correspond to the three common clinical fracture patterns: tuberosity avulsion, Jones fracture, and diaphyseal injuries, which are often stress fractures **(Fig. 62-15A)**.[35]

The importance of the blood supply of the fifth metatarsal and fracture healing has been well demonstrated (Fig. 62-15B).[36,37] The nutrient artery enters medially in the middle third of the bone and divides into a distal and proximal branch after penetrating the cortex. In addition, there is a rich plexus of metaphyseal vessels at each end. Injuries to the proximal diaphysis may disrupt the intraosseous vessel proximally, limiting the blood supply to the distal aspect of the proximal segment, with a resultant unfavorable effect on fracture healing.

The widespread use of the term "Jones fracture" to describe all fractures of the proximal fifth metatarsal has contributed to the controversy regarding the outcomes and preferred method of treatment.[38] This eponym should be reserved for a transverse fracture at the junction of the diaphysis and the metaphysis, without extension distal to the fourth-fifth intermetatarsal articulation **(Fig. 62-16A,B)**. Medial comminution is often present.[7] A true Jones fracture is not a "stress fracture"; it is an acute injury with no history of prodromal symptoms and no stress reaction visible on radiographs.

Diaphyseal stress fractures are the result of a summation of repetitive forces, any of which individually would be innocuous. DeLee[39] defined the criteria for a stress fracture of the proximal fifth metatarsal as a history of prodromal symptoms from the lateral aspect of the foot, radiographic signs of a stress reaction of the bone, and no

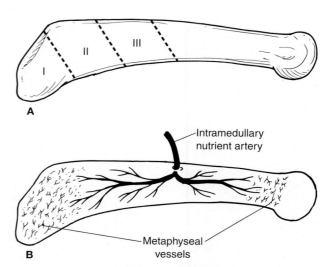

Fig. 62-15. A: The three anatomic and clinical zones for fractures of the proximal fifth metatarsal. **B:** The arterial blood supply of the fifth metatarsal.

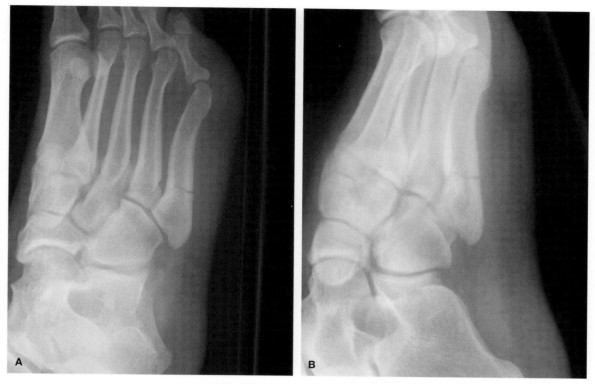

Fig. 62-16. A,B: Acute Jones fracture. The fracture line is at the junction of zones 1 and 2; there is no cortical hypertrophy or periosteal reaction.

history of previous treatment for a fracture. Torg et al.[40] divided diaphyseal stress fractures into three types. Type I acute fractures are characterized by a fracture line with sharp clear margins, no widening or radiolucency, no periosteal reaction, and minimal cortical widening; often the fracture involves only the lateral cortex. Type II is a delayed union with a history of previous injury or fracture; both cortices are usually disrupted and there is associated periosteal bone formation, widening at the fracture line, cortical hypertrophy, and intramedullary sclerosis. Type III is a nonunion exhibited by repetitive trauma and recurrent symptoms, bone resorption with radiolucency at the fracture line, and sclerotic bone formation at the fracture site that obliterates the medullary canal. There is obviously some overlap among these subtypes, and these classifications represent both a clinical and radiographic continuum **(Fig. 62-17A,B,C)**.

Treatment

The natural history and outcomes of nonoperative and operative treatment for proximal fifth metatarsal fractures is difficult to determine because many of the published reports include a mixture of acute Jones fractures and diaphyseal stress fractures.

Three studies have described the results of treatment for acute Jones fractures. In Torg's[40] series, 14 of 15 (93%) of acute Jones fractures healed after an average of 6.5 weeks in a non–weight-bearing short leg cast. Clapper et al.[41] reported union in 18 of 25 (72%) true Jones fractures treated non–weight bearing in a cast for 8 weeks and then weight bearing as tolerated in a cast or walker boot. The average time to union was 21.2 weeks. The single nonunion in Torg's series healed after medullary curettage and bone grafting. In the study of Clapper et al., there were seven clinical and radiographic nonunions at 25 weeks after injury; all healed with intramedullary screw fixation at an average of 12 weeks. Quill[35] reported 100% union in 11 true Jones fractures treated with immediate intramedullary screw fixation; the average time to union was 7.4 weeks.

The indications for surgery in acute Jones fractures remain unclear. High performance athletes may benefit from early intramedullary screw fixation, as this appears to be more predictable and shortens the recovery time. Acute displaced fractures are a relative indication for operative treatment.

The treatment options and decision-making variables for Torg type I diaphyseal stress fractures are similar to acute nondisplaced Jones fractures: non–weight-bearing cast immobilization for 6 to 8 weeks or intramedullary screw fixation. Torg types II and III diaphyseal stress fractures, as well as nonunion or delayed union of Jones fractures, are best managed with intramedullary screw fixation and/or inlay bone grafting.

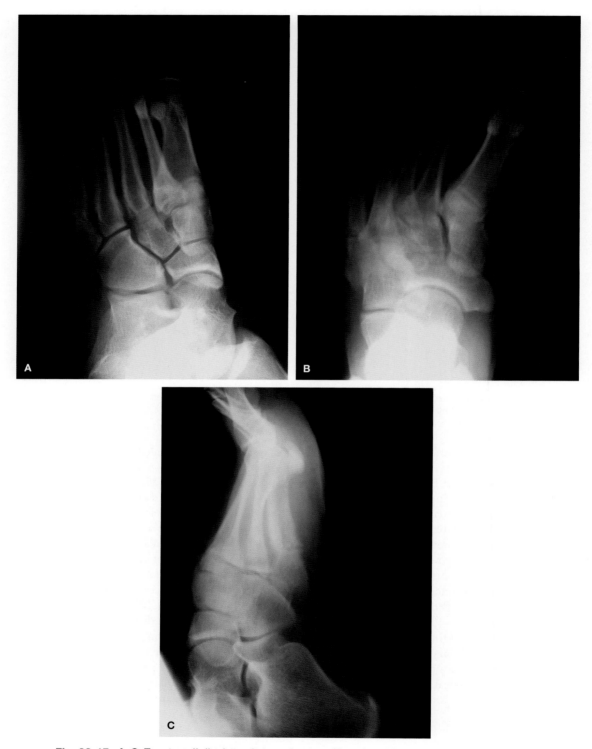

Fig. 62-17. A–C: Torg type II diaphyseal stress fracture. Note the widening of the fracture line and periosteal bone formation.

Torg[40] reported the results of corticocancellous bone grafting, without internal fixation, for diaphyseal stress fractures. The concept and method is similar to the classic Russe technique for scaphoid nonunions[42]; a rectangular graft is harvested from the ipsilateral distal tibia and inserted into a

trough on the lateral aspect of the fracture site after drilling of the medullary canal. In a series of 20 fractures, 19 healed with this technique, there was only 1 nonunion, and no complications. In a later report from the same institution, Glasgow et al.[43] described five patients with complications

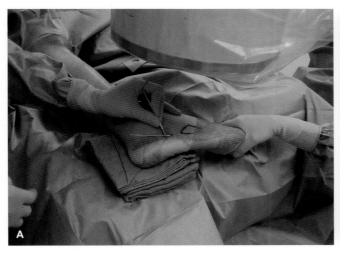 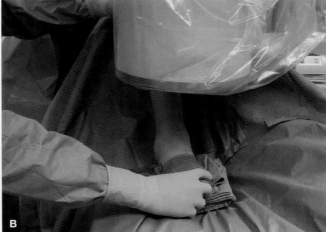

Fig. 62-18. **A,B:** Fluoroscopic control; flexion of the knee past 90 degrees allows AP imaging.

after this procedure: four refractures and one nonunion. The relative percentage of complications in relation to a defined treatment group was not specified.

The results of intramedullary screw fixation for nonunions of Jones fractures and diaphyseal stress fractures have been reported by several authors. In Quill's[35] series, nine of ten diaphyseal stress fractures treated with a cannulated intramedullary screw united at an average of 6.5 weeks. The single nonunion was felt to be due to osteogenesis imperfecta. Successful union was obtained at an average of 7.5 weeks in all ten athletes with diaphyseal stress fractures treated by DeLee[39] with closed intramedullary screw fixation. Pain over the screw head was present in 7 patients. Portland et al.[44] reported 100% union in 22 patients with acute Jones fractures and Torg type I and II diaphyseal stress fractures treated with early intramedullary screw fixation. Healing occurred at an average of 6.2 weeks for acute Jones fractures and type I diaphyseal stress fractures; the mean time to union was 8.3 weeks for type II stress fractures. The overall complication rate was 9.5%.

Three studies highlight the complications and potential pitfalls of intramedullary screw fixation for proximal fifth metatarsal fractures. In a series reported by Glasgow et al.,[43] refractures and nonunions were related to small diameter screws (less than 4.5 mm) and early weightbearing. Wright et al.[45] described six instances of refracture of clinically and radiographically united fractures of the proximal fifth metatarsal after intramedullary screw fixation. All patients were high-level competitive athletes who returned to full activities an average of 8.5 weeks after fixation. Fixation failure seemed to correlate with small diameter screws. Larson et al.[46] reported a failure rate of 40% following intramedullary cannulated screw fixation of proximal fifth metatarsal fractures. There were four refractures and two symptomatic nonunions in 15 patients. Failure was related to an earlier return to full activity (6.8 weeks versus 9 weeks) and an elite level of competitive athletics (83% division 1 college or

professional versus 11%) in the failure group compared to patients with a successful outcome.

Surgical Technique: Percutaneous Intramedullary Screw Fixation

The patient is placed in the supine position on a radiolucent table with a bolster beneath the ipsilateral buttock; general or regional anesthetic is employed. Image intensification with a C-arm is required. It is helpful to have the entire limb draped free so that the knee can be flexed past 90 degrees; this facilitates imaging of the foot **(Fig. 62-18A,B)**. A tourniquet is generally not utilized. A 2- to 3-cm incision is made parallel to the plantar surface of the foot, beginning 2 cm proximal to the tip of the tuberosity **(Fig. 62-19)**. The correct position for the incision is confirmed with C-arm. Blunt dissection is carried down to the tuberosity. A drill guide is used to protect the soft tissues and a 2.5-mm drill is utilized to open the entry portal **(Fig. 62-20A,B)**. The correct

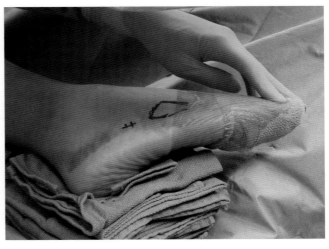

Fig. 62-19. Skin incision proximal to tuberosity.

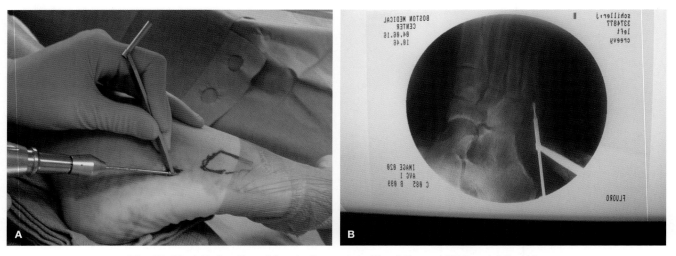

Fig. 62-20. A,B: Creation of the starting portal with a 2.5-mm drill bit and drill guide.

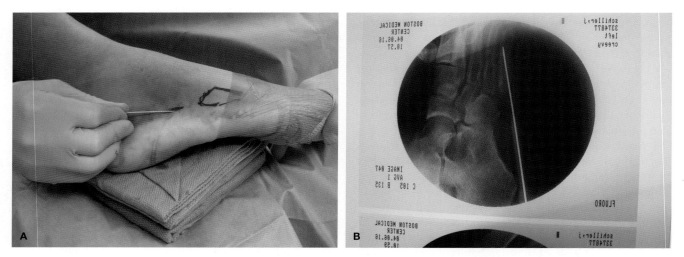

Fig. 62-21. A,B: Insertion of a flexible guidewire down the intramedullary canal.

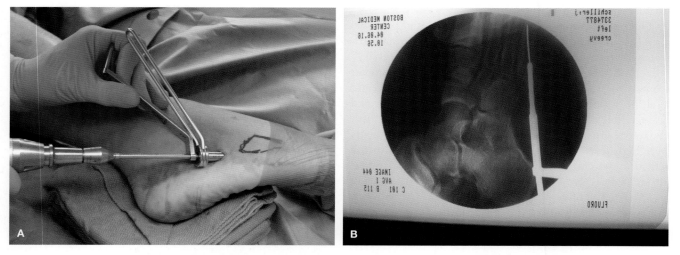

Fig. 62-22. A,B: Preparation of the intramedullary canal with a 3.2-mm cannulated drill and protective drill sleeves.

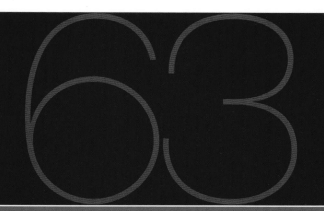

SURGICAL TREATMENT OF LIGAMENTOUS INJURIES ABOUT THE ANKLE

■ LISA WASSERMAN, MD, FRCS(C), ANNUNZIATO AMENDOLA, MD, FRCS(C)

■ HISTORY OF THE TECHNIQUE

Ligamentous injury and surgical repair about the foot and ankle may involve the lateral ligament complex, the syndesmosis ligaments, or the ligaments of the medial side of the ankle joint. This chapter details the indications and surgical technique of anatomic and nonanatomic lateral-sided reconstructions, treatment of syndesmosis injuries, and the management of the emerging entity of medial ankle instability.

There have been several modifications of the original procedure, described by Brostrom[1] in 1966, of direct repair of the lateral ankle ligaments. Gould et al.[2] recommended proximal advancement of the inferior extensor retinaculum to the distal fibula to reinforce the repair and to stabilize the subtalar component of recurrent instability. This modification has been shown to be biomechanically stronger in reducing anterior drawer and talar tilt when compared with the Watson-Jones and Chrisman-Snook procedures in a cadaver model.[3] Karlsson et al.[4] advocated shortening of the elongated lateral ligament complex and reattachment to the fibula through drill holes. More recently, suture anchors have become the preferred mode of reattachment of the ligaments.[5]

Nonanatomic reconstructions (Evans, Watson-Jones) have generated concern regarding excessive tightening of the subtalar joint and the sacrifice of the peroneus brevis, a dynamic stabilizer of the ankle.[6,7] These issues have contributed to the decrease in popularity of nonanatomic repairs as first-line procedures for lateral ligament instability. However, they remain useful in the setting of revision reconstructions for lateral instability.

■ INDICATIONS AND CONTRAINDICATIONS

Complaints of instability must be probed to determine whether true mechanical instability due to ligamentous laxity exists. This is differentiated from functional instability related to muscular weakness or pain inhibition reflexes from associated injury. If pain is not present between sprains, true mechanical instability may be the primary problem. Stress radiographs have repeatedly demonstrated low specificity due to the large variability in physiologic values and the lack of correlation with clinical symptoms and therefore may not be useful on a routine basis.[8] Initial treatment for all patients, regardless of the duration of the instability, involves a therapy program of peroneal muscle strengthening and proprioceptive training, combined with use of a lace-up brace for high-risk activities. This regimen is effective in the majority of patients. The remaining patients are candidates for operative stabilization, provided that they exhibit true symptoms of mechanical instability and have ligamentous laxity on physical examination.

■ SURGICAL TECHNIQUES

Anatomy

The lateral ligamentous complex of the ankle joint consists of the anterior talofibular ligament (ATFL), the calcaneofibular ligament (CFL), and the posterior talofibular ligament (PTFL). A fourth structure, the lateral talocalcaneal ligament (LTCL), is variable and may be found coalescing with the

ATFL and/or the CFL. The ATFL is the primary restraint to inversion in plantar flexion. It also resists anterolateral translation of the talus in the mortise. It originates 10 mm proximal to the tip of the fibula, just lateral to the margin of the articular cartilage. It is directed 45 degrees medially toward the talus in the coronal plane and inserts directly distal to the articular cartilage of the talar body, averaging 18 mm dorsal to the subtalar joint.[9] It is the weakest of the lateral ligaments.

The CFL is the primary restraint to inversion when the ankle is in the neutral or dorsiflexed position. The CFL originates on the anterior edge of the fibula, 9 mm proximal to the distal tip. It subtends an angle of 133 degrees from the posterior border of the fibula, inserting on the calcaneus 13 mm distal to the subtalar joint, deep to the peroneal tendon sheaths.[9] The PTFL is the strongest of the collateral ligaments and bridges the posterolateral tubercle of the talus to the posterior aspect of the lateral malleolus.

Gould Modification of Brostrom Technique

The skin incision begins at the tip of the distal fibula and is carried proximally in an inverted "J" along the anterior border of the fibula over a distance of 4 cm. Care is taken to avoid the intermediate dorsal cutaneous branch of the superficial peroneal nerve. The inferior extensor retinaculum is dissected free at its proximal border for later use **(Fig. 63-1)**. The peroneal sheath is opened distally to allow retraction of the peroneal tendons. The CFL is identified under the tendons and the ATFL is identified within the capsule more anteriorly **(Fig. 63-2)**. The ligaments and capsule are then sharply incised 2 mm distal to the fibula, and a periosteal flap is raised proximally off the bone. A burr is used to roughen the fibula anteriorly and distally. Three suture anchor drill holes are then placed, two at the anterior border of the fibula, 1 cm from the tip, and the third slightly more distally **(Fig. 63-3)**. The suture anchors are inserted. Alternatively, transfibular drill holes may be used instead of suture anchors. These are made with a 2.0-mm drill bit and small, sharp, bone-holding forceps are

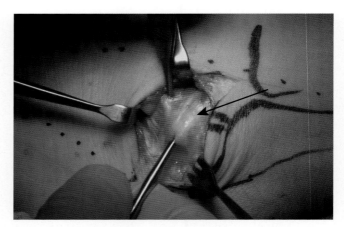

Fig. 63-2. The ATFL is exposed *(arrow)* and the metal probe identifies the distal tip of the fibula.

passed through the drill holes to complete the tunnels. This is technically more difficult and time-consuming and risks breakage through the tunnel sites. Next, redundancy of the capsuloligamentous complex is excised and the ligaments are reefed, beginning posteriorly with the CFL. The sutures are tied with the foot held in dorsiflexion and eversion, and this position is maintained throughout the remainder of the case. The periosteal flap of the distal fibula is then sutured down over the newly reattached ligaments. Finally, the inferior extensor retinaculum is mobilized proximally **(Fig. 63-4)** and secured over the repaired ligaments with absorbable suture **(Fig. 63-5)**. The skin is closed with an absorbable monofilament subcuticular stitch followed by surgical tapes. A non–weight-bearing fiberglass cast is applied with the foot maintained in its dorsiflexed and everted position.

Nonanatomic Reconstruction

Colville et al.[7] developed a reconstruction using a split peroneus brevis tendon graft that reproduces the orientation of the native ATFL and CFL. The advantage of this configu-

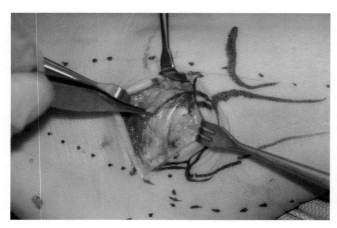

Fig. 63-1. The inferior extensor retinaculum *(held in forceps)* is mobilized for use later in the repair.

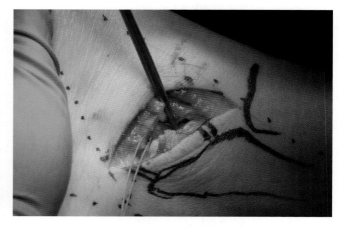

Fig 63-3. A suture anchor has been placed in the tip of the fibula. A second anchor is being placed more anteriorly.

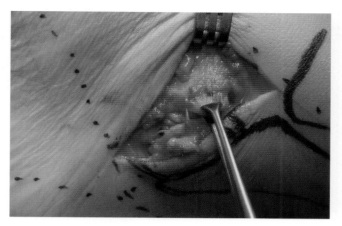

Fig. 63-4. The inferior extensor retinaculum is reefed over the capsuloligamentous repair.

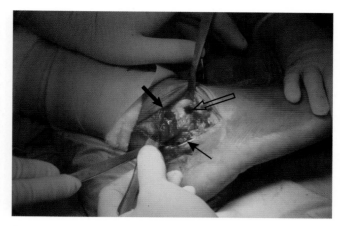

Fig 63-6. The bony tunnel in the fibula is visible *(open arrow)*, as are the drill holes in the talus distally *(small arrow)* and in the calcaneus inferiorly *(large arrow)*.

ration is that subtalar laxity will be limited only to the physiologic amount allowed by the intact CFL. This technique may be modified by using an Achilles tendon bone-block allograft in place of sacrificing the peroneus brevis tendon.

Modified Technique Using Achilles Bone-Block Allograft

The patient is positioned supine with a bump under the ipsilateral hip. A tourniquet is used on the thigh. A longitudinal incision is made on the anterior border of the distal fibula, curving posteriorly around the tip in a backward "J." Care is taken to avoid the intermediate dorsal cutaneous nerve. The peroneal tendons are identified by opening their sheath and are retracted posteriorly to reveal the calcaneal attachment site of the CFL. The attachment site of the ATFL on the talus is exposed, 18 mm dorsal to the subtalar joint, and a drill hole for a tendon-securing screw is made in this location. The fibular site of attachment of the ATFL is located 9 mm proximal to the tip on its anterior border. At this starting point, a tunnel is drilled with a 6-mm drill bit,

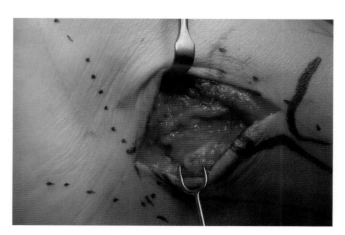

Fig. 63-5. The inferior extensor retinaculum sewn in place with absorbable suture.

aiming directly posteriorly and ending halfway through the width of the fibula. A second 6-mm drill hole is begun in the fibula at its tip and continued until it meets the first drill hole, forming a tunnel. The site of attachment of the native CFL to the calcaneus is identified, 13 mm distal to the subtalar joint, at the previously described angle of approximately 45 degrees to the fibula. A drill hole is made here to accept eventual placement of the Achilles bone-block **(Fig. 63-6)**. The donor Achilles tendon is then sewn with a baseball stitch using heavy nonabsorbable suture. The graft is then placed through the tunnel from posterior to anterior with the aid of an arthroscopic suture passer. The bone block of the allograft is secured to the calcaneus through the drill hole with a bone-tendon screw **(Fig. 63-7A,B)**. The anterior arm of the graft is secured under tension through the talar drill hole with a soft-tissue screw, taking care to hold the foot everted while the graft is fixated **(Fig. 63-8)**. The skin is closed with an absorbable monofilament subcuticular suture and a below-knee, non-weight bearing cast is applied with the foot held everted.

Syndesmosis Injury

The distal tibiofibular articulation is secured by the anterior and posterior inferior tibiofibular ligaments (AITFL and PITFL, respectively), the transverse tibiofibular ligament, and the interosseous membrane. Syndesmotic ankle sprain, also referred to as a "high ankle sprain," results from an external rotation or abduction force at the ankle. Less commonly, a severe inversion force may be the cause. Syndesmosis injury is estimated to be involved in 1% to 10% of all ankle sprains. Cases that are refractory to conservative treatment, those displaying diastasis on stress radiographs, and patients presenting longer than 3 months since the time of injury should be managed with surgical treatment. In the case of chronic diastasis, the medial ankle joint is opened and any interposed soft tissues in the medial gutter are debrided to allow reduction of the talus within the mortise.

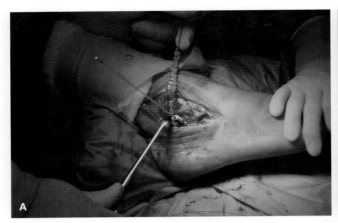 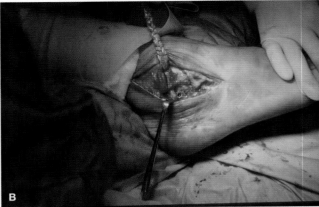

Fig. 63-7. **A:** The graft has been placed through the fibular tunnel and the bone block is being secured through the calcaneal drill hole. **B:** Completed fixation of the calcaneal side of the graft.

A large reduction clamp is used to reduce the syndesmosis while two 4.5-mm syndesmosis screws are placed through four cortices. The postoperative plaster splint is removed after 2 weeks, however, non–weight-bearing status is maintained for 6 weeks. The screws are routinely removed after 12 weeks. Postsprain impingement lesions of the syndesmosis may occur. These result from a fascicle of the AITFL that becomes trapped intra-articularly.[10] Treatment involves arthroscopic removal of the fascicle.

■ TECHNICAL ALTERNATIVES AND PITFALLS

The Role of Arthroscopy in Lateral Ankle Ligament Reconstruction

Successful operative stabilization of lateral ankle laxity is followed by persistence of ankle pain in up to 35% of

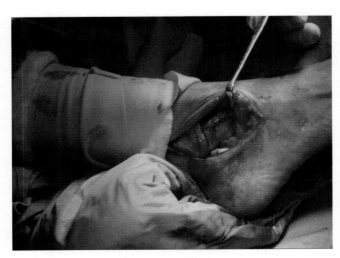

Fig. 63-8. The completed graft, with fixation at both the calcaneal and talar ends.

patients.[11] Intra-articular lesions occurring at the time of initial injury or during subsequent instability episodes may be responsible for this continuation of pain. Taga et al.[12] found osteochondral lesions (OCL) in 95% of chronically unstable ankles. Even high-grade lesions were not noted radiographically, requiring arthroscopy to make the diagnosis. Kibler[13] found OCLs in 83%, while Komenda and Ferkel[11] demonstrated intra-articular pathology in 93%, with a 25% incidence of OCLs. Other abnormalities included loose bodies, synovitis, adhesions, and osteophytes. Injuries were treated with common arthroscopic procedures, yielding good or excellent results in 96%. Hintermann et al.[14] discovered cartilage lesions in 66% of chronically unstable ankle joints, as well as deltoid ligament injury in 40%, and rotational instability in 25%.

Based on the findings of the literature, it is prudent to address all intra-articular pathology at the time of ligamentous stabilization for chronic ankle instability. If the patient has isolated recurrent instability without symptoms between episodes, we do not perform arthroscopy prior to stabilization. If the patient is having symptoms such as pain, catching, or swelling between instability episodes, our preference is to carry out arthroscopic evaluation prior to proceeding to ligamentous repair, under the same anesthetic. Swelling from fluid extravasation is present but usually is not an impediment to identifying anatomy and performing the procedure.

Additional Procedures

Peroneal tendon exploration and repair may be required in conjunction with lateral ligament reconstruction. Tears in the tendons are found in up to 10% of patients with recurrent ankle sprains and may be identified preoperatively by magnetic resonance imaging (MRI) if suspected clinically. This pathology can be attributed to overuse of the tendons as they try to compensate for inadequate lateral ligamentous support. The lateral incision may be modified to address both problems by

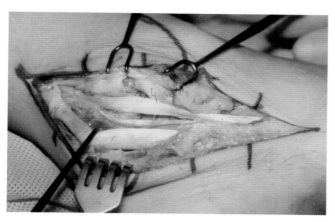

Fig. 63-9. Modification of the incision to accommodate repair of the peroneus brevis tendon split.

using a straight incision placed slightly more posteriorly and extending the incision proximally or distally as dictated by the location of the peroneal tendon tear **(Fig. 63-9)**.

Finally, if recurrent ankle instability occurs in association with a varus-aligned hindfoot, a lateral closing wedge osteotomy of the calcaneus may be indicated, in addition to further correction of the forefoot deformity as is deemed necessary **(Fig. 63-10)**.

■ REHABILITATION AND RETURN TO PLAY RECOMMENDATIONS

Following anatomic and nonanatomic repairs, a below-knee cast maintains immobilization for a total of 6 weeks. The cast is changed at 2 weeks postoperatively to allow inspection of the incision and to reposition the foot from an everted position to a neutral position. Non–weight-bearing status is maintained for the first 2 weeks, followed by weight bearing

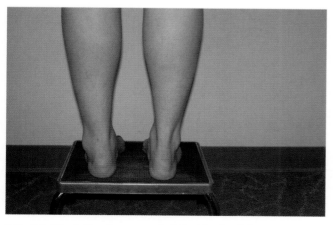

Fig. 63-10. A Brostrom repair failed in the left ankle of this woman with a varus hindfoot who may have benefited from a lateral calcaneal closing wedge osteotomy at the time of her lateral ligamentous repair.

as tolerated in the cast for the next 4 weeks. Physical therapy, with an early emphasis on range of motion, is then begun at 6 weeks postoperatively. A soft, lace-up brace is used during the immediate postoperative period including physical therapy sessions. Therapy is progressed to include peroneal and global muscular strengthening as well as proprioceptive training. At 10 weeks after surgery, functional, sport-specific exercises and light jogging are begun, and full activity with a brace is resumed at 12 weeks postoperatively. A lace-up brace is recommended indefinitely for sporting activities.

■ OUTCOMES AND FUTURE DIRECTIONS

The anatomic Brostrom–type repair has been shown to have excellent outcomes in the majority of published studies. A 91% good or excellent functional result was reported by Messer et al.[5] in 20 patients at a mean follow-up of 34.5 months after use of a Gould modification of the Brostrom procedure with suture anchors. Similarly, Hamilton et al.[15] found that 93% of 28 repairs with drill holes had an excellent result at an average of 64.3 months. Fifty-four percent of these patients were professional ballet dancers.

Colville and Grondel[16] found no failures in their series of 12 patients who underwent their technique of augmented reconstruction as originally described using a split peroneus brevis tendon graft.

Medial Ankle Instability

Medial ankle ligamentous instability has recently been described by Hintermann.[17] This entity is suspected when the patient complains of recurrent "giving way" of the ankle, pain in the medial gutter, and a valgus deformity of the hindfoot that can typically be corrected by active recruitment of the posterior tibial muscle. Lesions are diagnosed by arthroscopy in symptomatic individuals and are classified into three types. Proximal avulsions from the medial malleolus are designated as type 1. Intrasubstance tears are type 2, while distal avulsions are type 3 lesions. Treatment involves surgical exploration of the tibionavicular and tibiospring ligaments via a medial longitudinal incision, with reattachment or imbrication of the ligaments as necessary using suture anchors. The posterior tibial tendon is examined and debrided or shortened if required. The lateral ankle ligaments are reconstructed as well if clinically indicated. Postoperatively, type 1 repaired lesions are treated with functional mobilization in a stabilizing shoe for 6 weeks, while types 2 and 3 lesions are allowed to weight bear in a below-knee cast for 6 weeks. Hintermann et al.[18] has reported on a series of 54 patients treated in this manner. At an average of 4.4 years, results were good or excellent in 48 cases (89%), fair in 4 cases (7%), and poor in 1 case (2%). Further study of this emerging diagnosis is warranted.

■ SUGGESTED READINGS

Burks RT, Morgan J. Anatomy of the lateral ankle ligaments. Am J Sports Med. 1994;22(1):72–77.

Colville MR, Marder RA, Zarins B. Reconstruction of the lateral ankle ligaments: a biomechanical analysis. Am J Sports Med. 1992;20(5):594–600.

Hintermann, B. Medial ankle instability. Foot Ankle Clin North Am. 2003;8:723–738.

Hintermann B, Boss A, Schafer D. Arthroscopic findings in patients with chronic ankle instability. Am J Sports Med. 2002;30(3):402–409.

Krips R, van Dijk CN, Halasi T, et al. Long-term outcome of anatomical reconstruction versus tenodesis for the treatment of chronic anterolateral instability of the ankle joint: a multicenter study. Foot Ankle Int. 2001;22(5):415–421.

Messer TM, Cummins CA, Ahn J, et al. Outcome of the modified Brostrom procedure for chronic lateral ankle instability using suture anchors. Foot Ankle Int. 2000;21(12):996–1003.

■ REFERENCES:

1. Brostrom L. Sprained ankles. VI. Surgical treatment of "chronic" ligament ruptures. Acta Chir Scand. 1966;132(5):551–565.
2. Gould N, Seligson D, Gassman J. Early and late repair of lateral ligament of the ankle. Foot Ankle. 1980;1(2):84–89.
3. Liu SH, Baker CL. Comparison of lateral ankle ligamentous reconstruction procedures. Am J Sports Med. 1994;22(3):313–317.
4. Karlsson J, Bergsten T, Lansinger O, et al. Reconstruction of the lateral ligaments of the ankle for chronic lateral instability. J Bone Joint Surg Am. 1988;70(4):581–588.
5. Messer TM, Cummins CA, Ahn J, et al. Outcome of the modified Brostrom procedure for chronic lateral ankle instability using suture anchors. Foot Ankle Int. 2000;21(12):996–1003.
6. Krips R, van Dijk CN, Halasi T, et al. Long-term outcome of anatomical reconstruction versus tenodesis for the treatment of chronic anterolateral instability of the ankle joint: a multicenter study. Foot Ankle Int. 2001;22(5):415–421.
7. Colville MR, Marder RA, Zarins B. Reconstruction of the lateral ankle ligaments: a biomechanical analysis. Am J Sports Med. 1992;20(5):594–600.
8. Frost SC, Amendola A. Is stress radiography necessary in the diagnosis of acute or chronic ankle instability? Clin J Sport Med. 1999;9(1):40–45.
9. Burks RT, Morgan J. Anatomy of the lateral ankle ligaments. Am J Sports Med. 1994;22(1):72–77.
10. Bassett FH III, Gates HS III, Billys JB, et al. Talar impingement by the anteroinferior tibiofibular ligament: a cause of chronic pain in the ankle after inversion sprain. J Bone Joint Surg Am. 1990;72(1):55–59.
11. Komenda GA, Ferkel RD. Arthroscopic findings associated with the unstable ankle. Foot Ankle Int. 1999;20(11):708–713.
12. Taga I, Shino K, Inoue M, et al. Articular cartilage lesions in ankles with lateral ligament injury: an arthroscopic study. Am J Sports Med. 1993;21(1):120–126.
13. Kibler WB. Arthroscopic findings in ankle ligament reconstruction. Clin Sports Med. 1996;15(4):799–804.
14. Hintermann B, Boss A, Schafer D. Arthroscopic findings in patients with chronic ankle instability. Am J Sports Med. 2002;30(3):402–409.
15. Hamilton WG, Thompson FM, Snow SW. The modified Brostrom procedure for lateral ankle instability. Foot Ankle. 1993;14(1):1–7.
16. Colville MR, Grondel RJ. Anatomic reconstruction of the lateral ankle ligaments using a split peroneus brevis tendon graft. Am J Sports Med. 1995;23(2):210–213.
17. Hintermann B. Medial ankle instability. Foot Ankle Clin. 2003;8(4):723–738.
18. Hintermann B, Valderrabano V, Boss A, et al. Medial ankle instability: an exploratory, prospective study of fifty-two cases. Am J Sports Med. 2004;32(1):183–190.

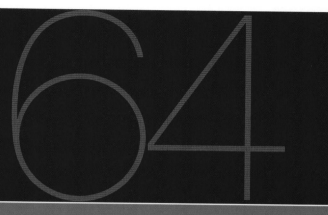

JONATHAN B. FEIBEL, MD, DANE K. WUKICH, MD, BRIAN G. DONLEY, MD

TENDON INJURIES AROUND THE FOOT AND ANKLE

Tendon injuries around the foot and ankle are a common cause of disability in athletic individuals and a frequent reason for seeking orthopedic consultation. Some of these injuries are chronic, occurring over a period of time or with recurrent injuries, and others are acute, resulting from a single traumatic incident. Treatment requires a thorough understanding of the pathology surrounding each of these tendon injuries. Many can be treated with conservative methods, while others require operative intervention.

■ ACHILLES TENDON DISORDERS

Achilles tendon problems are common in those playing both competitive and recreational sports and can be caused by overuse that results in chronic tendon problems such as tendonitis or tendinosis or by trauma that results in acute or chronic Achilles tendon rupture. Factors that often contribute to Achilles tendon problems include training errors such as a sudden increase in activity, a sudden increase in training intensity (distance or frequency), resuming training after a long period of inactivity, running on uneven or loose terrain, postural problems (such as foot pronation), poor footwear (generally poor hindfoot support), or a tight gastroc-soleus complex.

Achilles Tendonitis

Introduction
Achilles tendonitis is a condition that develops over time and is associated with degeneration of the tendon and inflammation that causes pain. Achilles tendonitis is described as noninsertional or insertional, depending upon its location. The treatments of these two entities are very different.

Pathophysiology
The etiology of Achilles tendonitis is overuse. A hypovascular zone, 4 cm proximal to the tendon insertion on the calcaneus, is the most common location of noninsertional Achilles tendonitis. Microtears develop and lead to collagen degeneration, fibrosis, and calcifications within the tendon.[1–4]

Three subgroups of Achilles tendonitis have been identified: paratendinitis, which is inflammation of the tendon lining; tendinosis, which is more advanced and has intrasubstance degeneration; and paratendinitis with tendinosis, which has components of both.[1,5]

Diagnosis
Patients often complain of pain posteriorly over the Achilles tendon. Fusiform swelling often is associated with the tendon degeneration. Activity-related pain is a common presenting complaint. Initially the pain is not debilitating, but as the degeneration continues, the pain becomes more severe.

With insertional Achilles tendonitis, the pain is directly over the posterior aspect of the calcaneus rather than over the Achilles tendon. More swelling is usually present, and often the calcaneus is prominent and inflamed.

A history and physical examination should rule out a stress fracture or an Achilles tendon rupture. Patients who have Achilles tendonitis have a reactive (normal) Thompson test. The Thompson test is done with the patient prone, with both feet extended off the end of the table. Both calf muscles are squeezed by the examiner. If the tendon is intact the foot will plantarflex when the calf is squeezed (reactive). If the tendon is ruptured, normal plantarflexion will not occur (nonreactive). Patients with an Achilles tendon rupture are unable to do a single heel rise. In patients with paratendinitis, tenderness remains in one position when the foot is moved from dorsiflexion to plantar flexion; in patients with tendinosis, the "painful arc" sign is positive (the point of tenderness moves) because the thickened portion of the tendon moves with active plantarflexion and dorsiflexion of the ankle.

Routine ankle radiographs should be taken to rule out other pathology or to show a spur associated with insertional Achilles tendonitis. Radiographs also can show calcification that often is present within the tendon. Magnetic resonance imaging (MRI) can also help to confirm the diagnosis of Achilles tendonitis and should be used if the history and physical examination do not clearly indicate the diagnosis. Ultrasonography has been reported to be effective in evaluating Achilles tendon pathology, but this technique is very dependent on a skilled ultrasonographer.

Treatment

The initial treatment of Achilles tendonitis should always be conservative. Initially, a nonsteroidal anti-inflammatory drug can be used in conjunction with a stretching program. Often a formal physical therapy program is helpful. An off-the-shelf heel lift that fits inside the shoe can take stress off the tendon. Corticosteroid injection rarely should be used in or around the tendon because of the reported association between corticosteroid injection and spontaneous Achilles tendon rupture.[6] A recent retrospective cohort study, however, reported no ruptures in 43 patients at an average of 37 months after fluoroscopically guided, low-volume corticosteroid injections into the peritendinous space. If these modalities are unsuccessful, or the patient presents with severe pain, a removable walking boot or a short leg cast can be worn for 6 weeks to decrease inflammation. Because a walking boot can be removed for showering, patients generally are more willing to accept it than a cast.

If immobilization in the walking boot is successful, its use can be gradually decreased and the patient can resume activities. A posterior heel pad sock can be used to decrease friction on the calcaneal prominence.

A newer noninvasive treatment for Achilles tendonitis is extra corporeal shock wave therapy (ESWT). The same technology used to dissolve kidney stones has been reported to be effective for the treatment of a number of orthopedic disorders. It is done as an outpatient procedure with only a local block for anesthesia, and some sort of immobilization is needed for approximately 3 weeks to protect the tendon from rupture. The use of ESWT is currently not FDA approved for treatment of Achilles tendonitis, but some studies have reported its effectiveness. If conservative methods are unsuccessful in relieving symptoms, surgery is indicated.

■ SURGICAL INTERVENTION

Noninsertional Tendonitis

Surgery for noninsertional Achilles tendonitis can be done percutaneously or through an open approach. Maffulli et al.[7] reported better functional and cosmetic results and quicker return to activities after percutaneous longitudinal tenotomy than after open procedures.

Percutaneous Technique

The patient is placed prone on the operating table, and the area of maximal tenderness and swelling is marked. A no. 11 blade is placed longitudinal to the tendon fibers through the skin and the tendon. The blade is pointed proximally and is kept still as the ankle is moved into full dorsiflexion. The blade is then turned 180 degrees and the ankle is moved into plantarflexion. The procedure is repeated four times approximately 2 cm proximal (medial and lateral) and distal (medial and lateral) to the first incision. The wounds are closed with Steri-strips. An aggressive rehabilitation program is begun, with passive range of motion 2 or 3 days after surgery and a jogging program at 2 weeks.[7]

Maffulli et al.[7] reported excellent subjective results in 25 of 48 middle- and long-distance runners, good results in 12, fair results in 7, and poor results in 4. Strength increased about 10% after the operation, and endurance improved almost 50%.

Open Technique

A posterior-based incision is made medial to the tendon at the area of maximal swelling or pain. Sharp dissection is carried to the paratenon. The paratenon is opened and the degenerative tendon segment is debrided with care taken to protect the integrity of the tendon and keep it in continuity. After debridement, the tendon is repaired using interrupted 0 nonabsorbable sutures, the paratenon is closed with 0 absorbable sutures, the subcutaneous tissue is closed with 3-0 absorbable sutures, and the skin is closed with vertical nylon mattress sutures. A compressive dressing and an anterior-based splint are applied. No anesthetic is used locally in the incision to decrease the chance of wound healing problems. If extensive debridement is required (more than 50% of the tendon, a flexor hallucis longus (FHL) tendon transfer can be used for augmentation.

Rehabilitation

The amount and duration of postoperative immobilization depends on the extent of the debridement. The more structural integrity lost, the longer the immobilization should be continued. Certainly the ankle should be immobilized until the incision heals. Stitches usually are removed at 3 weeks, and a rehabilitation program is begun as soon as wound healing allows.

Insertional Tendonitis

Decompression for insertional Achilles tendon has been described using a posterior central splitting incision, a hockey stick incision, transverse incisions, an isolated medial or lateral incision, or combined medial and lateral incisions.[1,8,9] We prefer an isolated lateral incision if full decompression can be accomplished through this approach; a medial incision can be added if necessary for complete decompression.

Surgical Technique

A longitudinal incision is made on the lateral aspect of the calcaneus extending proximally along the lateral aspect of the Achilles. Care must be taken to avoid injury to the sural nerve, which is very close to the surgical dissection. Sharp dissection is carried to the paratenon, and the Achilles tendon and its insertion are inspected. Any degenerative tissue is débrided as described for noninsertional tendonitis. The Haglund deformity that usually is present is isolated with a Homén retractor. Care is taken to protect the Achilles tendon insertion as well as the medial structures. A microsagittal saw is used to remove enough bone to effectively decompress the posterior prominence that contributes to the tendonitis. After adequate decompression is confirmed with a fluoroscopic lateral view, the insertion of the Achilles tendon is inspected. If the tendon is detached or is significantly weakened, two suture anchors should be used to attach it to the calcaneus in the resected area. Closure and splinting are as previously described.

Rehabilitation

Again, the amount of disruption of the tendon and its insertion determines postoperative care. If suture anchors are used, immobilization for up to 6 weeks in a cast followed by 3 weeks in a removable boot is not unreasonable. Weight bearing, range of motion, and gentle strengthening exercises are allowed in the boot.

Achilles Tendon Ruptures

Achilles tendon ruptures can occur in men or women of any age, but are most common in 30- to 40-year-old men, especially "weekend warriors," those middle-aged athletes who play high demand sports on a recreational basis.[10,11] Achilles tendon ruptures usually occur in people with no or few symptoms of tendonitis. Corticosteroid injection into or around the Achilles tendon has been implicated as a factor in spontaneous tendon rupture,[6] as has the use of fluoroquinolones.

Diagnosis

Patients with Achilles tendon ruptures often describe a feeling of being shot or kicked in the back of the leg, followed by an inability to bear weight or difficulty with bearing weight. Often a palpable defect is present and the Thompson test is nonreactive.

It is important to differentiate an Achilles tendon rupture from a gastrocnemius tear or strain. A gastrocnemius tear or strain usually is more proximal, is associated with a reactive Thompson test, and can be treated nonoperatively. If the diagnosis is in question, MRI can be helpful. Plain radiographs should be obtained to identify a bony avulsion or calcification in the tendon, which can make repair more difficult. However, the diagnosis is most often based on the history and physical examination.

Nonoperative Treatment

Whether to treat Achilles tendon ruptures operatively or nonoperatively remains a matter of controversy. Advocates of nonoperative treatment cite wound healing issues and perioperative morbidity as reasons to avoid surgical treatment.[12] Those who advocate operative treatment cite higher chances of rerupture, decreased range of motion, and decreased strength as disadvantages of nonoperative treatment.[12–14] Nonoperative methods still have a definite role in the treatment of Achilles tendon ruptures, especially in elderly or high-risk patients such as those with diabetes.

Surgical Intervention

Many surgical approaches have been described for repair of Achilles tendon ruptures, some for acute tears (those that are diagnosed and treated within 6 weeks of injury) and others for chronic tears (those present longer than 6 weeks).

Repair of Acute Rupture

Although percutaneous techniques using devices have been developed, we prefer an open technique for repair of Achilles tendon ruptures. Sural nerve complications have been reported to be more frequent after percutaneous techniques.[15]

Open Repair

Surgical Technique

A longitudinal incision is made medial to the tendon to reduce the risk of sural nerve injury. Sharp dissection is carried directly to the paratenon, which is incised sharply and left in a position that allows it to be repaired after the tendon is repaired.

Opening the paratenon exposes the Achilles tendon rupture. Usually the Achilles tendon is torn in a jagged fashion, with frayed ends resembling the end of a mop. These ends should be freshened with a scalpel, removing just enough of the frayed tendon to achieve a clean, sharp edge; removing too much tendon increases the size of the gap to be closed. The tendon is now ready for repair. A modified Bunnell stitch is used to place two no. 2 FiberWire sutures, one in the proximal stump and one in the distal stump of the tendon. Each end of the tendon can now be securely grasped.

The suture is tied to repair the tendon while the foot is held in the same plantarflexion as the opposite foot. This mimics the resting tension of the uninjured Achilles tendon. This is a very important step to decrease the chance of weakness caused by incorrect tensioning of the Achilles tendon. If necessary, the repair can be supplemented with a horizontal mattress suture to achieve four strands across the repair, taking care not to cut the other stitches.

The paratenon is closed with 2-0 absorbable sutures. If this repair is too tight, a relaxing incision can be made in the

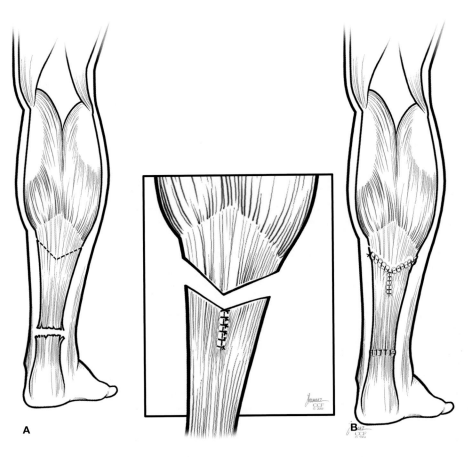

A

B

Fig. 64-1. **A:** Demonstrates the V-Y lengthening. The figure on the left shows the proposed cut (V) portion in the proximal aspect of the tendon, which allows the tendon to lengthen. The figure on the right shows the lengthened tendon proximally, which demonstrates how the V has now turned into a Y. The distal aspect of the Y is already sutured. **B:** Demonstrates the lengthened tendon after repair of the Y limb and repair of the torn tendon.

anterior aspect of the paratenon to allow the posterior aspect to cover the tendon without tension (Fig. 64-1). It is important to obtain a good repair of the paratenon. The subcutaneous tissue is closed with 3-0 absorbable sutures, and the skin is closed with 3-0 nylon vertical mattress sutures.

A Robert Jones compressive dressing is applied and an anterior-based splint is placed to hold the foot in plantarflexion to take stress off the repair. No local anesthetic is used to decrease the chance of flap necrosis. The patient is instructed to keep all pressure off the posterior aspect of the distal leg to decrease the chance of wound healing problems.

Repair of Chronic Rupture

For chronic ruptures, we prefer to attempt a primary repair, but this often is not possible. If a primary repair is not attainable, we use a step-wise approach. First a V-Y advancement of the tendon is done, which usually gains approximately 3 cm of tendon length.[16] If this is not adequate, an FHL transfer is added.

Surgical Technique

After exposure of the tendon as previously described, the tendon is débrided of devitalized tissue and the gap between the tendon ends is evaluated. This gap can be lessened or completely eliminated by using a grasping suture to place

gentle traction on the proximal stump of the tendon for 10 to 15 minutes.

If adequate length is not obtained, a generous V-Y lengthening is done at the musculotendinous junction **(Fig. 64-1A,B)**. The apex of the inverted V is made in the central part of the aponeurosis. The arms of the V should be at least one and one half times the length of the defect. The arms of the incision extend through the aponeurosis and underlying muscle tissue. The flap is then pulled distally until the ruptured ends of the tendons are approximated. A standard Achilles tendon repair is then done as described above. The V-Y portion is then approximated.[14]

If this does not allow the gap to be bridged, an FHL tendon transfer is added. Once the tendon is exposed, dissection is carried anteriorly through the fascia overlying the deep posterior compartment of the leg. The FHL tendon, the most lateral in the deep posterior compartment, is exposed. The FHL can further be identified because its muscle belly is the most distal of the three muscles. Movement of the big toe and confirming excursion of the tendon posteriorly further verifies that it is the FHL. Once the FHL is identified, care must be taken with any dissection medial to the tendon because the neurovascular bundle is quite close. The FHL tendon is traced as far distal as possible. It is cut in a medial to lateral direction to protect the neurovascular bundle and is delivered into the posterior aspect of the leg. The tendon can then be attached with either a suture anchor or with an interference fit using an Arthrex Biotenodesis (Arthrex, Inc, Naples, Fla) screw. The FHL is tensioned to approximate the resting tension of the uninjured Achilles tendon. We often drape out the contralateral leg to use as a template during this tensioning process. The FHL tendon can be further sutured to the proximal and distal limbs of the tendon to improve the strength of the repair.[17] Pedobarographic analysis has proven that FHL transfer causes clinically insignificant changes in the pressures distributed to the forefoot.[18]

Rehabilitation

The wound is checked at 1 week and a cast is applied with the foot in some degree of plantarflexion. The stitches are removed at 3 weeks. A cast is used for 6 weeks. The patient is then allowed to bear weight in a removable boot. Immobilization is discontinued at approximately 10 weeks. Sometimes a small heel insert is used to help decrease stress on the repair.

■ POSTERIOR TIBIAL TENDON

Historical Perspective

Although some posterior tibial tendon problems are the result of acute trauma, most are chronic overuse conditions. These chronic conditions occur most frequently in females over the age of 40, especially those who stand or walk for prolonged periods. In addition to increasing age and repetitive microtrauma, other contributing factors include obesity, diabetes, hypertension, seronegative spondyloarthropathies, and rheumatoid arthritis. The severity of posterior tibial tendon insufficiency (PTTI) generally is a continuum rather than separate discrete entities, but classification is helpful in treatment decision making. Johnson and Strom[19] described three stages based on clinical symptoms and severity of foot deformity. Stage I is tendonitis with a competent tendon and normal foot alignment. Stage II is elongation of the tendon with flexible hindfoot valgus. In stage III the hindfoot deformity becomes rigid and the deformity is no longer passively correctable. Often arthritic changes are present in the hindfoot. Stage IV, added by Myerson,[20] includes ankle arthritis, with or without valgus talar tilt and loss of competence of the deltoid ligament complex. Younger athletic individuals usually present with stage I or II PTTI because they are less likely to neglect the condition and usually seek treatment sooner than older, nonathletic individuals who often do not seek treatment until involvement reaches stage III or IV. Acute traumatic posterior tibial injuries usually occur in younger, more athletic individuals and can be much more difficult to treat, making it more difficult to return to a preinjury level of activities.

Anatomy/Function

The posterior tibial tendon arises from the interosseous membrane, fibula, and tibia. It is the tendon that traverses closest to the medial malleolus. It curves more acutely around the medial side than the FHL tendon or the flexor digitorum longus (FDL) tendon. The posterior tibial tendon passes posterior to the axis of the ankle joint and medial to the axis of the subtalar joint.[21] It attaches to the tuberosity of the navicular and then continues to its attachments on the cuneiforms and the bases of the second, third, and fourth metatarsals.[22] It also has multiple other attachments,[23] including multiple ligaments on the medial side as well as the plantar fascia and peroneus longus tendon. A 4-cm zone of relative hypovascularity in the midportion of the posterior tibial tendon extends proximally from the navicular insertion. This relatively hypovascular zone, combined with the acuity of the course of the tendon around the medial malleolus, makes it susceptible to injury.[21]

The posterior tibial tendon is a strong inverter and plantar flexor of the foot and is responsible for initiating heel rise.[24] Without a functioning posterior tibial tendon, a single limb heel rise is impossible. Over time, the unopposed peroneus brevis tendon, which is the antagonist to the posterior tibial tendon, will pull the foot into a valgus and abducted position.

Diagnosis

The diagnosis of a traumatic rupture or attenuation of the posterior tibial tendon is difficult and requires a high index of suspicion. Often the medial side of the ankle is swollen out of proportion to the injury. No bony injury is visible on three-view radiographs of the ankle. With an acute injury, assessing the competence of the posterior tibial tendon is difficult. If rupture is suspected, an MRI should be obtained, which will reveal a traumatic rupture of the tendon. Often a small fleck of bone is present just medial to the medial malleolus; this may be a "soft" sign of a posterior tibial tendon injury.

Posterior tibial tendonitis or a chronic rupture is easier to diagnose. In the early stages, pain and often swelling is medially based overlying the posterior tibial tendon. Early in the process, when the tendon is still functioning competently, patients are able to do a single limb heel rise, but it causes pain on the medial side. Later in the process, after tendon rupture, pain and swelling migrate to the lateral side because of subfibular impingement.

MRI can be used as an adjunct to diagnosis of these chronic disorders; when tendonitis is present, fluid is visible in the tendon sheath. Later, MRI can confirm a tendon rupture.[25]

Treatment

Nonoperative

For tendonitis (stage I), conservative care is the initial treatment. Anti-inflammatory medication is combined with immobilization in a cast or removable boot, usually for 6 weeks. If inflammation resolves and the patient is relatively asymptomatic, an off-the-shelf medial-posted orthotic or a custom orthotic is used. If the pain recurs, or if complete tendon rupture occurs, operative intervention should be

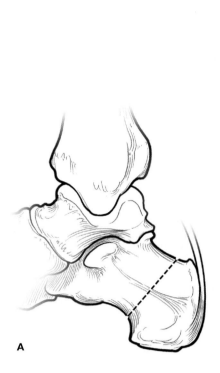
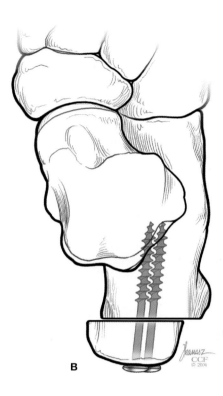

Fig. 64-2. A: Proposed calcaneal osteotomy from lateral to medial. **B:** Calcaneal osteotomy after 1-cm displacement. Note position of screws. Screws start lateral to ensure purchase in distal aspect of calcaneus.

considered for athletic individuals. For nonathletic individuals with stage II PTTI, an AFO or University of California at Berkeley Laboratory (UCBL) brace can be used.[26]

Operative

Many operative approaches have been described for posterior tibial tendonitis (stage I) or posterior tibial tendon rupture (stage II). Procedures recommended for stage I PTTI include debridement of the tendon, tendon transfer combined with a calcaneal osteotomy or lateral column lengthening or both, and tendon transfer combined with subtalar fusion. Lateral column lengthening is associated with stiffness and chronic lateral foot pain,[27] and subtalar fusion is debilitating for an athletic individual. A medial displacement osteotomy combined with an FDL transfer usually is the best option for an athletic individual because it generally spares motion and adequately substitutes for the incompetent posterior tibial tendon. Good results have been reported with isolated debridement and repair of the posterior tibial tendon in athletes with isolated stage I tendonitis.

Some[28] have advocated using the FHL tendon for transfer because its strength is closer to that of the posterior tibial tendon than is that of the FDL.[29]

Surgical Technique

An oblique incision is made posterior to the lateral malleolus at approximately a 45-degree angle to the foot. This incision is made posterior to the sural nerve and the peroneal tendons. Sharp dissection is carried down to the periosteum,

which is elevated a few millimeters in each direction. Eighteen-gauge needles are placed on the superior and inferior aspects of the calcaneus in line with the proposed osteotomy **(Fig. 64-2A,B)**. A fluoroscopic lateral heel view confirms that the proposed osteotomy is anterior to the insertion of the Achilles tendon and posterior to the posterior facet. Homén retractors are placed superiorly and inferiorly to protect surrounding structures. An oscillating saw is used to complete the osteotomy. Care is taken not to avoid medial penetration with the saw because the neurovascular structures are in close proximity to the osteotomy. A lamina spreader is placed into the osteotomy. This puts the medial periosteum on stretch. A Freer elevator can be used to release the periosteum medially, allowing the osteotomy to be displaced medially approximately a centimeter. A 6.5-mm cannulated screw system is then used to hold the osteotomy in place. The guide wires are placed parallel to the inferior border of the foot starting laterally in the calcaneus to make sure that the screws will remain in the calcaneus. Lateral and axial radiographs of the calcaneus are necessary to confirm correct placement of the guide wires and appropriate medial displacement. Care should be taken to make sure that both screws avoid the posterior facet. The screws are placed parallel to each other on the lateral view.[30]

Next, attention is turned medially. A gently curved incision is made on the medial aspect of the foot and ankle, from the medial malleolus to the plantar border of the medial cuneiform. The posterior tibial tendon is excised with care taken to preserve a portion of the flexor retinaculum. The FDL is identified proximally and followed distally to where it dives below the medial cuneiform. At this level it is sharply transected under direct observation. A no. 2 nonabsorbable braided suture (FiberWire, Arthrex, Inc, Naples, Fla) is placed in the FDL end using a whipstitch. The FiberWire has a Kevlar core that gives it the strength of a no. 5 nonabsorbable braided suture with the size of a no. 2 suture. This minimizes the bulk of the suture and the suture knots. A 0.062-in Kirschner wire guide pin is drilled into the navicular from medial to lateral corresponding to the anatomic insertion of the posterior tibial tendon. An image is obtained to confirm correction orientation for the drill hole. Next, a 5.5-mm cannulated drill from the Biotenodesis set is used to create a 5.5-mm hole that is 17-mm deep **(Fig. 64-3A,B)**. The 5.5-mm screw is of optimal size for the navicular bone and transfer of the FDL tendon. For this transfer we do not overdrill or underdrill the screw hole. With a forceps, the tendon end is placed into the depth of the drill hole while held firmly to the end of the Biotenodesis screwdriver with tension on the suture end that is passed through the screwdriver. The tip of the screwdriver, with the screw on it, is used to assist in keeping the tendon in the 17-mm drill hole and also serves to hold the tendon in place while the screw is tightened. The foot is plantarflexed and inverted while the screw is inserted. Fixation with a Biotenodesis screw has several advantages over bone tunnel fixation through a vertical hole. Because the FDL is secured through an interference fit, less of the tendon is required and less distal dissection is needed, resulting in less venous bleeding, a smaller incision, and a shorter operative time. The transferred FDL can be attached at a more anatomic site on the navicular tuberosity, and less subperiosteal stripping of the navicular bone is required. Iatrogenic fracture of the navicular is less likely because no bone bridge is created. A Robert Jones compressive dressing with a splint is placed with the foot inverted and plantar flexed.

Rehabilitation

The wound is checked at 1 week, and a non–weight-bearing short-leg cast is applied with the foot in inversion and plantarflexion. At 3 weeks after surgery, stitches are removed, and a weight-bearing short-leg cast is applied with the foot in neutral position. Three weeks later, an Aircast boot is fitted and worn for another 4 weeks. After the Aircast boot, a Hapad medial wedge orthotic is used to take stress off the tendon repair. Gradual return to athletic activity is allowed after a formal physical therapy program.

■ PERONEAL TENDON DISORDERS

Historical Perspective

Peroneal tendon problems are common in athletic individuals and if neglected can cause significant disability. If treated correctly, function often can be maintained. Peroneal tendon

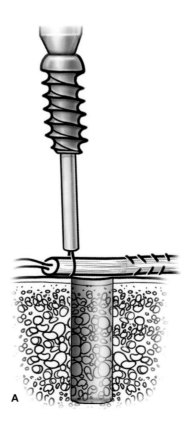
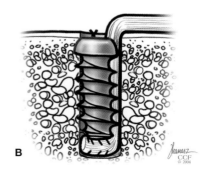

Fig. 64-3. **A:** FDL tendon prior to placing it into drill hole in navicular. **B:** FDL tendon held in drill hole by Biotenodesis screw.

disorders include tendonitis, longitudinal splits, frank tendon rupture, and peroneal tendon subluxation.

Anatomy

Two peroneal tendons occupy the lateral compartment of the leg. They are contained within a fibro-osseous tunnel in a common synovial sheath on the posterior aspect of the fibula.[31] Both the peroneus longus and brevis traverse the lateral side of the leg and pass just posterior to the lateral malleolus. The peroneus longus proceeds under the fifth metatarsal to insert on the first metatarsal base. In this way, it acts as a plantar flexor and evertor of the foot as well as a supporter of the arch. Its antagonist is the anterior tibial tendon. The peroneus brevis has the lower lying muscle belly of the two and inserts onto the base of the fifth metatarsal. The function of this muscle is eversion and plantarflexion of the foot. Its antagonist is the posterior tibial tendon. The main restraint to peroneal tendon subluxation is the superior peroneal retinaculum, as well as the posterolateral ridge of the fibula.[32,33] The superficial peroneal retinaculum, which is a factor in traumatic peroneal tendon subluxation, is located from the tip of the fibula proximally by approximately 1 to 2 cm. It is formed by a confluence of the superficial fascia of the leg and the sheath of the peroneal tendons.[32] The superficial peroneal retinaculum has a variable insertion in cadaveric studies.[34] In any peroneal tendon surgery, it is important to preserve or repair this structure.

Peroneal Tendonitis

Diagnosis

Peroneal tendons, like other tendons around the foot and ankle, are susceptible to inflammation. Often the diagnosis is easy to make. Patients usually have pain and swelling posterolaterally around the lateral malleolus. Pain can be elicited by resisted peroneal tendon stretch. Plain radiographs of the ankle are necessary to rule out any other pathology. If the diagnosis is in doubt or if there is concern about tendon tear or subluxation, an MRI can be obtained. The usual mechanism causing longitudinal splits in the peroneal tendons is ankle plantarflexion and inversion.[35]

Nonoperative Management

Peroneal tendon inflammation often can be resolved with a combination of nonsteroidal anti-inflammatory drugs and temporary activity modification. If symptoms persist, 6 weeks of immobilization usually will decrease the inflammation.

Operative Treatment

If nonoperative management fails, operative exploration is warranted. Repair of longitudinal splits in the tendon should be anticipated, because MRI often underestimates the level of tendon involvement.[36,37] Also, longitudinal splits, which are more common in the peroneus brevis,[35] are often associated with tendonitis.

Surgical Technique

A longitudinal incision is made in line with the peroneal tendons. Care should be taken to protect the sural nerve, which is just posterior to the plane of dissection. The peroneal tendon sheath is opened, taking care to keep the superior peroneal retinaculum intact. Any inflamed areas are débrided, and any longitudinal splits are débrided and tubularized. Tubularization of the tendon is done to allow a smooth outer border to be reestablished, giving it more of an appearance of an uninjured tendon. If more than 50% of the tendon is débrided, a tenodesis to the other intact tendon, as described by Krause and Brodsky,[36] can be done. A no. 2 nonabsorbable suture is used for tenodesis. After debridement and repair, the tendon sheath is closed before subcutaneous and skin closure. A Robert Jones compressive splint is applied with the foot in slight eversion.

Rehabilitation

The wound is checked in a week, and a non–weight-bearing cast is applied. At 3 weeks after surgery, the stitches are removed and a weight-bearing short-leg cast is applied and worn for 3 weeks. Six weeks after surgery, an Aircast boot is fitted and worn for another 3 weeks, after which activities can be resumed.

Peroneal Tendon Rupture

Diagnosis

The diagnosis of peroneal tendon rupture is similar to that of peroneal tendonitis, with the exception of weakness with manual muscle testing. MRI also can aid significantly in making the diagnosis. Usually a patient with a frank tendon rupture can relate it to a specific traumatic event.

Treatment

Unlike longitudinal peroneal tendon tears, which can be treated nonoperatively, frank peroneal tendon ruptures generally require operative treatment. Treatment of a peroneal tendon rupture usually depends on the competency of both of the tendons. A primary repair is attempted if possible. If one of the tendons is competent, but the other is not, a tenodesis of both the proximal and distal ends to the competent tendon, as described in the previous section, can be done.

Peroneal Tendon Subluxation

Diagnosis

With peroneal tendon subluxation or dislocation, usually a snapping sensation is followed by immediate pain in the posterolateral ankle.[38] After this acute event, swelling and pain usually subside, and the diagnosis of peroneal tendon subluxation can be difficult. Often the patient complains of the feeling of an unexplained snapping associated with pain at the site of the snapping.[31] This subluxation often can be elicited on physical exam. Sometimes strength of the peroneal tendons is decreased. Often a longitudinal split is associated with subluxation as the tendon is pulled across the sharp border of the fibula. Plain ankle radiographs should be obtained to rule out any associated pathology. A characteristic radiographic sign that is pathognomonic of peroneal tendon dislocation is a thin cortical rim of avulsed bone from the lateral aspect of the distal fibula seen on the mortise view.[39] MRI also may be helpful if the diagnosis is in question.

Nonoperative Treatment

Several studies have reported successful nonoperative treatment of acute peroneal tendon dislocations with 6 weeks of immobilization in a non–weight-bearing short-leg cast with the foot in midplantarflexion.[38,40,41]

Operative Treatment

Operative treatment is the mainstay for traumatic peroneal tendon subluxation. Surgical intervention is preferred because of (a) the high incidence of failure with nonoperative management,[31,38,40,41] (b) the frequency of this injury in athletic individuals who desire rapid return to activity,[31,42] (c) the frequency of peroneus brevis longitudinal splits requiring repair with chronic subluxation,[31,32,39] and (d) the good results obtained with surgical repair.[31,38,43] For acute subluxation or dislocation, direct repair of the superficial peroneal retinaculum is indicated. Soft-tissue reconstruction with[31] or without[31,42] fibular groove deepening is most often recommended for chronic subluxation or dislocation. We prefer fibular groove deepening with repair of the superficial peroneal retinaculum if possible. Whether groove deepening is planned or not, the distal posterior fibula should be carefully inspected intraoperatively. If it is convex, without a natural concave groove, a groove deepening procedure should be performed.

Surgical Technique

A longitudinal incision is made just posterior to the fibula. Care is taken to protect the sural nerve, which should be posterior to the area of dissection. The peroneal tendon sheath is entered and the peroneal tendons are retracted posteriorly. The tip of the fibula is exposed. A guide wire from a 6.5-mm cannulated screw set is placed under fluoroscopy from the tip of the fibula into the intramedullary cavity. After position is confirmed with image intensification, a drill from this set is used to make a large hole in the intramedullary cavity of the fibula, incorporating as much of the distal fibula as possible without violating the cortex. A bone tamp is used to gently tamp the posterior aspect of the distal fibula to deepen the groove. This helps to keep the smooth cortical border of the posterior fibula intact to decrease the chance of an attritional rupture. The groove is deepened enough to keep the peroneal tendons reduced through a range of motion. The deepening is then supplemented with repair of the superficial peroneal retinaculum to the distal fibula using no. 0 nonabsorbable sutures or Mitek suture anchors. The subcutaneous tissue is closed,

followed by a nylon vertical style mattress suture closure of the skin. A Robert Jones compressive dressing is applied with a U-shaped splint with the foot everted to take pressure off the peroneal tendons.

Rehabilitation

A wound check is performed at 1 week, at which time a short-leg cast is applied with the foot in slight eversion. At 2 weeks, a weight-bearing short leg cast is applied with the foot in slight eversion. At 3 weeks, the stitches are removed and a weight-bearing short-leg cast is applied with the foot in neutral position. This cast is worn for 3 weeks, followed by the use of a removable Aircast boot walker for 3 to 4 weeks. During the time in a boot walker, gentle range of motion exercises are begun. At 9 to 10 weeks after surgery, a formal physical therapy program is started for strengthening and range of motion exercises.

■ REFERENCES

1. Myerson M, McGarvey W. Disorders of the Achilles tendon insertion and Achilles tendonitis. J Am Acad Orthop Surg. 1999;48:211–218.
2. Fox JM, Blazina ME, Jobe FW, et al. Degenerative and rupture of the Achilles tendon. Clin Orthop. 1975;107:201–224.
3. Gould N, Korson R. Stenosing tenosynovitis of the pseudosheath of the tendo Achilles. Foot Ankle. 1980;1:179–187.
4. Lotke PA. Ossification of the Achilles tendon: report of seven cases. J Bone Joint Surg. 1970;52A:157–160.
5. Puddu G, Ippolito E, Postacchini F. A classification of Achilles tendon disease. Am J Sports Med. 1976;4:145–150.
6. Mahler F. Fritschy D. Partial and complete ruptures of the Achilles tendon and local corticosteroid injections. Br J Sports Med. 1992;26:7–14.
7. Maffulli N, Testa V, Capasso G, et al. Results of percutaneous longitudinal tenotomy for Achilles tendinopathy in middle- and long-distance runners. Am J Sports Med. 1997;25:835–840.
8. Schepsis AA, Leach RE. Surgical management of Achilles tendon overuse injuries. Am J Sports Med. 1987;15:308–315.
9. Digiovanni BF, Gould JS. Achilles tendinitis and posterior heel disorders. Foot Ankle Clin. 1997;2:411–428.
10. Jozsa L, Kvist M, Balint BJ, et al. The role of recreational sport activity in Achilles tendon rupture: a clinical, pathoanatomical, and sociological study of 292 cases. Am J Sports Med. 1989;17:338–343.
11. Levi N. The incidence of Achilles tendon rupture in Copenhagen. Injury. 1997;28:311–313.
12. Wills CA, Washburn S, Caiozzo V, et al. Achilles tendon rupture: a review of the literature comparing surgical versus nonsurgical treatment. Clin Orthop. 1986;207:156–163.
13. Helgeland J, Odland P, Hove LM. Achilles tendon rupture: surgical or non-surgical treatment. Tidsskr Nor Laegeforen. 1997;117: 1763–1766.
14. Feibel J, Bernacki B. A review of salvage procedures after failed Achilles tendon repair. Foot Ankle Clin North Am. 2003;8:105–114.
15. Lim J, Dalal R, Waseem M. Percutaneous vs. open repair of the ruptured Achilles tendon: a prospective randomized controlled study. Foot Ankle. 2001;22:559–566.
16. Bosworth DM. Repair of defects in the tendo Achilles. J Bone Joint Surg. 1956;38:111–114.
17. Den Hartog B. Flexor hallucis longus transfer for chronic Achilles tendonosis. Foot Ankle. 2003;24:233–237.

18. Coull R, Flavin R, Stephens M. Flexor hallucis longus tendon transfer: evaluation of postoperative morbidity. Foot Ankle. 2003;24:931–993.

19. Johnson KA, Strom DE. Tibialis posterior tendon dysfunction. Clin Orthop. 1989;239:196–206.

20. Myerson MS. Adult acquire flat foot deformity: treatment of dysfunction of the posterior tibial tendon. J Bone Joint Surg. 1996; 78A:780–792.

21. Mosier S, Pomeroy G, Manoli A II. Pathoanatomy and etiology of posterior tibial tendon dysfunction. Clin Orthop. 1999;365: 12–22.

22. Johnson KA. Tibialis posterior tendon rupture. Clin Orthop. 1983;177:140–147.

23. Mueller TJ. Acquired flatfoot secondary to tibialis posterior dysfunction: biomechanical aspects. J Foot Surg. 1991;30:2–11.

24. Funk DA, Cass JR, Johnson KA. Acquired flat foot secondary to posterior tibial-tendon pathology. J Bone Joint Surg. 1986;68A: 95–102.

25. Feighan J, Towers J, Conti S. The use of magnetic resonance imaging in posterior tibial tendon dysfunction. Clin Orthop. 1999;365:23–38.

26. Wapner K, Chao W. Nonoperative treatment of posterior tibial tendon dysfunction. Clin Orthop. 1999;365:39–45.

27. Choung S, Inda D, Deland J. Evans procedure vs. medial displacement calcaneal osteomy for the treatment of adult acquired flatfoot deformity. Paper presented at 34th Annual Meeting of American Orthopedic Foot and Ankle Society: 2004; San Francisco.

28. Parekh S, Lowry T, Pedowitz D, et al. Reconstruction of chronic tendon disorders: randomized prospective comparison of FHL and FDL tendon transfer. Paper presented at 34th Annual Meeting of American Orthopedic Foot and Ankle Society: 2004; San Francisco.

29. Silver R, Garza J, Rang M. The myth of muscle balance. J Bone Joint Surg Br. 1985;67-B(3):432–437.

30. Trnka H, Easley M, Myerson M. The role of calcaneal osteotomies for correction of adult flatfoot. Clin Orthop. 1999;365:50–64.

31. Mason R, Henderson I. Traumatic peroneal tendon instability. Am J Sports Med. 1996;24:652–658.

32. Geppert MJ, Sobel M, Bohne WHO. Lateral ankle instability as a cause of superior peroneal retinacular laxity: an anatomic and biomechanical study of cadaveric feet. Foot Ankle. 1993;14:330–334.

33. Martens MA, Noyez JF, Mulier JC. Recurrent dislocation of the peroneal tendons: results of rerouting the tendons under the calcaneofibular ligament. Am J Sports Med. 1986;14:148–150.

34. Davis W, Sobel M, Deland J, et al. The superior peroneal retinaculum: an anatomic study. Foot Ankle. 1994;5:271–275.

35. Bassett III F, Speer K. Longitudinal rupture of the peroneal tendons. Am J Sports Med. 1993;21:354–357.

36. Krause J, Brodsky J. Peroneus brevis tendon tears: pathophysiology, surgical reconstruction and clinical results. Foot Ankle. 1998;19: 271–279.

37. Brandes C, Smith R. Characterization of patients with primary peroneus longus tendinopathy: a review of twenty two cases. Foot Ankle Int. 2000;21(6):462–468.

38. Eckert WR, David EA Jr. Acute rupture of the peroneal retinaculum. J Bone Joint Surg. 1976;58A:670–673.

39. Arrowsmith SR, Fleming LL, Allman FL. Traumatic dislocations of peroneal tendons. Am J Sports Med. 1983;11:142–146.

40. Stover CN, Bryan DR. Traumatic dislocation of the peroneal tendons. Am J Surg. 1962;103:180–186.

41. Escalas F, Figueras JM, Merino JA. Dislocation of the peroneal tendons. J Bone Joint Surg. 1980;62A:451–453.

42. Clanton TO, Schon LC. Athletic injuries to the soft tissues of the foot and ankle. In: Mann RA, Coughlin MJ, eds. *Surgery of the Foot and Ankle*. 6th ed. St. Louis: CV Mosby Co; 1993:1095–1224.

43. Marti R. Dislocation of the peroneal tendons. Am J Sports Med. 1977;5:19–22.

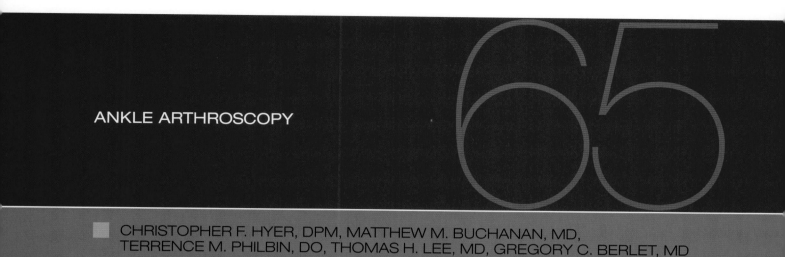

65

ANKLE ARTHROSCOPY

CHRISTOPHER F. HYER, DPM, MATTHEW M. BUCHANAN, MD,
TERRENCE M. PHILBIN, DO, THOMAS H. LEE, MD, GREGORY C. BERLET, MD

■ HISTORY OF THE TECHNIQUE

Ankle arthroscopy derives from early 1900s Japan when Takagi began adapting endoscopes for use in joints in the lower extremity, beginning in the knee.[1] In 1925, arthroscopy was introduced in the United States, but it was not until later in the 1950s when arthroscopy technical manuals were published.[2,3] In the past 30 years, however, there has been a dramatic increase in the indications and use of ankle arthroscopy as the technology and skill level of the surgeon have evolved.

■ INDICATIONS AND CONTRAINDICATIONS

Anterior ankle arthroscopy is both diagnostic and therapeutic for many ankle disorders. Diagnostic indications for ankle arthroscopy include unexplained symptoms of pain, swelling, or stiffness as well as in patients with symptoms unresponsive to conservative therapies. Therapeutic indications include ankle synovitis, anterolateral ankle impingement lesion, anterior bony impingement, osteochondral lesions of the talus or tibia, intra-articular loose bodies, arthrofibrosis, ankle fractures, and degenerative joint disease. Ankle arthroscopy also has a role in lateral ankle stabilization procedures and arthrodesis, as well as for irrigation and débridement of septic arthritis.

Overlying soft tissue infection is a contraindication to ankle arthroscopy. Severe degenerative joint disease and ankle malalignment are relative contraindications as they can influence the ability to establish arthroscopic portals into the ankle.

The specific conditions of ankle synovitis, anterolateral impingement lesion, anterior bony impingement, osteochondral lesions of the talus, and lateral ankle instability are specifically addressed.

Ankle Synovitis

Patients with ankle synovitis complain of global ankle pain. Most commonly, this pain is perceived across the anterior ankle joint line, but posterior pain is possible. Symptoms can be relieved with oral anti-inflammatories and with intra-articular injections, which are used to aid diagnosis as well as for symptomatic treatment. Patients may relate a history of a previous significant ankle injury that seemed to incite the current complaints. Co-morbid medical conditions such as rheumatoid arthritis often present with synovitis in the ankle.

On physical exam, there is pain with palpation along the anterior joint line and with end ranges of motion. Joint motion is typically smooth without any popping or catching. Joint laxity may be present from previous injury and an anterior drawer should be attempted. Radiographs are typically negative for synovitis, but magnetic resonance imaging (MRI) can detect inflammation of the joint lining **(Fig. 65-1)**. Ankle arthroscopy with synovectomy is indicated if conservative therapies such as cortisone injection, physical therapy, and oral anti-inflammatories are unsuccessful and the patient continues to have pain and disability.

Anterolateral Impingement Lesion

A soft tissue impingement lesion can develop in the anterior lateral corner of the ankle joint, often after injuries such as

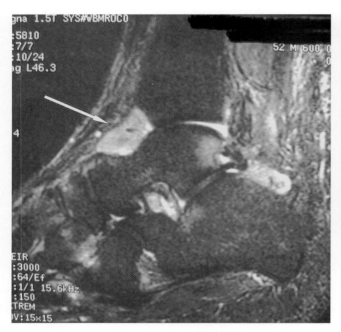

Fig. 65-1. T2 MRI. Sagittal plane image of anterior ankle synovitis with joint effusion. White arrow indicates area of effusion.

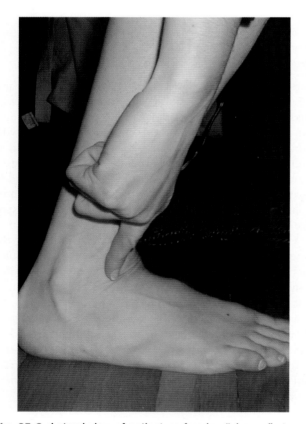

Fig. 65-2. Lateral view of patient performing "charger" stance. While weight bearing, patient bends knees, which maximally dorsiflexes the ankle. The heel is kept flat on the floor. This maneuver causes pain in the anterolateral corner of the ankle in cases of anterolateral impingement lesions.

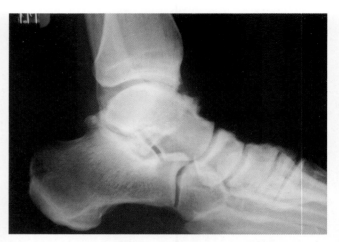

Fig. 65-3. Lateral radiograph of anterior ankle impingement spurs. The talar spur in this example spans across the anterior joint line.

fracture or severe ankle sprain. Patients may point specifically to this area as the source of pain and often will perceive a catching or clicking. On exam, maximal dorsiflexion and deep palpation to the anterior lateral corner of the ankle joint reproduces the pain. The "charger" stance, with the patient weight bearing, flexing the knee, and keeping the heel flat on the ground, also will produce pain in this corner of the ankle (Fig. 65-2). Radiographs are typically negative for soft tissue impingement lesions. MRI can detect a focal impingement lesion at the anterolateral corner, particularly on the T2 or SPIN images, when fluid outlines the abnormal soft-tissue structure.[4] Ankle arthroscopy with débridement of the anterolateral impingement lesion is indicated if conservative therapies such as cortisone injection, physical therapy, and oral anti-inflammatories are unsuccessful and the patient continues to have pain and disability.

Anterior Ankle Bony Impingement

Often called "footballers ankle," this bony impingement is a source of decreased ankle dorsiflexion and anterior ankle pain.[5] Limited ankle dorsiflexion is found on exam with a "bony end feel" or abrupt end to the range of motion (Fig. 65-3). Anterior bony impingement lesions occur most commonly in the athletic population, particularly dancers, soccer, football, and basketball players.[6] Anterior ankle capsular strain from forced plantarflexion with resultant calcific deposits or repetitive dorsiflexion, resulting in subchondral injury and new bone formation, are both possible mechanisms of anterior exostoses.[6,7] The chronically unstable ankle often develops anterior bony exostoses, which may represent capsular strain from rotational instability. These spurs are offset with the talar spur anteromedial and the tibia spur anterolateral[8] (Fig. 65-4). "Kissing" spurs can occur with degenerative joint disease with the tibial and talar spurs directly impinging, although there is no conclusive evidence that chronic ankle

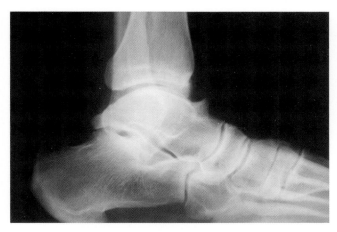

Fig. 65-4. Lateral radiograph of anterior ankle impingement spurs. The talar spur in this example is focused medial and is consistent with chronic ankle instability. Decompression of this spur may unmask ankle instability.

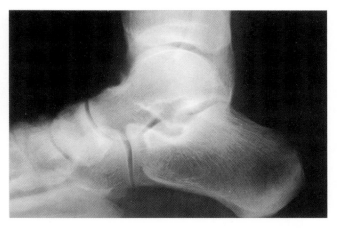

Fig. 65-6. Lateral radiograph of intact anterolateral OLT. The lesion is a subtle finding in this view.

instability leads to degenerative joint disease.[9] Radiographs can illustrate the orientation of the spurs, particularly if an oblique lateral view is used.[10] If further workup is necessary, computed tomography (CT) scan is recommended to fully evaluate the orientation of the bony impingement. Ankle arthroscopy with decompression of the anterior bony impingement is indicated if conservative therapies such as cortisone injection, physical therapy, and oral anti-inflammatories are unsuccessful and the patient continues to have pain and disability. Large exostoses are a relative contraindication due to the technical difficulty associated with a minimally invasive procedure.

Osteochondral Lesions of the Talus

Osteochondral lesions of the talus (OLT) are most commonly attributed to trauma either acute or remote in nature.[11–13] Lateral and medial talar dome lesions are unique and distinct from one another. Lateral talar dome lesions are

more likely from acute trauma.[14,15] The mechanisms of injury of lateral lesions are dorsiflexion and inversion, in which the anterolateral aspect of the talus impacts the fibula (Figs. 65-5, 65-6, 65-7). These anterolateral lesions typically are thin and waferlike in appearance.

Medial lesions result from combined inversion, plantar flexion, and external rotational forces. The medial lesion is caused by the posteromedial talar dome impacting the tibial articular surface and is typically deep and cup-shaped. The results of several biomechanical studies indicate that a

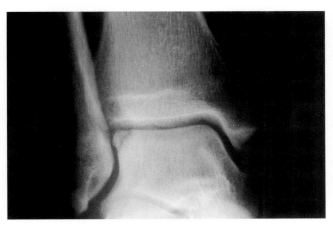

Fig. 65-5. Anterior-posterior (AP) radiograph of intact anterolateral osteochondral lesion of the talus (OLT).

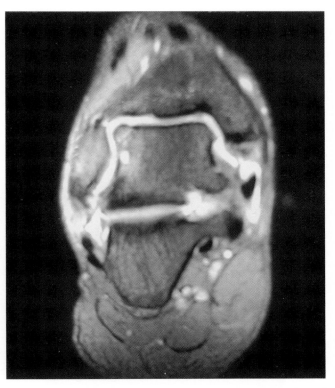

Fig. 65-7. T2 MRI. Coronal plane image of intact anterolateral OLT from Fig. 65-5. Marrow edema is noted beneath the lesion within the talus.

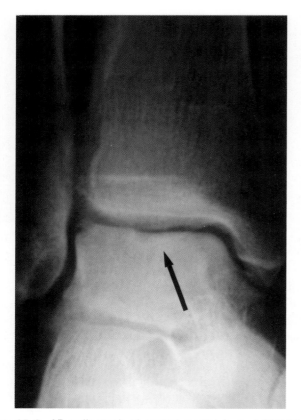

Fig. 65-8. AP radiograph of central-medial *(arrow)* OLT. This demonstrates the sometime subtle findings seen on plain film studies.

repetitive overuse syndrome may also be responsible for medial lesions.[16]

Patients may complain of generalized ankle tenderness that is worse with weight bearing and activity. A history of prior injury may be given, but often is not recalled by the patient. A catching or locking sensation may be perceived if there is a loose chondral flap or free floating loose body. Often, there is the overlying pain of ankle synovitis or an anterolateral impingement lesion that can cloud the diagnosis. Radiographic evaluation of the ankle can reveal osteochondral lesions, but findings can be subtle. MRI is helpful in identifying injuries of the subchondral bone and cartilage and precisely locating the lesion **(Figs. 65-8, 65-9, 65-10, 65-11)**. Staging of the lesion is performed according to one of several classification systems published previously.[17,18] The classification described by Hepple et al.[18] incorporates MRI findings. Stage 1 represents articular cartilage damage only. Stage 2a is cartilage injury with underlying fracture and edema. Stage 2b is the same as stage 2a without the edema. In Stage 3, the fragment is detached (rim signal) but not displaced. In stage 4, the fragment is displaced, and stage 5 shows subchondral cyst formation.

Arthroscopic treatment of OLT depends on the lesion itself. In acute chondral fractures, where significant bone remains attached to the chondral flap, securing the OLT back to the talar dome using absorbable fixation can be performed with arthroscopic visualization and débridement of interposed tissue.

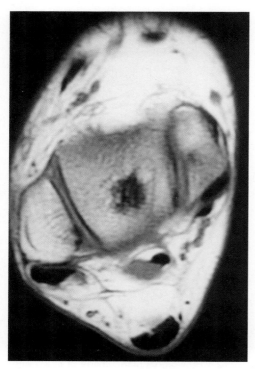

Fig. 65-9. T1 MRI. Axial plane image of central-medial OLT from Fig. 65-8.

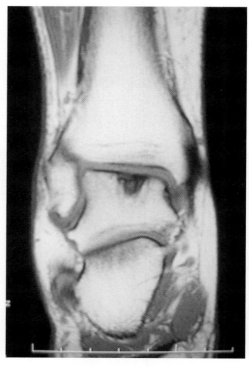

Fig. 65-10. T1 MRI. Coronal plane image of central-medial OLT from Fig. 65-8.

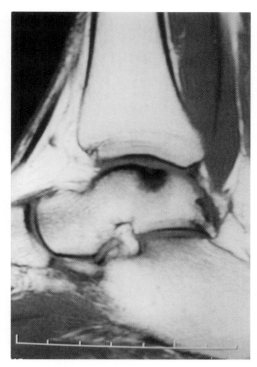

Fig. 65-11. T1 MRI. Sagittal plane image of central-medial OLT from Fig. 65-8.

In older lesions, removal of loose bodies with débridement and microfracture techniques stimulate development of fibrocartilage. The microfracture technique entails perforating subchondral bone and creating vascular access channels to release substances such as mesenchymal stem cells and growth factors to promote new tissue formation. Ultimately, fibrocartilage can form and fill the original defect. The excision, curettage, and microfracture technique has a success rate of 85% in a meta-analysis of the literature.[19]

In OLTs with an intact cartilage cap and subchondral cystic formation, retrograde drilling of the defect may be possible **(Figs. 65-12, 65-13)**. For medial lesions, the drilling begins laterally from the sinus tarsi and is used to perforate the subchondral cyst. The drill path supplies a route for revascularization and the cyst is back filled with bone graft or bone graft substitute. A cannulated system facilitates easy and accurate positioning of the drill hole and provides a delivery cannula for bone graft substitute or autograft. Arthroscopy is used to monitor the integrity of the cartilage cap during the procedure and ensure that bone graft does not enter the joint. As the bone fills the cystic void, the cartilage cap is anchored to the subchondral plate.

Ankle arthroscopy with treatment of the OLT is indicated if conservative therapies such as immobilization, physical therapy, and oral anti-inflammatories are unsuccessful and the patient continues to have pain and disability. Surgical treatment is also indicated in stage 3 and 4 lesions in which loose bodies or chondral flaps are already present.

Chronic Ankle Instability

Ankle sprains are common injuries, occurring in an estimated one out of 10,000 persons per day.[20] The anterior talofibular ligament (ATFL) is the most commonly injured ligament during ankle sprains. It serves as the primary restraint to inversion and translation of the talus within the ankle mortise. During an inversion ankle sprain, the anterolateral capsule is typically injured first, followed by the ATFL, calcaneal fibular ligament (CFL), and posterior talofibular ligament (PTFL).

The majority of acute ankle sprains heal with physical therapy/ankle rehabilitation; however, approximately 29% to 42% of patients experience chronic functional ankle instability.[21] Chronic lateral ankle instability is defined as instability for greater than 6 months with repeated episodes of "giving out," persistent pain, and inability to resume preinjury activity levels.[22] Physical exam will reveal laxity of the ATFL with a positive anterior drawer on the affected ankle as compared to the contralateral side. An anterior drawer maneuver that reveals anterior subluxation of the talus on the tibia

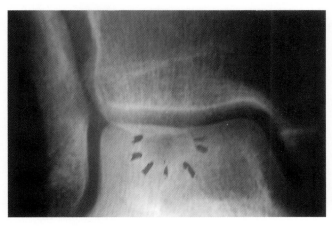

Fig. 65-12. AP ankle radiograph of cystic OLT with an apparent intact cartilage cap.

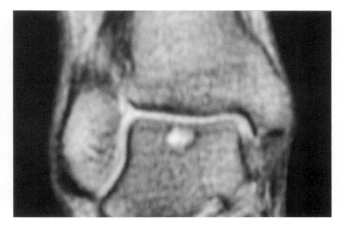

Fig. 65-13. T1 MRI. Coronal image of cystic OLT with an apparent intact cartilage cap from Fig. 65-12.

greater than 4 mm as compared with the contralateral side is considered indicative of ATFL laxity or rupture. Diminished ankle proprioception is frequently seen in chronic instability. To test proprioception, have the patient in a single limb stance close his or her eyes for 20 seconds and maintain balance. The patient should be able to do this without assistance and recover balance if you lightly push him or her. Functional instability fails to demonstrate gross ankle laxity, but the patient perceives instability and is unable to trust the ankle. Neuromuscular deficits are present in proprioception, muscle strength, muscle reaction time, and postural control.

The thermal-assisted capsular shift (TACS) procedure for chronic lateral ankle instability has been reported, and early results are encouraging.[23,24] Thermal energy is applied between 65°C and 70°C, which shrinks the collagen that comprises the joint capsule and ligaments. Patients who continue to have pain and instability despite aggressive physical therapy, proprioceptive training, and bracing are considered for TACS procedure. The decision to use TACS for lateral ligament reconstruction is influenced by the patient's body habitus, activity pattern, and degree of ligament injury. Indications include patients with moderate build, intra-ligament stretching (not avulsed from bone), generalized ligamentous laxity with functional ankle instability, a commitment to adhere to the postoperative rehabilitation protocol, and no previous ankle ligament reconstructive surgery. Contraindications include muscle weakness, tendon tears, neurological disorders, subtalar instability, and tibiofibular joint instability.

■ SURGICAL TECHNIQUES

For each of the five pathologies described above, the same surgical approach and anatomic considerations are used. Anesthesia is dependent on surgeon preference and anesthetist recommendations. Regional popliteal nerve block with a saphenous nerve augmentation work very well for all of these arthroscopic procedures and is our first choice.

Preoperatively, the ankle anatomy is drawn on the skin. Standard anteromedial and anterolateral ankle arthroscopy portals are utilized. The anteromedial portal is located in line with the joint, just medial to the anterior tibialis tendon. The saphenous vein and nerve run along the anterior border of the medial malleolus and are at risk with this approach. Keeping the portal just off the edge of the anterior tibialis tendon keeps these structures at a safe distance from the portal.

The anterolateral portal is placed again in line with the ankle joint, just lateral to the peroneus tertius tendon, entering the joint between the fibula and the talus **(Fig. 65-14)**. Structures at risk with the lateral portal include the lateral and medial branches of the superficial peroneal nerve. Placing the medial portal first and transilluminating the lateral soft tissue may reveal these nerve branches. Also, flexion of the fourth toe can accentuate the subcutaneous course of the superficial peroneal nerve and aid in avoidance.[25]

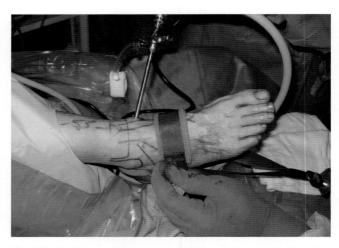

Fig. 65-14. Intraoperative image of ankle arthroscopy. Noninvasive ankle distractor is in place. Anatomic structures are drawn with ink on anterior ankle. Medial portal is already established. Spinal needle is inserted in proposed later portal, lateral to peroneus tertius tendon.

A well-padded thigh tourniquet is applied and the operative extremity is placed in a thigh holder with the knee flexed at approximately 45 degrees to 60 degrees, allowing the foot to rest 3 to 4 inches above the operating table. Care is taken to pad the holder sufficiently to ensure there is no pressure on the peroneal nerve **(Fig. 65-15)**. The tourniquet is rarely inflated during these procedures unless hemostasis and visualization are concerns.

After sterile preparation and drape of the ankle, a noninvasive ankle distractor is applied. A spinal needle is introduced into the ankle joint through the planned anteromedial portal. The joint is then insufflated with approximately 15 cc of local anesthetic with epinephrine. Reflux of joint fluid is noted into the syringe confirming correct placement into the joint. A small, superficial skin incision is made with a no. 11 blade. Blunt dissection of the subcutaneous tissue and

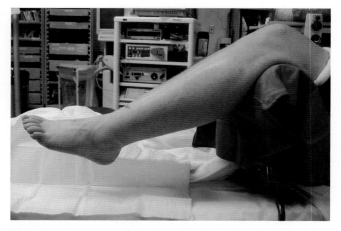

Fig. 65-15. Optimal placement of leg is stirrup holder. Note well padded at thigh with tourniquet in place. Heel should hang several inches above the operative table.

TABLE 65-1	Anatomic Points to Review During Arthroscopic Ankle Exam

Medial portal exam	Lateral portal exam
Medial gutter (talar-malleolar joint)	Lateral ankle gutter
Medial malleolus	Lateral malleolus
Deep fibers of deltoid ligament	ATFL
Anterior joint line/anterior tibia	Anterior joint line/ anterior tibia
Talar dome	Talar dome
Tibiofibular joint/tibiofibular ligaments	Medial malleolus
Lateral ankle gutter (talar-fibular joint)	Medial ankle gutter

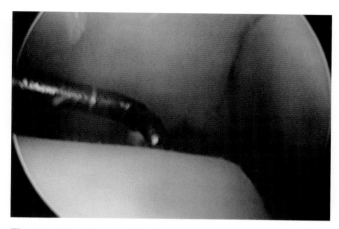

Fig. 65-17. Arthroscopic view of normal lateral talar dome. Probe indicates intact cartilage surface. Tibiofibular articulation is seen in background.

penetration of the joint capsule are performed with a curved hemostat. Next, a 30-degree, 4.0-mm arthroscope is introduced with a blunt trocar and cannula. Care is taken to use controlled pressure with the trocar and not plunge into the joint and create cartilage damage. Articular cartilage is visualized through the arthroscope before saline inflow is started to avoid extracapsular extravasation. A positive pressure inflow system is used for saline inflow and can be adjusted to the surgeon's preference.

The anterolateral region of the ankle joint is transilluminated with the arthroscope and the fourth toe is plantarflexed to visualize the superficial neurovascular anatomy. A spinal needle is once again introduced at the planned anterolateral portal just lateral to the peroneus tertius tendon. The identical steps are taken to introduce a blunt trocar through the lateral portal, and this should be visualized by the arthroscope. A 3.5-mm resector is then placed through the lateral portal.

The midline of the talar dome should be visualized and kept horizontal in the field of view for orientation. A thorough sequential exam of the joint is performed from the medial portal, taking care to note several anatomic landmarks **(Table 65-1)**. Care is taken to assess the integrity of the cartilage using a

blunt probe on the medial and lateral talar shoulders, the talar dome, and the tibial plafond **(Figs. 65-16, 65-17, 65-18)**. Any pathology encountered is addressed with instrumentation through the lateral portal. Then the arthroscope is placed in the lateral portal and another exam is performed. Any additional pathology is treated now with instrumentation from the medial portal.

Synovectomy/Anterolateral Impingement Resection

Synovitis can be found throughout the joint, but is typically thickest along the anterior joint line and in the medial and lateral ankle gutters. The 3.5-mm aggressive resector is used to remove the hypertrophic synovitis **(Fig. 65-19)**. Careful control of suction through the wand can facilitate débridement by drawing in the synovium without collapse of the capsular envelope. Resection of hemorrhagic synovium can compromise visualization due to bleeding and may necessitate use of the thigh tourniquet or intra-articular cautery.

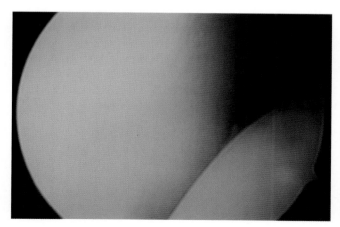

Fig. 65-16. Arthroscopic view of normal medial ankle gutter. The medial malleolus is seen on the left and the medial talar shoulder on the right.

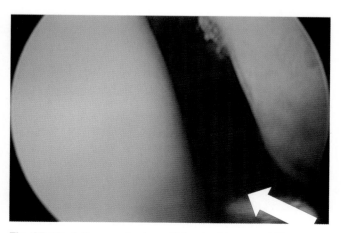

Fig. 65-18. Arthroscopic view of lateral ankle gutter. White arrow indicates location of ATFL deep within the ankle gutter.

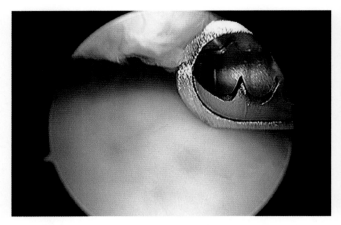

Fig. 65-19. Arthroscopic view of aggressive resector. Careful control is required to prevent iatrogenic cartilage damage.

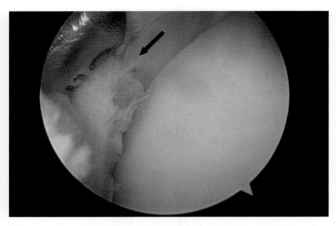

Fig. 65-21. Arthroscopic view of impingement lesion resection. Arthroscopic biters are often needed to transect the lesion.

Débridement of synovium should first begin in the medial gutter, then along the anterior joint line, and finally at the lateral gutter. Complete débridement will require switching portals for full access of the joint. Care should be taken to protect the cartilage from the teeth of the resector. Any loose bodies encountered can be débrided with the resector or removed using a variety of arthroscopic graspers and biters. The capsule has a white to pinkish coloration and should be maintained during débridement procedures **(Fig. 65-20)**.

The anterolateral impingement lesion appears at the corner of the joint, with a whitish, thick, scar-tissue consistency **(Fig. 65-21)**. This impingement lesion may represent hypertrophy of the anterior inferior tibiofibular ligament.[26] Often this is difficult to débride with the resector alone and often requires the use of arthroscopic biters as well. Once transected into two discrete ends, the resector is more efficient at removal.

After synovectomy and impingement resection is completed through both portals, a final survey of the joint is made. The inflow is stopped and the suction is used to remove any

excess fluid. The instrumentation is removed and the joint and soft tissues are manually compressed to remove fluid.

Our standard closure and dressings consist of simple interrupted nylon sutures and a sterile dressing as well as a posterior splint with a cold care unit built into the padding. Care is taken to ensure several layers of cotton padding are between the skin and the cold unit to prevent skin injury. The patient is instructed to remain non–weight bearing on the surgical extremity and is seen in the office 10 days postoperatively.

Anterior Bony Impingement Decompression

Often in cases of anterior bony impingement, another intra-articular pathology such as synovitis or soft tissue impingement exists. The same joint survey and synovectomy procedures are used as described above. Attention is then directed to the anterior joint line. Gentle blunt reflection of the anterior ankle capsule is performed using the resector as a probe. The capsule is elevated superiorly off the anterior tibia and inferiorly off the neck of the talus. Release of the distractor facilitates this procedure and eases traction of the anterior capsule.

Typically the tibial spur is wide and may span the entire anterior lip. The talar spur is more discrete and protrudes medially off the medial edge of the talar neck. It is sometimes difficult to accurately gauge the extent of the tibia spur. It is important to find the medial or lateral margin of the spur to determine the interval between normal tibia and exostosis.

A 4.0-mm burr is used to remove the exostoses. It is important to keep the burr facing the bone during this procedure and not at the anterior ankle soft tissue. The anterior neurovascular bundle is potentially at risk for injury. The burr can be run on reverse for less aggressive resection and is useful for final smoothing or for less experienced arthroscopists. Find either the medial or lateral interval between normal tibia and exostosis. Débride the bone back to the normal margin and then work across the joint. This ensures complete decompression of the anterior spur. After careful

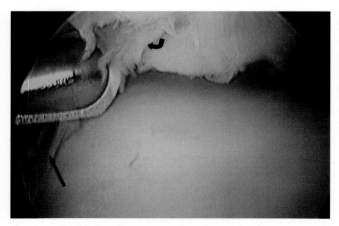

Fig. 65-20. Arthroscopic view of synovectomy *(curved arrow)*. Normal, pink colored capsule *(straight arrow)* is noted and protected.

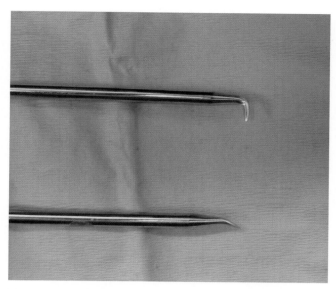

Fig. 65-22. Table-side view of arthroscopic awls or picks—90 degree and 30 degree awls are pictured and commonly used.

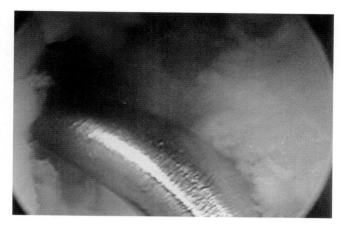

Fig. 65-24. Arthroscopic view of débrided OLT. A 30-degree awl is in use for microfracture technique. Tip of the pick is perforating subchondral bone.

resection of the exostoses, the resector is reintroduced into the joint and any residual debris is removed. Standard closing and splint dressing is used. The patient is kept non–weight bearing and is seen 10 days postoperatively.

Treatment for Osteochondral Lesions of the Talus

Débridement and Microfracture
The noninvasive ankle distractor is used and standard arthroscopic portals are established. A full joint survey is performed and any hypertrophic synovitis or loose debris is removed. The OLT is located and evaluation of the corresponding tibial side is performed as well. For medial lesions, it is often necessary to plantarflex the ankle to gain additional visualization. The blunt angled probe is used to assess the integrity of the cartilage. It is important to determine the stability of the

surrounding cartilage rim. Often what appears to be intact cartilage is actually undermined and loose.

Using a combination of resectors, ring curettes and graspers, the nonviable cartilage is removed and the base of the bed exposed. The bed is débrided back to bleeding bone and the edges should be trimmed to viable cartilage. The surgeon must maintain control of the loose debris and not allow it to travel to other portions of the joint. A crisp, firm edge around the OLT is created with the ring curettes. It is important to come straight down with the ring curette and not create skived margins.

Arthroscopic awls of various angles are used to microfracture or perforate the bed and create the vascular access channels (Fig. 65-22). The perforations are made approximately 3 to 4 mm apart in the subchondral bone while maintaining the integrity of the bone plate (Figs. 65-23, 65-24, 65-25). After thorough débridement, punctate bleeding and lipid droplets should be visualized from the bed when inflow pressure is decreased.

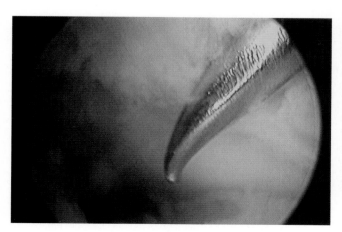

Fig. 65-23. Arthroscopic view of débrided OLT. A 30-degree awl seen is in view for microfracture technique.

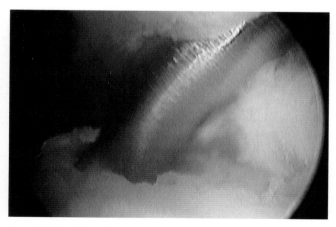

Fig. 65-25. Arthroscopic view of débrided OLT. A 30-degree awl is in use for microfracture technique. The entire tip of the awl should penetrate the subchondral bone to create vascular access channels.

After completion of the OLT débridement and microfracture, a joint survey is again performed from both portal sites to ensure removal of all debris. Standard closure and splint dressings are used. The patient is kept non–weight bearing on the operative leg and seen back at 10 days postoperatively.

Chondral Flap Repair

Standard anteromedial and anterolateral portals are used along with the noninvasive distractor. A complete joint survey is performed and the chondral flap is identified. It is important to look for loose bodies associated with the flap. An acute, discrete chondral fracture that is completely detached is still potentially amenable to internal fixation. This is dependant on the size and integrity of the osteochondral fragment. If the fragment is small or comminuted, it is excised and the débridement and microfracture technique is used at the donor site.

The blunt probe is used to assess the integrity of the flap and the surrounding cartilage. Any nonviable and interposing tissue is resected and the flap is held in place with the blunt probe. Traditional antegrade bone screws damage the intact articular cartilage and are not appropriate. Kirschner wires can be placed via a retrograde insertion through a nonarticular portion of the talus and advanced immediately below the articular surface to capture the fragment. The wire is cut off at the skin for later removal. The use of bioabsorbable pins, such as the Chondral Dart (Arthrex, Naples, Fla), eliminates the need for future removal and many are small enough to be used antegrade without damaging the cartilage. Once the flap or fragment is secured, the joint is again inspected for any additional injuries.

Standard closure with nylon suture and sterile dressing with posterior splint and cold unit is applied. The patient is kept non–weight bearing and seen 10 days postoperatively.

Retrograde Drilling of Osteochondral Lesions of the Talus

The standard arthroscopy set up and portal placement is used with the noninvasive distractor in place. Intraoperative fluoroscopy is needed and should be available. Preoperative MRI is used to accurately locate the lesion. A full arthroscopic inspection of the joint is performed. An intact cartilage cap must be present for the retrograde drilling procedure to be used. Plain film radiograph and MRI are useful tools, but arthroscopy is definitive to assess cap viability **(Figs. 65-26, 65-27)**. If the cap has been violated, the débridement and microfracture protocol should be followed.

The blunt tipped probe is used to gently palpate the cap. With subchondral cystic formation, the cap will feel very soft as compared to the firm feeling of the surrounding healthy cartilage **(Fig. 65-28)**. If the cartilage cap is intact, the retrograde drilling procedure continues.

A novel cannulated retrograde drilling set is used. A small stab incision is created laterally over the sinus tarsi. Bluntly dissect the subcutaneous tissue with hemostat and introduce the guide wire. Fluoroscopy confirms the guide

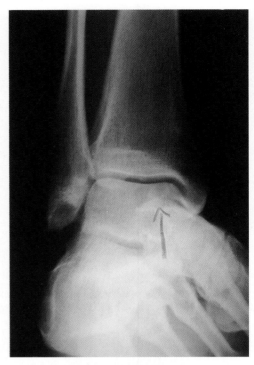

Fig. 65-26. AP ankle radiograph detailing medial OLT with apparent intact cartilage cap *(arrow)*.

wire is in the sinus tarsi, specifically the nonarticular junction of the talar body and neck **(Fig. 65-29)**. Advance the wire from inferior-lateral to superior-medial to the rim of the subchondral cyst. Multiple views using the fluoroscopy are taken to confirm precise location of the guide wire. It is critical not to penetrate or damage the cartilage cap.

Once optimal wire placement is ensured, advance the 6.0-mm cannulated drill over the wire toward the lesion **(Fig. 65-30)**. Again, use the fluoroscopy to monitor the depth of the drill. It is only necessary to penetrate the sclerotic rim

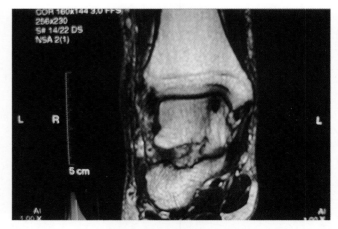

Fig. 65-27. Coronal T1 MRI image of medial OLT from Fig. 65-26. OLT appears cystic with intact cartilage covering. MRI is more sensitive to determine status of cartilage cap.

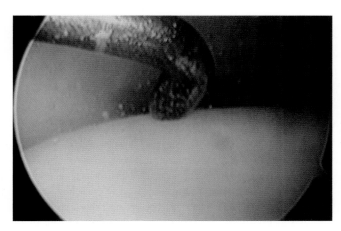

Fig. 65-28. Arthroscopic view of medial OLT from Figs. 65-26 and 65-27. Blunt probe confirms cartilage cap is intact and OLT is amenable to retrograde drilling.

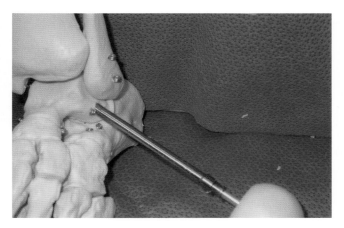

Fig. 65-31. The cannula and plunger are now in place on this bone model demonstration. Allograft bone gel is carefully back filled into the OLT using the plunger.

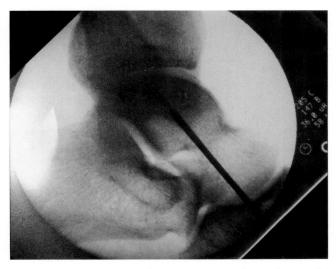

Fig. 65-29. Intraoperative fluoroscopic view of lateral to medial drilling of OLT. Combinations of arthroscopic and fluoroscopic views are used to prevent injury to cartilage cap.

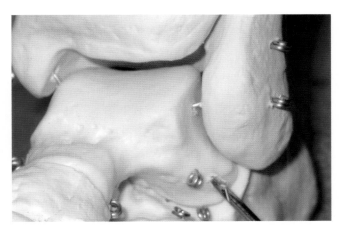

Fig. 65-30. The cannulated retrograde drill is demonstrated on a bone model. Drilling is started on nonarticular portion of lateral talus and directed medial and superior toward the OLT.

of the cyst. Next, removed the drill and place the cannula over the guide wire. Once the cannula is secured, remove the guide wire. Inject approximately 1 cc of allograft bone gel into the cannula and slowly advance with the plunger **(Fig. 65-31)**. Take care not to generate too much pressure during this back filling, which could disrupt the cartilage cap. Use the arthroscope to ensure the cartilage is maintained and bone graft remains extra-articular.

Standard closure with nylon suture and sterile dressing with posterior splint and cold unit is applied. The patient is kept non–weight bearing and seen 10 days postoperatively.

Thermal-Assisted Capsular Shift Procedure

Standard anteromedial and anterolateral arthroscopy portals are established, again with the aid of the noninvasive ankle distractor. A complete arthroscopic joint exam is performed and any concomitant hypertrophic or hemorrhage synovitis or anterolateral impingement lesions are addressed as appropriate. Care is taken to adequately decompress the lateral gutter of synovitis and debris without being overly aggressive. The ankle capsule is maintained.

A temperature-controlled thermal probe is placed in the anterolateral portal. An end effect probe is used and set on desiccation mode to obliterate any redundant synovitis or fibrous bands. It is important to identify the ATFL off the anterior distal portion of the fibula deep in the lateral ankle gutter. The thermal wand is placed on the ATFL and the ankle distractor is disengaged. The thermal wand is set for a maximum of 65°C. The temperature-controlled wand is a bipolar device that constantly regulates the energy delivered at the tip to maintain the desired temperature.

Beginning deep in the lateral gutter against the ATFL, the thermal wand is activated and used in a "corn-row" sweeping technique. As tissue shrinkage and a subtle color change are observed, the probe is moved in a straight line from deep to superficial. The thermal wand is used to gently probe the tissue in order to assess the tension of the ligament and capsular shrinkage. The probe is then placed adjacent to the previous line of shrinkage and the maneuver is repeated. It is imperative that a slow but constant sweeping motion is used to minimize tissue ablation. This shrinkage technique is repeated until all areas of the ligament and anterolateral capsule are treated. Keep the treatment area below the horizon of the talar dome to prevent iatrogenic creation of an impingement lesion.

The thermally modified joint capsule and ATFL are structurally weakened during the TACS procedure and even physiologic loads during this time period can produce significant laxity of these structures. It is imperative that the ankle be protected from inversion stress during application of the dressings and splint.

Standard portal closure with nylon interrupted sutures and a sterile dressing is applied. A well-padded cold care unit and posterior splint are applied. A medial to lateral stirrup is also built into the splint for inversion/eversion protection of the ankle. The patient is kept non–weight bearing on the operative limb and seen 10 days postoperatively.

■ TECHNICAL ALTERNATIVES AND PITFALLS

Synovectomy/Anterolateral Impingement Resection

Arthroscopic débridement of synovitis and anterolateral impingement is quite successful and has a low incidence of complication or morbidity. As with all ankle arthroscopic procedures, the surgeon should exercise care in protecting the anterior neurovasculature and superficial nerves as described.

Some arthroscopists do not use distraction of the ankle. This limits access of the joint and allows only a partial synovectomy. The noninvasive distractor can be safely used to gently distract the ankle without the morbidity of previous invasive models. Distraction with up to 30 lb (135 N) of traction can safely be applied for up to 1 hour.[27] It is potentially possible to overdistract the ankle and cause traction injury to the neurovasculature. Greater traction or longer distraction is associated with increased nerve conduction abnormalities.[27]

For hemorrhagic synovitis, use of the thigh tourniquet or cautery is recommended to maintain visibility within the joint. If possible, address other pathologies first and then perform the synovectomy. The anterolateral impingement lesion is often quite thick and often requires transection with the arthroscopic biter. The resector is then used to débride the cut ends.

Some surgeons may prefer open arthrotomy for synovectomy and débridement, and this is certainly an option. Open

arthrotomy is limited in terms of the joint exposure, ability to perform a full joint inspection, and thorough débridement, unless a larger dissection is used. This could increase the likelihood of soft tissue complications as compared to arthroscopy.

Anterior Bony Impingement Decompression

The critical points in successful arthroscopic anterior decompression are: (a) adequate blunt elevation of the anterior joint capsule off the anterior tibia and dorsal talar neck, (b) relaxation of ankle distraction, and (c) visualization of exostosis-normal bone interval. Following these three tenets allows successful and reproducible decompression of anterior ankle exostoses.

Some surgeons may prefer open arthrotomy for decompression of anterior spurs. Open decompression is necessary with extremely large spurs to allow complete resection. As the surgeon's skill and comfort with ankle arthroscopy advances, the use of open arthrotomy decreases.

The decompression of large bony impingement may unmask marked ankle instability. This should be considered during procedure selection. If it is felt that ankle instability will be created with large spur decompression, the addition of an ankle stabilization procedure is indicated. Spurs associated with instability tend to be medial on the talus as compared to global anterior spurring with degenerative joint disease.

Treatment for Osteochondral Lesions of the Talus

Arthroscopy is ideal for OLT débridement and microfracture techniques. It allows access to the majority of the joint, and posterior portals can be placed as needed for total access. There is, however, a significant learning curve associated with using the various instruments for débridement and microfracture. The skill of triangulating the camera and instrumentation does take time, but this is not unique to ankle arthroscopy.

Some surgeons may prefer open treatment for OLTs, especially for posterior medial lesions. Open arthrotomy with possible malleolar osteotomy certainly has a role in the operative treatment of OLTs and is used by the authors. Large lesions, which have previously failed débridement and microfracture, may require osteochondral grafting, which necessitates opening the joint.

Retrograde drilling of select OLTs has the potential pitfall of disrupting the intact cartilage cap. This can happen any time during the drilling procedure. When drilling over the wire, the wire can slightly advance and perforate the cartilage. The authors recommend drilling under live fluoroscopic imaging to monitor the advance of both the drill bit and the wire tip. Also, care is taken when plunging the graft through the cannula to prevent cap displacement. If the cap is violated,

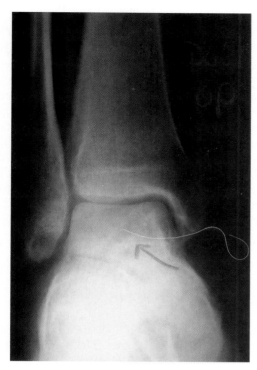

Fig. 65-32. Postoperative retrograde drilling AP ankle radiograph. Bone canal is subtly noted traversing inferior-lateral to superior-medial *(arrow)*.

graft could enter the joint and the débridement and microfracture protocol may be necessary. The incorporation of bone graft can be monitored with radiographs and MRI if needed **(Figs. 65-32, 65-33)**.

Thermal-Assisted Capsular Shift Procedure

The TACS procedure works well in functional and chronic ankle instability. The procedure is not indicated in trau-

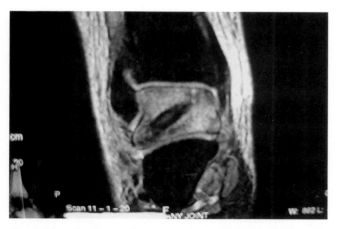

Fig. 65-33. Coronal T2 MRI image of postoperative retrograde drilling. Bone edema is noted. Bone canal seen from inferior-lateral to superior-medial. Note cartilage cap remains intact.

matic rupture or avulsion of the ATFL. The advantages of this procedure are a decreased risk of complications inherent to open procedures and the ability to fully assess and treat any associated intra-articular ankle pathology. Between February 1999 and December 2001, the authors performed 42 arthroscopic thermal-assisted capsular modifications of the anterolateral capsule and the ATFL. The American Orthopaedic Foot and Ankle Society Hindfoot scores improved significantly: scores averaged 29.57 preoperatively (SD 15.6) and improved to 55.36 (SD 13.56) at an average follow-up of 14.1 months ($p < .001$).[24]

The alternative many surgeons are familiar with is the open modified Brostrom procedure. This is an excellent procedure that consistently yields good to excellent results. The modified Brostrom is used in patients with mechanical instability beyond the normal physiological range and in patients with concomitant large distal fibula loose bodies.

In performing TACS, there are several tenets to remember. First, distraction of the joint should be released before thermal treatment of the tissues. The thermal energy causes shrinkage of the ligament and capsule by breaking crosslinks within the collagen of the tissue. This weakens the tissue and if distraction is applied, the lateral tissues will lengthen, not shorten. Second, it is imperative to treat only capsular and intracapsular tissues with a deliberate paint-brushing or checkerboard patterning. It is possible to cause soft tissue thermal injury and skin slough if the tissues are overexposed or if the thermal probe is activated within the subcutaneous envelope. Third, start deep in the lateral gutter and work your way out anteriorly, keeping below the talar dome level. The tissue will tighten as the treatment progresses, and if you start superiorly, it is difficult to reach the deep portions of the lateral gutter. Also, keep below the horizon of the talar dome to lessen the chance of creating an iatrogenic anterolateral soft tissue impingement lesion.

■ REHABILITATION/RETURN TO PLAY RECOMMENDATIONS

Synovectomy/Anterolateral Impingement Resection

The operative ankle is immobilized in a posterior splint and the patient is non–weight bearing immediately after surgery. At 10 days postoperatively, the sutures are removed and the patient is placed in a removable boot walker. The patient is to wear the boot at all times other than bathing and sleeping. Beginning at 2 weeks postoperatively, formal physical therapy is begun to enhance range of motion, proprioception, and strength of the ankle. The patient is allowed to migrate out of the boot and into normal shoe gear with the help of the therapist. Typically patients are rapidly advanced out of the boot pending healing of the portal sites. Athletic patients can quickly return into sport by the third week postoperatively.

Anterior Bony Impingement Decompression

The rehabilitation protocol for bony decompression is identical to the synovectomy/anterolateral impingement resection protocol. Again, it is important to get the ankle moving by the second week postoperatively with the aid of formal physical therapy. This time is tailored to the healing status of the portal sites.

Treatment of Osteochondral Lesions of the Talus

Débridement/Microfracture for Osteochondral Lesions of the Talus

For all of our OLT treatments, the same postoperative and rehabilitation protocol is used. The operative ankle is immobilized in a posterior splint with medial/lateral stirrup and the patient is non–weight bearing immediately after surgery. At 10 days postoperatively, the sutures are removed and the patient is placed in a non–weight bearing boot walker. The patient is kept non–weight bearing but instructed to perform gentle range of motion exercises. Early motion may "train" mesenchymal cells to reform cartilage. Between weeks 4 and 8, the patient is allowed to bear weight as tolerated in the boot walker. Formal physical therapy is begun at 8 weeks to enhance range of motion, proprioception, and strength of the ankle. For athletes, sport-specific training is ordered with the therapist with an anticipated return to sport at 14 to 16 weeks.

Chondral Flap Repair

Our standard OLT treatment postoperative and rehabilitation protocol is used for chondral flap repair. Occasionally, the patient may be kept non–weight bearing for a total of 6 weeks and then advanced into a boot walker. This may be done in cases of tenuous fixation of the fragment or other concerns of healing.

Retrograde Drilling of Osteochondral Lesions of the Talus

Our standard OLT treatment postoperative and rehabilitation protocol is used after retrograde drilling. Typically these patients rapidly advance through the protocol and rarely need additional non–weight bearing casting.

Thermal-Assisted Capsular Shift Procedure

The operative ankle is immobilized in a posterior splint with medial/lateral stirrup and the patient is non–weight bearing immediately after TACS surgery. It is critically important to protect the ankle while applying the postoperative dressing and splint. The ankle should be positioned in neutral to slightly dorsiflexed/everted position.

At 10 days postoperatively, the sutures are removed and the patient is placed in a non–weight bearing below the knee cast. The patient is kept non–weight bearing for an additional 3 weeks. The cast is changed to a walking cast for an additional 3 weeks and then a removable boot walker for another 3 weeks. The boot is worn at all times other than bathing and sleeping. Once in the boot walker, formal physical therapy is begun to enhance range of motion, proprioception, and strength of the ankle. Physical therapy is ordered for 3 times a week for 3 weeks. The patient is allowed to migrate out of the boot and into normal shoe gear with the help of the therapist. For athletes, sport-specific training is ordered with the therapist with an anticipated return to competitive sport at 4 months. A lace-up ankle brace with figure-8 straps is used during "at risk" activities beginning at month 4. This protection is continued for the remainder of the postoperative year.

■ OUTCOMES AND FUTURE DIRECTIONS

Ankle arthroscopy is a reliable and safe means of treating a variety of ankle joint pathologies. The minimally invasive nature of arthroscopy versus open procedures translates into fewer complications and quicker recovery times. Complications are rare and the steps outlined above can reduce them even more. There is a learning curve to the arthroscopic procedures discussed, but adept arthroscopists are quickly able to become efficient.

Innovative arthroscopic techniques such as TACS and retrograde drilling of OLTs are promising. A long-term follow-up study as well as a prospective comparison between TACS and the open Brostrom are currently under way. Second-look arthroscopy on TACS patients has shown a smooth remodeling and maintenance of the anterolateral capsule and ATFL tension at 1 year **(Fig. 65-34)**. The indications for ankle arthroscopy will likely continue to expand as instrumentation and surgeon skill are advanced.

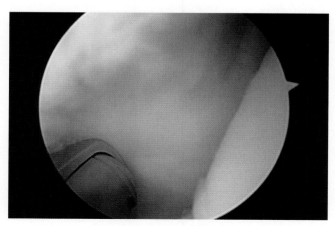

Fig. 65-34. Arthroscopic view of anterolateral capsule/ATFL 1-year status post-TACS. Appropriate tension is maintained as seen by stress force with resector.

■ SUGGESTED READINGS

Barnes CL, Ferkel RD. Arthroscopic débridement and drilling of osteochondral lesions of the talus. Foot Ankle Clin. 2003;8(2):243–257.

Berberian WS, Hecht PJ, Wapner KL, et al. Morphology of tibiotalar osteophytes in anterior ankle impingement. Foot Ankle Int. 2001;22(4):313–317.

Berlet GC, Anderson RB, Davis WH. Chronic lateral ankle instability. Foot Ankle Clin. 1999;4(4):713–728.

Berlet GC, Saar WE, Raissi A, et al. Thermal-assisted capsular modification for chronic lateral ankle instability. Tech Foot Ankle Surg. 2002;1(2):138–144.

Berlet GC, Saar WE, Ryan A, et al. Thermal-assisted capsular modification for functional ankle instability. Foot Ankle Clin. 2002;7:567–576.

Ferkel RD, Whipple TL, Brust SE. *Arthroscopic Surgery: The Foot and Ankle.* Philadelphia: Lippincott, Williams & Wilkins; 1996.

Parisien JS. Arthroscopic treatment of osteochondral lesions of the talus. Am J Sports Med. 1986;14:211–217.

Parkes JC, Hamilton WG, Patterson AH, et al. The anterior impingement syndrome of the ankle. J Trauma. 1980;20(10):895–898.

Scranton PE Jr, McDermott JE. Anterior tibial spurs: a comparison of open versus arthroscopic débridement. Foot Ankle. 1992;13:125–129.

Sledge SL. Microfracture techniques in the treatment of osteochondral injuries. Clin Sports Med. 2001;20:365–377.

Thordarson DB. Retrograde drilling of osteochondral lesions in the mediotalar dome. Foot Ankle Int. 2000;21(5):434–435.

Tol JL, Struijs PA, Bossuyt PM, et al. Treatment strategies in osteochondral defects of the talar dome: a systematic review. Foot Ankle Int. 2000;21(2):119–126.

Tol JL, Verhegen CP, van Dijk CN. Arthroscopic treatment of anterior impingement in the ankle. J Bone Joint Surg Br. 2001;83(1):9–13.

■ REFERENCES

1. Watanabe M, Bechtol RC, Nottage WM. The history of arthroscopy. In: Shahriaree H, ed. *O'Connor's Textbook of Arthroscopic Surgery*, 2nd ed. Philadelphia: JB Lippincott Co; 1992:213–217.
2. Watanabe M, Takeda S. The number 21 arthroscope. Nippon Seikeigeka Gakkai Zasshi. 1960;34:1042.
3. Kreuscher PH. Semilunar cartilage disease: a plea for early recognition by means of the arthroscope and early treatment of this condition. Ill Med J. 1925;47:290–292.
4. Rubin DA, Tishkoff NW, Britton CA, et al. Anterolateral soft-tissue impingement in the ankle: diagnosis using MR imaging. Am J Roentgenol. 1997;169(3):829–835.
5. McMurray TP. Footballer's ankle. J Bone Joint Surg. 1950;32-B:68.
6. Stoller SM, Hekmat F, Kleiger B. A comparative study of the frequency of anterior impingement exostoses of the ankle in dancers and nondancers. Foot Ankle. 1984;4:201–203.
7. Parkes JC, Hamilton WG, Patterson AH, et al. The anterior impingement syndrome of the ankle. J Trauma. 1980;20(10):895–898.
8. Berberian WS, Hecht PJ, Wapner KL, et al. Morphology of tibiotalar osteophytes in anterior ankle impingement. Foot Ankle Int. 2001;22(4):313–317.
9. DeMaio M, Paine R, Drez D Jr. Chronic lateral ankle instability—inversion sprains: part II. Orthopedics. 1992;15(2):241–248.
10. van Dijk CN, Wessel RN, Tol JL, et al. Oblique radiograph for the detection of bone spurs in anterior ankle impingement. Skeletal Radiol. 2002;31(4):214–221.
11. Parisien JS. Arthroscopic treatment of osteochondral lesions of the talus. Am J Sports Med. 1986;14:211–217.
12. Pettine KA, Morrey BF. Osteochondral fractures of the talus: a long-term follow-up. J Bone Joint Surg. 1987;69B:89–92.
13. Van Buecken K, Barrack RL, Alexander AH, et al. Arthroscopic treatment of transchondral talar dome fractures. Am J Sports Med. 1989;17:350–355.
14. Canale ST, Belding RH. Osteochondral lesions of the talus. J Bone Joint Surg. 1980;62A:97–102.
15. Flick AB, Gould N. Osteochondritis dissecans of the talus (transchondral fractures of the talus): review of the literature and new surgical approach for medial dome lesions. Foot Ankle. 1985;5:165–185.
16. Bruns J, Rosenbach B, Kahrs J. Etiopathogenetic aspects of medial osteochondrosis dissecans tali. Sportverletz Sportschaden. 1992;6:43–49.
17. Berndt AL, Harty M. Transchondral fractures (osteochondritis dissecans) of the talus. J Bone Joint Surg. 1959;41A:988–1020.
18. Hepple S, Winson IG, Glew D. Osteochondral lesions of the talus: a revised classification. Foot Ankle Int. 1999;20(12):789–793.
19. Tol JL, Struijs PA, Bossuyt PM, et al. Treatment strategies in osteochondral defects of the talar dome: a systematic review. Foot Ankle. 2000;21(2):119–126.
20. Trevino SG, Davis P, Hecht PJ. Management of acute and chronic lateral ligament injuries of the ankle. Orthop Clin North Am. 1994;25:1–16.
21. Berlet GC, Anderson RB, Davis WH. Chronic lateral ankle instability. Foot Ankle Clin. 1999;4(4):713–728.
22. Messer TM, Cummins CA, Ahn J, et al. Outcome of the modified Brostrom procedure for chronic lateral ankle instability using suture anchors. Foot Ankle. 2000;21(12):996–1003.
23. Ryan AH, Lee TH, Berlet GC. Arthroscopic thermal assisted capsular shrinkage in anterolateral ankle instability: a retrospective review of 13 patients. Paper presented at: American Orthopaedic Foot and Ankle Society Annual Summer Meeting; July 2000; Vail, Colo.
24. Berlet GC, Saar WE, Ryan A, et al. Thermal-assisted capsular modification for functional ankle instability. Foot Ankle Clin. 2002;7:567–576.
25. Stephens MM, Kelly PM. Fourth toe flexion sign: a new clinical sign for identification of the superficial peroneal nerve. Foot Ankle. December 2000;21(12):995–998.
26. Nikolopoulos CE, Tsirikos AI, Sourmelis S, et al. The accessory anterointerior tibiofibular ligament as a cause of talar impingement: a cadaveric study. Am J Sports Med. 2004;32(2):389–395.
27. Dowdy PA, Watson BV, Amendola A, et al. Noninvasive ankle distraction: relationship between force, magnitude of distraction, and nerve conduction abnormalities. Arthroscopy. 1996;12(1):64–69.

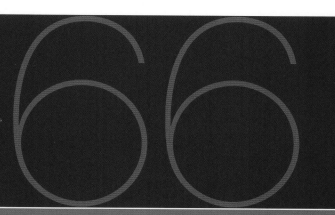

66

POSTERIOR ANKLE ARTHROSCOPY AND TENDOSCOPY

C. NIEK VAN DIJK, MD, PhD, HELEEN SONNEVELD, MD,
PETER A. J. DE LEEUW, MSc, ROVER KRIPS, MD, PhD

■ HISTORY OF THE TECHNIQUE

Over the past 20 years arthroscopy of the ankle joint has become an important diagnostic and therapeutic procedure for chronic and posttraumatic complaints of the ankle joint. Burman,[1] in 1931, regarded the ankle joint as unsuitable for arthroscopy because of its anatomy. Tagaki,[2] in 1939, described systematic arthroscopic assessment of the ankle joint.[2] Watanabe[3] published a series of 28 ankle arthroscopies in 1972 followed by Chen[4] in 1976. In the 1980s several publications followed.[5–11] Some authors recommend routine placement of posterior portals in ankle arthroscopy.[7,8] In these cases, a posterolateral portal is recommended. Because of the potential for serious complications, most authors feel the posteromedial portal is contraindicated in all but the most extreme situations.[7,8,12,13] Arthroscopy of the subtalar joint was first described by Parisien and Vangsness[11] in 1985. Endoscopic access to the posterior tibial tendons, including treatment of pathology, was first described by van Dijk et al.[14] in 1997, followed by tendoscopy of the peroneal tendons[15] in 1998 and endoscopic release of the flexor hallucis longus tendon in 2000.[16]

Hindfoot endoscopy has been demonstrated to give excellent access to the posterior ankle compartment, the subtalar joint, as well as extra-articular structures such as the os trigonum, the deep portion of the deltoid ligament, the posterior syndesmotic ligaments, and the tendons of the tarsal tunnel.[16]

Nagai[17] was the first author to use the arthroscope to access the retrocalcaneal recess. He reported a case in which he identified the Achilles tendon and an avulsed portion of its insertion at the calcaneus. A description of the entry portals and the surgical approach to the retrocalcaneal bursa

appeared in 1997.[18] The results of a first cohort of 22 consecutive patients, with a minimal follow-up of 2 years, was published in 2000.[16]

■ INDICATIONS AND CONTRAINDICATIONS

Indications can be divided according to the location of the pathology.

Articular Pathology

Posterior Compartment Ankle Joint
The main indications are the débridement and drilling of posteriorly located osteochondral defects of the ankle joint, removal of loose bodies from the posterior compartment, removal of ossicles, posttraumatic calcifications, avulsion fragments, resection of posterior tibial rim osteophytes, treatment of chondromatosis, and treatment of chronic synovitis.

Posterior Compartment Subtalar Joint
The main indications are osteophyte removal and débridement of degenerative changes in the subtalar joint, removal of loose bodies, treatment of an intraosseous talar ganglion by drilling, curetting and bone grafting, and subtalar arthrodesis (Fig. 66-1A,B,C,D).

Periarticular Pathology

Posterior Ankle Impingement
Posterior ankle impingement is a pain syndrome. The patient experiences posterior ankle pain that is mainly present on

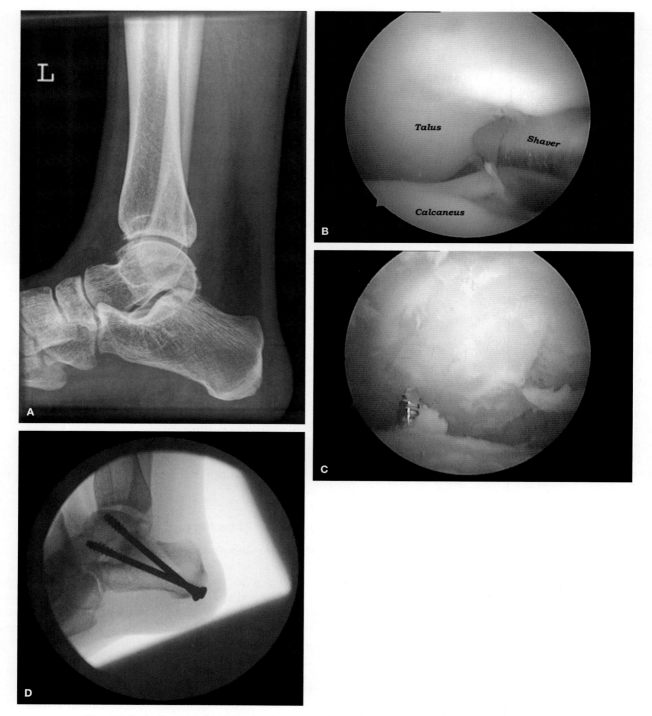

Fig. 66-1. A: Preoperative lateral x-ray of a patient with degeneration of the left subtalar joint (**B–D** refer to the same patient). **B:** Arthroscopic débridement of the degenerated cartilage of the subtalar joint by means of posterior ankle arthroscopy. With the shaver the superficial cartilage layer is removed in order to gain access to the subtalar joint and to create a working area. **C:** The deeper cartilage layers from talus and calcaneus are removed using a shaver and curette. The screws are percutaneously inserted at the tuber calcanii. **D:** Postoperative lateral x-ray demonstrating subtalar fusion.

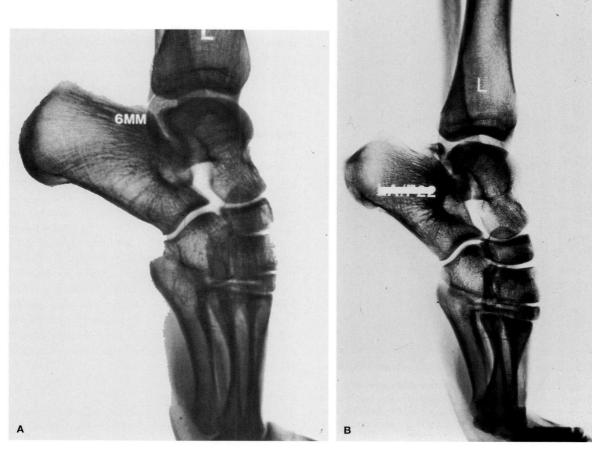

Fig. 66-2. A: Lateral x-ray of a ballet dancer in demi-pointe position leading to compression at the posterior aspect of the left ankle. **B:** Lateral x-ray of a ballet dancer who experiences pain of the left ankle in the demi-pointe position. The pain is produced by compression of the avulsed os trigonum.

forced plantarflexion. Posterior ankle impingement can be caused by overuse or trauma. Distinction between these two seems important since posterior impingement through overuse has a better prognosis.[19] A posterior ankle impingement syndrome through overuse is mainly found in ballet dancers and runners.[20–22] Running that involves forced plantarflexion such as downhill running can put repetitive stress on the posterior aspect of the ankle joint.[23] In ballet dancers the forceful plantar flexion during the en pointe position or the demi-pointe position produces compression at the posterior aspect of the ankle joint. The joint mobility and range of motion (ROM) gradually increase through exercise. In the presence of a prominent posterior talar process or an os trigonum, this can lead to compression of these structures **(Fig. 66-2A,B)**.

The presence of an os trigonum itself does not seem to be relevant.[20] This anatomic anomaly must be combined with a traumatic event such as a supination trauma, a hyperplantarflexion trauma, dancing on hard surfaces, or pushing beyond anatomic limits. The forced hyperplantarflexion test

is most important for the diagnosis **(Fig. 66-3)**. A negative test rules out a posterior impingement syndrome. A positive test is followed by a diagnostic infiltration of local anesthetic. If the pain on forced hyperplantarflexion disappears, the diagnosis is confirmed.

Deep Portion of the Deltoid Ligament

Eversion or hyperdorsiflexion trauma can result in avulsion fragments, posttraumatic calcification, or ossicles in the deep portion of the deltoid ligament. Patients experience posteromedial ankle pain especially on running and walking on uneven ground.

Flexor Hallucis Longus

A flexor hallucis longus tendonitis is often present in patients with a posterior ankle impingement syndrome. The pain is located posteromedial. In ballet dancers, it is present in plié and especially grand plié. The flexor hallucis longus tendon can be palpated behind the medial malleolus. By

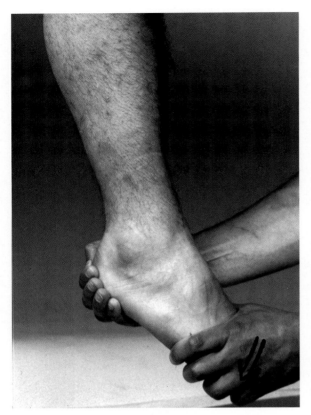

Fig. 66-3. The forced hyperplantarflexion test is performed with patient sitting with the knee flexed in 90 degrees. The test should be performed with repetitive quick passive hyperplantarflexion movements. The test can be repeated in slight external rotation or slight internal rotation of the foot relative to the tibia. The investigator can apply to this rotational movement on the point of maximal plantar flexion, thereby "grinding" the posterior talar process/os trigonum between tibia and calcaneus.

asking the patient to repetitively flex the big toe with the ankle in 10 to 20 degrees of plantarflexion, the flexor hallucis longus tendon can be palpated in its gliding channel behind the medial malleolus. The tendon glides up and down under the palpating finger of the examiner. In case of stenosing tendonitis or chronic inflammation, crepitus and recognizable pain can be provoked. Sometimes a nodule in the tendon can be felt to move up and down under the palpating finger.

Peroneal Tendons

Tenosynovitis of the peroneal tendons, dislocation, rupture, and snapping of one of the peroneal tendons account for the majority of symptoms at the posterolateral side of the ankle joint.[24,25] A differentiation must be made with (fatigue) fractures of the fibula, lesions of the lateral ligament complex, and posterolateral impingement (os trigonum syndrome).

Peroneal tendon disorders are often associated and secondary to chronic lateral ankle instability. As the peroneal muscles act as lateral ankle stabilizers, more strain is placed on these tendons in chronic lateral instability, resulting in hypertrophic tendinopathy, tenosynovitis, and ultimately in (partial) tendon tears.[26–28] Postsurgery and postfracture adhesions and irregularities in the posterior aspect of the fibula (sliding channel) can be responsible for symptoms in this region.[15]

Posterior Tibial Tendon

The posterior tibial tendon plays an important roll in normal hindfoot function.[29] Several investigators have described development of posterior tibial dysfunction as the disease progresses from peritendinitis to elongation, degeneration, and rupture[27–31] **(Fig. 66-4A,B)**. Tenosynovitis is often seen in

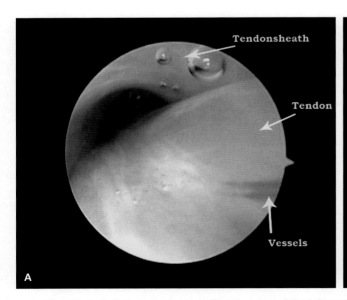
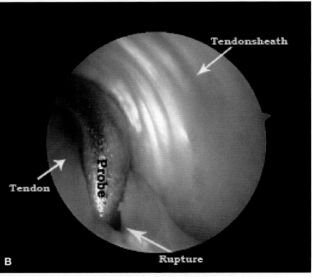

Fig. 66-4. **A:** Arthroscopic view of tendoscopy of the left posterior tibial tendon. The blood vessels are pathognomic for tenosynovitis of the posterior tibial tendon. The view is from distal to proximal in the tendon sheath. **B:** Arthroscopic view of a rupture of the left posterior tibial tendon at the level of its groove in the posterior aspect of the medial malleolus.

association with flat feet and psoriatic and rheumatic arthritis. In the early stage of posterior tibial dysfunction, tenosynovitis is the main symptom. Tenosynovectomy can be performed if conservative treatment fails.[32] Postsurgery and postfracture adhesions and irregularity of the posterior aspect of the tibia (sliding channel) can be responsible for symptoms in this region.

Achilles Tendon and Retrocalcaneal Bursa

Chronic retrocalcaneal bursitis is accompanied with deep pain and swelling of the posterior soft tissue just in front of the Achilles tendon. The prominent bursa can be palpated medial and lateral from the tendon at its insertion. The lateral radiograph demonstrates the characteristic prominent superior calcaneal deformity. Operative treatment involves removal of the bursa and resection of the lateral and medial posterosuperior aspect of the calcaneus **(Fig. 66-5A,B,C,D)**. Retrocalcaneal bursitis is often accompanied by midportion insertional tendinosis. Often a partial rupture of the midportion of the tendon at its insertion is present. In case of insertional tendinosis, there is pain at the bone-tendon junction, which is worsened after exercise. The tenderness is specifically located directly posterior.

Neurovascular Bundle

Entrapment of the posterior tibial nerve within the tarsal tunnel is commonly known as a tarsal tunnel syndrome.[33] Clinical examination should be sufficient to differentiate these disorders from an isolated posterior tibial tendon disorder.

■ OPERATIVE TECHNIQUES

Posterior Ankle Arthroscopy

The posterior ankle arthroscopy is generally carried out as outpatient surgery under general anesthesia or epidural anesthesia. The patient is placed in a prone position. A tourniquet is applied around the upper leg and a small support is placed under the lower leg, making it possible to move the ankle freely **(Fig. 66-6)**. We use a soft-tissue distraction device when indicated.[34] No antibiotics are given.

For irrigation we use normal saline although glycine, or ringers solution can also be used. We use one saline bag with gravity flow. A 4.0-mm arthroscope with 30 degrees is routinely used for posterior ankle arthroscopy. Apart from the standard excisional and motorized instruments for treatment of osteophytes and ossicles, a 4-mm chisel and periosteal elevator can be useful.

The landmarks on the ankle are the lateral malleolus, medial and lateral border of the Achilles tendon, and the foot sole. The ankle should be kept in a neutral position. We draw a line from the tip of the lateral malleolus to the Achilles tendon, parallel to the foot sole.

At the medial side of the talus we find the flexor hallucis longus, flexor digitorum longus, posterior tibial tendon, and the neurovascular bundle. The neurovascular bundle is the most important structure at risk. On the lateral side the peroneal tendons are located.

The posterolateral portal is made just above this line, just in front of the Achilles tendon **(Fig. 66-7)**. After making a vertical stab incision, the subcutaneous layer is split by a mosquito clamp. The mosquito clamp is directed anteriorly, pointing in the direction of the interdigital webspace between the first and second toe **(Fig. 66-8)**. When the tip of the clamp touches the bone, it is exchanged for a 4.5-mm arthroscope shaft with the blunt trocar pointing in the same direction. By palpating the bone in the sagittal plane, the level of the ankle joint and subtalar joint can be distinguished since the prominent posterior talar process or os trigonum can be felt as a posterior prominence between the two joints. The trocar is situated extra-articulary at the level of the ankle joint. The trocar is exchanged for the 4.0-mm arthroscope; the direction of view is to the lateral side **(Fig. 66-9)**.

The posteromedial portal is made at the same level, just above the line from the tip of the lateral malleolus, but just in front of the medial aspect of the Achilles tendon **(Fig. 66-10)**. After making a vertical stab incision, a mosquito clamp is introduced and directed toward the arthroscope shaft in a 90-degree angle. When the mosquito clamp touches the shaft of the arthroscope, the shaft is used as a guide to travel anteriorly in the direction of the ankle joint, all the way down touching the bone. The arthroscope is now pulled slightly backward and slides over the mosquito clamp until the tip of the mosquito clamp comes to view. The clamp is used to spread the extra-articular soft tissue in front of the tip of the camera. In situations where scar tissue or adhesions are present, the mosquito clamp is exchanged for a 5-mm full radius shaver.[16] The tip of the shaver is directed in a lateral and slightly plantar direction toward the lateral aspect of the subtalar joint.

The joint capsule and fatty tissue can be removed. After removal of the very thin joint capsule of the subtalar joint, the posterior compartment of the subtalar joint can be visualized. At the level of the ankle joint, the posterior tibiofibular ligament can be recognized as well as the posterior talofibular ligament. The posterior talar process can be freed of scar tissue, and the flexor hallucis longus tendon can be identified. The flexor hallucis longus tendon is an important landmark to prevent damage to the more medially located neurovascular bundle **(Fig. 66-11)**. After removal of the thin joint capsule of the ankle joint, the ankle joint can be entered and inspected.

On the medial side, the tip of the medial malleolus can be visualized as well as the deep portion of the deltoid ligament. By opening the joint capsule from inside out at the level of the medial malleolus, the tendon sheath of the posterior tibial tendon can be opened and the arthroscope can be introduced into the tendon sheath **(Fig. 66-12)**. The posterior tibial tendon can be inspected. The same procedure can be followed for the flexor digitorum longus tendon.

By applying manual distraction to the os calcis, the posterior compartment of the ankle opens up and the shaver

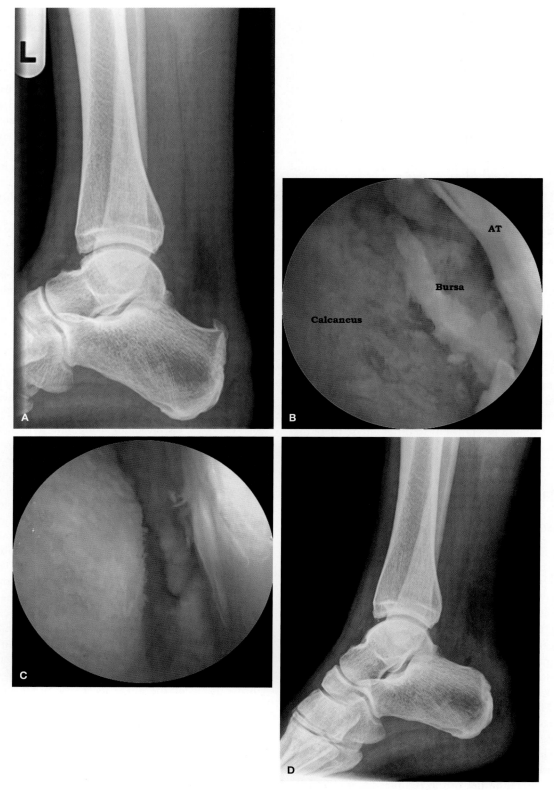

Fig. 66-5. A: Lateral x-ray of the left ankle showing the characteristic prominent superior cal-caneal deformity (Haglund exostosis) in a patient with chronic retrocalcaneal bursitis. **B:** Arthroscopic view of the inflamed retrocalcaneal bursa (AT = Achilles Tendon). **C:** The bursa has been removed and the lateral and medial posterosuperior aspects of the calcaneus have been resected. **D:** Lateral x-ray showing the postoperative result.

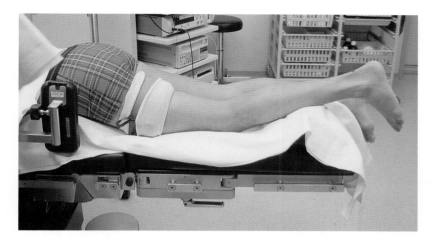

Fig. 66-6. For posterior ankle arthroscopy the patient is placed in a prone position. A tourniquet is applied around the upper leg, and a small support is placed under the lower leg, making it possible to move the ankle freely.

can be introduced into the posterior ankle compartment. We prefer to apply a soft-tissue distractor, which is attached to a belt around the waist of the surgeon **(Fig. 66-13)**.[34] A total synovectomy or capsulectomy can be performed. The talar dome can be inspected over almost its entire surface as well as the complete tibial plafond. An osteochondral defect or subchondral cystic lesion can be identified, débrided, and drilled. The posterior syndesmotic ligaments are inspected and, if hypertrophic, partially resected.

Removal of a symptomatic os trigonum, a nonunion of a fracture of the posterior talar process, or a symptomatic large posterior talar prominence involves partial detachment of the posterior talofibular ligament and release of the flexor retinaculum, which both attach to the posterior talar prominence **(Fig. 66-14A,B)**. Removal of the pathological bony process can be done by reduction from medial to lateral with a bur or by use of a 4-mm osteotome or a small rasp. When using the osteotome it is important not to start too far anteriorly to prevent damage to the subtalar joint.

Release of the flexor hallucis longus tendon involves detachment of the flexor retinaculum from the posterior talar process. Adhesions surrounding the flexor tendon can be removed. On the lateral side, the peroneal tendons can be inspected.

When a tight and thickened crural fascia is present, this can hinder the free movement of instruments. It can be helpful to enlarge the hole in the fascia by means of a punch or shaver. Bleeding is controlled by electrocautery at the end of the procedure.

After removal of the instruments the stab incisions are closed with 3.0 Ethilon to prevent sinus formation. A sterile compression dressing is applied.

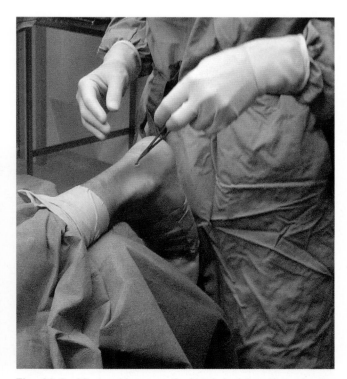

Fig. 66-8. After making a vertical stab incision, the subcutaneous layer is split by a mosquito clamp. The mosquito clamp is directed anteriorly, pointing in the direction of the interdigital webspace between the first and second toes.

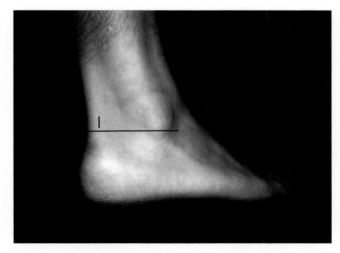

Fig. 66-7. The posterolateral portal is made just above the line from the tip of the lateral malleolus to the Achilles tendon, parallel to the foot sole, just in front of the Achilles tendon.

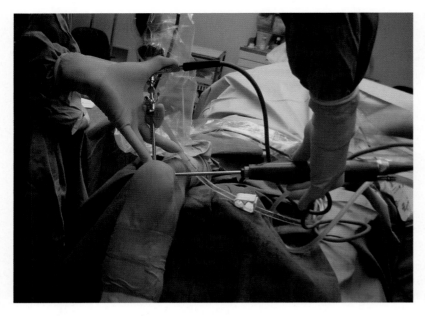

Fig. 66-9. The scope is situated extra-articulary at the level of the ankle joint. The scope points to the webspace between the first and second toe; the direction of the view is to the lateral side. The shaver is introduced through the posteromedial portal at the 90 degree angle in relation to the scope. Once it has touched the shaft of the scope, the shaft is used as a guide for the tip of the shaver to be brought to the tip of the scope.

Postoperative treatment consists of weightbearing as tolerated on crutches for 2 or 3 days. The dressing can be taken off after 3 days. As soon as possible after the surgery the patient is advised to start ROM exercises, as tolerated.

Posterior Tibial Tendoscopy

Posterior tibial tendoscopy is generally carried out as outpatient surgery under general anesthesia or epidural anesthesia. The patient is placed in the lateral decubitus position, with the nonoperative side up. A tourniquet is applied around the upper leg and a small support is placed under the lower leg, making it possible to move the ankle freely. The important landmarks are the medial malleolus and the posterior tibial tendon.

Access to the posterior tibial tendon can be obtained anywhere along the tendon. The two main portals for posterior tibial tendoscopy are located directly over the involved tendon, 2 cm distal and 2 cm proximal to the posterior edge of the medial malleolus. We start with the distal portal by making an incision through the skin. After blunt dissection with a mosquito clamp the trocar is introduced. The trocar is exchanged for a 2.7-mm arthroscope with an inclination angle of 30 degrees **(Fig. 66-15)**. After introduction of a spinal needle under direct vision, an incision is made through the skin into the tendon sheath to create a proximal portal. Instruments like a probe, disposable cutting knife, scissors, or shaver can be introduced through this portal. A complete overview of the posterior tibial tendon can be obtained, from its insertion (navicular bone) to some 6 cm above the level of the tip of the medial malleolus. By rotating the scope over the tendon the complete tendon sheath can be inspected.

In a cadaver study van Dijk et al.[14] found that a vincula was present in all specimens. During tendoscopy a pathological

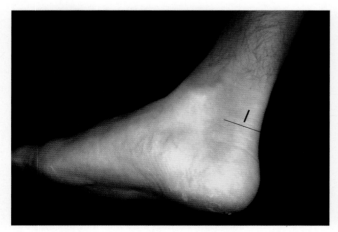

Fig. 66-10. The posteromedial portal is made at the same level as the posterolateral portal, just above the line from the tip of the lateral malleolus, but just in front of the medial aspect of the Achilles tendon.

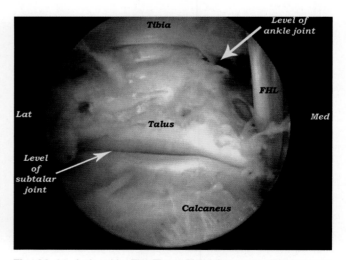

Fig. 66-11. Left ankle. The Flexor Hallucis Longus (FHL) tendon is an important landmark to prevent damage to the more medially located neurovascular bundle (Lat = Lateral, Med = Medial).

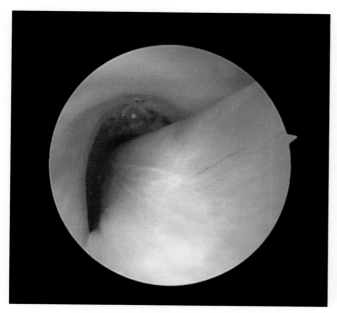

Fig. 66-12. Left ankle. Inspection of the posterior tibial tendon is possible during routine posterior ankle arthroscopy.

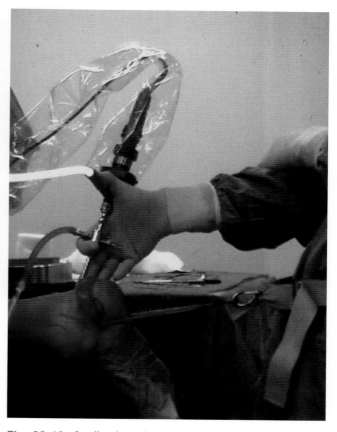

Fig. 66-13. Application of a soft-tissue distractor in order to open up the posterior ankle compartment. The talar dome can be inspected over almost its entire surface as well as the complete tibial plafond.

thickened vincula can be excised. The tendon sheath can be released and adhesions can be removed. When a total synovectomy is to be performed, we create a third portal more distally from the previous described portals. To prevent sinus formation, the portals are closed with a monofil suture. Postoperative treatment consists of a pressure bandage (Klinigrip® Ideal, Oud-Bijerland, The Netherlands) and partial weightbearing for 2 to 3 days. Active ROM is advised immediately postoperative.[14,15]

Peroneal Tendoscopy

Peroneal tendoscopy is generally carried out as outpatient surgery under general anesthesia or epidural anesthesia. The

patient is placed in the lateral decubitus position, with the operative side up. A tourniquet is applied around the upper leg, and a small support is placed under the lower leg, making it possible to move the ankle freely. The important landmarks are the lateral malleolus and the peroneal tendons.

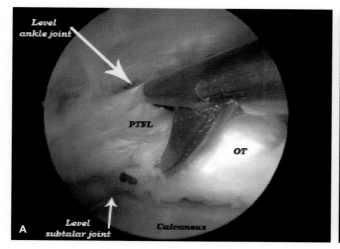
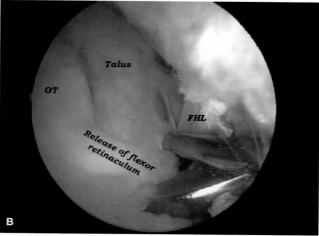

Fig. 66-14. Left ankle. Partial detachment of the posterior talofibular ligament **(A)** and release of the flexor retinaculum **(B)**, both of which attach to the posterior talar prominence, is necessary to remove a symptomatic os trigonum (OT = Os Trigonum, FHL = Flexor Hallucis Longus, PTFL = Posterior Talofibular Ligament).

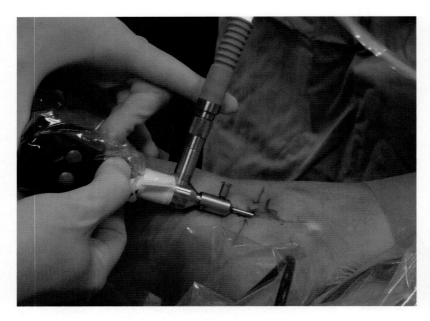

Fig. 66-15. For tendoscopy of the posterior tibial tendon a distal portal is made 2 cm distal and 2 cm proximal to the posterior edge of the medial malleolus. An arthroscope with an inclination angle of 30 degrees is used. A proximal portal is created under direct vision.

Access to the peroneal tendons can be obtained anywhere along the tendons. The two main portals for the peroneal tendoscopy are located directly over the involved tendons, 2 cm distal and 2 cm proximal to the tip of the lateral malleolus. We start with the distal portal by making an incision through the skin. After blunt dissection with a mosquito clamp, the arthroscope shaft with blunt trocar is introduced into the tendon sheath. A 2.7-mm arthroscope with an inclination angle of 30 degrees is introduced. The proximal portal is made under direct vision, after introduction of a spinal needle. Instruments like the probe, disposable cutting knife, scissors, or shaver system can be introduced. Through the distal portal, a complete overview can be obtained of both peroneal tendons. The inspection starts some 6 cm proximal from the posterior tip of the lateral malleolus, where a thin membrane splits the tendon compartment into two tendon chambers **(Fig. 66-16)**. More distally, both tendons lie in one compartment. By rotating the endoscope over and in between both tendons, the complete compartment can be inspected.

We found that a vincula is consistently present in both peroneal tendons over their full length.[15] The vincula attaches both tendons to each other and to the tendon sheath. By tendoscopy a pathological thickened vincula or tendon sheath can be released, adhesions can be removed, and a symptomatic prominent tubercle can be resected. A rupture of the peroneal longus or brevis tendon can be sutured. When a total synovectomy of the tendon sheath is to be performed, it is advisable to create a third portal more distally or more proximally from the previous described portals. In case of treatment for recurrent peroneal tendon dislocation, it is possible to deepen the groove of the peroneal tendons with a bur.[40] To prevent sinus formation, the portals are closed with a monofil suture. Postoperative treatment consists of a pressure bandage and partial weightbearing for 2 to 3 days. Active ROM is advised immediately postoperative.

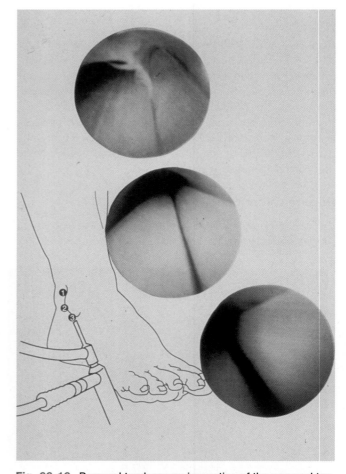

Fig. 66-16. Peroneal tendoscopy: inspection of the peroneal tendons starts some 6 cm proximal from the tip of the lateral malleolus, where a thin membrane splits the tendon compartment into two separate tendon chambers *(1)*. More distally, both tendons lie in one compartment *(2 and 3)*. By rotating the scope over and in between both tendons, the complete compartment can be inspected.

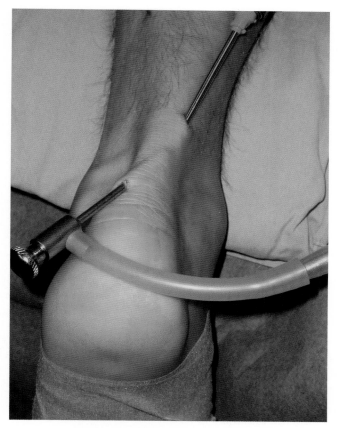

Fig. 66-17. In case of peritendinitis of the Achilles tendon, the portals are created 2 cm proximal and 2 cm distal of the lesion. The distal portal is made first through the skin only. After introduction of a spinal needle under direct vision, an incision is made at the location of the proximal portal. Instruments like a probe or a small shaver can be introduced.

Retrocalcaneal Endoscopy

Endoscopy for retrocalcaneal bursitis and Haglund deformity is generally carried out as outpatient surgery under general anesthesia or epidural anesthesia. The endoscopic calcaneoplasty procedure is performed in the prone position.[35] A tourniquet is applied around the upper leg and a small support is placed under the lower leg, making it possible to move the ankle freely.

Two portals are created on the medial and lateral sides of the Achilles tendon, at the level of the superior border of the os calcis. After a vertical stab incision is made at the posterolateral side, a blunt trocar is introduced for blunt dissection and opening of the retrocalcaneal space. The trocar is exchanged for a 4.0-mm arthroscope with a 30-degree angle. After localization of the posteromedial portal with a needle, a stab incision is made under direct vision. A probe and subsequently a 5-mm full radius resector are introduced through the posteromedial portal. After the removal of the bursa and inflamed soft tissue, the calcaneal prominence is removed with the full radius resector and small acromionizer. Portals should be changed to remove the posterolateral side of the superior calcaneal rim and for final inspection.

In case of peritendinitis of the Achilles tendon, the portals are created 2 cm proximal and 2 cm distal of the lesion **(Fig. 66-17)**. The distal portal is made first: an incision is made through the skin only. The arthroscope shaft with a blunt trocar penetrates the crural fascia. A 2.7-mm arthroscope with an inclination angle of 30 degrees is introduced. After introduction of a spinal needle under direct vision, an incision is made at the location of the proximal portal. Instruments like a probe or a small shaver are introduced. The pathologic paratenon is removed by shaver. The Achilles tendon can be inspected by rotating the scope over the tendon. The plantaris tendon can be recognized and released or resected when indicated.

When a total synovectomy of the tendon sheath is to be performed, it is advisable to create a third portal more distally or more proximally from the previous described portals. To prevent sinus formation, the portals are closed with a monofil suture. Postoperative treatment consists of a pressure bandage and partial weightbearing for 2 to 3 days. Active ROM is advised immediately postoperative.

■ TECHNICAL ALTERNATIVES AND PITFALLS

Peroneal Tendons

For routine tendoscopy of the peroneal tendons we use a 2.7-mm scope. It is possible, however, to use a 4.0-mm arthroscope. This greater diameter scope gives better flow. In cases where a lot of debris is expected, such as groove deepening procedures for recurrent peroneal tendon dislocation, this is an advantage.

Tendoscopy for the Posterior Tibial Tendon

It is important to identify the location of the posterior tibial tendon before creating the portals. Ask the patient to actively invert the foot, identify the tendon, and mark the location of the portals on the skin. The tendon sheath between the posterior tibial tendon and the flexor digitorum longus is quite thin. Always check to ensure that you are inspecting the correct tendon. In cases where you have entered the tendon sheath of the flexor digitorum longus, you can easily see tendon move up and down when you passively flex and extend the toes. If you remain in the tendon sheath of the posterior tibial tendon, the neurovascular bundle is not in danger.

Tendoscopy Achilles Tendon and Endoscopic Calcaneoplasty

An alternative to perform an endoscopic calcaneoplasty is to use a 2.7-mm scope instead of a 4.0-mm scope. We prefer the 4.0-mm scope, however, since this gives a better flow. By placing the scope between the Achilles tendon and calcaneus, the arthroscope shaft lifts the tendon of the bone, thus creating a working space. This is another advantage of using a larger diameter scope.

It can be useful to use fluoroscopy in order to check if enough bone has been removed. It is important to go down to the insertion of the Achilles tendon.

Hindfoot Endoscopy and Posterior Ankle Arthroscopy

In the hindfoot the crural fascia can be quite thick. This local thickening is called the ligament of Rouviere. It can be attached to the posterior talar process. It can be helpful to enlarge the entry through the crural fascia **(Fig. 66-18)**. We use an arthroscopic punch or scissors.

The position of the arthroscope is important. Always check if the direction of your view is lateral. If your scope points into the direction of the webspace between the first and second toes, the scope is in a safe area. Stay lateral to the flexor hallucis longus tendon. Use the flexor hallucis longus tendon as a landmark (Fig. 66-11). Always check if the direction of your view is lateral. Go medial from the flexor hallucis longus tendon only in cases where a release of the neurovascular bundle is required (posttraumatic tarsal tunnel syndrome). When you remove a hypertrophic posterior talar process by using a chisel, take care not to place the chisel too far anterior. Start at the posterosuperior edge of the posterior talar process and chisel away the inferoposterior part of the process **(Fig. 66-19)**. Use a shaver (bone cutter) to remove the remnant of the process. If you initially position your chisel too far anterior, you might take away too much at the level of the subtalar joint.

The advantage of a two-portal procedure with the patient in the prone position is the working space that you can create in between the Achilles tendon and the back of the ankle and subtalar joint. The position is ergonomic for the orthopedic

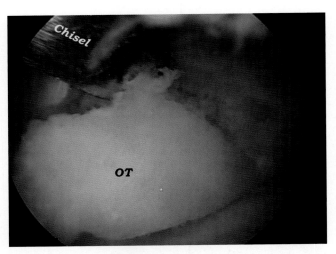

Fig. 66-19. Right ankle. When removing a hypertrophic posterior talar process by using a chisel, care must be taken not to place the chisel too far anteriorly in order to prevent damage to the subtalar joint. It is best to start at the posterosuperior edge of the posterior talar process and chisel away the inferoposterior part of the process. Remnants can be taken away by a shaver or bone cutter.

surgeon. Soft-tissue distraction can easily be applied. We use the distraction system that we described earlier (Fig. 66-13).[34]

An alternative is to use two posterolateral portals with the patient in the lateral decubitus position.[36] We have no experience with this approach.

Subtalar Arthroscopy

An alternative access to the subtalar joint has been described by several authors.[11,13,37,38] The patient is in the lateral decubitus position, and a combination of anterolateral and posterolateral portals are used. Other authors prefer a supine position.[39]

■ REHABILITATION

The postoperative treatment for most arthroscopic procedures consists of functional treatment. Most patients are advised to start practicing ROM immediately after surgery, as tolerated, and protected weightbearing for the first 3 days. One week postoperatively we will see them in the outpatient department. If necessary, physiotherapy can be prescribed for ROM, strengthening, and stability.

In case of a peroneal tendon rupture treated with suture repair, we will apply a plaster cast for 4 weeks, with 3 weeks of full weightbearing.

■ OUTCOMES AND FUTURE DIRECTIONS

Tenosynovectomy, screw removal, and exostosis removal were performed successfully by means of posterior tibial

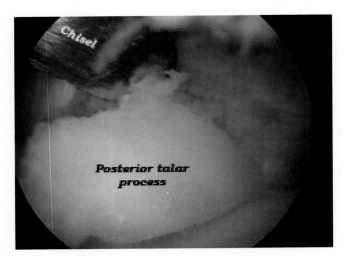

Fig. 66-18. Left ankle. In the hindfoot the crural fascia can be quite thick. This local thickening is called the ligament of Rouviere. It can be helpful to enlarge the entry through the crural fascia with an arthroscopic punch or scissors.

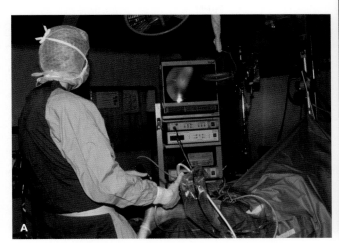
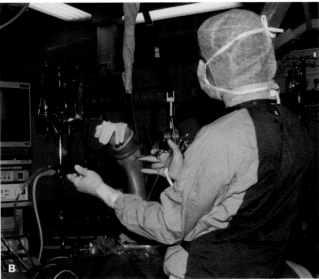

Fig. 66-20. A,B: In patients with both anterior and posterior ankle problems, the posterior ankle arthroscopy is performed first, in the prone position. Subsequently, the anterior ankle arthroscopy is performed with the foot hanging upside down.

tendoscopy and peroneal tendoscopy.[14,15] In case of a longitudinal rupture of the peroneus brevis tendon, by means of a small incision, the ruptures were sutured.[15] Recurrent peroneal tendon dislocation was successfully treated by deepening of the groove.[40] A pathologic thickened posterior tibial vincula was successfully removed in four patients.[14] Removal of an inflamed retrocalcaneal bursa, together with the prominent posterosuperior part of the calcaneus by means of endoscopic calcaneal plasty, was associated with a good or excellent result in over 80% of cases.[35] Resection of an inflamed peritendineum, in cases of localized Achilles tendonitis, gave promising early results. Removal of a pathologic os trigonum or a painful posterior soft-tissue impediment did not cause any technical problems and was successful in most patients. At a follow-up of 36 months postoperative, the mean American Orthopaedic Foot and Ankle Society Hindfoot score raised from 71 preoperative to 90 postoperative in 57 consecutive patients. Return to work was on average 3 weeks, and return to sports activities was on average 9 weeks. Patients with a bony impingement had a better outcome when compared with patients with a soft-tissue impingement.

In patients in whom a total synovectomy was performed, there was no recurrence of the synovitis. All loose bodies were successfully removed. Of the 14 débrided/drilled osteochondral defects, 10 had good or excellent results. Four patients were treated for an intraosseous talar ganglion. All patients were without symptoms at the last follow-up. Patients treated for degenerative changes in the subtalar joint experienced clear alleviation of their symptoms. None of these patients had deterioration of their results over time.

We have gained experience with patients, especially ballet dancers and soccer players, with anterior and posterior ankle problems. We performed a posterior arthroscopy first, in the prone position. Subsequently, we performed an anterior ankle arthroscopy by flexing the knee to a 90 degree position (Fig. 20A,B).

In the near future, procedures for arthroscopic arthrodesis will be refined (Fig. 66-1A,B,C,D). This includes optimization of the mechanical axis and optimization of the arthrodesed joint position. Probably computer-aided surgery will play a role to achieve the desired position. Another future possibility is the arthroscopic-assisted or minimally invasive joint replacement.

■ REFERENCES

1. Burman MS. Arthroscopy of direct visualization of joints. An experimental cadaver study. J Bone Joint Surg. 1931;13:669–695.
2. Tagaki K. The arthroscope. Jpn J Orthop Assoc. 1939;14:359.
3. Watanabe M. Selfoc-Arthroscope (Watanabe no 24 arthroscope). Monograph. Tokyo: Teishin Hospital, 1972.
4. Chen DS, Wertheimer SJ. Centrally located osteochondral fracture of the talus. J Foot Surg. 1992;31:134–140.
5. Biedert R. Anterior ankle pain in sports medicine: aetiology and indications for arthroscopy. Arch Orthop Trauma Surg. 1991; 110(6):293–297.
6. Feder KS, Schonholtz GJ. Ankle arthroscopy: review and long-term results. Foot Ankle. September 1992;13(7):382–385.
7. Ferkel RD, Scranton PE. Current concepts review: arthroscopy of the ankle and foot. J Bone Joint Surg Am. 1993;75:1233–1242.
8. Guhl JF. Foot and Ankle Arthroscopy. New York: Slack; 1993.
9. Jerosch J, Schneider T, Strauss JM, et al. Arthroscopy of the upper ankle joint. List of indications from the literature—realistic expectations—complications. Unfallchirurg. 1993;96(2):82–87.
10. Martin DF, Baker CL, Curl WW, et al. Operative ankle arthroscopy: long-term follow-up. Am J Sports Med. 1989;17(1): 16–23; discussion 23.

11. Parisien JS, Vangsness T. Arthroscopy of the subtalar joint: an experimental approach. Arthroscopy. 1985;1:53–57.

12. Andrews JR, Timmerman LA. *Diagnostic and Operative Arthroscopy.* Philadelphia: WB Saunders; 1997.

13. Ferkel RD. Arthroscopic surgery. In: Whipple TL, ed. *The Foot and Ankle.* New York: Lippincott-Raven; 1996: Chapter 6, 103–116.

14. Van Dijk CN, Kort N, Scholten P. Tendoscopy of the posterior tibial tendon. Arthroscopy. 1997;13:692–698.

15. Van Dijk CN, Kort N. Tendoscopy of the peroneal tendons. Arthroscopy. 1998;14(5):471–478.

16. Van Dijk CN, Scholten PE, Krips R. A 2-portal endoscopic approach for diagnosis and treatment of posterior ankle pathology. Arthroscopy. 2000;16(8):871–876.

17. Nagai H. Tunnel endoscopy. In: Watanabi M, ed. *Arthroscopy of Small Joints.* New York: Igaku-shoin; 1985:163–164.

18. Lundeen RO. Arthroscopic resection of Haglund's deformity and retrocalcaneal bursae. Paper presented at the American Orthopaedic Foot and Ankle Society (AOFAS) Annual Meeting, 1997; Palm Springs.

19. Stibbe AB, van Dijk CN, Marti RK. The os trigonum syndrome. Acta Orthop Scand. 1994;(suppl 262):59–60.

20. Van Dijk CN, Lim LSL, Poortman A, et al. Degenerative joint disease in female ballet dancers. Am J Sports Med. 1995;23(3): 295–300.

21. Hamilton WG, Geppert MJ, Thompson FM. Pain in the posterior aspect of the ankle in dancers. J Bone Joint Surg Am. 1996;87: 1491–1500.

22. Hedrick MR, McBryde AM. Posterior ankle impingement. Foot Ankle Int. 1994;15:2–8.

23. Funk DA, Cass JR, Johnson KA. Acquired adult flatfoot secondary to posterior tibial tendon pathology. J Bone Joint Surg Am. 1986; 68(1):95–102.

24. Roggatz J, Urban A. The calcareous peritendinitis of the long peroneal tendon. Arch Orthop Traum Surg. 1980;96:161–164.

25. Schweitzer GJ. Stenosing peroneal tenovaginitis. Case reports. S Afr Med J. 1982;4:521–523.

26. Yao L, Tong JF, Cracchiolo A, et al. MR findings in peroneal tendopathy. Comput Assist Tomogr. 1995;19:460–464.

27. Myerson MS, McGarvey W. Disorders of the insertion of the Achilles tendon and Achilles tendinitis. J Bone J Surgery Am. 1998;80(12):1814–1824.

28. Richardson EG. Disorders of tendons. In: Grenshaw AH, ed. *Campbell's Operative Orthopaedics.* St. Louis: Mosby; 1992: 2851–2873.

29. Cosen L. Posterior tibial tenosynovitis secondary to foot strain. Clin Orthop. 1965;42:101–102.

30. Johnson KA, Strom DE. Tibialis posterior tendon dysfunction. Clin Orthop. 1989;239:196–206.

31. Williams R. Chronic non-specific tendovaginitis of tibialis posterior. J Bone Joint Surg Br. 1963;45:542–549.

32. Trevino S, Gould N, Korson R. Surgical treatment of stenosing tenosynovitis at the ankle. Foot Ankle. 1981;2:37–45.

33. Coughlin MJ, Mann RA. Tarsal tunnel syndrome. In: Surgery of the Foot and Ankle. Ed. 6, Vol 1. St. Louis: Mosby-Year Book; 1993:554.

34. Van Dijk CN, Verhagen RA, Tol HJ. Technical note: Resterilizable noninvasive ankle distraction device. Arthroscopy. 2001;17(3):E12.

35. Van Dijk CN, van Dyk E, Scholten P, et al. Endoscopic calcaneoplasty. Am J Sports Med. 2001;29(2):185–189.

36. Lundeen RO. Arthroscopic excision of the os trigonum. In: Guhl JF, Parisien JS, Boyton MD, eds. *Foot and Ankle Arthroscopy.* 3rd ed. New York: Springer-Verlag; 2004:191–199.

37. Guhl JF, Parisien JS, Boyton MD. *Foot and Ankle Arthroscopy.* 3rd ed. New York: Springer-Verlag; 2004.

38. Frey C, Gasser S, Feder K. Arthroscopy of the subtalar joint. Foot Ankle Int. 1994;15(8):424–428.

39. Parisien JS. Posterior subtalar joint arthroscopy. In: Guhl JF, Parisien JS, Boyton MD, eds. *Foot and Ankle Arthroscopy.* 3rd ed. New York: Springer-Verlag; 2004:175–182.

40. Scholten P, Breugem S, van Dijk CN. Tendoscopic treatment of peroneal tendon dislocation. Submitted to European Society of Knee Surgery, Sports Traumatology and Arthroscopy. 2006.

Note: After a page number an "*f*" stands for figure and a "*t*" stands for table.